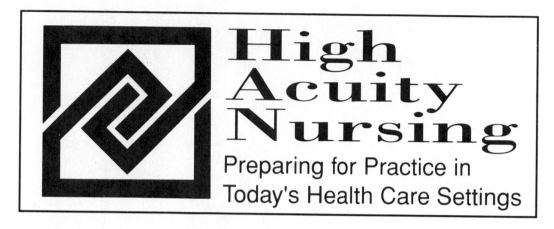

High Acuity Nursing

Preparing for Practice in
Today's Health Care Settings

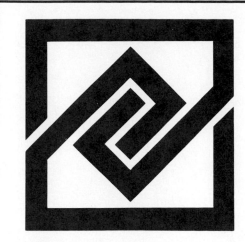

High Acuity Nursing

Preparing for Practice in Today's Health Care Settings

Pamela Stinson Kidd, RN, PhD, CEN
Assistant Professor
University of Kentucky College of Nursing
University Hospital
Lexington, Kentucky

Kathleen Dorman Wagner, RN, MSN
Critical Care Clinical Nurse Specialist
Instructor
University Hospital
University of Kentucky College of Nursing
Lexington, Kentucky

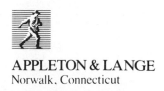

APPLETON & LANGE
Norwalk, Connecticut

0-8385-1054-X

92 93 94 95 96 / 10 9 8 7 6 5 4 3 2

Prentice Hall International (UK) Limited, *London*
Prentice Hall of Australia Pty. Limited, *Sydney*
Prentice Hall Canada, Inc., *Toronto*
Prentice Hall Hispanoamericana, S.A., *Mexico*
Prentice Hall of India Private Limited, *New Delhi*
Prentice Hall of Japan, Inc., *Tokyo*
Simon & Schuster Asia Pte. Ltd., *Singapore*
Editoria Prentice Hall do Brasil Ltda., *Rio de Janeiro*
Prentice Hall, *Englewood Cliffs, New Jersey*

Library of Congress Cataloging-in-Publication Data

Kidd, Pamela S. (Pamela Stinson)
    High acuity nursing : preparing for practice in today's health
care settings / Pamela S. Kidd, Kathleen D. Wagner.
        p.   cm.
    Includes index.
    ISBN 0-8385-1054-X
    1. Intensive care nursing.   I. Wagner, Kathleen D. (Kathleen
Dorman)   II. Title.
    [DNLM: 1. Critical Care—methods.   2. Nursing Process—methods.
WY 154 K46h]
RT120.I5K53   1992
610.73'61—dc20
DNLM/DLC
for Library of Congress   91-44123
                                                                 CIP

Executive Editor: William Brottmiller
Production: CRACOM Corporation
Designer: Steve Byrum

PRINTED IN THE UNITED STATES OF AMERICA

Contents

Contributors

Robyn Cheung, RN, MSN, CCRN
Critical Care Clinical Nurse Specialist
Trauma Case Manager
University Hospital, University of Kentucky
Lexington, Kentucky

Beatrice DiCostanzo, RN, C, MN
St. Vincent's Medical Center of Richmond
Staten Island, New York

Evelyn Dantzic Geller, RN, MSN, MED
University of Kentucky
College of Nursing
Lexington, Kentucky

Helen F. Hodges, RN, MSN
RN-BSN Program Coordinator
Georgia Baptist College of Nursing
Atlanta, Georgia

Paula Hogsten, RN, MSN, CS, CCRN
Critical Care Clinical Nurse Specialist
King's Daughters' Medical Center
Ashland, Kentucky

Linda M. Holtzclaw, RN, MSN, CCRN
Staff Development Specialist
University Hospital, University of Kentucky
Lexington, Kentucky

Karen L. Johnson, RN, MSL, CCRN
Critical Care Clinical Nurse Specialist
Instructor
University Hospital
University of Kentucky College of Nursing
Lexington, Kentucky

Pamela Stinson Kidd, RN, PhD, CEN
Assistant Professor
University of Kentucky College of Nursing
University Hospital
Lexington, Kentucky

Alice Saint MacPhail, RN, BSN
Formerly Nutrition Support Coordinator
University Hospital, University of Kentucky
Lexington, Kentucky

James P. McGraw, RN, MN, CCRN, CEN
Trauma Clinical Nurse Specialist
Harris Methodist Fort Worth
Fort Worth, Texas

Catherine Paradiso, RN, MSN
St. Vincent's Medical Center of Richmond
Staten Island, New York

Michelle Rountree, RN, ADN
Medical University of South Carolina
Charleston Hospital
Nephrology/Kidney-Pancreas Transplant Unit
Charleston, South Carolina

Jane G. E. Silver, MSN, RN
Zone Clinical Manager
Tokos Medical Corporation
Santa Ana, California

Colleen H. Swartz, RN, MSN, CCRN
Trauma Nurse Coordinator
University Hospital, University of Kentucky
Lexington, Kentucky

Paula Vernon-Levett, MS, RN, CCRN
Pediatric Critical Care Clinical Nurse Specialist
St. Luke's Hospital
Cedar Rapids, Iowa

Kathleen Dorman Wagner, RN, MSN
Critical Care Clinical Nurse Specialist
Instructor
University Hospital
University of Kentucky College of Nursing
Lexington, Kentucky

Reviewers

Michele Gerwick, RN, MSN
Assistant Professor
Indiana University of Pennsylvania
School of Nursing
Indiana, Pennsylvania
and
Doctoral Candidate
University of Pittsburgh
Pittsburgh, Pennsylvania

Elizabeth Hennemann, RN, MS, CCRN
Clinical Nurse Specialist—Medical ICU
UCLA Medical Center
Los Angeles, California

Gayle Johnson, RN, BSN, CCRN, EMT
Vanderbilt University Medical Center
Nashville, Tennessee

Rebecca Katz, RN, MA, CCRN
Critical Care Clinical Nurse Specialist
Director, Staff Development
Grant Medical Center
Columbus, Ohio

Cecilia Kinsel, PhD, RNC
San Antonio College
School of Nursing
San Antonio, Texas

Deborah Klein, RN, MSN, CCRN, CS
Clinical Nurse Specialist
Trauma/Critical Care Nursing
MetroHealth Medical Center
Cleveland, Ohio

Gail Lewis, RN, MSN
Associate Professor
Barnes College
School of Nursing
St. Louis, Missouri

Kathy Lindsay, RN, BA, CCRN, CEN
The Methodist Hospital
Houston, Texas

Dee Malchow, RN, BSN
Limb Viability Service Coordinator
Harborview Medical Center
Seattle, Washington

Nancy Nuwer-Konstantinides, RN, MS, CANP, CNSN
Metabolic Nurse Specialist
University of Minnesota Hospital
Minneapolis, Minnesota

Linda Robinson, MN, RN, RRT, CCRN
Los Angeles Veterans Administration Hospital
Los Angeles, California

Susan Rush, RN, MSN
Instructor, Obstetrical Nursing
Fairleigh Dickinson University
Teaneck, New Jersey

Frances Watson, RN, BSN, CCRN
Head Nurse, ICU/CCU
Lee Hospital
Johnstown, Pennsylvania

Marion Winfrey, EdD, RN
University of Massachusetts at Boston
College of Nursing
Boston, Massachusetts

Preface

The term *high acuity* as used in this text refers to a level of patient complexity that falls beyond uncomplicated acute illness on a health-illness continuum. Today, high acuity patients are increasingly found outside of critical care units. The patient population is older and sicker upon entering the health care system, and they are being discharged earlier, in a poorer state of health. In the home health setting, we see mechanical ventilators, central intravenous lines, large wounds, and IV antibiotic therapy. While critical care units are considered specialty areas within the hospital walls, much of the knowledge base required to work within that specialty is generalist in nature. The majority of this knowledge base is needed by all novice nurses in today's acute care market to better assure a competent and safe nursing practice.

Purpose of the Text

This text was conceived when we were assigned the responsibility of teaching senior baccalaureate students how to apply in a clinical setting the knowledge previously learned in the junior year medical-surgical nursing course. In searching for resources to assist with the teaching task, we found that existing medical-surgical texts and critical care texts were too detailed, too complex, or lacked sufficient reality-based clinical application. To address this problem, an experimental teaching design was developed incorporating self-directed modular learning. Self-directed study focuses on adult learning principles, placing the responsibility on the learner for mastery of content. The modules allow redirecting of educational energies and resources towards application of module principles and problem-solving exercises, using the nursing process. Thus, faculty serve as facilitators and translators to illuminate problem solving.

A series of self-study modules focusing on the relationship between the nursing process and pathophysiology were developed with the following goals in mind:

1. Revisit and translate critical pathophysiologic concepts pertaining to the high acuity patient in a clinically applicable manner
2. Examine the interrelationships between physiologic concepts
3. Enhance clinical decision-making skills
4. Free class time to focus on clinical application
5. Hold learners accountable for their own learning
6. Provide immediate feedback to the learner regarding *assimilation* of concepts and principles

This book is appropriate for use by multiple audiences, such as nursing students, novice nurses, and novice critical care nurses. It is also a review book for the experienced nurse wanting to update knowledge in acute care nursing (e.g., re-entry programs, or general interest). Hospital staff development departments may find it useful as a supplement or required reading for critical care orientation, as a review mechanism for per diem and traveler (mobile) nurses, or as an orientation program for small groups of nurses for whom a classroom orientation program was not economically feasible.

Text Construction

The book consists of seven parts: Ventilation, Perfusion, Trauma, Metabolism, Psychosocial Concepts, Caring for Special Patients, and Clinical Simulations. Case studies are frequently included within the modules to reinforce problem solving. Normal laboratory values used throughout the book are not necessarily consistent between modules but all are within valid parameters and acceptable norms. This resembles the variance encountered in the clinical setting.

Parts I Through IV

The first four parts are comprised of modules that are written in a consistent format for reading ease. Each basic concepts module focuses on physiology and pathophysiology related to a particular topic. Topics have been chosen based on disorders commonly dealt with in high acuity patients. Basic concepts modules all include an introduction, glossary, abbreviations list, objectives, pretest, sections with review questions, and a posttest. The learner is able to receive immediate feedback because all questions in the modules include answers. Each of the first four parts ends with a nursing care module designed to integrate the concepts presented within that part, to develop nursing care strategies. The structure of the nursing care modules differs from the basic concepts modules: rather than being divided into small sections, they are more integrated, focusing on the nursing process using a case study approach. Nursing diagnoses are assimilated primarily in the nursing care modules. The NANDA framework has been used whenever possible for formulation of nursing diagnoses. However, nursing diagnoses are also included that are not NANDA approved yet are clinically meaningful to the high acuity patient.

Part V

Psychosocial Concepts, the fifth part, addresses the psychosocial needs of high acuity patients, their families, and the nurses who care for them. It is an overview of pertinent concepts that should be addressed in the provision of nursing care.

Part VI

The sixth part, Caring for Special Patients, addresses a void in existing medical-surgical and critical care texts: high acuity pediatrics and obstetrics concepts. In reality, nurses often encounter high acuity pediatric patients who have been integrated into adult settings because of a lack of pediatric bed availability. Obstetric patients who become acutely ill may also be admitted onto a nonobstetric hospital area. This patient population has special needs related to the physiologic changes encountered in pregnancy that must be addressed in planning and implementing nursing care. Module structure in this part uses an integrative approach, incorporating multiple physiologic concepts, as well as the nursing process.

Part VII

The book ends with Part VII, a series of three Clinical Simulations. The simulations are designed to apply selected aspects of modular content. They are *not* intended to serve as a comprehensive review. The simulations reinforce principles and concepts by focusing on a reality-based situation requiring clinical problem solving. The simulations have been designed to teach rather than to test. Answers are provided with rationales, and a scoring mechanism is included.

Summary

This textbook is a series of reality-based modules that translates concepts frequently encountered in the high acuity patient. It is not designed as a comprehensive review of pathophysiology or medical-surgical nursing. Nursing has been criticized in the past for "eating our young," in part because of inadequate preparation of novice nurses for the reality of the practice environment. Reality-based learning strategies, including case studies, essential "need-to-know" physiology and pathophysiology, and clinical problem solving, are some of the means by which this text nurtures novice nurses in facilitating adequate preparation. This book has as its ultimate goal the enhancement of learning the high acuity nursing concepts to facilitate adequate preparation of the novice nurse for practicing in today's health care setting.

CEU Credits: Earn continuing education credits. See last book page for information.

Pamela Stinson Kidd
Kathleen Dorman Wagner

Acknowledgments

Development of this textbook has touched the lives of many people, both professionally and personally. We would like to give particular thanks to

- The University of Kentucky Hospital and College of Nursing for believing in the book and supporting our efforts.
- The contributors who gave so much time and effort for so little "glory."
- Our comrade in teaching, Karen L. Johnson, for supporting development of the book and maintaining the home front.
- The NUR 877 students who acted as "guinea pigs" in module development. Their strong enthusiasm was instrumental in module development. Their patience in using drafts as a textbook was much appreciated.
- Linda Nold for helping to create the structure, expand the idea, and nurture the editors.
- Sally Taylor for recognizing the potential of the modules and acting on it.
- Butch Kidd for convincing me to not take life so seriously and believing in my potential. You are my best friend and agent.
- Elizabeth Kidd for learning how to cook and to live with a mom who is "working on the book." You have been very patient and I love you for it.
- My family who lived without me (physically and/or mentally) at family functions for the last 2 years. I feel your presence in the pages of this book because of the support you have given me.
- Don, Becky and Debby Wagner who took over control of family life when the deadlines drew near.
- The Respiratory Therapy Program at Lexington Community College, especially Tri, Jim and Ron, for sharing their expertise.
- A special thank you goes to Julia Hempenstall Fultz, RN, and Franketta Zalaznik, RN, from the University of Kentucky Aeromedical Service for their case study contributions. It took a lot of time to write those cases up and even though the cases were modified, you provided the "guts."
- Many thanks to Jim McGraw for stimulating and supporting the editors to take an idea and run with it. It was your original module that provided the initial format.

PART I

Ventilation

Module 1

Respiratory Process

Kathleen Dorman Wagner

The focus of this module, *Respiratory Process,* is on physiologic as well as pathophysiologic processes involved in pulmonary ventilation and respiration. Nursing management is addressed in a separate self-study module, *Nursing Care of the Patient with Altered Respiratory Function.* The module is composed of nine sections. Sections One through Four consider the underlying general principles involved in the respiratory process, including respiration and ventilation, pulmonary diffusion, the relationship between ventilation and perfusion, and pulmonary shunting. Section Five gives a brief overview of evaluation of pulmonary function. Section Six differentiates pulmonary diseases on the basis of restrictive vs obstructive processes. Sections Seven through Nine describe the pathophysiologic basis of selected pulmonary disorders, including chronic obstructive pulmonary disease, acute respiratory failure, and adult respiratory distress syndrome. Each section includes a set of review questions to help the learner evaluate understanding of the section content before moving on to the next section. All Section Reviews and the Pretests and Posttests in the module include answers. It is suggested that the learner review those concepts that were missed in the review questions before proceeding to the next section.

Objectives

On completion of this module, *Respiratory Process,* the learner will be able to

1. Explain the concept of ventilation
2. Discuss pulmonary diffusion
3. Explain the relationship between ventilation and perfusion
4. Describe the physiologic basis of right-to-left shunt
5. Describe various tests used for evaluation of pulmonary function
6. Explain the basic difference between restrictive and obstructive pulmonary diseases
7. Describe the pathophysiologic processes involved in chronic obstructive pulmonary disease (COPD) in the adult
8. Discuss the pathophysiologic basis of respiratory failure
9. Describe the pathophysiologic basis of adult respiratory distress syndrome (ARDS)

Pretest

1. Ventilation is best defined as
   A. movement of gases across the alveolar–capillary membrane
   B. mechanical movement of gases in and out of the lungs
   C. transport of gases through the blood to and from the tissues
   D. movement of gases down a pressure gradient

2. During inspiration, air is drawn into the lungs because intrapulmonary pressure is
   A. above alveolar–capillary pressure
   B. equal to intraabdominal pressure
   C. below atmospheric pressure
   D. above intrathoracic pressure

3. All of the following factors affect pulmonary diffusion EXCEPT
   A. gradient
   B. thickness
   C. surface area
   D. barometric pressure

4. If the ventilation-perfusion ($\dot{V}/\dot{Q}$) ratio is low, it will affect arterial blood gases in which way?
   A. decreased Pao_2
   B. decreased $Paco_2$
   C. increased Pao_2
   D. increased pH

5. Physiologic shunt refers to which of the following?
   A. blood that bypasses the heart
   B. blood that bypasses the lungs
   C. blood that does not take part in diffusion
   D. blood that does not release carbon dioxide

6. The primary ventilatory problem associated with obstructive pulmonary disease is
   A. obstruction to perfusion
   B. decreased diffusion of gases
   C. delay of airflow out of the lungs
   D. inability to achieve normal tidal volumes

7. Pure pulmonary emphysema affects the lungs in which of the following ways?
   A. decreases alveolar size
   B. destroys alveoli
   C. causes bronchospasm
   D. increases production of mucus

8. Chronic bronchitis affects airway cilia by
   A. destroying cilia
   B. increasing ciliary activity
   C. decreasing ciliary activity
   D. causing hypertrophy of ciliary epithelium

9. The nurse would expect a person who has respiratory insufficiency to have which of the following blood gas conditions?
   A. pH below normal
   B. $Paco_2$ below normal
   C. pH normal
   D. $Paco_2$ normal

10. Symptoms of a person with a high $Paco_2$ would include
    A. weak, thready pulse
    B. flushed, wet skin
    C. decreased blood pressure
    D. slow, shallow breathing

11. Adult respiratory distress syndrome (ARDS) is primarily a problem of
    A. oxygenation
    B. ventilation
    C. perfusion
    D. pressure

Pretest answers: 1, B. 2, C. 3, D. 4, A. 5, C. 6, C. 7, B. 8, A. 9, C. 10, B. 11, A.

Glossary

Absolute (true) shunt. The sum of anatomic shunt and capillary shunt

Adult respiratory distress syndrome (ARDS). A type of respiratory failure caused by diffuse injury to the alveolar–capillary membrane, resulting in noncardiogenic pulmonary edema

Anatomic shunt. Movement of blood from the right heart and back into the left heart without coming into contact with alveoli

Capillary shunt. Normal flow of blood past completely unventilated alveoli

Chronic bronchitis. A chronic obstructive pulmonary disease of the larger airways that is defined clinically as the presence of chronic productive cough that occurs daily for at least 3 months per year for at least 2 years in succession

Chronic obstructive pulmonary disease (COPD) (chronic airflow limitation diseases). A group of pulmonary diseases that cause obstruction to expiratory airflow

Compliance (C_L). Measurement of the ability of the lungs and thorax to expand

Cor pulmonale. Right ventricular hypertrophy and dilation secondary to pulmonary disease

Diffusion. Movement of gases down a pressure gradient from an area of high pressure to an area of low pressure

Emphysema. A pathologic pulmonary process characterized by enlargement of alveoli and destruction of alveoli and surrounding capillary beds

External respiration. Movement of gases across the alveolar–capillary membrane

Forced expiratory volumes (FEVs). Measure of how rapidly a person can forcefully exhale air after a maximal inhalation; a measurement of dynamic lung function

Internal respiration. Movement of gases across systemic capillary–cell membrane, in the tissues

Minute ventilation ($\dot{V}_E$). The total volume of expired air in 1 minute

Obstructive disease. Pulmonary disorders that are associated with decreased or delayed airflow during expiration

Physiologic shunt. Movement of blood from the right heart, through the lungs, and on into the left heart without taking part in alveolar–capillary diffusion

Respiration. The process by which the body's cells are supplied with oxygen and carbon dioxide is eliminated from the body

Respiratory failure. A state of pulmonary decompensation in which the body is no longer able to maintain normal gas exchange. It can be expressed as Pa_{O_2} <60 mm Hg or Pa_{CO_2} > 50 mm Hg at pH <7.30

Respiratory insufficiency. A state of pulmonary compensation in which a normal blood pH is maintained only at the expense of the cardiopulmonary system

Restrictive disease. Pulmonary disorders associated with a decrease in lung volume

Sepsis. A pathologic state in which microorganisms, or their toxins, are present in the bloodstream

Shuntlike effect. Effect created by an excess of perfusion in relation to alveolar ventilation

Surfactant. A lipoprotein produced by type II alveolar cells; reduces the surface tension of the alveolar fluid lining

Tidal volume (TV or V_T). The amount of air that moves in and out of the lungs with each normal breath

Total lung capacity (TLC). The amount of gas present in the lungs after maximal inspiration

Venous admixture. The effect that a physiologic shunt has on the contents of the blood as it drains into the left heart

Ventilation. The mechanical movement of airflow to and from the atmosphere and the alveoli

Vital capacity (VC). The maximum amount of air expired after a maximal inspiration; a measurement of lung capacity

$\dot{V}/\dot{Q}$ ratio. A ratio expressing the relationship of ventilation to perfusion

Abbreviations

ABG. Arterial blood gas

ARDS. Adult respiratory distress syndrome

C_L. Lung compliance, expressed in cm H_2O/mL

CO_2. Carbon dioxide

COPD. Chronic obstructive pulmonary disease

f. Frequency, rate of breathing, expressed in breaths per minute

FEV. Forced expiratory volume

IPPB. Intermittent positive pressure breathing

$\dot{Q}$. Pulmonary capillary perfusion

P_{CO_2}. Partial pressure of carbon dioxide or carbon dioxide tension, expressed in mm Hg; variations:
  PA_{CO_2}. Specifies alveolar carbon dioxide tension
  Pa_{CO_2}. Specifies arterial carbon dioxide tension
  $P\bar{v}_{CO_2}$. Specifies venous carbon dioxide tension

P_{O_2}. Partial pressure of oxygen or oxygen tension, expressed in mm Hg; variations:

PAO$_2$. Specifies alveolar oxygen tension
PaO$_2$. Specifies arterial oxygen tension
PvO$_2$. Specifies venous oxygen tension

V̇. Ventilation

VC. Vital capacity

V̇E. Minute ventilation

V̇/Q̇ ratio. Ventilation-perfusion ratio

VT (TV). Tidal volume, expressed in milliliters or liters

Section One: Ventilation

At the completion of this section, the learner will be able to explain the concept of ventilation.

The respiratory process consists of two distinct concepts, respiration and ventilation. Respiration is the process by which the body's cells are supplied with oxygen and carbon dioxide (cellular waste product) is eliminated from the body. Respiration can be further divided into external and internal respiration. External respiration refers to the movement of gases across the alveolar–capillary membrane. Internal respiration refers to the movement of gases across systemic capillary–cell membranes in the tissues. External respiration is discussed throughout this module.

Ventilation is defined as the mechanical movement of airflow to and from the atmosphere and the alveoli. Ventilation involves the actual work of breathing and requires adequate functioning of the lungs and conducting airways, thorax, ventilatory muscles, and nervous system control. Decreased functioning of any one of these factors will affect the body's ability to ventilate properly.

Ventilation is accomplished through a bellowslike action. Air is able to move in and out of the lungs as a result of the changing size of the thorax caused by ventilatory muscle activity. When the thorax enlarges, the intrapulmonary pressure drops to below atmospheric pressure. Air then moves from the area of higher pressure to the area of lower pressure, resulting in air flowing into the lungs (inspiration) until the pressure in the lungs becomes slightly higher than atmospheric pressure. At this point, air flows back out of the lungs (expiration) until once again pressures are equalized.

Lung tissue has a constant tendency to collapse due to several important properties. First, the fluid lining of the alveoli has a naturally high surface tension, creating a tendency for the alveolar walls to collapse. To prevent this, special cells in the alveoli secrete a lipoprotein called surfactant. Surfactant has a detergentlike action, reducing the surface tension of the fluid lining the alveolar sacs and thereby decreasing the tendency toward collapse. Second, the lungs are composed of elastic fibers. The elastic force of these fibers constantly seeks to return to their resting state, causing a collapsed lung. To maintain the lungs in an inflated state, the elastic forces must constantly be overcome by opposing forces (Figure 1–1).

The primary opposing force that maintains the lung in an expanded state is the thorax, which, with its associated respiratory muscles, naturally moves outward, thus expanding during inspiration. The thoracic bony structure provides a cagelike framework to maintain the lungs in a baseline inflated state even at rest.

What causes the lungs to adhere to the thoracic walls? An attraction exists between the visceral and parietal pleura. The pleurae are slick-surfaced moist

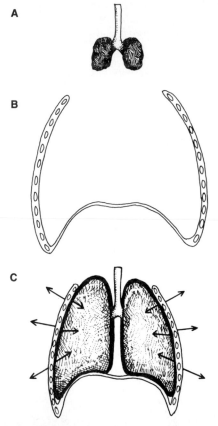

Figure 1–1. Opposing elastic forces of the lungs and thorax. **A.** The resting state of normal lungs when removed from the chest cavity. Elasticity causes total collapse. **B.** Resting state of normal chest wall and diaphragm when apex is open to the atmosphere, and the thoracic contents are removed. **C.** End expiration in the normal, intact thorax. Note that the elastic forces of the lung and chest wall are in opposite directions. The pleural surfaces link these two opposing forces. (*From* Clinical application of respiratory care, *4th ed., p. 22, by B.A. Shapiro et al, 1991, St. Louis, MO: Mosby Year Book.*)

membranes. The parietal pleura adheres to the thoracic walls, diaphragm, and mediastinum, and the visceral pleura adheres to the lung parenchyma. To understand the pleural attraction, it may help to think of placing two moistened sheets of smooth glass together. Although it would be relatively easy to glide one sheet over the other in a parallel fashion, it would be very difficult to pull them directly apart at a 180-degree angle. The glass sheets represent the two pleurae. Under normal circumstances (a negative intrapleural state), the parietal and visceral pleura act as one membrane. Therefore, as the thorax increases and decreases in volume, so will the lungs.

Compliance

The ease with which the lungs are able to be expanded is measured in terms of lung compliance. For example, it is much more difficult to blow up a small balloon than a large balloon. To inflate the small balloon, you would need to blow much harder (exert more pressure force) to obtain the same volume that you would be able to obtain with much less force in the large balloon. The small balloon is less compliant than the large balloon. Compliance is defined in terms of lung volume (mL) and pressure (cm H_2O) as

$$C_L = \frac{\Delta V}{\Delta P}$$

where C_L is lung compliance, ΔV is change in volume (mL), and ΔP is change in pressure (cm H_2O).

Like a bag of assorted size balloons, alveoli also come in many sizes. Each size of alveolus has a certain filling capacity beyond which it becomes overexpanded and may even burst. As the alveoli approach their filling capacity, they become less compliant, that is, it takes more force to completely expand the alveoli and even greater force to hyperexpand them. Patients with adult respiratory distress syndrome

(ARDS) require moderate to high levels of positive end-expiratory pressure (PEEP) to open, expand, or hyperexpand alveoli that have become significantly noncompliant due to the disease process. Use of PEEP ideally increases lung compliance. However, if too much PEEP (measured in centimeters H_2O pressure) is used, alveoli become so hyperexpanded that compliance decreases dramatically and the alveoli are at risk of rupture, causing pneumothorax. (PEEP is explained in detail in Mechanical Ventilation Module.)

Many pulmonary and extrapulmonary problems can influence compliance. Compliance is very sensitive to any condition that affects the lung's tissues, particularly if the disorder causes a reduction in pulmonary surfactant, which is crucial to maintenance of functional alveoli. When there is a deficiency of surfactant, compliance is decreased. Decreased compliance is sometimes referred to as "stiff lungs," meaning that it now takes more force (pressure) to increase lung volume. For example, whereas a person with normal lungs can inhale 50 to 100 mL of air for every 1 cm H_2O of pressure exerted, a person with decreased compliance might be able to inhale 30 to 40 mL/cm H_2O of pressure. Decreased compliance increases the work of breathing and causes a decreased tidal volume. Breathing rate increases to compensate for the decreased tidal volume. Pulmonary problems causing decreased compliance are called restrictive pulmonary disorders (Section Six), and examples of conditions associated with decreased compliance can be found in Table 1-2.

In summary, the respiratory process has two major components: respiration and ventilation. Lung tissue has to constantly overcome the tendency to collapse. The substance surfactant is crucial in maintaining the alveoli in an open state. Lung compliance is decreased by many intrapulmonary and extrapulmonary disorders affecting the volume of air moved in and out of the lungs.

Section One Review

1. The elastic force of lung tissue seeks to
   A. keep lungs expanded
   B. make lungs collapse
   C. flatten the diaphragm
   D. decrease thorax size
2. During expiration, air flows out of the lungs because the intrapulmonary pressure
   A. increases to above atmospheric pressure
   B. is equal to perfusion pressure
   C. drops to below atmospheric pressure
   D. is equal to alveolar pressure
3. The purpose of surfactant is to
   A. decrease lung compliance
   B. increase alveolar surface tension
   C. cleanse the alveoli
   D. decrease alveolar surface tension

4. The lungs adhere to the thoracic walls because of
   A. elastic forces
   B. pulmonary surfactant
   C. hydraulic traction
   D. lung compliance
5. As alveoli near their filling capacity, they become
   A. less compliant
   B. less elastic
   C. more compliant
   D. hyperexpanded

6. External respiration refers to
   A. movement of air from the atmosphere to the alveoli
   B. diffusion of gases across the alveolar–capillary membrane
   C. movement of air from the alveoli to the atmosphere
   D. Diffusion of gases across the tissue–capillary membranes

Answers: 1, B. 2, A. 3, D. 4, C. 5, A. 6, B.

Section Two: Diffusion

At the completion of this section, the learner will be able to discuss pulmonary diffusion.

Oxygenation of tissues is dependent on the process of diffusion as the vital mechanism for both external and internal respiration. Diffusion is the movement of gases down a pressure gradient from an area of high pressure to an area of low pressure. There are three factors that affect diffusion through the alveolar–capillary membrane: gradient, area, and thickness.

Gradient

A pressure gradient (difference) exists between the atmosphere and the alveoli and between the alveoli and the pulmonary capillaries. The greater the pressure difference, the more rapid the flow of gases. Several factors that increase the gradient include exercise, positive pressure mechanical ventilation, and intermittent positive pressure breathing (IPPB).

Air enters the alveoli from the atmosphere because the atmospheric air pressure is slightly higher than alveolar pressure. A pressure gradient also exists between the alveoli and the pulmonary capillaries, causing flow of gases across the alveolar–capillary membrane. This process is called external respiration. Atmospheric air is composed of molecules of nitrogen, oxygen, carbon dioxide, and water vapor. The combination of all of these gases exerts about 760 mm Hg of pressure. The respiratory process, however, does not actively involve use of the water vapor or nitrogen. It is concerned with exchange of oxygen and carbon dioxide (Figure 1–2).

Oxygen and carbon dioxide both exert a certain percentage of the total air pressure. Oxygen in the alveoli exerts approximately 100 mm Hg pressure, and this partial pressure of oxygen is called P_{O_2} or oxygen tension. When the P_{O_2} refers to oxygen in the alveoli, it is more precisely referred to as $P_{A_{O_2}}$. When it refers to arterial blood, it is abbreviated as $P_{a_{O_2}}$, and when it refers to venous blood, it is specified as $P_{v_{O_2}}$. Carbon dioxide in the alveoli exerts approximately 40 mm Hg of pressure. This partial pressure is called P_{CO_2}. The abbreviation alterations of A, a, and v used for describing P_{O_2} also apply to P_{CO_2}.

Venous blood returning to the lungs from the tissues is oxygen poor (P_{O_2} of $\approx$ 40 mm Hg). This is because the blood has dropped off its load of oxygen for use by the tissues. Venous blood is rich in carbon dioxide (P_{CO_2} of $\approx$ 45 mm Hg) due to transport of the cellular waste product, carbon dioxide (CO_2), for removal from the lungs.

The alveolar–capillary membrane is very thin. Oxygen and carbon dioxide molecules move easily across the membrane by diffusion. Alveolar oxygen moves into the capillaries, and carbon dioxide moves out of the capillaries into the alveoli. Oxygen and carbon dioxide do not diffuse at the same rate. Carbon dioxide is able to diffuse about 20 times more rapidly than oxygen. Therefore, when a person has

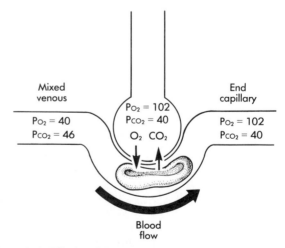

Figure 1–2. Diffusion of oxygen and carbon dioxide. Gas exchange occurs solely by diffusion from a region of relatively high gas pressure to one of relatively low gas pressure. (*From* Pulmonary physiology in clinical practice: The essentials in clinical practice, *p. 39, by L. Martin, 1987, St. Louis: C.V. Mosby.*)

diseased lung tissue, severe tissue hypoxia may exist long before carbon dioxide levels are affected. Figure 1-2 shows the movement of gases during diffusion.

In internal respiration, the process is reversed. The arterial blood is rich in oxygen and poor in carbon dioxide, whereas the cells are poor in oxygen and rich in carbon dioxide. The pressure differences between the Pao_2 and $Paco_2$ in the blood and cells cause oxygen to move from the circulating hemoglobin into the cells. The cells release carbon dioxide back into the bloodstream for transport back to the lungs for excretion.

Surface Area

The total surface area of the lung is very large. The greater the available alveolar–capillary membrane surface area, the greater the amount of oxygen and carbon dioxide that can diffuse across it during a specific period of time. Emphysema is a major pulmonary disorder that destroys the alveolar–capillary membrane. This greatly reduces surface area and consequently impairs gas exchange. Many pulmonary conditions, including severe pneumonia, lung tumors, pneumothorax, and pneumonectomy, can reduce functioning surface area significantly.

Thickness

The thickness of the alveolar–capillary membrane is of major importance. The thinner the membrane, the more rapid the rate of diffusion of gases. Several conditions can increase membrane thickness, thereby decreasing the rate of diffusion.

- Fluid in the alveoli or interstitial spaces or both (e.g., pulmonary edema)
- An inflammatory process involving the alveoli (e.g., pneumonia)
- Lung conditions that cause fibrosis (e.g., adult respiratory distress syndrome or pneumoconiosis)

In summary, diffusion is the process by which gases are exchanged in the lungs and in the tissues. The factors of gradient, surface area, and thickness all greatly influence the effectiveness of diffusion. Should a pulmonary disorder cause a problem with any one of these factors, gas exchange becomes impaired, resulting in an increase in arterial carbon dioxide levels, a decrease in arterial oxygen levels, or both.

Section Two Review

1. Pressure gradient affects diffusion of gases in which of the following ways?
   A. the more rapid the ventilatory rate, the greater the gradient
   B. the greater the difference, the more rapid the gas flow
   C. the less rapid the ventilatory rate, the greater the gradient
   D. the smaller the difference, the more rapid the gas flow
2. Which of the following factors increases the diffusion pressure gradient?
   A. increased exercise
   B. decreased activity
   C. negative pressure ventilation
   D. amount of lung surface area
3. The normal partial pressure of alveolar oxygen is approximately
   A. 60 mm Hg
   B. 80 mm Hg
   C. 100 mm Hg
   D. 110 mm Hg

4. Surface area as a factor affecting diffusion refers to
   A. size of the alveoli
   B. the conducting airways
   C. the functional capillary perfusion
   D. the functional alveoli and surrounding capillaries
5. An example of a disease process that would increase the thickness of the alveolar–capillary membrane is
   A. pneumonia
   B. pneumothorax
   C. lung tumor
   D. pneumonectomy
6. Which of the following statements regarding diffusion is appropriate?
   A. gas flows down a pressure gradient
   B. diffusion refers to alveolar pressure
   C. gas flows up a pressure gradient
   D. diffusion refers to capillary pressure

Answers: 1, B. 2, A. 3, C. 4, D. 5, A. 6, A.

Section Three:
Ventilation-Perfusion Relationship

At the completion of this section, the learner will be able to explain the relationship between ventilation and perfusion.

Normal diffusion of gases requires a certain balance of alveolar ventilation (movement of gas into the alveoli) and pulmonary perfusion (blood flow through the pulmonary capillaries). Should an imbalance in this relationship develop, normal gas exchange cannot take place in the affected areas. For this reason, it is important to gain a basic understanding of the relationship of ventilation ($\dot{V}$) to perfusion ($\dot{Q}$). This relationship is expressed as a ratio of alveolar ventilation to pulmonary capillary perfusion ($\dot{V}/\dot{Q}$ ratio).

For ideal gas exchange to occur, one would expect that for every liter of fresh air coming into the alveoli, 1 L of blood would flow past it, creating a 1:1 ratio of ventilation to perfusion. In reality, for approximately every 4 L of air flowing into the alveoli, about 5 L of blood flows past (an average ratio of 4:5, or 0.8) (Figure 1–3).

To facilitate discussion of the $\dot{V}/\dot{Q}$ ratio, P_{AO_2} and P_{ACO_2} must be described further. P_{AO_2} refers to alveolar oxygen, and P_{ACO_2} refers to alveolar carbon dioxide. The balance of ventilation to perfusion is greatly affected by the P_{AO_2} and P_{ACO_2}. Des Jardins (1988) explains that P_{AO_2} is "determined by the balance between (1) the amount of oxygen ventilated into the alveoli and (2) its removal by capillary blood flow." P_{ACO_2} is "determined by the balance between (1) the amount of carbon dioxide that diffuses into the alveoli from the capillary blood and (2) its removal out of the alveoli by means of ventilation" (p. 202).

Though normal values are given for P_{AO_2} (100 mm Hg) and P_{ACO_2} (40 mm Hg), these numbers only express an average. The actual partial pressures of oxygen and carbon dioxide vary throughout the lungs. Ventilation is not distributed evenly throughout the lungs. In an upright person, alveolar ventilation is only moderate in the apices of the lungs because of increased negative pleural pressures in the apices in relation to the lung bases. This makes the alveoli in the lung apices more resistant to airflow during inspiration. When breathing spontaneously, airflow naturally moves toward the diaphragm, resulting in more air movement into the bases and peripheral lung during inspiration (airflow follows the path of least resistance). Pulmonary capillary perfusion is gravity dependent. Perfusion is greatest in the dependent areas of the lungs (the bases in an upright person). Consequently, since ventilation and perfusion are both greatest in the bases of the lungs, the greatest amount of gas exchange occurs in this portion of the lung fields.

In the upper lungs, there is moderate alveolar ventilation and very reduced perfusion, making an excess of ventilation to available perfusion. This may be expressed as a high $\dot{V}/\dot{Q}$ ratio (>0.8). In the lower lungs, there is a moderate increase in ventilation with a great increase in perfusion. This may be expressed as a low $\dot{V}/\dot{Q}$ ratio, since there is a relatively moderate increase in ventilation associated with a significant increase in perfusion.

The clinical significance of ventilation-perfusion balance becomes apparent when considering its implications in acutely ill patients. When an acutely ill person is placed in bed, he or she is kept in a relatively horizontal position. Since perfusion is gravity dependent, it will shift from the lung bases to whichever lung area is now in the dependent position (Figure 1–4).

Keeping the principles of $\dot{V}/\dot{Q}$ ratio in mind, what could happen if a patient is positioned on the right side if there is significant pneumonia in the right lung fields? Since the patient is lying on the right side, maximum pulmonary capillary perfusion will be on the right. Pneumonia is associated with secretions and other factors that cause obstruction to airflow into the affected right lung alveoli. Therefore, since airflow follows the path of least resistance, it will decrease in the diseased right lung area. This

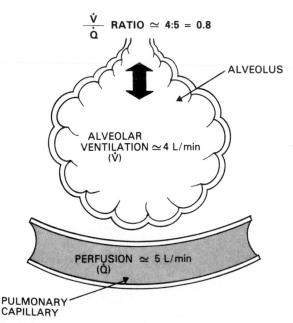

$$\frac{\dot{V}}{\dot{Q}} \text{ RATIO} \simeq 4:5 = 0.8$$

ALVEOLUS

ALVEOLAR VENTILATION $\simeq$ 4 L/min ($\dot{V}$)

PERFUSION $\simeq$ 5 L/min ($\dot{Q}$)

PULMONARY CAPILLARY

Figure 1–3. The relationship of ventilation to perfusion. The normal ventilation-perfusion ratio ($\dot{V}/\dot{Q}$ ratio) is about 0.8. (*Reproduced by permission. From* Cardiopulmonary anatomy & physiology: Essentials for respiratory care, p. 201, by Terry R. Des Jardins. Albany, NY: Delmar Publishers. Copyright 1988.)

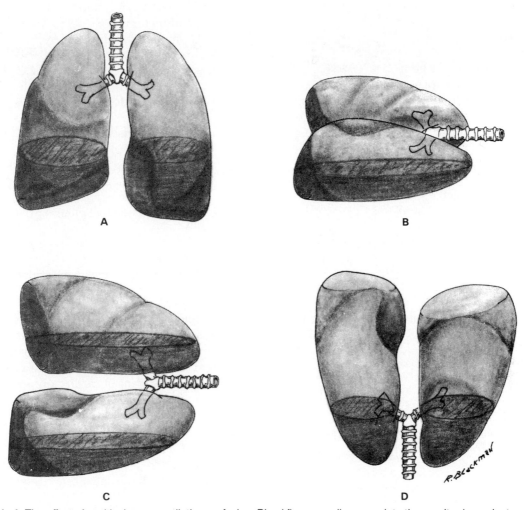

A

B

C

D

Figure 1–4. The effect of positioning on ventilation-perfusion. Blood flow normally moves into the gravity-dependent areas of the lungs. Thus, body position affects the distribution of the pulmonary blood flow as illustrated in the erect (**A**), supine (**B**), lateral (**C**), and upside-down (**D**) positions. (*Reproduced by permission. From* Cardiopulmonary anatomy & physiology: Essentials for respiratory care, *p. 137, by Terry R. Des Jardins. Albany, NY: Delmar Publishers. Copyright 1988.*)

combination of significant decrease in ventilation in the presence of normal to increased perfusion causes a mismatching of ventilation to perfusion, creating a low $\dot{V}/\dot{Q}$ ratio. If sufficient mismatching occurs, Pao_2 and oxygen saturation levels could drop significantly. Positioning this patient on the left side would be tolerated better, since $\dot{V}/\dot{Q}$ matching would be improved. This, then, is one reason why some acutely ill patients tolerate being turned on one side

more than another. Table 1–1 compares high and low $\dot{V}/\dot{Q}$ ratios.

In summary, the relationship of ventilation to perfusion ($\dot{V}/\dot{Q}$ ratio) varies throughout the lung. An overall balance in this relationship must be maintained to optimize proper diffusion of gases. Pulmonary disorders may create a mismatching of ventilation and perfusion, creating problems associated either with a high $\dot{V}/\dot{Q}$ ratio or a low $\dot{V}/\dot{Q}$ ratio.

Section Three Review

1. Which of the following statements is true regarding the relationship of ventilation to perfusion in an upright person?
   A. it varies throughout the lung

   B. ventilation is best in the apices
   C. perfusion is best in peripheral lung areas
   D. it maintains a 1:1 relationship

2. During spontaneous breathing, air flows toward
   A. the apices
   B. the diaphragm
   C. higher pressure gradient
   D. higher resistance areas
3. Mr. M. has a left lower lobe pneumonia. His remaining lung fields are clear. It is time to reposition Mr. M. in bed. Of the following positions, which is most likely to optimize the ventilation-perfusion relationship?
   A. place him on his right side
   B. place him on his back
   C. place him on his left side
   D. place him flat in the bed
4. When ventilation-perfusion mismatching occurs, it can be detected by which of the following parameters?
   A. hemoglobin (Hg) level
   B. oxygen saturation level (Sao_2)
   C. partial pressure of arterial CO_2 ($Paco_2$)
   D. arterial sodium bicarbonate level (HCO_3)
5. What causes a decrease of airflow to the apices of the lungs?
   A. increased natural airflow toward lung periphery
   B. increased negative pleural pressure in bases
   C. increased negative pleural pressure in apices
   D. increased positive pleural pressure in apices

Answers: 1, A. 2, B. 3, A. 4, B. 5, C.

TABLE 1–1. COMPARISON OF HIGH AND LOW $\dot{V}/\dot{Q}$ RATIO

High $\dot{V}/\dot{Q}$ Ratio	Low $\dot{V}/\dot{Q}$ Ratio
Normal to increased ventilation associated with decreased perfusion	Decreased alveolar ventilation associated with normal to increased perfusion
Alveolar gas effect Increased cardiac output Decreased alveolar CO_2	Alveolar gas effect Decreased oxygen in alveoli Increased carbon dioxide in alveoli
Exists normally in upper regions of lung	Normally exists in lower lung fields
Caused abnormally by Decreased cardiac output Pulmonary emboli Pneumothorax Destruction of pulmonary capillaries	Abnormally exists with Hypoventilation Obstructive lung diseases Restrictive lung diseases
Arterial blood gas effects Increased Pao_2 Decreased $Paco_2$, increased pH	Arterial blood gas effect Decreased Pao_2 Increased $Paco_2$, decreased pH

Section Four: Right-to-Left Shunt

At the completion of this section, the learner will be able to describe the physiologic basis of right-to-left shunt.

Pulmonary shunting is a major cause of hypoxemia in acutely ill patients. Shunting also helps explain how problems in ventilation and perfusion originate. Not all blood that flows through the lungs participates in gas exchange. Physiologic shunt is the term used to describe the blood that moves from the right heart through the lungs and into the left heart without taking part in alveolar–capillary diffusion.

Physiologic shunt can be divided into three types: anatomic, capillary, and shuntlike effect (Figure 1–5). Total physiologic shunting normally ranges from 5 percent to 20 percent of cardiac output. Shunting of more than 20 percent of cardiac output represents a threat to adequate oxygenation. Formulas to calculate shunt are beyond the scope of a basic concepts module and, therefore, are not discussed.

Anatomic Shunt

Anatomic shunt refers to blood that moves from the right heart and back into the left heart without coming into contact with alveoli. Normally, this is approximately 2 percent to 5 percent of blood flow. Normal anatomic shunting occurs as a result of emptying of the bronchial and several other veins into the lung's own venous system. Abnormal anatomic shunting can occur because of heart or lung problems. For example, a ventricular septal defect allows shunting of venous blood from the right heart directly into the arterial blood in the left heart. Traumatic injury to pulmonary blood vessels and tissues and certain types of lung tumors also can cause abnormal anatomic shunting.

Capillary Shunt

Capillary shunt is the normal flow of blood past completely unventilated alveoli. Capillary shunt results from such conditions as consolidation or collapse of alveoli, atelectasis, or fluid in the alveoli. Anatomic shunt and capillary shunt together are called absolute (true) shunt. The amount of absolute shunt has important clinical implications. Lung tissue that is

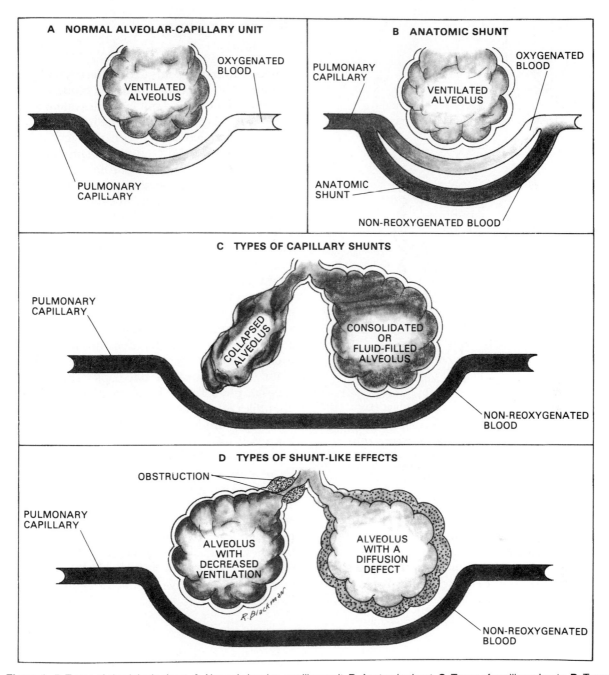

Figure 1–5. Types of physiologic shunt. **A.** Normal alveolar–capillary unit. **B.** Anatomic shunt. **C.** Types of capillary shunts. **D.** Types of shuntlike effects. (*Reproduced by permission. From* Cardiopulmonary anatomy & physiology: Essentials for respiratory care, *p. 175, by Terry R. Des Jardins. Albany, NY: Delmar Publishers. Copyright 1988.*)

affected by absolute shunt is unaffected by oxygen therapy, since it involves nonfunctioning alveoli. No matter how much oxygen is administered, diffusion cannot take place if alveoli are completely bypassed or nonfunctioning. For example, patients with ARDS generally have a shunt of over 20 percent of cardiac output. The hallmark of ARDS is refractory hypoxemia (hypoxemia that is not significantly affected by administration of increasing levels of oxygen, which is consistent with the clinical picture of absolute shunt). Typical therapy for ARDS consists of recruit-

ment of more alveoli into a more functional state through use of PEEP on a mechanical ventilator.

Shuntlike Effect

A third type of physiologic shunt is referred to as shuntlike effect. Shuntlike effect is not complete shunting but occurs when there is an excess of perfusion in relation to alveolar ventilation. Such a condition exists when alveolar ventilation is reduced but

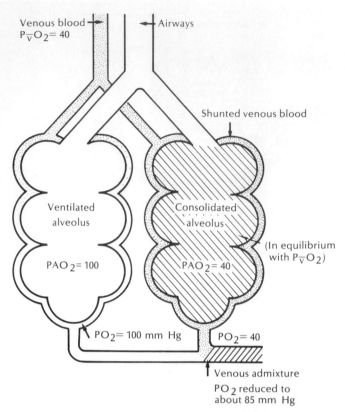

Venous blood → Pv̄O₂= 40

← Airways

Shunted venous blood

Ventilated alveolus

Consolidated alveolus

(In equilibrium with Pv̄O₂)

$PAO_2= 100$

$PAO_2= 40$

$PO_2= 100$ mm Hg

$PO_2= 40$

Venous admixture
PO_2 reduced to about 85 mm Hg

Figure 1–6. Venous admixture. Venous admixture occurs when reoxygenated blood mixes with nonreoxygenated blood distal to the alveoli. (*From* Clinical manifestations of respiratory disease, 2nd ed., p. 22, by T.R. Des Jardins, 1990 Chicago: Year Book Medical Publishers.)

Venous Admixture

Venous admixture refers to the effect that physiologic shunt has on the contents of the blood as it drains into the left heart and out into the system as arterial blood. Venous admixture is "the mixing of shunted, non-reoxygenated blood with reoxygenated blood distal to the alveoli (i.e., downstream in the pulmonary venous system)" (Des Jardins, 1988, p. 176).

As the reoxygenated and unoxygenated blood combine in the bloodstream beyond the shunt area, the blood seeks to gain an equilibrium of oxygen molecules. The oxygen molecules remix in the combined blood to establish a new balance. The end resulting Pao_2 will be higher than that which existed in the shunted (unoxygenated) blood but lower than what it was in the reoxygenated (nonshunted) blood (Figure 1–6).

In summary, oxygenation is greatly affected by the amount of blood that does not take part in gas exchange in the lungs. Physiologic shunt helps explain how hypoxemia develops. There are three types of physiologic shunt: anatomic, capillary, and shuntlike effect. The combination of anatomic and capillary shunt is called absolute shunt, which is refractory to oxygen therapy, since it involves nonfunctioning alveoli. Shuntlike effect, however, is very correctable using oxygen therapy, since the alveoli are still functioning to some extent. The end result of shunting is called venous admixture, which represents the final oxygen content of the blood as it moves into arterial circulation. It is composed of the blending of the reoxygenated and unoxygenated (shunted) blood. An arterial blood gas specimen gives a representative sample of venous admixture blood.

not totally absent. This may be created by conditions that cause such problems as bronchospasm, hypoventilation, or pooling of secretions. Fortunately, since the alveoli are still functioning, hypoxemia secondary to shuntlike effect is very responsive to oxygen therapy.

Section Four Review

1. Which of the following best describes the term *physiologic shunt?*
    A. alveoli that have no air flow
    B. alveoli that have air trapped in them
    C. blood that does not take part in pulmonary gas exchange
    D. blood entering the right heart without being oxygenated
2. Normal physiologic shunt ranges from
    A. 0–5 percent

    B. 5–20 percent
    C. 10–30 percent
    D. 20–40 percent
3. Of the following, anatomic shunt would most likely exist associated with
    A. pneumonia
    B. pulmonary edema
    C. tuberculosis
    D. ventricular septal defect

4. Normal blood flow past completely unventi-
   lated alveoli is the definition of
   A. physiologic shunt
   B. anatomic shunt
   C. capillary shunt
   D. venous admixture
5. Oxygen therapy is most effective in treating
   which of the following?

A. shuntlike effect
B. anatomic shunt
C. capillary shunt
D. absolute shunt

Answers: 1, C. 2, B. 3, D. 4, C. 5, A.

Section Five: Pulmonary Function Evaluation

At the completion of this section, the learner will be
able to briefly describe various tests used to evaluate
pulmonary function.

The medical team generally initiates orders for
pulmonary function testing to assist in diagnosing a
pulmonary problem or updating or evaluating a patient's pulmonary status. Actual implementation and
interpretation of the tests often become an interdisciplinary undertaking.

Pulmonary Function Tests

Ventilation is measured in a variety of ways using
pulmonary function studies. Pulmonary function
studies provide baseline data and also provide a
means to monitor the progress of pulmonary diseases. They also help differentiate a restrictive pulmonary problem from an obstructive problem.
Farzan (1985, p. 28) explains that pulmonary function
tests (PFTs)

> are especially useful for identifying various pat-
> terns of functional impairment, assessing the se-
> verity of functional defects, evaluating disability,
> determining suitability for certain jobs or ac-
> tivities, and following the progress of disease
> and its response to therapeutic measures.

Total Lung Capacity

Total lung capacity (TLC) is the amount (volume) of
gas present in the lungs after maximal inspiration,
which is equal to about 6,000 mL in an adult. TLC is
composed of four separate volumes, each of which
can be measured separately. These volume are called
inspiratory reserve volume (IRV), tidal volume (TV),
expiratory reserve volume (ERV), and residual volume (RV). Volumes also can be measured in combinations called lung capacities. Lung capacities include
inspiratory capacity (IC), vital capacity (VC), func-

tional residual capacity (FRC), and total lung capacity
(TLC).

Bedside Pulmonary Function Measurements

Patients who are acutely ill with or without direct
pulmonary involvement run a risk of developing pulmonary complications associated with immobility
and respiratory muscle fatigue. Pulmonary function
may be monitored in patients who are at particular
risk for ventilatory decompensation. Of particular interest are TV and VC and minute ventilation ($\dot{V}E$). TV
(or V_T) is the amount of air that moves in and out of
the lungs with each normal breath. Normal tidal volume is approximately 7 to 9 mL/kg (Des Jardins,
1988), about 500 mL in the average sized man. When
tidal volume drops below 4 mL/kg, a state of alveolar
hypoventilation develops. If the hypoventilation is
severe enough, acute respiratory failure results. VC
is the maximum amount of air expired after a maximal inspiration. Normal VC is approximately 4,800
mL in the average sized man. Both TV and VC help
monitor respiratory muscle strength. As the patient
experiences respiratory muscle fatigue, these values
will decrease. Both of these pulmonary function tests
can be measured using a respiratory spirometer.

Minute Ventilation

Minute ventilation ($\dot{V}E$) is the total volume of expired
air in 1 minute. It is used as a rapid method of measuring total lung ventilation changes, but it is not
considered to be an accurate measure of alveolar ventilation. Minute ventilation is not a direct measurement but a simple calculation

$$\dot{V}E = V_T \times f$$

where f = frequency, breaths per minute. Normal
minute ventilation is 5 to 10 L/minute. When it increases to over 10 L/minute, the work of breathing
is significantly increased. Minute ventilation below
5 L/minute indicates that the patient is at risk for
problems associated with hypoventilation.

Forced Expiratory Volumes

Forced expiratory volumes (FEVs) are important diagnostic measurements that help differentiate restrictive pulmonary problems from obstructive problems and measures airway resistance. FEVs measure how rapidly a person can forcefully exhale air after a maximal inhalation, measuring volume (in liters) over time (in seconds). Patients who have a restrictive airway problem will be able to push air forcefully out of their lungs at a normal rate, whereas persons who have an obstructive problem will have a delayed emptying rate (a reduced rate of air flow).

In summary, there is a wide variety of methods by which pulmonary function can be evaluated. Pulmonary function tests, such as tidal volume, vital capacity, and total lung capacity, help measure the effects of a disease process on ventilation. Assessment of gas exchange is discussed in depth in the module, *Gas Exchange and Blood Gas Analysis*.

Section Five Review

1. In the acutely ill patient, pulmonary function testing helps monitor for
   A. impending ventilatory failure
   B. acute hypoxemia
   C. acute metabolic acidosis
   D. impending oxygenation failure
2. Minute ventilation $\dot{V}_E$ is calculated as
   A. $\dot{V}_E = VC \times f$
   B. $\dot{V}_E = TV/f$
   C. $\dot{V}_E = VC \times TV$
   D. $\dot{V}_E = TV \times f$
3. Patients who have obstructive pulmonary disease, will have which of the following patterns of forced expiratory volumes (FEVs)?
   A. increased FEVs
   B. delayed FEVs
   C. normal FEVs
   D. variable FEVs

4. Total lung capacity (TLC) is defined as
   A. the rate at which air can be forcefully exhaled after a maximal inspiration
   B. the amount of air that moves in and out of the lungs with each normal breath
   C. the volume of gas present in the lungs after a maximal inspiration
   D. the maximum amount of air expired after a maximal inspiration
5. Normal tidal volume in an average sized adult male would be ___ mL/kg
   A. 3–4
   B. 4–5
   C. 5–7
   D. 7–9

Answers: 1, A. 2, D. 3, B. 4, C. 5, D.

Section Six: Restrictive vs Obstructive Pulmonary Disorders

At the completion of this section, the learner will be able to explain the basic difference between restrictive and obstructive pulmonary diseases.

Pulmonary diseases may be divided into acute and chronic problems. Acute problems have a rapid onset and are episodic. Acute pulmonary problems frequently are confined to the lungs. Chronic problems have a slow, often insidious onset. The pulmonary impairment either does not change or slowly worsens over an extended period of time. Chronic pulmonary problems generally involve other organs as part of the disease process. Patients with chronic pulmonary problems, such as emphysema, may develop an acute restrictive problem (e.g., pneumonia) that may further stress their pulmonary status.

Pulmonary diseases may be divided further into problems of inflow of air (restrictive) and problems of outflow of air (obstructive).

Restrictive Pulmonary Disorders

Restrictive diseases are associated with decreased lung expansion, and, thus, decreased lung compliance is present. Restrictive disorders may be caused by a decrease in functioning alveoli, as in pneumonia, by a lung tissue loss, as in pneumonec-

TABLE 1–2. EXAMPLES OF RESTRICTIVE DISORDERS

■ External Problems	■ Internal (Parenchymal) Problems
Obesity	Pneumonia
Extensive chest burns	Atelectasis
Flail chest	Congestive heart failure
Neuromuscular diseases	Pulmonary edema
Myasthenia gravis	Pulmonary fibrosis
Muscular dystrophy	Pulmonary tumors
Guillain-Barré syndrome	
Spinal cord trauma	

tomy or lung tumors, or by external problems, such as chest burns or obesity (Table 1–2 provides a more complete listing of restrictive disorders).

Restrictive disorders are problems of volume, not airflow. The term volume refers to the amount of air that can be moved in and out of the lung with either normal breathing or maximal breathing. Total lung capacity (TLC) is a measurement of lung volume (see Section Five). TLC is decreased in individuals who have a restrictive disorder. Air cannot move into the alveoli as readily as it should because of limited expansion, causing alveolar hypoventilation. Alveolar hypoventilation causes hypoxemia, and if severe enough, it can cause retention of carbon dioxide.

Restrictive disorders do not interfere with airflow (the rate of movement of air in or out of the lungs). The volume of air the person is able to get into the lungs can be exhaled at a normal rate of flow. The relationship of ventilation to perfusion ($\dot{V}/\dot{Q}$ ratio) may be disturbed as a result of restrictive problems. In mild to moderate restrictive disease, the $\dot{V}/\dot{Q}$ ratio may stay normal, since both ventilation and perfusion may be fairly equally disturbed. In many acute restrictive diseases, perfusion can be diminished through edema resulting from the inflammatory process or from reduced or absent blood flow due to compression or blockage of capillaries. In severe disease, a low $\dot{V}/\dot{Q}$ ratio may develop because ventilation is greatly diminished, whereas perfusion may be fairly normal or moderately disturbed. A low $\dot{V}/\dot{Q}$ ratio is associated with hypoxemia with a decreasing pH and increasing Pa_{CO_2}.

Obstructive Pulmonary Disorders

Obstructive diseases involve problems causing a decreased or delayed airflow during expiration. Lung volumes remain normal. Examples of obstructive disorders are pulmonary emphysema, chronic bronchitis, and asthma. Asthma differs from the other two diseases in that it is episodic rather than continuous obstruction. Air is able to flow into the lungs but then becomes trapped, making it very difficult to rid the lungs of the inspired air. The inability to exhale rapidly causes a prolongation of expiratory time. If expiratory time is severely prolonged, the lungs may never be able to empty before the person must inhale again. Expiratory times can be measured using forced expiratory volumes (FEV) studies (Section Five).

Obstructive problems may be caused by airway narrowing, such as in bronchospasm and bronchoconstriction, or by airway obstruction, such as is seen with pooling of secretions or destruction of bronchioles and alveoli. Obstructive disorders cause increased lung compliance accompanied by a loss of elastic recoil. The $\dot{V}/\dot{Q}$ ratio also may be disturbed with this group of disorders. In disease processes that do not destroy alveoli (chronic bronchitis), a low $\dot{V}/\dot{Q}$ ratio may exist. Ventilation is reduced, whereas perfusion remains normal. If lung tissue is actually destroyed (emphysema), the $\dot{V}/\dot{Q}$ ratio may remain normal because both ventilation and perfusion are equally destroyed. A normal $\dot{V}/\dot{Q}$ ratio does not indicate healthy lungs. It indicates only that a balance exists between ventilation and blood flow. Obstructive diseases are discussed in further detail in Section Seven.

In summary, restrictive diseases are those that interfere with lung expansion. They cause a decrease in lung volumes while expiratory airflow remains normal. They are associated with decreased compliance. Restrictive diseases can be measured by pulmonary function tests, particularly TLC. Obstructive diseases are those that interfere with expiratory airflow. Airflow is reduced or delayed, whereas lung volume remains normal. Obstructive diseases are associated with increased lung compliance. They can be evaluated by measuring FEV flow rates.

Section Six Review

1. Restrictive pulmonary diseases are associated with
   A. increased lung expansion

   B. increased lung compliance
   C. decreased lung expansion
   D. decreased air flow into lungs

2. Which of the following is considered a restrictive disease?
   A. pneumonia
   B. asthma
   C. emphysema
   D. chronic bronchitis
3. Obstructive pulmonary diseases are associated with
   A. decreased lung expansion
   B. decreased lung compliance
   C. decreased air flow into lungs
   D. decreased expiratory airflow
4. An example of an obstructive pulmonary disease is
   A. multiple sclerosis
   B. asthma
   C. tuberculosis
   D. pneumonia
5. Lung compliance is increased with which disorder?
   A. emphysema
   B. pneumonia
   C. pneumothorax
   D. chest burns

Answers: 1, C. 2, A. 3, D. 4, B. 5, A.

Section Seven: Chronic Obstructive Pulmonary Disease

At the completion of this section, the learner will be able to describe the pathophysiologic processes involved in chronic obstructive pulmonary disease (COPD) in the adult.

Chronic obstructive pulmonary disease (COPD) refers to a group of pulmonary diseases causing obstruction to expiratory airflow. There are three major diseases that are most commonly considered COPDs, chronic bronchitis, pulmonary emphysema, and asthma.

Chronic Bronchitis

Chronic bronchitis is a pulmonary disease of the larger airways that is characterized by hypersecretion of mucus in the bronchial tree. Chronic bronchitis is closely associated with cigarette smoking and is reversible if smoking is terminated.

Chronic bronchitis is diagnosed on the basis of clinical history. It is defined as, "the presence of chronic cough with sputum production on a daily basis for a minimum of 3 months per year for not less than 2 successive years" (Neagley, 1991, p. 91). The typical clinical presentation is a pattern of increasing sputum and cough, an increasing pattern of shortness of breath, symptoms of chronic hypoxia, and a well-nourished appearance.

Pathogenesis

Cilia are a crucial part of the mucociliary escalator that moves secretions from the lower airway to the upper airway, where they can be swallowed or expectorated. Smoking interferes with the mucociliary escalator and damages the ciliated epithelium. As ciliated cells are destroyed, they are replaced by mucus-secreting cells. The resulting increase in mucus, associated with decreased ability to move it, causes pooling of secretions. Coughing becomes the primary means for moving pooled secretions out of the lower airway. Thus, the hallmark of chronic bronchitis is excessive mucous secretions and chronic cough.

Hypoxemia develops due to the obstructed airway. Pooling of secretions increases the risk for development of pulmonary infections. The presence of infection can overtax an already heavily burdened pulmonary defense system, possibly precipitating acute respiratory failure.

Pulmonary Emphysema

Emphysema is "an anatomic alteration of the lung parenchyma characterized by abnormal enlargement of the alveoli and alveolar ducts and destruction of the alveolar walls" (Price and Wilson, 1986, p. 522). The hallmark of emphysema is permanent enlargement of airspaces and destruction of alveoli and surrounding capillaries. These destructive changes are irreversible. The primary etiology of emphysema is cigarette smoking, although a very small percentage of the disease is thought to be caused by a genetic deficiency of a particular enzyme, alpha$_1$-trypsin.

The typical presentation of a person with pure emphysema is shortness of breath, minimal sputum production, barrel-shaped chest, thin, often emaciated appearance, and tripod sitting position (leaning forward with elbows on knees).

Pathogenesis

The pathogenesis of emphysema is not clearly understood. Lung tissue is composed largely of elastin and collagen. The protease-antiprotease hypothesis suggests that "the major factor resulting in alveolar disruption in emphysema is the elastin-attacking enzyme (elastase) released from phagocytic cells, unopposed by its inhibitor" (Farzan, 1985, p. 89). In other words, an overabundance of circulating neutrophils in the lungs actually destroys the alveoli. Alveoli provide a supporting structure for the small bronchioles. Once the alveoli are destroyed, the small bronchioles collapse. Bronchiolar collapse primarily occurs during expiration, causing air trapping.

Emphysema is a relentlessly progressive disease. As more tissue is destroyed, the lungs lose their elasticity, which results in permanent hyperinflation of the lungs. The hyperinflated lungs increase compliance significantly, as previously discussed.

The most common type of emphysema affects the central lobules (usually in the upper lobes) and is called centrilobular emphysema. Centrilobular emphysema most commonly occurs with chronic bronchitis. Therefore, patients with centrilobular emphysema generally have clinical manifestations of both emphysema and chronic bronchitis.

Asthma

Asthma is a reversible chronic pulmonary disease caused by hyperreactivity of the trachea and bronchi to extrinsic or intrinsic stimuli. It differs from the other COPDs in its reversibility once the triggering factor has been removed or reversed. Approximately 50 percent of asthma cases begin before the age of 10, and approximately one third of the cases have a family history of asthma (Farzan, 1985).

Asthma is manifested by a triad of symptoms causing narrowing of the airways.

- Hypersecretion of tenacious, thick mucus
- Bronchospasm
- Mucosal edema

Clinically, this triad translates into dyspnea and wheezing, which may be mild or severe depending on the severity of the physiologic response to the trigger.

There are two categories of asthma based on etiology: extrinsic and intrinsic. Extrinsic (allergic) asthma is caused by an allergic response to external environmental triggers (allergens), such as pollen, dust, food, or food additives, and is most clearly demonstrated in childhood asthma (Farzan, 1985). Intrinsic (nonallergic) asthma is caused by triggers within the internal environment of the body. Common causes of intrinsic asthma include such factors as respiratory infection (particularly viral), inhalation

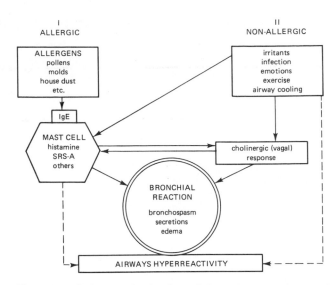

Figure 1–7. Pathogenesis of asthma. Schematic demonstration of the pathogenic mechanisms of asthma in both allergic and non-allergic forms. Note their close interrelationship. (*From A concise handbook of respiratory diseases, 2nd ed., p. 98, by S. Farzan, 1985, Reston, Virginia: Reston Publishing Co.*)

of irritants, exercise, and strong emotions. Intrinsic asthma is seen most commonly in adults.

Pathogenesis

The ultimate sequence of events involved in an acute asthma attack remains the same regardless of the etiologic triggering factor once hyperreactivity is initiated (Figure 1–7).

Status Asthmaticus

Status asthmaticus is a severe asthmatic attack that fails to respond to the usual acute asthma therapy. If not adequately treated, it can cause acute respiratory failure. During status asthmaticus, airway patency becomes compromised as airways become plugged with mucus and mucosal edema continues to increase. Treatment primarily consists of higher doses of regular asthmatic therapy and often includes hydration, aminophylline (IV), corticosteroids (IV), oxygen therapy, and possibly adrenergic agents via nebulizer or systemically. Mechanical ventilation may be required if the patient becomes too exhausted or the arterial blood gas levels become critically deranged.

Cor Pulmonale

Cor pulmonale refers to right ventricular hypertrophy and dilation secondary to pulmonary disease. It

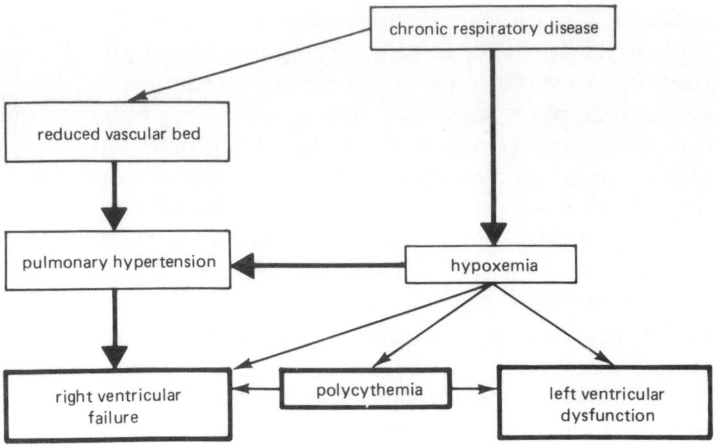

Figure 1–8. Cor pulmonale. Schematic demonstration of the effect of chronic respiratory disorders on the heart. (*From* A concise handbook of respiratory diseases, *2nd ed., p. 188, by S. Farzan, 1985, Reston, VA: Reston Publishing Co.*)

is a complication of both restrictive and obstructive pulmonary diseases. Cor pulmonale can cause right heart failure and is a major cause of death in the COPD patient.

Cor pulmonale is the result of a sequence of events precipitated by pulmonary hypertension. Pulmonary vessels function in a low pressure system. Many pulmonary conditions, both acute and chronic, cause pressures to increase in the vascular bed, creating a state of pulmonary hypertension. When this occurs, pulmonary vascular resistance increases. Pressure in the pulmonary artery is increased, making it more difficult to push blood out of the right heart during systole. The right heart becomes congested because less blood is moved out

with each contraction. Over time, this congestion causes the right heart chambers to dilate. The right heart muscle hypertrophies to compensate for the required increased work of contraction. Figure 1–8 is a diagram showing how the heart is affected by chronic respiratory disorders.

In summary, three pulmonary diseases comprise the primary COPD disorders originating during adulthood. These include chronic bronchitis and emphysema, which often occur together and are most commonly the result of cigarette smoking, and asthma. Although chronic bronchitis is a reversible disease process, emphysema is permanently destructive to both alveoli and surrounding capillaries.

Section Seven Review

1. The primary symptom of chronic bronchitis is
   A. dry, persistent, hacky cough
   B. excessive mucous secretions
   C. malnourished appearance
   D. shallow, rapid respirations
2. In chronic bronchitis, hypoxemia is caused by
   A. alveolar destruction
   B. decreased diffusion
   C. increased CO_2 retention
   D. airway obstruction
3. Pulmonary emphysema is characterized by
   A. bronchoconstriction
   B. excessive mucous secretions
   C. alveolar wall destruction
   D. decreased tidal volume

4. When a patient has pulmonary emphysema, the bronchioles
   A. collapse during expiration
   B. enlarge during expiration
   C. collapse during inspiration
   D. spasm during inspiration
5. A patient who has cor pulmonale will have
   A. left heart dilation
   B. right heart hypertrophy
   C. pulmonary fibrosis
   D. left ventricular dilation

Answers: 1, B. 2, D. 3, C. 4, A. 5, B.

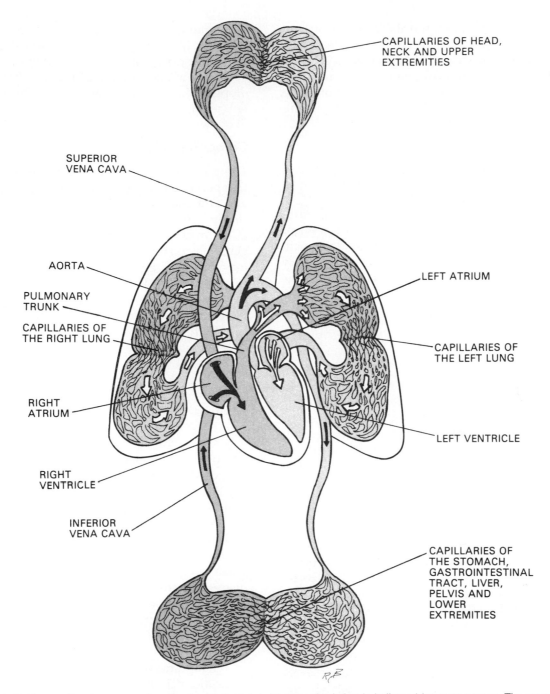

Figure 1–9. The cardiopulmonary and systemic circuit. The pulmonary circulation is indicated by open arrows. The systemic circulation is indicated by solid arrows. (*Reproduced by permission. From* Cardiopulmonary anatomy & physiology: Essentials for respiratory care, *p. 129, by Terry R. Des Jardins. Albany, NY: Delmar Publishers. Copyright 1988.*)

Section Eight: Acute Respiratory Failure

At the completion of this section, the learner will be able to discuss the basis of respiratory failure.

Cardiopulmonary System

It is helpful to think of the heart and lungs as a complex integrated cardiopulmonary system. Since the heart and lungs and systemic circulation share a common circuit (Figure 1–9), whatever affects one part of the system potentially affects the whole. The cardiopulmonary system is very sensitive to pressure changes within it, requiring compensatory adjustments to maintain homeostasis. Problems of cardiac origin can create secondary pulmonary problems. For example, left heart failure can cause cardiogenic pulmonary edema. Pulmonary problems can affect cardiac status, for example, cor pulmonale. If a pulmonary disorder decreases the ability of the lungs to adequately maintain an acid-base balance and oxygenation, the heart will work harder to make more blood available for diffusion, causing a compensatory increase in vital signs (increased blood pressure and pulse). The lungs will work harder by altering the breathing rate to better meet the need.

Insufficiency vs Failure

Respiratory disorders vary greatly in the way in which they affect lung function. The amount of diffusion surface area that becomes impaired is a major factor in altering gas exchange. The extent of impairment paired with the rate of onset contribute greatly to the ability of the body to cope adequately. The terms chronic respiratory insufficiency and acute respiratory failure are used to differentiate the level of compensation of the lungs.

Chronic Respiratory Insufficiency

Respiratory insufficiency is "the circumstance in which gas exchange is maintained at an acceptable level only at the expense of significantly increased work of the cardiopulmonary system" (Shapiro et al, 1991, p. 253). Chronic pulmonary problems have a slow onset and often are progressive in nature. The body has time to compensate for growing pulmonary deficits, thus maintaining an adequate level of oxygenation and acid-base balance. A person can lead a relatively normal life in a state of chronic respiratory insufficiency. Arterial blood gases would reflect a normal pH, though the $Paco_2$ may be abnormal (a compensated respiratory acidosis) with a correspondingly high bicarbonate level, and the Pao_2 might reflect some degree of hypoxemia. This compensated state, however, is not normal. A person in chronic respiratory insufficiency is always in a state of impending respiratory failure. Should a new stress overtax the ability of the body to compensate to meet an even greater demand, the person will develop acute respiratory failure.

Acute Respiratory Failure

Respiratory failure is the "direct life-threatening inability of the cardiopulmonary system to maintain adequate gas exchange at the pulmonary level" (Shapiro et al, 1991, p. 253). More specifically, it can be defined clinically as

$$Paco_2 \geq 50 \text{ mm Hg at a pH of } \leq 7.30 \text{ and/or}$$
$$Pao_2 \leq 60 \text{ mm Hg}$$

Acute respiratory failure is caused by an imbalance in supply and demand. Normally, the cardiopulmonary system is able to meet the demands of the body, increasing its work to supply adequate oxygen and ridding the body of carbon dioxide. If the body's demands become higher than the cardiopulmonary system can supply, the system will fail, precipitating acute respiratory failure.

Components of Acute Respiratory Failure

The term acute respiratory failure is a general one that pertains to both gas exchange components, oxygen and carbon dioxide. To better understand and clarify respiratory failure, it is helpful to break it down into its two component parts, failure of oxygenation and failure of ventilation. Both components may occur together initially, the patient suffering from both a low Pao_2 and a high $Paco_2$, with accompanying low pH. At the onset of failure, however, the primary problem is often one or the other rather than both. For this reason, it is important to be able to differentiate the two failure components.

Failure of Oxygenation

Oxygenation failure can be clinically defined as

$$Pao_2 \text{ of } \leq 60 \text{ mm Hg}$$

The primary problem is one of hypoxemia. Carbon dioxide (CO_2) is able to diffuse across the alveolar–capillary membrane approximately 20 times more rapidly than is oxygen. For this reason, CO_2 levels may remain normal when diffusion is interfered with, even though the patient is showing signs of moderate to severe hypoxemia. Conditions that can cause oxygenation failure include adult respiratory distress syndrome (ARDS), pulmonary embolus, acute asthmatic attack, pneumonia, and others. Should these conditions worsen or should the patient fatigue, the ventilatory component can be initiated.

Symptoms of oxygenation failure reflect hypoxemia and include

- Pulmonary: Dyspnea, tachypnea
- Cardiovascular: Increased blood pressure and pulse, cardiac arrhythmias, cyanosis, and pulmonary vasoconstriction (increased pulmonary vascular resistance)
- Central nervous system: Altered level of responsiveness, restlessness

Failure of Ventilation

Ventilatory failure can be clinically defined as

$$Paco_2 \text{ of } \geq 50 \text{ mm Hg with a pH of } \leq 7.30$$
$$(\text{acute respiratory acidosis})$$

Ventilatory failure (acute respiratory acidosis) is caused by alveolar hypoventilation, that is, the inability to move air adequately in and out of the alveoli, allowing a buildup of carbon dioxide. Ventilatory failure can be caused by any problem that interferes with adequate movement of air flow (i.e., neuromuscular disorders, respiratory muscle fatigue, COPD, and many others).

Symptoms of ventilatory failure reflect hypercapnia and include

- Pulmonary: Tachypnea
- Vascular: Headache, flushed, wet skin
- Cardiovascular: Bounding pulse, increased blood pressure and pulse
- Central nervous system: Anesthetic effects of carbon dioxide: Lethargy, drowsiness, coma

Most of the symptoms associated with hypercapnia are due to the strong vasodilator effect of carbon dioxide. The term "CO_2 narcosis" is sometimes used to describe ventilatory failure based on its anesthetic effects.

Complications of Respiratory Failure

Acute respiratory failure can affect virtually all body systems by causing organ hypoxia. If the respiratory failure is coupled with decreased cardiac output, the patient is at particular risk for development of hypoperfusion/hypoxic organ shock complications, such as those seen with multisystem organ failure (MSOF). Typical problems triggered by this mechanism include ARDS, acute tubular necrosis (acute renal failure), and many others. (MSOF is presented in a different self-study module.)

Pathogenesis of Respiratory Failure

The sequence of events that leads to the development of respiratory failure is a complicated one. It is initiated by the presence of a respiratory disease (acute or chronic) that interferes with the relationship of ventilation to perfusion ($\dot{V}/\dot{Q}$ ratio) and decreases Pao_2. The body recognizes increased oxygen demand and responds by increasing the rate and depth of respirations to move more air in and out of the alveoli (compensation). This compensatory mechanism increases the Pao_2 and decreases the $Paco_2$ to regain an adequate level of oxygenation and acid-base balance. Compensatory mechanisms, however, increase the metabolic rate by increasing the work of breathing. When the metabolic rate is increased, more oxygen is consumed by the tissues and more carbon dioxide is produced. The overall effect of the sequence is a progressive increase in arterial carbon dioxide and a decrease in arterial oxygen. A state of acute respiratory failure exists when the patient meets the clinical criteria of $Paco_2 \geq 50$ mm Hg with a pH of ≤ 7.30 and/or a Pao_2 of ≤ 60 mm Hg (Kersten, 1989).

Should the sequence of events that precipitated the acute respiratory failure not be managed adequately, the level of respiratory failure worsens, causing a further increase in the work of breathing. As the work of breathing increases, the patient develops respiratory muscle fatigue. Once muscle fatigue sets in, the patient will quickly decompensate, worsening both ventilation and oxygenation. If this sequence of events is allowed to continue, arterial blood gases will worsen steadily, leading to death of the patient (Kersten, 1989).

In summary, respiratory failure is a potential complication of respiratory insufficiency. Acute respiratory failure can be divided into two components: failure to oxygenate and failure to ventilate. Respiratory failure can cause dysfunction of all organs due to tissue hypoxia, possibly leading to MSOF.

Section Eight Review

1. Of the following, which arterial blood gas pH results would best reflect respiratory insufficiency?
   A. pH within normal limits
   B. pH above normal range
   C. pH below normal range
   D. variable pH

2. Of the following, which arterial blood gas pH results would best reflect acute respiratory failure?
   A. normal pH
   B. pH higher than normal
   C. pH lower than normal
   D. variable pH

3. Failure to oxygenate refers to which of the following primary problems?
   A. ventilation
   B. hypoxemia
   C. arterial pH
   D. carbon dioxide
4. Which of the following symptoms is typical of failure to oxygenate?
   A. bounding pulse
   B. headache
   C. flushed skin
   D. restlessness
5. The primary problem associated with failure to ventilate is
   A. alveolar hypoventilation
   B. capillary hypoperfusion

C. alveolar hyperventilation
D. capillary hyperperfusion
6. The symptoms that are typical of ventilatory failure are primarily the result of
   A. vasoconstriction
   B. hypoxemia
   C. vasodilation
   D. acidosis
7. The result of increased metabolic demand is
   A. decreased oxygen consumption
   B. decreased carbon dioxide production
   C. increased oxygen consumption
   D. increased carbon dioxide consumption

Answers: 1, A. 2, C. 3, B. 4, D. 5, A. 6, C. 7, C.

Section Nine: Adult Respiratory Distress Syndrome

At the completion of this section, the learner will be able to describe the pathophysiologic basis of adult respiratory distress syndrome (ARDS).

Adult respiratory distress syndrome (ARDS) is a distinct type of respiratory failure caused by diffuse injury to the alveolar–capillary membrane, resulting in noncardiogenic pulmonary edema. It is estimated that there are more than 150,000 cases of ARDS per year (Brannin, 1990). ARDS is not a disease but a pattern of pathophysiologic lung changes resulting in a corresponding pattern of clinical manifestations.

Etiologic Factors

ARDS can be triggered by direct or indirect pulmonary injury. Patients who are at highest risk for developing ARDS are those experiencing serious infections (particularly sepsis), oxygen toxicity, shock, and multiple trauma. A complete list of potential causes of ARDS would be an extensive one. The underlying factor that is common to all precipitating insults is hypoperfusion of the lung parenchyma.

Pathogenesis

No matter what insult triggers the onset of ARDS, the subsequent sequence of events remains relatively predictable. Figure 1–10 shows this sequence of events.

Clinical Presentation

ARDS usually develops within 24 to 48 hours after an initial event. An increasing pattern of dyspnea and tachypnea develops. As ARDS progresses, cyanosis and accessory muscle use may be noted. A cough develops, frequently producing sputum that is typical of pulmonary edema (blood-tinged and frothy). Laboratory findings show a pattern of increasing hypoxemia that is refractory to increasing concentrations of oxygen. The hallmark of ARDS is oxygenation failure, with a Pao$_2$ of <50 mm Hg at oxygen concentrations of >50 percent. Chest x-ray findings may be normal during the early stages of ARDS but will show diffuse, fluffy infiltrates in the later stages. Pulmonary function tests will be consistent with decreased lung compliance and decreased functional residual capacity (FRC).

The mortality rate associated with ARDS is about 50 percent (Farzan, 1985). For those who survive, however, there is often no significant permanent lung damage. Treatment of ARDS centers on supportive measures to maintain the patient until the alveolar–capillary membrane regains its integrity and the syndrome resolves.

In summary, ARDS is a severe form of acute respiratory failure that is resistant to oxygen therapy. It can be initiated by many events that either directly or indirectly injure the lungs. Lung tissue hypoperfusion seems to be the triggering mechanism common to all events. Severe hypoxemia that is refractory to oxygen therapy is the hallmark of ARDS. People who survive the syndrome often may have no significant permanent residual lung damage.

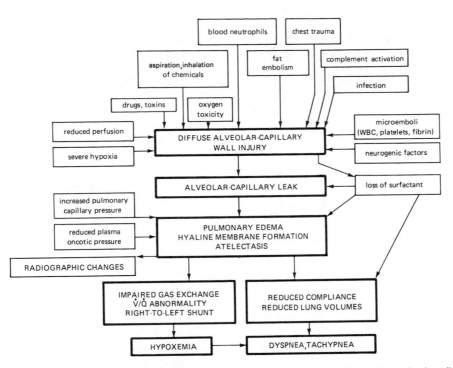

Figure 1–10. Pathogenesis and pathophysiology of adult respiratory distress syndrome. (*From* A concise handbook of respiratory diseases, *2nd ed., p. 252, by S. Farzan, 1985, Reston, VA: Reston Publishing Co.*)

Section Nine Review

1. Which of the following statements is true about adult respiratory distress syndrome (ARDS)?
   A. it is a distinct disease process
   B. it results from hypoperfusion of lung tissue
   C. it is associated with increasing levels of CO_2
   D. it has a mortality rate of over 90 percent
2. The pulmonary edema associated with ARDS is caused by
   A. capillary microembolism
   B. left ventricular failure
   C. loss of surfactant
   D. increased membrane permeability
3. The clinical hallmark of ARDS is
   A. $Paco_2$ of <50 mm Hg at >50 percent oxygen concentration
   B. $Paco_2$ of <50 mm Hg on room air
   C. $Paco_2$ of >50 mm Hg at >50 percent oxygen concentration

   D. $Paco_2$ of >50 mm Hg on room air
4. The refractory (resistant) nature of ARDS to oxygen therapy is based on the amount of
   A. capillary shunt
   B. venous admixture
   C. absolute shunt
   D. shuntlike effect
5. When recovered from ARDS, the patient generally has
   A. permanent chronic obstructive disease
   B. little permanent lung damage
   C. severe permanent lung damage
   D. permanent restrictive lung disease

Answers: 1, B. 2, D. 3, A. 4, C. 5, B.

Posttest

The following Posttest is constructed in a case study format. A patient is presented, and questions are asked based on available data. New data are presented as the case study progresses.

James Smith is a 55-year-old construction worker. He is active and considers himself fairly healthy. He has a history of smoking one pack of cigarettes per day for 20 years.

1. When Mr. Smith inhales, air moves into his lungs because
   A. intrapulmonary pressure has dropped below atmospheric pressure
   B. intrapleural pressure has dropped below atmospheric pressure
   C. intrapulmonary pressure has risen above atmospheric pressure
   D. intrapleural pressure has risen above atmospheric pressure
2. If his surfactant production would cease, how would it effect the alveoli?
   A. alveoli would hyperinflate
   B. alveoli would be destroyed
   C. alveoli would collapse
   D. alveoli would have decreased surface tension
3. Should Mr. Smith develop a pulmonary problem that decreases his lung compliance, it would
   A. increase his tidal volume
   B. decrease his carbon dioxide level
   C. decrease his oxygen consumption
   D. increase his work of breathing

Mr. Smith becomes ill. He develops a cough and fever and is producing greenish sputum. He is diagnosed as having right middle lobe pneumonia.

4. His pneumonia can affect pulmonary diffusion by increasing membrane thickness due to
   A. inflammation
   B. atelectasis
   C. bronchial secretions
   D. surfactant deficiency
5. Ventilation will decrease in the affected lung area because

A. pressure gradient is increased
B. gas follows the path of least resistance
C. decreased perfusion causes decreased ventilation
D. gas moves from low pressure to high pressure areas

6. Mr. Smith has a low ventilation-perfusion ($\dot{V}/\dot{Q}$) ratio. This means that there is
   A. decreased ventilation in relation to perfusion
   B. increased ventilation with decreased perfusion
   C. decreased ventilation with decreased perfusion
   D. increased ventilation in relation to perfusion
7. Mr. Smith has developed a physiologic shunt of 25 percent. One would anticipate which of the following resulting clinical manifestations?
   A. stupor, bounding pulse
   B. warm, wet skin, cyanosis
   C. headache, flushed appearance
   D. restlessness, cardiac arrhythmias

Mr. Smith's shunt is a capillary shunt. Oxygen therapy has been initiated per Venti-mask.

8. Considering his type of shunt, the nurse can anticipate what kind of response to oxygen therapy?
   A. hypoxemia will remain the same
   B. hypoxemia will worsen
   C. hypoxemia will be relieved
   D. hypoxemia will initially improve and then worsen

Mr. Smith has pulmonary mechanics tests performed. Both his tidal volume and vital capacity are below normal.

9. Inadequate volumes of tidal volume and vital capacity most likely indicate which of the following?
   A. respiratory muscle fatigue
   B. increased atelectasis
   C. loss of pulmonary surfactant
   D. worsening of his pneumonia

10. If Mr. Smith had an underlying chronic problem of emphysema, his pneumonia condition would be considered
    A. an acute ventilatory failure
    B. an acute obstructive disease
    C. an acute oxygenation failure
    D. an acute restrictive disease

End Mr. Smith situation.

11. A restrictive pulmonary disorder affects air flow in which way?
    A. increases
    B. no effect
    C. decreases
    D. increases or decreases
12. Obstructive pulmonary disorders are associated with
    A. decreased tidal volumes
    B. increased inspiratory times
    C. decreased inspiratory air flow
    D. increased expiratory times
13. The chronic bronchitis patient will exhibit which of the following primary symptoms?
    A. frequent productive cough
    B. prolonged inspiratory time
    C. frequent dry hacky cough
    D. shortened expiratory time
14. The patient with pure emphysema will undergo which pulmonary parenchymal changes?
    A. destruction of cilia
    B. increased goblet cells
    C. alveolar destruction
    D. bronchiolar constriction

15. The patient who develops heart failure secondary to cor pulmonale would most likely experience
    A. dependent edema
    B. left ventricular enlargement
    C. low blood pressure
    D. pulmonary edema
16. A person in chronic respiratory insufficiency would most likely exhibit which of the following?
    A. decreased respiratory rate
    B. increased blood pressure
    C. increased temperature
    D. decreased pulse rate
17. When caring for a patient in acute ventilatory failure, you would anticipate which of the following arterial blood gas findings?
    A. $Pao_2 < 60$ mm Hg
    B. $Paco_2 > 50$ mm Hg
    C. $Pao_2 > 100$ mm Hg
    D. $Paco_2 < 35$ mm Hg
18. According to the module, respiratory failure is clinically defined as
    A. $Paco_2 \geq 50$ mm Hg with a pH of ≤ 7.30 and/or $Pao_2 \leq 60$ mm Hg
    B. $Paco_2 \geq 60$ mm Hg with a pH of ≤ 7.30 and $Pao_2 \leq 60$ mm Hg
    C. $Paco_2 \geq 45$ mm Hg with a pH of ≤ 7.35 and/or $Pao_2 \leq 80$ mm Hg
    D. $Paco_2 \geq 60$ mm Hg with a pH of ≤ 7.35 and $Pao_2 \leq 80$ mm Hg
19. Adult respiratory distress syndrome (ARDS) is a pulmonary disorder that initially causes
    A. lung destruction
    B. ventilatory failure
    C. alveolar hypoventilation
    D. oxygenation failure

Posttest Answers

Question	Answer	Section	Question	Answer	Section
1	A	One	11	B	Six
2	C	One	12	D	Six
3	D	One	13	A	Seven
4	A	Two	14	C	Seven
5	B	Three	15	A	Seven
6	A	Three	16	A	Eight
7	D	Four	17	B	Eight
8	C	Four	18	A	Eight
9	A	Five	19	B	Nine
10	D	Six			

REFERENCES

Brannin, P.K. (1990). Adult respiratory distress syndrome (ARDS). In C.M. Hudak, B.M. Gallo, and J.J. Benz (eds). *Critical care nursing: A holistic approach*, 5th ed., pp. 386–389. Philadelphia: J.B. Lippincott Co.

Des Jardins, T.R. (1988). *Cardiopulmonary anatomy & physiology: Essentials for respiratory care*. Albany, NY: Delmar Publishers.

Des Jardins, T.R. (1990). *Clinical manifestations of respiratory disease*, 2nd ed. Chicago: Year Book Medical Publishers.

Farzan, S. (1985). *A concise handbook of respiratory diseases*, 2nd ed. Reston, VA: Reston Publishing Co.

Kersten, L.D. (1989). *Comprehensive respiratory nursing: A decision making approach*. Philadelphia: W.B. Saunders.

Martin, L. (1987). *Pulmonary physiology in clinical practice: The essentials for patient care and evaluation*. St. Louis: C.V. Mosby Co.

Neagley, S.R. (1991). The pulmonary system. In J.G. Alspach (ed). *American association of critical-care nurses: Core curriculum for critical care nursing*, 4th ed., pp. 1–131. Philadelphia: W.B. Saunders Co.

Price, S.A., and Wilson, L.M. (1986). *Pathophysiology: Clinical concepts of disease processes*, 3rd ed. New York: McGraw-Hill Book Co.

Shapiro, B.A., Kacmarek, R.M., Cane, R.D., Peruzzi, W.T., and Hauptman, D. (1991). *Clinical application of respiratory care*, 4th ed. St. Louis: Mosby Year Book.

Module 2

Gas Exchange and Blood Gas Analysis

Linda M. Holtzclaw

The self-study module, *Gas Exchange and Blood Gas Analysis*, focuses on the concepts of gas exchange and arterial blood gas analysis rather than on management of the patient with dysfunction. The module is composed of eight distinct sections. Section One reviews factors affecting gas exchange. In Sections Two through Six, the focus shifts to acid-base physiology and compensation, normal arterial blood gas values, acid-base disturbances, and interpretation of arterial blood gases. Sections Seven and Eight briefly describe invasive and noninvasive methods used in monitoring gas exchange. Each section includes a set of review questions or exercises to help the learner evaluate understanding of each section content before moving on to the next section. All Section Reviews and Pretests and Posttests in the module include answers. It is suggested that the learner review those concepts that have been missed in the review questions before proceeding to the next section.

Objectives

Following completion of the module, *Gas Exchange and Blood Gas Analysis,* the learner will be able to

1. Briefly discuss factors involved in gas exchange
2. Identify mechanisms that the body uses to compensate for acid-base imbalances
3. Identify normal values for arterial blood gases
4. Differentiate between respiratory acidosis and alkalosis

5. Differentiate between metabolic acidosis and alkalosis
6. Interpret arterial blood gases for abnormalities of oxygenation, acid-base, and degree of compensation
7. List noninvasive methods of monitoring gas exchange and applications
8. Describe the purpose of mixed venous oxygen saturation monitoring ($S\bar{v}o_2$) and clinical applications

Pretest

1. Factors affecting gas exchange include all except
   A. acid-base balance
   B. diffusion
   C. pulse oximetry
   D. ventilation-perfusion matching
2. The body initially compensates for an acute respiratory imbalance by
   A. blowing off carbon dioxide
   B. excreting bicarbonate
   C. retaining carbon dioxide
   D. shifting to anaerobic metabolism
3. Select a normal arterial blood gas (ABG)
   A. pH = 7.30, $Paco_2$ = 49 mm Hg, HCO_3 = 24 mEq/L, Pao_2 = 99 mm Hg, Sao_2 = 98 percent
   B. pH = 7.40, $Paco_2$ = 35 mm Hg, HCO_3 = 24 mEq/L, Pao_2 = 98 mm Hg, Sao_2 = 97 percent
   C. pH = 7.54, $Paco_2$ = 48 mm Hg, HCO_3 = 32 mEq/L, Pao_2 = 100 mm Hg, Sao_2 = 100 percent
   D. pH = 7.15, $Paco_2$ = 70 mm Hg, HCO_3 = 18 mEq/L, Pao_2 = 60 mm Hg, Sao_2 = 75 percent
4. Respiratory acid-base disturbances are reflected by changes in
   A. $Paco_2$
   B. Pao_2
   C. HCO_3
   D. base excess
5. Metabolic acid-base disturbances are reflected by changes in
   A. $Paco_2$, Pao_2
   B. $Paco_2$, HCO_3
   C. HCO_3, base excess
   D. HCO_3, Sao_2

Questions 6, 7, 8
   Interpret the following arterial blood gas
   pH = 7.37, $Paco_2$ = 50 mm Hg, HCO_3 = 30 mEq/L, Pao_2 = 80 mm Hg, Sao_2 = 96 percent
6. Acid-base interpretation
   A. metabolic acidosis
   B. metabolic alkalosis
   C. respiratory acidosis
   D. respiratory alkalosis
7. Identify type of compensation
   A. complete metabolic compensation
   B. complete respiratory compensation
   C. partial metabolic compensation
   D. partial respiratory compensation
8. Oxygenation status
   A. high
   B. inadequate
   C. low
   D. normal
9. Noninvasive monitoring techniques include
   A. ABG, end tidal CO_2
   B. ABG, $S\bar{v}o_2$
   C. end tidal CO_2, pulse oximetry
   D. pulse oximetry, $S\bar{v}o_2$
10. $S\bar{v}o_2$ monitoring reflects
   A. alveolar O_2 levels
   B. arterial capillary O_2 levels
   C. O_2 supply/demand
   D. tissue O_2 extraction
11. What is the most important factor that you ALWAYS evaluate?
   A. hemodynamics
   B. laboratory values
   C. oximetry
   D. patient

Pretest answers: 1, C. 2, A. 3, B. 4, A. 5, C. 6, C. 7, A. 8, D. 9, C. 10, C. 11, D.

Glossary

Acids. Substances that dissociate or lose ions

Bases. Substances capable of accepting ions

Buffer. A substance reacting with acids and bases to maintain a neutral environment of stable pH

Capnogram. Graphic representation of carbon dioxide levels during respiration

Capnometry. Measurement of carbon dioxide in expired gas

Compensated. A state in which the pH is within normal limits with the acid-base imbalance being neutralized but not corrected

Corrected. A state in which all acid-base parameters have returned to normal ranges after a state of acid-base imbalance

Diffusion. Movement of gas molecules from an area of high to an area of low partial pressure

2,3-DPG (diphosphoglycerate). A molecule produced by red blood cells

End tidal carbon dioxide (P_{ETCO_2} or $EtCO_2$). Concentration of carbon dioxide at the end of exhalation

Mixed venous oxygen saturation ($S\bar{v}o_2$). Measurement of the oxygen saturation of hemoglobin returning to the heart

Nonvolatile acids. Metabolic acids that cannot be converted to a gas, requiring excretion through the kidneys

Oxyhemoglobin dissociation curve. A graphic representation of the relationship between oxygen saturation of hemoglobin (Sao_2) and the partial pressure of oxygen (Pao_2) in the plasma

Oxygen consumption extraction. The amount of oxygen used by the tissues

Partially compensated. A state in which the pH is abnormal but the body buffers and regulatory mechanisms have started to respond to the imbalance

Partial pressure. Pressure each gas exerts in a total volume of gases

pH. Represents free hydrogen ion concentration

Pressure gradient. Difference between pressures exerted by different gases

Pulse oximetry. Noninvasive technique for monitoring arterial capillary oxygen saturation

Volatile acids. Acids that can convert to a gas form for excretion

Uncompensated. An acid-base state in which the pH is abnormal because other buffer and regulatory mechanisms have begun to correct the imbalance

---

Abbreviations

ABG. Arterial blood gas

BE. Base excess

CO_2. Carbon dioxide

H^+. Hydrogen ion

H_2CO_3. Carbonic acid

Hb (Hgb). Hemoglobin

HCO_3. Bicarbonate

K^+. Potassium

mEq/L. Milliequivalents per liter

mm Hg. Millimeters of mercury

O_2. Oxygen

$Paco_2$. Partial pressure of arterial carbon dioxide

Pao_2. Partial pressure of arterial oxygen

P_{ETCO_2}. Partial pressure of end tidal carbon dioxide

pH. Free hydrogen ion concentration

$P\bar{v}co_2$. Partial pressure of venous carbon dioxide

$P\bar{v}o_2$. Partial pressure of venous oxygen

Sao_2. Saturation of arterial oxygen

$S\bar{v}o_2$. Saturation of venous oxygen

Section One: Factors Affecting Gas Exchange

At the completion of this section, the learner will be able to briefly discuss factors involved in gas exchange.

Many factors affect gas exchange. This process occurs between the alveoli and pulmonary capillaries and between the capillaries and tissues. Concepts to be considered are partial pressure, diffusion, ventilation perfusion matching, oxyhemoglobin dissociation, and acid-base mechanisms. Several of these concepts have been covered in other modules and are reviewed briefly in this module.

Partial Pressure

Partial pressure, or tension, is the pressure each individual gas exerts in a total volume of gases. "Dalton's law states the total pressure of a volume of gases is equal to the sum of partial pressures" (Kinney et al, 1988, p. 170). For example, atmospheric pressure (the total pressure of gases) is 760 mm Hg at sea level, and oxygen (O_2) comprises 21 percent of room air. To determine the partial pressure of oxygen

$$0.21 \text{ (percent of oxygen)} \times 760 \text{ mm Hg}$$
$$\text{(atmospheric pressure)} = 158 \text{ mm Hg (Pao}_2\text{)}$$

As the percentage of oxygen is increased, the pressure it exerts also increases.

Henry's law states that when a gas is exposed to liquid, some of it will dissolve in the liquid. The partial pressure of the gas and its solubility determine the amount of gas that dissolves. Oxygen is not very soluble in plasma. Only 3 percent of the total oxygen content dissolves in blood. It is the partial pressure of gases (oxygen and carbon dioxide) moving out of the plasma that is measured in a blood gas sample (Kinney et al, 1988).

Diffusion

Diffusion of gas refers to the transfer of gas molecules from an area of high partial pressure to an area of lower partial pressure. The difference between the partial pressures is called the pressure gradient. Diffusion occurs at the alveolar and tissue levels to exchange oxygen and carbon dioxide. At the alveolar level, oxygen moves into blood, and carbon dioxide moves out. At the tissue level, oxygen leaves the blood to nourish the tissues, and carbon dioxide (waste) shifts into the capillaries for removal from the body by the lungs.

The alveolar–capillary membrane is very thin (0.5 μm), offering little resistance to diffusion in normal circumstances. The membrane can thicken when pulmonary pathologic processes exist, reducing diffusion (e.g., pulmonary edema, adult respiratory distress syndrome). Since carbon dioxide diffuses 20 times faster than oxygen, the carbon dioxide tension may remain at normal levels initially, but the oxygen tension decreases.

Ventilation-Perfusion Relationship

The relationship between ventilation and perfusion ($\dot{V}/\dot{Q}$ ratio) also affects gas exchange. Normally, ventilation is the greatest where perfusion is the greatest, thus optimizing gas exchange. Many pulmonary disorders interfere with this relationship, decreasing ventilation to the alveoli (pneumonia, atelectasis), decreasing perfusion of capillary blood flow by the alveoli (pulmonary embolus), or both (emphysema). The relationship of ventilation to perfusion is discussed in detail in Module 1, *Respiratory Process*.

Oxyhemoglobin Dissociation Curve

Hemoglobin is the primary carrier of oxygen in the blood. It has an affinity or attraction for oxygen molecules. In the pulmonary capillaries, oxygen binds loosely and reversibly to hemoglobin, forming oxyhemoglobin for transport to the tissues, where it can be released. The amount of oxygen that loads onto hemoglobin is expressed as a percentage of hemoglobin saturation by oxygen (% Sao_2). The affinity of hemoglobin for oxygen varies, depending on certain physiologic factors. A graph has been developed to represent the relationship of the partial pressure of arterial oxygen (Pao_2) and hemoglobin saturation (Sao_2). This graph is called the oxyhemoglobin dissociation curve (Figure 2–1), which is depicted as an S-curve rather than a straight line, showing that the percentage saturation of hemoglobin does not maintain a direct relationship with the Pao_2.

The top portion of the curve (Pao_2 of $\geq$ 60 mm Hg) is flattened into a horizontal position. In this portion of the curve, a large alteration in Pao_2 produces only small alterations in percentage of hemoglobin saturation (% Sao_2). For example, note that a

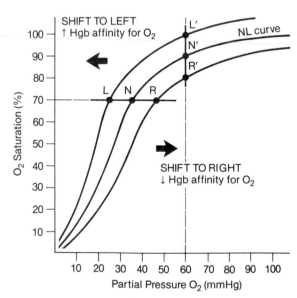

Figure 2–1. The oxyhemoglobin dissociation curve. Right and left shifts of the oxyhemoglobin dissociation curve. Hgb, hemoglobin; NL, normal. (*From* Comprehensive respiratory nursing: A decision making approach, *p. 48, by L.D. Kersten, 1989, Philadelphia: W.B. Saunders Co.*)

10 mm Hg decrease of a patient's Pao_2 from 80 mm Hg to 70 mm Hg would produce very little change in Sao_2 (Figure 2–1). Clinically, this means that although administering supplemental oxygen may significantly increase the patient's Pao_2, the resulting Sao_2 increase will be small in proportion. The patient's oxygenation status is better protected at the top of the curve.

The bottom portion of the curve (Pao_2 of ≤ 60 mm Hg) is steep. In this portion, any alteration in Pao_2 yields a large change in percentage of hemoglobin saturation (Sao_2). For example, a 10 mm Hg decrease in Pao_2 from 60 mm Hg to 50 mm Hg drops the Sao_2 from about 85 percent to about 75 percent (a decrease of approximately 10 percent Sao_2). Clinically, this means that administration of supplemental oxygen sufficient to increase the Pao_2 should yield large increases in Sao_2. However, abnormalities in the ventilation-perfusion relationship may exist, interfering with reoxygenation.

Low Pao_2 at the tissue level stimulates oxygen release from hemoglobin to the tissue. High Pao_2 at the pulmonary capillary level stimulates hemoglobin to bind with more oxygen. Other factors can change the curve. Acidosis, hyperthermia, hypercarbia, and increased 2,3-DPG (diphosphoglycerate) causes a shift of the curve to the right. A right shift prevents hemoglobin from binding as readily with oxygen, although oxygen is able to be released at the tissue level more readily. Alkalosis, hypothermia, hypocarbia, and decreased 2,3-DPG cause a shift of the curve to the left. A left shift causes hemoglobin to bond more readily with oxygen in the lungs, but inhibits release at the tissue level. Slight shifts are adaptive. For example, an increased body temperature increases oxygen demand, causing a slight right shift, which increases release of oxygen to the tissues to meet increasing tissue oxygen demand. Severe or rapid shifts, however, can produce life-threatening tissue hypoxia.

In summary, many factors affect gas exchange, including the partial pressure of a gas, ability to diffuse across the alveolar–capillary membrane, $\dot{V}/\dot{Q}$ ratio, and oxyhemoglobin dissociation. An understanding of these concepts assists in determining alternatives for clinical interventions.

Section One Review

1. Factors affecting gas exchange include all of the following EXCEPT
   A. partial pressure
   B. oxyhemoglobin dissociation
   C. mixed venous saturation
   D. diffusion
2. Partial pressure is defined as
   A. the difference between concentrations of gases
   B. the amount of pressure exerted by each gas
   C. the atmospheric pressure at sea level
   D. the amount of diffusion across alveolar membranes
3. Which of the following reflects the natural movement of gas diffusion?

A. from low to high pressure
B. from high to low pressure
C. from equal to unequal pressure
D. from negative to positive pressure

4. The oxyhemoglobin dissociation curve represents hemoglobin ability to
   A. transport heme
   B. react with carbon dioxide
   C. form oxyhemoglobin molecules
   D. chemically bind and release oxygen

Answers: 1, C. 2, B. 3, B. 4, D.

Section Two: Acid-Base Physiology and Compensation

At the completion of this section, the learner will be able to identify mechanisms that the body uses to compensate for acid-base imbalances.

Acid-base balance is crucial to the effective functioning of our body systems (Figure 2–2). Severe imbalances can be lethal to the patient. The body contains many acid or base substances. Acids are substances that dissociate or lose ions. Bases are substances capable of accepting ions. The pH represents the free hydrogen ion (H^+) concentration. An increase in H^+ concentration lowers pH and increases acidity. A decrease in H^+ concentration increases pH and increases alkalinity.

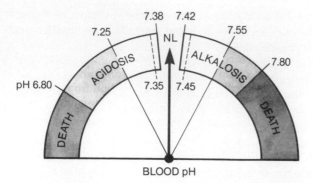

Figure 2–2. The pH scale. Blood pH defines acidotic and alkalotic states. The normal range for pH is 7.38 to 7.42. The dotted lines demarcate the less sensitive but commonly used normal range of 7.35 to 7.45. The light gray area represents potentially life-threatening ranges for pH. The dark gray areas are ranges of pH that are incompatible with life. (*From* Comprehensive respiratory nursing: A decision making approach, *p. 358, by L.D. Kersten, 1989, Philadelphia: W.B. Saunders Co.*)

The body's acids include volatile acids and non-volatile acids. Volatile acids can convert to a gas form for excretion (carbonic acid). Carbonic acid rapidly converts to carbon dioxide for excretion from the lungs. The lungs excrete a very large amount of acid each day in this manner. Nonvolatile (metabolic) acids cannot be converted to gas, so they must be excreted through the kidneys. Examples of metabolic acids include lactic acid and ketones. Unlike the lungs, the kidneys are capable of excreting only a small amount of acid each day and respond slowly to changes. Hydrogen ions are excreted in the proximal and distal tubules of the kidneys in exchange for sodium.

Buffer Systems

The body is not tolerant of wide changes in pH and is working constantly to maintain the pH range between 7.35 and 7.45. A normal pH is maintained if the ratio of bicarbonate (HCO_3) to carbon dioxide (CO_2) remains at approximately a 20:1 (HCO_3/CO_2) ratio. The body has three mechanisms to maintain acid-base balance: the buffering mechanism, the respiratory compensation mechanism, and the metabolic compensation mechanism.

The buffering mechanism represents chemical reactions between acids and bases to maintain a neutral environment. Bases react with excess hydrogen ions (H^+) to prevent shifts in pH, and acids react with excess HCO_3. This process starts immediately. The bicarbonate buffer system is the major buffering system in the body. Its components are regulated by the lungs (CO_2) and kidneys (HCO_3). The following reversible reaction represents the shifts that occur as

carbonic acid (H_2CO_3) is shifted depending on body needs.

$$H^+ + HCO_3 \rightleftharpoons H_2CO_3 \rightleftharpoons CO_2 + H_2O$$

Additional nonbicarbonate buffers include hemoglobin, serum proteins, and the phosphate system, which is mainly a function of the kidneys.

The respiratory compensation mechanism increases or decreases alveolar ventilation. Hyperventilation excretes carbon dioxide, ridding the system of excessive acid (often called blowing off CO_2). Hypoventilation results in the retention of carbon dioxide, which increases the amount of acid available to combine with excess bicarbonate to form carbonic acid. Compensation begins rapidly in minutes but may take several hours for maximum effect.

The metabolic compensation mechanism controls the rate of elimination or reabsorption of hydrogen and bicarbonate ions in the kidney. In situations of increased acid loads (acidosis), there is increased H^+ elimination and increased bicarbonate reabsorption. In alkalosis, H^+ is reabsorbed and HCO_3^- is excreted. Metabolic compensation is slow. It begins in hours but takes days to reach maximum compensation.

Levels of Compensation

- Uncompensated: The pH is abnormal because buffer and regulatory mechanisms have not kicked in to correct the imbalance. In these situations, the acid or base component is abnormal.
- Partially compensated: The pH is abnormal, but the body buffers and regulatory mechanisms have started to respond to the imbalance. In these situations, the acid and base components are abnormal.
- Compensated: The pH is within normal limits. The acid-base imbalance has been neutralized but not corrected. In this situation, the acid and base components are abnormal but balanced.
- Corrected: The pH is within normal limits. All acid-base parameters have returned to normal ranges after a state of acid-base imbalance.

The body corrects imbalances with continual slight adjustments. However, it does not overcompensate for acid-base abnormalities. Thus, pH reflects the primary problem of acidosis or alkalosis. Clinically, when drugs are administered to correct an acid-base imbalance, the larger dose or adjustment may overshoot the neutral target point. For example, the administration of large amounts of sodium bicarbonate in a cardiac arrest (metabolic acidosis) situation can overshoot the neutral target pH and place the patient in metabolic alkalosis.

In summary, the body attempts to maintain pH within a narrow range. Compensatory mechanisms include buffering, excretion or retention of carbon dioxide (respiratory), and excretion or retention of H^+/HCO_3^- (metabolic).

Section Two Review

1. The body compensates for acid-base imbalance by all of the following mechanisms EXCEPT
   A. buffering
   B. hepatic compensation
   C. respiratory compensation
   D. excretion of HCO_3
2. Respiratory compensation involves excretion or retention of
   A. CO_2
   B. HCO_3
   C. H_2O
   D. K^+
3. Metabolic compensation involves changes in excretion or reabsorption of

A. H^+, CO_2
B. HCO_3, H^+
C. glucose, HCO_3
D. CO_2, HCO_3

4. The body's buffering system continually works toward maintenance of a bicarbonate/carbon dioxide ratio of
   A. 1:5
   B. 1:20
   C. 5:1
   D. 20:1

Answers: 1, B. 2, A. 3, B. 4, D.

Section Three: Normal Values for Arterial Blood Gases

At the completion of this section, the learner will identify normal values for arterial blood gases.

Indicators for Determination of Acid-Base State

pH

The pH represents the amount of free H^+ available in the blood (normal value 7.35 to 7.45). The body's normal state is slightly alkaline, and the body strives to maintain this range. Extreme deviation for long periods of time is incompatible with survival. pH reflects the body's total acid-base balance. It is shifted by changes in hydrogen (H^+) or bicarbonate (HCO_3^-) ion concentration. Gain of acid or loss of base shifts the acid-base balance to the acid side. Loss of acid or gain in base or both shift the balance to the alkaline side.

Paco₂

The $Paco_2$ is the partial pressure of carbon dioxide in arterial blood (normal value 35 to 45 mm Hg). $Paco_2$ represents the respiratory component of the arterial blood gases (ABG). The lungs control the excretion or retention of carbon dioxide through alveolar ventilation. Elevated $Paco_2$ indicates hypoventilation of the alveoli. Decreased $Paco_2$ represents alveolar hyperventilation.

HCO₃

HCO_3 represents the concentration of bicarbonate in the blood (normal value 22 to 28 mEq/L). HCO_3 represents the renal or metabolic component of the arterial blood gases. It is influenced by metabolic processes.

Base Excess

The level of base excess (BE) can be measured as an indirect reflection of bicarbonate concentration in the body (normal value ± 2 mEq/L). Base excess is considered a purely nonrespiratory measurement because it is not affected by carbonic acid concentrations. A base deficit is present if BE is greater than −2 mEq/L, reflecting an excess of fixed acids or a deficit in base. A base excess is present if the BE is greater than +2 mEq/L, reflecting either an excess of base or a deficit of fixed acids. BE measurement is not considered an essential step in basic arterial blood gas interpretation, since HCO_3 is a sufficient metabolic measurement (Kersten, 1989).

Indicators of Oxygenation Status

Pao_2

Pao_2 represents the partial pressure of the oxygen dissolved in arterial blood (3 percent of total oxygen) (normal value 80 to 100 mm Hg), not the total amount of oxygen available. Though it comprises only a small percentage of total oxygen in the blood, it is an important indicator of oxygenation, since Pao_2 and oxygen saturation (Sao_2) maintain a relationship. This relationship is reflected in the oxyhemoglobin dissociation curve, making it an important indicator of oxygenation status.

Sao_2

Oxygen saturation (Sao_2) is the measure of percentage of oxygen combined with hemoglobin compared to the total amount it could carry (normal value 95 to 100 percent). The degree of saturation is important in determining the amount of oxygen available for delivery to the tissues.

Hemoglobin

Hemoglobin (Hb or Hgb) is the major component of red blood cells (normal values 12 to 16 g/dL in women, 13.5 to 18 g/dL in men). It is composed of protein and heme, which contains iron. Oxygen binds to the iron atoms located on the four heme groups of each hemoglobin molecule. Hemoglobin is the major carrier of oxygen in the blood and is, therefore, an important factor in tissue oxygenation.

Arterial Blood Gas

Arterial blood gas (ABG) normal values typically are reported as normal at sea level (760 mm Hg) partial pressures, room air (21 percent oxygen), and a blood temperature of 37C (98.6F). Changes in these factors need to be considered during interpretation. Age also affects the normal values. Newborns have a lower Pao_2 (40 to 70 mm Hg), as do elderly people, whose Pao_2 decreases approximately 10 mm Hg per decade (in the 60 to 90 year age range). Normal ABG values are ranges for normal healthy adults. It is important to establish a baseline for the individual, since abnormal values are normal for some individuals. A patient with chronic lung disease may have a Pao_2 of 60 mm Hg with a $Paco_2$ of 50 mm Hg as a normal baseline. Attempts to return ABG values to those of a normal, healthy individual would have serious consequences.

A person receiving supplemental oxygen also can be evaluated without determining room air gas. The Pao_2 should rise approximately 50 mm Hg for each 10 percent rise in oxygen concentration. A simple way to estimate what the Pao_2 should be is to multiply 5 times the percent of oxygen. If the Pao_2 is less than this value, the patient would probably be inadequately oxygenated on room air. For example, 5 × 50% O_2 = 250 mm Hg Pao_2 (Shapiro et al, 1989).

In summary, indicators of acid-base and oxygenation states have been presented. Included in the discussion were normal values and a brief description of each indicator. The concept of arterial blood gases was presented in regard to the basis of normal values, age considerations, and alterations in normal blood gas values associated with the pathophysiologic changes of chronic obstructive pulmonary disease.

Section Three Review

1. Normal values for arterial blood gases include
   A. pH 7.5
   B. $Paco_2$ 20 mm Hg
   C. HCO_3 26 mm Hg
   D. Sao_2 75 mm Hg
2. An increase in bicarbonate would cause the pH to become more
   A. acidic
   B. alkaline
   C. neutral
   D. no change
3. $Paco_2$ is the _____ component, and HCO_3 is the _____ component.

A. oxygenation, metabolic
B. respiratory, metabolic
C. metabolic, respiratory
D. hepatic, oxygenation
4. According to the oxyhemoglobin dissociation curve, at a Pao_2 of less than 60 mm Hg, a large decrease in Pao_2 should produce what kind of change in the Sao_2?
   A. small increase
   B. large increase
   C. small decrease
   D. large decrease

5. What factor must you always evaluate to place ABGs in the proper context?
   A. laboratory values
   B. oxygen supplemental therapy
   C. mode of ventilation
   D. patient

Section Four: Respiratory Acid-Base Disturbances

At the completion of this section, the learner will be able to differentiate between respiratory acidosis and alkalosis.

Primary respiratory disturbances are reflected by changes in the $Paco_2$ (partial pressure of arterial carbon dioxide), being either above normal, as in respiratory acidosis, or below normal as in respiratory alkalosis.

Respiratory Acidosis

Respiratory acidosis occurs when the $Paco_2$ moves above 45 mm Hg and the pH drops below 7.35. The elevated carbon dioxide (CO_2) indicates alveolar hypoventilation. The lungs are not excreting, or blowing off, enough CO_2, causing a carbonic acid excess. Carbon dioxide is considered an acid because it combines with water to form carbonic acid. It is essential to determine the cause of hypoventilation and then to correct it when possible. Table 2–1 shows sequences of events that can cause acute respiratory acidosis.

A chronic acid-base state means that a state of compensation exists. Chronic respiratory acidosis usually is associated with a chronic obstructive pulmonary disease, such as chronic bronchitis or em-

TABLE 2–2. COMPARISON OF ACUTE AND CHRONIC RESPIRATORY ACIDOSIS

| Parameter | Uncompensated | Compensated | |
	Acute	Chronic	Partial
pH	↓	Normal	↓
$Paco_2$	↑	↑	↑
HCO_3	Normal	↑	↑

physema. The elevation of carbon dioxide occurs gradually over many years. Thus, the body is able to compensate to maintain a normal pH by elevating the bicarbonate. Since these individuals have little respiratory reserve, additional stressors can cause decompensation, producing respiratory failure. Table 2–2 compares acute and chronic acidosis. (Respiratory failure is discussed in depth in Module 1, *Respiratory Process.*)

Respiratory Alkalosis

Respiratory alkalosis occurs when the $Paco_2$ falls below 35 mm Hg with a corresponding rise in pH to >7.45. The decreased carbon dioxide indicates alveolar hyperventilation. The lungs are eliminating too much carbon dioxide, causing a carbonic acid deficit. There are inadequate amounts of carbon dioxide available to combine with water to form carbonic acid (H_2CO_3). The key to effective treatment of respiratory alkalosis is to determine the cause of the hyperventilation and provide the intervention necessary to correct the problem. Common causes of acute respiratory alkalosis are listed in Table 2–3 as sequences of events.

TABLE 2–1. CAUSES OF ACUTE RESPIRATORY ACIDOSIS

Oversedation (narcotics, anesthetics, tranquilizers) → increased respiratory depression → hypoventilation

Overdose → increased/toxic drug levels → increased respiratory depression → hypoventilation

Head injury → increased pressure or damage to respiratory center → respiratory depression → hypoventilation or ineffective breathing patterns

Neuromuscular diseases → impaired functioning of respiratory muscles → decreased ventilation → hypoventilation

Pulmonary edema → decreased diffusion across alveolar capillary membrane → hypoventilation

Pneumonia, atelectasis → decreased ventilation → ventilation-perfusion mismatching → hypoventilation

Mechanical ventilation → inadequate (low) rate, tidal volume → decreased ventilation → hypoventilation

TABLE 2–3. COMMON CAUSES OF ACUTE RESPIRATORY ALKALOSIS

Anxiety, pain, fear → increased stimulation → hyperventilation

Head injury → damage to respiratory center → change in breathing pattern → hyperventilation

Mechanical ventilation → overventilation with high rate, tidal volume or minute volume → hyperventilation

Hypoxia → decreased O_2 → increases stimulation of respiratory center → hyperventilation

Fever → increases O_2 demand → increased respiratory stimulation → hyperventilation

TABLE 2–4. COMPARISON OF ACUTE AND CHRONIC RESPIRATORY ALKALOSIS

| Parameter | Uncompensated | Compensated | |
	Acute	Chronic	Partial
pH	↑	Normal	↑
$Paco_2$	↓	↓	↓
HCO_3	Normal	↓	↓

Chronic respiratory alkalosis is uncommon. The same factors causing acute respiratory alkalosis could cause a chronic state if the problem remains uncorrected. Table 2–4 compares the effects of acute and chronic respiratory alkalosis on arterial blood gases.

In summary, to differentiate between primary respiratory acidosis and alkalosis, the $Paco_2$ and pH must be evaluated. The cause of respiratory acidosis is alveolar hypoventilation, and the cause of respiratory alkalosis is alveolar hyperventilation. Compensation of respiratory acid-base disturbances requires evaluation of changes in bicarbonate. Treatment includes correction of the underlying problem, when possible.

Section Four Review

1. Respiratory acidosis indicates which of the following?
   A. hyperventilation
   B. hypoventilation
   C. mechanical ventilation
   D. inadequate perfusion
2. Which of the following occurs as a result of acute respiratory acidosis?
   A. pH increases
   B. pH decreases
   C. CO_2 decreases
   D. HCO_3 decreases
3. Respiratory alkalosis indicates which of the following?
   A. hyperventilation
   B. hypoventilation
   C. mechanical ventilation
   D. inadequate perfusion
4. Patient situations associated with respiratory alkalosis include
   A. sedation
   B. neuromuscular blockade
   C. asthma
   D. anxiety

Answers: 1, B. 2, B. 3, A. 4, D.

Section Five: Metabolic Acid-Base Disturbances

At the completion of this section, the learner will be able to differentiate between metabolic acidosis and alkalosis.

Primary metabolic disturbances are reflected by changes in bicarbonate (HCO_3) levels and base excess (BE). Metabolic acidosis can be defined clinically as HCO_3 = <22 mEq/L, pH <7.35, with a base deficit. Metabolic acidosis can be caused by an increase in metabolic acids or excessive loss of base.

Conditions precipitating an increase in hydrogen ion (H^+) concentrations include

- Diabetic acidosis due to elevated ketones
- Uremia associated with increased levels of phosphates and sulfates
- Ingestion of acidic drugs, such as aspirin (salicylate) overdose
- Lactic acidosis caused by increased lactic acid production (anaerobic metabolism of shock)

Conditions precipitating a decrease in bicarbonate (HCO_3) levels include

- Diarrhea, which causes loss of alkalotic substances
- Gastrointestinal fistulas due to loss of alkaline substances
- Loss of body fluids from drains below the umbilicus (except urinary catheter) causing loss of alkaline fluids
- Drugs causing loss of alkali, such as laxative overuse

Table 2–5 compares the effects of acute and chronic metabolic acidosis on arterial blood gases.

TABLE 2–5. COMPARISON OF ACUTE AND CHRONIC METABOLIC ACIDOSIS

Parameter	Uncompensated	Compensated	
	Acute	Chronic	Partial
pH	↓	Normal	↓
$Paco_2$	Normal	↓	↓
HCO_3	↓	↓	↓

TABLE 2–6. COMPARISON OF ACUTE AND CHRONIC METABOLIC ALKALOSIS

Parameter	Uncompensated	Compensated	
	Acute	Chronic	Partial
pH	↑	Normal	↑
$Paco_2$	Normal	↑	↑
HCO_3	↑	↑	↑

Metabolic Alkalosis

Metabolic alkalosis can be defined clinically as a bicarbonate (HCO_3) >28 mEq/L, pH >7.45, and a base excess. Metabolic alkalosis occurs when the amount of alkali (base) increases or excessive loss of acid occurs.

A common cause of increased alkali is in the ingestion of alkaline drugs associated with the overuse of antacids or overadministration of sodium bicarbonate during a cardiac arrest emergency.

Conditions resulting in a decrease in acid include

- Loss of gastric fluids from vomiting or nasogastric suction

- Treatment with corticosteroids
- Diuretic therapy with certain drugs, such as furosemide (Lasix), causing loss of K^+

Table 2–6 compares the effects of acute and chronic metabolic alkalosis on arterial blood gases.

In summary, to differentiate between primary metabolic acidosis or alkalosis, the bicarbonate and pH must be evaluated. BE provides additional data. Conditions that cause each acid-base disturbance have been presented. Compensation of metabolic acid-base disturbance requires evaluation of the $Paco_2$.

Section Five Review

1. Metabolic disturbances are reflected by changes in which of the following?
   A. HCO_3, Fio_2
   B. Pao_2, Sao_2
   C. HCO_3, BE
   D. BE, Pao_2
2. Metabolic acidosis results in
   A. decreased pH
   B. decreased HCO_3
   C. increased BE
   D. increased HCO_3
3. A condition that may cause metabolic acidosis due to a decrease in bicarbonate levels is

   A. diarrhea
   B. uremia
   C. aspirin ingestion
   D. diabetic ketoacidosis
4. Metabolic alkalosis is caused by a _____ in acid or an _____ in base.
   A. increase, increase
   B. decrease, decrease
   C. decrease, increase
   D. increase, decrease

Answers: 1, C. 2, A. 3, A. 4, C.

Section Six: Arterial Blood Gas Interpretation

At the completion of this section, the learner will interpret arterial blood gases for abnormalities of oxygenation, acid-base, and degree of compensation.

A single arterial blood gas (ABG) measurement

represents only a single point in time. Arterial blood gases are most valuable when trends are evaluated over time, correlated with other values, and incorporated into the overall clinical picture. Interpretation of ABGs includes determination of acid-base state, level of compensation, and oxygenation status. The oxygenation status reflects alveolar ventilation, the amount of oxygen available in arterial blood for possible tissue use, oxygen-carrying capacity, and oxygen transport.

Arterial Blood Gas Analysis

A step-by-step process for ABG interpretation evaluates each component to determine acid-base balance and oxygenation status. For the purpose of organizing this section, acid-base balance determination is discussed first. However, oxygenation status often is analyzed first, based on the needs of the patient and the preference of the person performing the analysis.

Acid-Base Balance Determination

Evaluate pH

The normal pH is 7.35 to 7.45, with the midpoint being 7.40. For the purpose of interpretation, consider all values higher than 7.4 to be alkaline and all values less than 7.4 to be acidic.

Ask: Is the pH within normal range? Does the pH deviate to the acid or alkaline side?

Evaluate $Paco_2$

Normal $Paco_2$ is 35 to 45 mm Hg. If the $Paco_2$ is <35 mm Hg, consider it alkaline. If it is >45 mm Hg, consider it acidic. Remember that CO_2 is the respiratory component.

Ask: Is $Paco_2$ within the normal range? If not, does it deviate to the acid or the alkaline side?

Evaluate HCO_3

The normal HCO_3 value is 22 to 28 mEq/L. If the HCO_3 is <22 mEq/L, consider it acid. If it is >28 mEq/L, consider it alkaline. Remember that HCO_3 is the metabolic component.

Ask: Is HCO_3 within the normal range? If not, does it deviate to the alkaline or acid side?

Determine the Acid-Base Status

The acid-base status has now been determined for the individual components of $Paco_2$ and HCO_3.

Ask: Which individual component matches the pH acid-base state? The match determines the primary acid-base disturbance.

Example: pH 7.21 (acid), $Paco_2$ 60 mm Hg (acid), HCO_3 22 mEq/L (normal). Interpretation: pH and $Paco_2$ match (acidosis). $Paco_2$ is the respiratory component. Thus, the primary disturbance is respiratory acidosis.

Determination of Compensation

Once the acid-balance has been analyzed, it is necessary to determine if compensation for an acid-base disturbance is occurring and at what level. In discussing compensation, only three components need to be considered: pH, $Paco_2$, and HCO_3.

Determine Compensation

The pH indicates the degree of compensation. A normal pH indicates that either the ABG is normal or full compensation exists. In full compensation, the body has balanced the acid-base state. An abnormal pH indicates an uncompensated or partially compensated acid-base state.

Determine the Level of Compensation

Uncompensated (Acute). Abnormal pH plus one abnormal value plus a normal value.

Example: pH 7.20, $Paco_2$ 60 mm Hg, HCO_3 24 mEq/L. Interpretation: The pH and $Paco_2$ match (acid). HCO_3 is normal. No compensation is occurring. A state of uncompensated (acute) respiratory acidosis exists.

Partially Compensated. Abnormal pH plus two abnormal values ($Paco_2$ and HCO_3 are moving in opposite directions). The body has initiated neutralizing the imbalance but has not fully compensated for it.

Example: pH 7.30, $Paco_2$ 60 mm Hg, HCO_3 30 mEq/L. Interpretation: The pH and $Paco_2$ match (acid). HCO_3 is alkaline or moving in the opposite direction from the $Paco_2$. The pH is still abnormal. A state of partially compensated respiratory acidosis exists.

Compensated. Normal pH plus two abnormal values ($Paco_2$ and HCO_3 are moving in opposite directions).

Example: pH 7.38, $Paco_2$ 50 mm Hg, HCO_3 30 mEq/L. Interpretation: The pH and $Paco_2$ match (acid). HCO_3 is alkaline (opposite of $Paco_2$). pH is normal. A state of compensated respiratory acidosis exists.

Corrected. Normal pH and two normal values. No acid-base disturbance currently exists.

Example: pH 7.36, $Paco_2$ 43 mm Hg, HCO_3 26 mEq/L. Interpretation: If this is the current acid-base state in a patient who, until recently, had an acid-base disturbance, this ABG would be called a corrected acid-base state.

TABLE 2–7. COMPENSATION STATES OF RESPIRATORY ACIDOSIS

Parameter	Normal ABC	Uncompensated Respiratory Acidosis	Partially Compensated Respiratory Acidosis	Compensated Respiratory Acidosis
pH	Normal 7.35–7.45	<7.35 Acid	<7.35 Acid	Normal 7.35–7.45
Paco$_2$	Normal 35–45 mm Hg	>45 mm Hg Acid	>45 mm Hg Acid	>45 mm Hg Acid
HCO$_3$	Normal 22–28 mEq/L	Normal	>28 mEq/L Alkaline	>28 mEq/L Alkaline

In summary, analysis of the acid-base state has been described using a step-by-step approach. This approach allows problem solving without requiring memorization of all disturbance possibilities. Compensation states were classified as uncompensated (acute), partially compensated, compensated (chronic), or corrected (Table 2–7). An example using a respiratory acid-base disturbance was used to show ABG level changes in pH, Paco$_2$, and HCO$_3$ for each level of compensation.

Acid-Base Exercise

Take time to practice determining acid-base and compensation using the steps outlined in the module. Interpret the acid-base status as normal, metabolic or respiratory, alkalosis or acidosis. Indicate the state of compensation as being uncompensated (acute state), partially compensated, or compensated (chronic state).

1. pH = 7.58, Paco$_2$ = 38 mm Hg, HCO$_3$ = 30 mEq/L
   Interpretation:

   Compensation:

2. pH = 7.20, Paco$_2$ = 60 mm Hg, HCO$_3$ = 26 mEq/L
   Interpretation:

   Compensation:

3. pH = 7.39, Paco$_2$ = 43 mm Hg, HCO$_3$ = 22 mEq/L
   Interpretation:

   Compensation:

4. pH = 7.32, Paco$_2$ = 60 mm Hg, HCO$_3$ = 28 mEq/L
   Interpretation:

   Compensation:

5. pH = 7.5, Paco$_2$ = 50 mm Hg, HCO$_3$ = 38 mEq/L
   Interpretation:

   Compensation

6. pH = 7.45, Paco$_2$ = 30 mm Hg, HCO$_3$ = 20 mEq/L
   Interpretation:

   Compensation:

7. pH = 7.40, Paco$_2$ = 40 mm Hg, HCO$_3$ = 24 mEq/L
   Interpretation:

   Compensation:

Acid-Base Exercise Answers

1. pH 7.58 (alkaline) and HCO_3 30 mEq/L (alkaline) match. $Paco_2$ 38 mm Hg (normal).
   Interpretation: metabolic alkalosis. Compensation: uncompensated.
2. pH 7.20 (acid) and $Paco_2$ 60 mm Hg (acid) match. HCO_3 26 mEq/L (normal).
   Interpretation: respiratory acidosis. Compensation: uncompensated.
3. pH 7.39 (normal, slightly to acid side of 7.4), $Paco_2$ 43 mm Hg (normal), and HCO_3 22 mEq/L (normal)
   Interpretation: normal. Compensation: none required.
4. pH 7.32 (acid) and $Paco_2$ 60 mm Hg (acid) match. HCO_3 28 mEq/L (alkaline).
   Interpretation: respiratory acidosis. Compensation: partial compensation (HCO_3 trying to neu-

tralize CO_2; however, pH is not back to normal yet).
5. pH 7.5 (alkaline) and HCO_3 38 mEq/L (alkaline) match. $Paco_2$ 50 mm Hg (acid).
   Interpretation: metabolic alkalosis. Compensation: partial compensation (lungs hypoventilating to retain CO_2 in an attempt to neutralize the alkaline substance).
6. pH 7.45 (normal, alkaline side) and $Paco_2$ 30 mm Hg (alkaline) match. HCO_3 20 mEq/L (acid).
   Interpretation: respiratory alkalosis. Compensation: full compensation.
7. pH, $Paco_2$, and HCO_3 are all normal.
   Interpretation: normal. Compensation: none required.

Evaluation of Oxygenation Status

Evaluation of oxygenation has three components: partial pressure of arterial oxygen (Pao_2), percentage of hemoglobin saturation (Sao_2), and hemoglobin (Hb or Hgb). The following is a systematic approach to evaluating oxygenation status.

Evaluate the Pao₂

Ask: Is it normal (normal Pao_2 is 80 to 100 mm Hg)? What is baseline for this person? Is it within the acceptable range? If not, is it too low or too high?

Evaluate the Sao₂

Ask: Is it within the acceptable range? (Normal Sao_2 is 80 to 100 percent).

Evaluate the Hb

Ask: Are there enough oxygen carriers? (Normal Hb is 12 to 16 g/dL in women and 13.5 to 18 g/dL in men.)

Patient Assessment

Although arterial blood gas interpretation is an important adjunct to assessing a patient's status, it cannot take the place of direct evaluation of the patient. Does the patient's clinical picture match the acid-base and oxygenation interpretation? Many things can interfere with the validity of blood gas analysis and oximetric measurements, for example, a pulse oximetry sensor malfunction, a venous rather than an arterial blood sample, or incorrect arterial blood gas procedures. Does the patient have a chronic disorder that is associated with long-term alterations in arterial blood gases? Are there any acute processes occurring that need to be taken into consideration?

In summary, arterial blood gas analysis is a step-by-step process. Each component is evaluated individually and then in relationship to other components. Although acid-base state, compensation, and oxygenation status are important factors, the most important step is applying the results to the individual patient and the particular clinical situation.

Oxygenation and Acid-Base Analysis Exercise

Take time to practice determining acid-base state and oxygenation status using the steps outlined in the module. Interpret the acid-base status as normal, metabolic or respiratory, alkalosis or acidosis. Indicate the state of compensation as being uncompensated (acute state), partially compensated, or compensated (chronic state). Indicate the oxygenation status as adequate or inadequate.

1. pH = 7.37, $Paco_2$ = 48 mm Hg, HCO_3 = 28 mEq/L, Pao_2 = 80 mm Hg, Sao_2 = 95 percent
   Acid-base state:

   Oxygenation status:

2. pH = 7.52, $Paco_2$ = 30 mm Hg, HCO_3 = 24 mEq/L, Pao_2 = 90 mm Hg, Sao_2 = 98 percent
   Acid-base state:

   Oxygenation status:

3. pH = 7.48, $Paco_2$ = 33 mm Hg, HCO_3 = 25 mEq/L, Pao_2 = 68 mm Hg, Sao_2 = 98 percent

Acid-base state:

Oxygenation status:

4. pH = 7.38, $Paco_2$ = 38 mm Hg, HCO_3 = 23 mEq/L, Pao_2 = 269 mm Hg, Sao_2 = 100 percent
   Acid-base state:

   Oxygenation status:

5. pH = 7.17, $Paco_2$ = 18 mm Hg, HCO_3 = 7 mEq/L, Pao_2 = 239 mm Hg, Sao_2 = 99 percent
   Acid-base state:

   Oxygenation status:

Oxygenation and Acid-Base Exercise Answers

1. pH 7.37 (normal range, acid) and $Paco_2$ 48 mm Hg (acid) match. HCO_3 28 mEq/L (alkaline) is opposite. Pao_2 80 mm Hg and Sao_2 95 percent both are low normal.
   Acid-Base state: compensated respiratory acidosis (pH normal). Oxygenation status: adequate. The Hb is not known, but the relationship between Pao_2 and Sao_2 appears normal. Assessing trends is important. Is the $Paco_2$ continuing to increase and Pao_2 continuing to decrease? Continue to monitor.

2. pH 7.52 (alkaline) and $Paco_2$ 30 mm Hg (alkaline) match. HCO_3 24 mEq/L, Pao_2 90 mm Hg, and Sao_2 95 percent are all normal.
   Acid-base state: acute respiratory alkalosis (uncompensated). Oxygenation status: within normal limits and seems adequate. Look at your patient.

3. pH 7.48 (alkaline) and $Paco_2$ 33 mm Hg (alkaline) match. HCO_3 25 mEq/L is normal. Pao_2 68 mm Hg (low) and Sao_2 98 percent (normal).
   Acid-base state: acute respiratory alkalosis. Oxygenation status: low oxygen with high saturation. Hemoglobin is carrying a full load but needs more carriers. What is this patient's he-

moglobin? Nursing interventions may focus on decreasing oxygen demand. Is this patient tachypneic? Is supplemental oxygen available? Is a transfusion ordered?

4. pH 7.38, $Paco_2$ 38 mm Hg, HCO_3 23 mEq/L are all normal. Pao_2 269 mm Hg is high, and Sao_2 100 percent is high normal.
   Acid-base state: normal. Oxygenation status: too high! What oxygen percentage is this patient on? Oxygenation supplement needs to be decreased.

5. pH 7.17 (acid) and HCO_3 7 mEq/L (acid) match. $Paco_2$ 18 mm Hg (alkaline) is opposite. Pao_2 239 mm Hg is high, and Sao_2 99 percent is high normal.
   Acid-base state: severe metabolic acidosis with partial compensation. Oxygenation status: adequate oxygen provided, but it is doubtful that the patient can use what is available efficiently due to the state of severe acidosis. Cellular metabolism is compromised and cannot function efficiently in the acid environment. Cardiovascular status is very likely compromised. The reactivity and effectiveness of many drugs are altered severely in an acidic environment such as this.

Section Seven: Noninvasive Monitoring of Gas Exchange

At completion of this section, the learner will list noninvasive methods of monitoring gas exchange and applications.

Pulse Oximetry

Pulse oximetry is a noninvasive technique for monitoring arterial capillary hemoglobin saturation. It uses light wavelengths to determine oxyhemoglobin saturation. It also detects pulsatile flow to differentiate between venous and arterial blood. A sensor is placed on a finger, nose, or ear, and an oximeter provides a constant assessment of arterial oxygen saturation (Sao_2). Pulse oximetry is best used as an adjunct to a variety of assessment modalities in providing continuous information for evaluation of oxygenation status.

The continuous arterial oxygen saturation readings reflect the patient's oxygenation status and alert the clinician to subtle or sudden changes. In some patients, use of oximetry may decrease the frequency of invasive arterial blood gas measurements if acid-base and ventilation are not problems. When an acid-base imbalance exists, an acidosis may cause a lower saturation reading, and alkalosis may cause a higher reading due to shifts in the oxyhemoglobin dissociation curve. A patient with CO_2 retention may have an adequate Sao_2 but a declining respiratory status. Under these conditions, arterial blood gas determinations are necessary to provide information on pH and $Paco_2$.

Pulsatile flow is essential for the sensor to detect changes in capillary arterial oxygen saturation (Sao_2) of the peripheral circulation. In low flow states (shock, severe vasoconstriction, cardiac arrest, hypothermia), this factor may limit usefulness and accuracy. Excessive patient movement or improper sensor placement also can contribute to inaccurate readings.

End Tidal CO₂ Monitoring

Capnometry is the noninvasive measurement of carbon dioxide (CO_2) concentration in expired gas. Infrared analyzers measure CO_2 based on absorption of particular wavelengths. Capnography is the "concept of plotting the CO_2 concentration of respiratory gas throughout the ventilatory cycle" (Shapiro et al, 1989, p. 301). The capnogram or curve is then analyzed. The normal capnogram shows a $Petco_2$ within several millimeters of mercury of arterial $Paco_2$ at the end of the plateau phase (the end tidal CO_2). In a normal capnogram, the CO_2 concentration is zero at the beginning of expiration, gradually rising until it reaches a plateau. The end tidal CO_2 is the highest concentration at the end of exhalation.

End tidal CO_2 ($Petco_2$) monitoring is used in the clinical setting as a noninvasive indirect method of measuring $Paco_2$. It is typically 1 to 4 mm Hg below $Paco_2$ (St. John, 1989). It may be used for assessing ventilatory status to provide an early warning of changes in ventilation. An abnormally low $Petco_2$ (<36 mm Hg) most commonly is associated with hyperventilation. Increased $Petco_2$ (>44 mm Hg) is associated with increased production of CO_2 or problems causing hypoventilation (i.e., respiratory center depression, neuromuscular diseases, COPD). Use of the capnogram may help detect improper intubation, ventilation patterns, mechanical problems, or failure in ventilators. Certain capnographic patterns are associated with hyperventilation, incomplete exhalation, and a variety of disease states. Anesthesiologists have used this technique in the operating room, and new applications are being explored in critical care, emergency care, and prehospital care.

In patients with ventilation-perfusion abnormalities, the end tidal CO_2 may not accurately reflect $Paco_2$. However, it still may be helpful if a correlation between $Paco_2$ and $Petco_2$ can be established and used for trending. Unfortunately, critically ill patients commonly have ventilation-perfusion abnormalities, which may limit the usefulness of $Petco_2$ monitoring.

In summary, pulse oximetry and end tidal CO_2 monitoring are noninvasive tools to assist in monitoring oxygenation and ventilation parameters. They can be used singly, but dual use provides information on capillary arterial oxygen saturation (oxygenation) and $Paco_2$ (ventilation). Advantages of use include continuous readings to trend conditions and less invasive procedures.

Section Seven Review

1. Pulse oximetry measures
   A. arterial O_2 capillary saturation
   B. venous capillary saturation
   C. mixed venous saturation
   D. transcutaneous saturation
2. Conditions that impair the accuracy of pulse oximetry include all of the following EXCEPT
   A. excessive movement
   B. improper sensor placement
   C. hypothermia
   D. vasodilation

3. End tidal CO_2 is used as a reflection of
   A. arterial CO_2
   B. $\dot{V}/\dot{Q}$ ratio
   C. oxygenation status
   D. venous CO_2
4. The end tidal CO_2 is an indicator of alveolar

A. acid-base state
B. compensation
C. oxygenation
D. ventilation

Answers: 1, A. 2, D. 3, A. 4, D.

Section Eight: Mixed Venous Oxygen Saturation Monitoring

At completion of this section, the learner will describe the purpose of mixed venous oxygen saturation monitoring ($S\bar{v}o_2$) and its clinical implications.

Many factors affect oxygenation status. Assessment of oxygenation at the tissue level can be difficult, yet many interventions focus on improving tissue oxygenation. Fortunately, technology has provided a means to assist in measuring the consumption of oxygen at the tissue level more accurately. This is accomplished through monitoring of mixed venous blood saturation. For continuous monitoring, the flow-directed pulmonary artery catheter must have a module for fiberoptic oximetry. "The methodology is based on reflectance spectrophotometry where the light wavelength is flushed back down the fiberoptic path and reflected light from the hemoglobin is passed back through the optic fiber and converted to a saturation reading" (Shapiro et al, 1989, p. 226). This provides a continuous display of the oxygen saturation of hemoglobin returning to the heart.

The $S\bar{v}o_2$ reflects the balance of oxygen supply and demand relationships. These relationships depend on oxygen delivery (i.e., cardiac output), arterial oxygen saturation, hemoglobin, and oxygen consumption (Shapiro et al, 1989). Changes in these parameters alter the supply-demand balance, and the body attempts to compensate by increasing cardiac output or increasing oxygen extraction to meet oxygen need. Arterial blood gases give information regarding available oxygen supply. $S\bar{v}o_2$ provides information about oxygen use or consumption.

When the normal oxygen supply-demand is altered, the body attempts to compensate. This compensation is immediately reflected in the $S\bar{v}o_2$, which provides the nurse with an early warning signal of a change in the patient status or effects of treatment before other parameters, such as cardiac output, vital signs, and arterial blood gases, can respond.

The normal range of $S\bar{v}o_2$ is 60 percent to 80 percent. As with all values, the clinical picture is essential for correct interpretation of data. Values in the normal range tend to indicate adequate tissue perfusion. A falling $S\bar{v}o_2$ indicates an increased demand or a decreased supply. A rising $S\bar{v}o_2$ indicates increased supply, decreased demand, or decreased extraction. Deviations from the baseline of more than 10 percent for longer than 5 minutes should be considered significant. The factors affecting oxygen supply-demand should be examined, and interventions should be made as appropriate.

Clinical interventions can be monitored to determine if oxygenation is being enhanced or reduced. Suctioning, turning, and bathing can result in a decrease in saturation. $S\bar{v}o_2$ monitoring allows the nurse to determine accurately and rapidly the effect of interventions. Consequently, interventions can then be grouped or performed separately depending on patient tolerance. Time intervals can be planned between actions to allow a decreased saturation to return to baseline. Therapeutic effects of medications, ventilator changes, and treatments also can be monitored immediately. Calculations can be performed to determine predicted oxygen need, oxygen supply available, and oxygen extraction.

$S\bar{v}o_2$ monitoring has several limiting factors. Insertion of a $S\bar{v}o_2$ catheter is an invasive procedure that places the patient at risk for complications (infection, pneumothorax, hemorrhage). $S\bar{v}o_2$ percentages reflect the general oxygenation state only. They do not provide information specific to the condition of individual organs (heart, kidneys, brain). Values are sometimes difficult to interpret because certain patient conditions alter $S\bar{v}o_2$ readings. In sepsis, peripheral shunting occurs, preventing adequate oxygen extraction at the tissue level. This would produce a high $S\bar{v}o_2$ but tissue hypoxia. In hyperdynamic states, oxygen may not have time to release, thus producing a similar situation. Shifts in the oxyhemoglobin dissociation curve also affect $S\bar{v}o_2$ values via its influence on the Sao_2. A left shift increases the percent of $S\bar{v}o_2$, and a right shift decreases it.

In summary, continuous mixed venous oxygen saturation ($S\bar{v}o_2$) is an additional tool to help clinicians assess oxygen supply and demand accurately. This tool may provide an early warning signal to changes in the patient's condition. Clinical applica- tion requires careful analysis of trends based on the individual situation.

Section Eight Review

1. Factors that directly influence the relationship between oxygen supply and demand include all of the following EXCEPT
   A. oxygen delivery
   B. hemoglobin
   C. end tidal CO_2
   D. oxygen consumption
2. The amount of oxygen used by the body is referred to as
   A. oxygen content
   B. oxygen consumption
   C. oxygen supply
   D. oxygen need
3. Your patient begins shivering. The $S\bar{v}o_2$ drops from 70 percent to 60 percent. What is the significance of this situation?

   A. decreased oxygen consumption
   B. increased oxygen consumption
   C. decreased metabolic rate
   D. technical problem
4. Your patient's $S\bar{v}o_2$ decreases after suctioning and turning. What implications would this have for your nursing interventions?
   A. group activities together to provide longer rest periods
   B. hyperoxygenate patient before turning
   C. allow recovery time for $S\bar{v}o_2$ return to baseline
   D. no implications for nursing interventions

Answers: 1, C. 2, B. 3, B. 4, C.

Posttest

1. Factors affecting gas exchange include all the following EXCEPT
   A. acid-base balance
   B. diffusion
   C. pulse oximetry
   D. ventilation-perfusion matching
2. The lungs initially compensate for increasing acid levels by
   A. blowing off CO_2
   B. excreting HCO_3
   C. retaining CO_2
   D. shifting to anaerobic metabolism
3. Select a normal arterial blood gas (ABG)
   A. pH 7.30, $Paco_2$ 49 mm Hg, HCO_3 24 mEq/L, Pao_2 99 mm Hg, Sao_2 98 percent
   B. pH 7.40, $Paco_2$ 35 mm Hg, HCO_3 24 mEq/L, Pao_2 98 mm Hg, Sao_2 97 percent
   C. pH 7.54, $Paco_2$ 48 mm Hg, HCO_3 32 mEq/L, Pao_2 100 mm Hg, Sao_2 98 percent
   D. pH 7.15, $Paco_2$ 70 mm Hg, HCO_3 18 mEq/L, Pao_2 60 mm Hg, Sao_2 75 percent

4. Respiratory acid-base disturbances are reflected by changes in
   A. $Paco_2$
   B. Pao_2
   C. HCO_3
   D. base excess
5. Metabolic acid-base disturbances are reflected by changes in
   A. $Paco_2$, Pao_2
   B. $Paco_2$, HCO_3
   C. HCO_3, base excess
   D. HCO_3, O_2 saturation

Questions 6, 7, 8
   Interpret the following ABG: pH 7.37, $Paco_2$ 50 mm Hg, HCO_3 30 mEq/L, Pao_2 80 mm Hg, Sao_2 96 percent
6. Acid-base interpretation
   A. metabolic acidosis
   B. metabolic alkalosis
   C. respiratory acidosis
   D. respiratory alkalosis

7. Compensation
   A. complete metabolic
   B. complete respiratory
   C. partial metabolic
   D. partial respiratory
8. Oxygenation status
   A. high
   B. inadequate
   C. low
   D. normal
9. Select two noninvasive methods for monitoring gas exchange
   A. ABG, end tidal CO_2
   B. ABG, $S\bar{v}o_2$

C. End tidal CO_2, pulse oximetry
D. Pulse oximetry, $S\bar{v}o_2$
10. $S\bar{v}o_2$ monitoring reflects
    A. alveolar O_2 levels
    B. arterial capillary O_2 levels
    C. O_2 supply-demand relationships
    D. specific tissue extraction
11. What is the most important factor you must always evaluate?
    A. hemodynamics
    B. laboratory values
    C. oximetry
    D. patient

Posttest Answers

Question	Answer	Section	Question	Answer	Section
1	C	One	7	A	Six
2	A	Two	8	D	Six
3	B	Three	9	C	Seven
4	A	Four	10	C	Eight
5	C	Five	11	D	Six
6	C	Six			

REFERENCES

Kersten, L.D. (1989). *Comprehensive respiratory nursing: A decision making approach.* Philadelphia: W.B. Saunders Co.

Kinney, M.R., Packa, D.R., and Dunbar, S.B. (1988). *AACN's clinical reference for critical care nursing,* 2nd ed. New York: McGraw-Hill Book Co.

St. John, R.E. (1989). Exhaled gas analysis—Technical and clinical aspects of capnography and oxygen consumption. *Crit. Care Nursing Clin. North Am.* 1: 669–679.

Shapiro, B.A., Harrison, R.A., Cane, R.D., and Kozlowski, T.R. (1989). *Clinical application of blood gases,* 4th ed. Chicago: Year Book Medical Publishers.

American Edwards. (1986). *Understanding continuous mixed venous oxygen saturation ($S\bar{v}o_2$).* Santa Ana, CA: American Edwards.

Hudak, C.M., Gallo, B.M., and Lohr, T.S. (1986). *Critical care nursing: A holistic approach,* 4th ed. Philadelphia: J.B. Lippincott Co.

Langfitt, D.E. *Critical care: Certification preparation and review.* Bowie, MD: Brady Communication Co., 1984.

Rutherford, K.A. (1989). Principles and application of oximetry. *Crit. Care Nursing Clin. North Am.* 1: 649–657.

Shapiro, B.A., Harrison, R.A., Kacmarek, R.M., and Cane, R.D. (1985). *Clinical application of respiratory care,* 3rd ed. Chicago: Year Book Medical Publishers.

Springhouse. (1984). *Respiratory disorders,* Springhouse, PA: Springhouse Corp.

ADDITIONAL READING

Alspach, J.G., and Williams, S. (eds). (1985). *Core curriculum for critical care nursing,* 3rd ed. Philadelphia: W.B. Saunders Co.

Module 3

Mechanical Ventilation

Kathleen Dorman Wagner

The self-study module, *Mechanical Ventilation*, focuses on a variety of concepts related to initiation of mechanical ventilation rather than on management of the patient on a mechanical ventilator. Nursing management is addressed in a separate self-study module, *Nursing Care of the Patient with Altered Respiratory Function*. This module uses information covered in two other modules *Respiratory Process* and *Gas Exchange and Blood Gas Analysis*. It is suggested that the reader become familiar with the material in those two modules before reading this one.

Mechanical Ventilation is divided into nine sections. Sections One through Five include such topics as criteria used for determination of the need for mechanical ventilation, required equipment to initiate mechanical ventilation, various types of mechanical ventilators, and a brief discussion of the more commonly monitored ventilator settings. In Sections Six through Eight, the focus shifts to a discussion of how mechanical ventilation and artificial airways affect various parts of the body, including information about potential complications and methods to avoid them. The final section briefly describes several of the innovations in mechanical ventilation. Each section includes a set of review questions to help the reader evaluate understanding of section content before moving on to the next section. All Section Reviews and the Pretests and Posttests in the module include answers. It is suggested that the learner review those concepts that have been missed in the review questions before proceeding to the next section.

Objectives

Following completion of the module, *Mechanical Ventilation*, the learner will be able to

1. Correctly state why a mechanical ventilator is not a mechanical respirator
2. Identify criteria used for determination of the need for mechanical ventilator support
3. Discuss the equipment necessary for initiation of mechanical ventilation
4. Describe the types of mechanical ventilators, based on mechanism of force and cycling mechanism
5. Explain the commonly monitored ventilator settings
6. Discuss the effects of mechanical ventilation on various body systems
7. Discuss the major complications associated with mechanical ventilation

49

8. Explain the cause and prevention of artificial airway complications

9. Describe three innovations in mechanical ventilation

Pretest

1. Mechanical ventilators are responsible for
   A. diffusion
   B. ventilation
   C. perfusion
   D. respiration
2. The most common indication for use of a mechanical ventilator is
   A. pneumonia
   B. chronic obstructive pulmonary disease
   C. acute asthmatic attack
   D. acute ventilatory failure
3. Acute ventilatory failure is associated with
   A. alveolar hypoventilation
   B. severe hypoxemia
   C. alveolar hyperventilation
   D. severe hypocarbia
4. Acute respiratory acidosis can be defined clinically as
   A. pH >7.50, Pao_2 <60 mm Hg
   B. pH <7.30, $Paco_2$ >50 mm Hg
   C. pH >7.50, Pao_2 <60 mm Hg
   D. pH <7.30, $Paco_2$ <30 mm Hg
5. The primary purpose of the endotracheal tube cuff is to
   A. seal off the lower airway from the upper airway
   B. seal off the lower airway from the esophagus
   C. seal off the oropharynx from the nasopharynx
   D. seal off the oropharynx from the esophagus
6. The most common type of airway access used during an emergency is
   A. tracheostomy
   B. nasal intubation
   C. pharyngeal airway
   D. oral intubation
7. A major advantage of volume-cycled ventilators is that they
   A. apply negative pressure to the thorax
   B. overcome changes in lung compliance
   C. do not require an artificial airway
   D. automatically adjust volume of gas delivered
8. A low tidal volume is associated most closely with which of the following?
   A. hypoventilation
   B. hypocapnia
   C. hypoxia
   D. hypotension
9. The fraction of inspired oxygen (Fio_2) is correctly measured in
   A. decimals
   B. percentages
   C. centimeters of water pressure
   D. millimeters of mercury
10. Synchronized intermittent mandatory ventilation (SIMV) is sensitive to
    A. rate of airflow
    B. respiratory rate
    C. concentration of oxygen
    D. the patient's ventilatory cycle
11. A common side effect of positive end-expiratory pressure (PEEP) is
    A. increased blood pressure
    B. decreased cardiac output
    C. decreased lung compliance
    D. increased venous return to the heart
12. During positive pressure ventilation, airflow will be greatest
    A. in areas that are diseased
    B. in areas that are nondependent
    C. in the peripheral lung areas
    D. in the lung apices
13. In what way does positive pressure ventilation affect intracranial pressure (ICP)?
    A. it has no effect
    B. it decreases ICP
    C. it increases ICP
    D. its effects are unknown
14. What effects does positive pressure ventilation have on renal function?
    A. urine output is unaffected
    B. urine output is decreased
    C. urine output is increased
    D. its effects are unknown
15. The term barotrauma refers to
    A. injury caused by oxygen
    B. injury caused by friction
    C. injury caused by temperature
    D. injury caused by pressure

16. Oxygen toxicity has what effect on lung tissue?
    A. it increases surfactant production
    B. it decreases mucous production
    C. it increases macrophage activity
    D. it increases lung compliance
17. Endotracheal cuff trauma can be avoided by maintaining cuff pressures at which of the following ranges?
    A. 5–10 mm Hg
    B. 10–20 mm Hg
    C. 20–25 mm Hg
    D. 25–30 mm Hg

18. Which of the following statements is true regarding microprocessor ventilators?
    A. they perform functions similar to non-microprocessor ventilators
    B. they are less expensive than nonmicroprocessor ventilators
    C. they are more difficult to update than non-microprocessor ventilators
    D. They have fewer features than most non-microprocessor ventilators

Answers: 1, B. 2, D. 3, A. 4, B. 5, A. 6, D. 7, B. 8, A. 9, A. 10, D. 11, B. 12, B. 13, C. 14, B. 15, D. 16, B. 17, C. 18, A.

Glossary

Acute ventilatory failure (AVF). A state of respiratory decompensation in which the lungs are unable to maintain adequate alveolar ventilation, losing the ability to eliminate carbon dioxide

Airway resistance (R_{aw}). The amount of opposition to airway flow through the conducting system

Alveolar ventilation (V_A). The air that fills the alveoli and is available for gas exchange

Assist/control mode (A/C). A mechanical ventilation mode that combines two single modes: assist, a patient-sensitive mode, and control, a time-triggered mode

Barotrauma. Injury to pulmonary tissues due to excessive volumes or pressures

Compliance. The amount of force required to expand the lungs; measured in mL/cm H_2O; normal is 50 to 100 mL/cm H_2O

Cycle. The mechanisms by which the inspiratory phase is stopped and the expiratory phase is started

Deadspace ventilation (V_D). Air that fills the conducting airways and does not take part in gas exchange

Fraction of inspired oxygen (F_{IO_2}). That portion of the total gas being inspired that is composed of oxygen; expressed in decimals from 0.21 to 1.0

Intermittent mandatory ventilation (IMV). A mechanical ventilator mode that allows the patient to breathe spontaneously through ventilator circuitry while interspersing mandatory mechanical breaths at even intervals via a preset rate

Mean airway pressure ($\overline{PA}$ or MAP). The average airway pressure measured over multiple breathing cycles

Negative inspiratory force (NIF), also called maximum inspiratory force (MIF). The amount of negative pressure a person can exert during inspiration; normal is -50 to -100 cm H_2O

Pa_{CO_2}. The partial pressure of carbon dioxide as it exists in the arterial blood; normal range is 35 to 45 mm Hg

Pa_{O_2}. The partial pressure of oxygen as it exists in the arterial blood; normal range is 80 to 100 mm Hg

Peak airway pressure (PAP). Amount of pressure required to deliver a volume of gas

Positive end-expiratory pressure (PEEP). The application of positive pressure to the airway at the end of expiration such that the airway pressure never returns to ambient

Pressure support ventilation (PSV). A type of mechanical ventilatory support in which a preset level of positive pressure augments the inspiratory effort required to attain a tidal volume, thereby decreasing the work of breathing

Respiration. The exchange of oxygen and carbon dioxide across a semipermeable membrane

Shunting. The state in which pulmonary capillary perfusion is normal but alveolar ventilation is lacking

Spontaneous breath. A breath that uses the patient's own respiratory effort and mechanics

Spontaneous ventilation mode (SV). A mechanical ventilation mode in which the patient breathes using only spontaneous effort, through the ventilator circuit

Synchronous intermittent mandatory ventilation (SIMV). A newer form of intermittent mandatory ventilation (IMV) mode in which the mandatory breaths are synchronized to the patient's own breathing cycle

Tidal volume (V_T). The volume of air moved in and out of the lungs during normal breathing

Ventilation. The gross movement of air in and out of the lungs

Ventilation-perfusion ratio ($\dot{V}/\dot{Q}$). The relationship of pulmonary ventilation to pulmonary perfusion expressed as a ratio in liters/minute; normal is 4:5 (0.8)

Ventilator (mechanical) breath. A breath, either patient or machine triggered, that delivers gas at prescribed ventilator settings

Vital capacity (VC). The volume of air that can be exhaled after maximum inhalation; an indication of respiratory muscle strength; normal is 65 to 75 mL/kg

---

Abbreviations

ABG. Arterial blood gases

A/C. Assist/control mode

ARDS. Adult respiratory distress syndrome

AVF. Acute ventilatory failure

cm H$_2$O. Centimeters of water pressure

CNS. Central nervous system

CO$_2$. Carbon dioxide

COPD. Chronic obstructive pulmonary disease

CPAP. Continuous positive airway pressure

CPP. Cerebral perfusion pressure

CVP. Central venous pressure

E-T tube. Endotracheal tube

f. Respiratory rate

FIO$_2$. Fraction of inspired oxygen

HFJV. High-frequency jet ventilation

ICP. Intracranial pressure

ILV. Independent lung ventilation

IMV. Intermittent mandatory ventilation

MABP. Mean arterial blood pressure

MAP. Mean airway pressure

mm Hg. Millimeters of mercury

MPV. Microprocessor ventilator

NIF. Negative inspiratory force

O$_2$. Oxygen

$\overline{PA}$. Mean airway pressure

Pao$_2$. Partial pressure of arterial oxygen

PAP. Peak airway pressure; proximal airway pressure

PEEP. Positive end-expiratory pressure

pH. Hydrogen ion concentration

PIP. Peak inspiratory pressure

PPV. Positive pressure ventilation

PSV. Pressure support ventilation

Sao$_2$. Saturation of arterial oxygen

SILV. Synchronous independent lung ventilation

SIMV. Synchronous intermittent mandatory ventilation

SV. Spontaneous ventilation

SVR. Systemic vascular resistance

T-E. Tracheoesophageal

VA. Alveolar ventilation

VC. Vital capacity

VD. Deadspace ventilation

$\dot{V}$E. Minute ventilation

$\dot{V}/\dot{Q}$. Ventilation-perfusion ratio

VT. Tidal volume

Section One: Ventilator vs Respirator

At the completion of this section, the learner will be able to briefly explain why a mechanical ventilator is not a mechanical respirator.

To understand the concept of mechanical ventilation, one must first have a basic understanding of the difference between respiration and ventilation.

Ventilation refers to the gross movement of air in and out of the lungs. It is composed of deadspace ventilation (VD), the air that fills the conducting airways and does not take part in gas exchange, and alveolar ventilation (VA), the air that fills the alveoli and is available for gas exchange.

VD is easily measured, since it is equivalent to the ideal body weight of the person. For example, if the patient's ideal body weight is 150 pounds, the VD would be 150 mL. V_A is easily calculated as the person's tidal volume (V_T) minus V_D.

$$V_A = V_T - V_D$$

Adequate alveolar ventilation is necessary to maintain normal arterial blood gases. Respiration is the exchange of oxygen and carbon dioxide across a semipermeable membrane. Respiration occurs both in the lungs (external respiration) and in the tissues (internal respiration).

Mechanical ventilators are sometimes referred to as "respirators." This is a misnomer. Though the technology has become very sophisticated, the machines only cause gases to be moved in and out of the lungs, using negative or positive pressure. Although certain ventilator settings help maintain alveoli in an open state to facilitate respiration, the machines do not have the capability to diffuse gases. Respiration, then, remains dependent on adequate functioning of the lung tissues and pulmonary capillaries.

In summary, mechanical ventilation is a mechanical means by which the patient receives ventilatory support in maintaining adequate alveolar ventilation. Mechanical ventilators cannot cause diffusion of gases in the lungs. Rather they facilitate the ventilatory process. Improved ventilatory status will enhance the ability of the gases to diffuse across the alveolar–capillary membrane.

Section One Review

1. The primary purpose of mechanical ventilation is to
   A. support external respiration
   B. support alveolar ventilation
   C. prevent fatigue of the diaphragm
   D. prevent development of pneumonia
2. Deadspace ventilation refers to
   A. the amount of air left in the lungs after expiration
   B. the amount of carbon dioxide in venous blood
   C. the air in the lungs that does not take part in gas exchange
   D. the air in the lungs that leaks into the pulmonary interstitial space

3. Internal respiration refers to
   A. gas exchange between the blood and tissues
   B. gas exchange between the alveoli and blood
   C. the movement of air into the alveoli
   D. the movement of gases between alveoli
4. The term alveolar ventilation refers to
   A. gas exchange between the alveoli and the blood
   B. the intraalveolar movement of air
   C. air in the alveoli that does not take part in gas exchange
   D. air that fills the alveoli and is available for gas exchange

Answers: 1, B. 2, C. 3, A. 4, D.

Section Two: Determining the Need for Ventilatory Support

At the completion of this section, the learner will be able to identify criteria used for determination of the need for mechanical ventilatory support.

The decision to place a patient on a mechanical ventilator is a very serious one. The invasiveness of the artificial airway as well as the physiologic alterations associated with mechanical ventilation place the patient at substantial risk for development of serious complications. Therefore, the relative benefits and costs must be weighed.

Mechanical ventilation is a supportive intervention only. It is meant to support the patient's ventilatory status while curative interventions are initiated to correct the underlying problem. Shapiro (1991) suggests that ventilatory support is probably best initiated as a "semi-elective" procedure before the patient's condition is severely compromised (i.e., cardiopulmonary arrest). Early support is thought to improve the patient's outcome.

How then is the decision made to place a patient on a mechanical ventilator? A variety of criteria have been established by pulmonary experts to aid the health care team in establishing rapidly which patients may require ventilatory support. These criteria generally are not based on specific medical diagnoses but rather on respiratory function status.

Acute ventilatory failure (AVF) is probably the most common indication for ventilator support. AVF is the inability of the lungs to maintain adequate alveolar ventilation. AVF is diagnosed on the basis of the acid-base imbalance it creates—acute respiratory acidosis, which is expressed as $Paco_2$ >50 mm Hg and pH <7.30. A variety of problems can cause AVF, such as head trauma, apnea of any etiology, neuromuscular dysfunction, and drug-induced central nervous system (CNS) depression. Essentially, any problem that decreases movement of air to and from the alveoli can precipitate AVF.

Generally speaking, AVF is a direct indication for rapid intubation and mechanical ventilatory support. A possible exception is the chronic obstructive pulmonary disease (COPD, chronic airflow limitation) patient. COPD patients live in a state of chronic (long-term) ventilatory insufficiency. They are at particularly high risk for development of complications if placed on a ventilator. For this reason, physicians often are reluctant to intubate and mechanically ventilate these patients unless it is absolutely necessary. Other criteria may be used, such as level of consciousness or a particular degree of respiratory acidosis, in making the decision to initiate mechanical support for this group of patients.

The second major indication for mechanical ventilatory support is hypoxemia, which is frequently quantified as a Pao_2 of < 50 mm Hg. Luce et al (1984) state that a low ventilation-perfusion ($\dot{V}/\dot{Q}$) ratio is the most common cause of hypoxemia. A low $\dot{V}/\dot{Q}$ ratio refers to a state in which there is an excess of perfusion in relation to ventilation. The cause of a low $\dot{V}/\dot{Q}$ ratio often is an obstructing mucous plug in the distal airway, causing a reduction in alveolar ventilation (Kersten, 1989). Examples of conditions that are associated with a low $\dot{V}/\dot{Q}$ ratio include asthma, pneumonia, COPD, and atelectasis.

Low $\dot{V}/\dot{Q}$ ratio is associated with a phenomenon called shunting. Shunting refers to the state in which pulmonary capillary perfusion is normal but alveolar ventilation is lacking. Pulmonary capillary blood that runs by a nonfunctioning alveolar unit cannot pick up oxygen from that alveolus. Although some shunting is normal, if many alveolar units become nonfunctioning, a significant decrease in oxygen saturation (Sao_2) will occur, causing hypoxemia. Severe shunting, and thus severe hypoxemia, is associated with such conditions as respiratory distress syndromes of both the infant and adult and severe pneumonia.

Pulmonary function (pulmonary mechanics)

TABLE 3–1. CRITERIA FOR VENTILATOR SUPPORT

Acute ventilatory failure[a]	$Paco_2$ >50 mm Hg, pH <7.30.
Acute hypoxemia	$Paco_2$ <50 mm Hg
Pulmonary mechanics	
Respiratory rate (f)	f >35/minute
Vital capacity (VC)	VC <15 mL/kg
	(Normal 65–75 mL/kg)
Negative inspiratory	NIF < −20 cm/H_2O
force (NIF)	(Normal −50 to −100 cm H_2O)
Minute ventilation ($\dot{V}E$)	$\dot{V}E$ >10 L/minute
	(Normal 5–10 L/minute)

[a] Refer to glossary for definitions.

testing may be used to decide if mechanical ventilatory support is needed. Such testing provides the clinician with crucial information about respiratory muscle strength and airflow. When evaluating the need for mechanical ventilation, pulmonary function tests can provide data regarding evidence of hypoventilation. Several of the more common tests used as criteria are vital capacity (VC), negative inspiratory force (NIF), and respiratory rate (f). Table 3–1 summarizes some criteria that may be used for establishing a need for mechanical ventilatory support.

In summary, the decision as to whether or not to place a patient on a mechanical ventilator is a complex one, based on analysis of a variety of data. A major consideration is the patient's respiratory status. AVF is a common problem requiring mechanical ventilation. AVF is associated with prolonged alveolar hypoventilation and is expressed as acute respiratory acidosis ($Paco_2$ >50 mm Hg with a pH of < 7.30). Hypoxemia (Pao_2 of less than 50 or 60 mm Hg) is a second important indication for mechanical ventilation. Hypoxemia frequently is associated with a ventilation-perfusion mismatch in which shunting is occurring (low $\dot{V}/\dot{Q}$ ratio). Shunting is a phenomenon in which airflow to the alveoli is reduced or lacking, but blood flow is relatively normal. Poor pulmonary mechanics are frequently used in evaluating the need for mechanical ventilation. Pulmonary mechanics provides the clinician with crucial information about the patient's work of breathing and ventilatory status. A patient need not be in AVF or in severe hypoxemia to be placed on mechanical ventilation. If the clinician believes that the patient is in impending ventilatory failure, mechanical ventilation may be initiated as a semielective procedure.

Section Two Review

1. The term ventilatory failure refers to
   A. the inability of the lungs to expand
   B. the inability of the lungs to diffuse gases
   C. the inability of the lungs to use oxygen and carbon dioxide
   D. the inability of the lungs to maintain adequate alveolar ventilation
2. Acute respiratory acidosis is defined clinically as
   A. $Paco_2$ of > 50 mm Hg and pH of < 7.30

B. Pao_2 of < 60 mm Hg

C. $Paco_2$ of > 45 mm Hg and pH of < 7.35

D. Pao_2 of < 80 mm Hg.

3. Common causes of acute ventilatory failure include all of the following EXCEPT
   A. apnea
   B. head trauma
   C. mechanical ventilation
   D. neuromuscular dysfunction

4. A low $\dot{V}/\dot{Q}$ ratio exists when
   A. ventilation is in excess of perfusion
   B. perfusion is in excess of ventilation
   C. blood is shunted away from the alveoli

D. there is an obstruction in the pulmonary capillaries

5. The term pulmonary shunt refers to
   A. movement of air directly from one alveolus to another
   B. normal pulmonary capillary perfusion, lacking alveolar ventilation
   C. an opening between the pulmonary artery and the heart
   D. normal alveolar ventilation, lacking pulmonary capillary perfusion

Answers: 1, D. 2, A. 3, C. 4, B. 5, B.

Section Three: Required Equipment for Mechanical Ventilation

At the completion of this section, the learner will be able to describe the equipment necessary for proper mechanical ventilation.

Mechanical ventilation is a complex intervention that requires a protocol of procedures and equipment. Adequate preparation before placement of the patient on the mechanical ventilator will facilitate smooth implementation.

Initial Equipment Necessary for Establishment of a Patent Airway

Mechanical ventilation requires the use of special cuffed artificial airways. Artificial airways can be divided into two groups: endotracheal tubes and tracheostomy tubes.

Endotracheal Tubes

The endotracheal (E-T) tube is a specially designed semirigid radiopaque tube. Its slightly curved shaft is designed for ease of passage through the curved upper airway. In adults, the tubes require a cuff if positive pressure ventilation is to be initiated. The cuff is a balloon that is attached to the outside wall on the distal end of the E-T tube. When inflated, the cuff seals off the lower airway from the upper airway and holds the tube in a stable position. Neonatal and small pediatrics E-T tubes do not have cuffs, since below the age of 5, the cricoid cartilage offers a sufficient seal once the tube is inserted (Kersten, 1989).

Choice of Endotracheal Tube Size. The size of the E-T tube to be inserted will depend primarily on the age of the person to be intubated. E-T tube sizes range from 2 mm to 11 mm, which reflects the diameter of the inside lumen. Table 3–2 lists the recommended E-T tube size by age.

In the adult, the route of entry also determines E-T tube size. A smaller sized tube is required if it is to be inserted nasally, since the nasal airway passage is significantly smaller than the oral airway passage. Many brands of E-T tubes designate, on the tube, which route is appropriate for each size tube (i.e., nasal, nasal/oral, or oral).

Nasal intubation generally is performed blindly, that is, without viewing the vocal cords through a laryngoscope. It is most frequently performed when the procedure is a semielective (nonemergency) intubation. The nasal route is more comfortable for the patient once it is in place, and the tube is very stable. Oral intubation is most frequently used during an emergency, since direct visualization of the vocal cords assures rapid proper placement in the lower airway. Figure 3–1 shows what a cuffed endotracheal tube looks like in the trachea.

TABLE 3–2. RECOMMENDED SIZES FOR ENDOTRACHEAL TUBES

Age	Endotracheal Tube Internal Diameter (mm)
Newborn	3.0
6 months	3.5
18 months	4.0
3 years	4.5
5 years	5.0
6 years	5.5
8 years	6.0
12 years	6.5
16 years	7.0
Adult (female)	8.0–8.5
Adult (male)	8.5–9.0

(Adapted from National Steering Committee. Standards for cardiopulmonary resuscitation and emergency cardiac care. *JAMA.* 227:852, 1974. Copyright 1974, American Medical Association.)

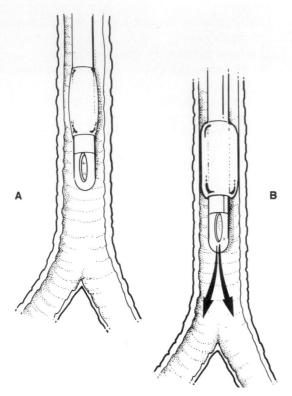

Figure 3–1. Endotracheal tube in the trachea. **A.** Balloon deflated. **B.** Balloon inflated. Air that is pushed through the tube enters the lungs, since it cannot escape around the tube when the balloon is inflated. (*From Pulmonary physiology in clinical practice: The essentials for patient care and evaluation, p. 198, by L. Martin, 1987, St. Louis, MO: C.V. Mosby Co.*)

Intubation Equipment. The endotracheal tube is inserted by a specially trained member of the health care team. The following items need to be gathered before intubation.

- Soft cuffed E-T tubes
- Stylet
- Topical anesthetic
- Laryngoscope handle with blade attached
- Magill forceps
- Yankauers pharyngeal (tonsil) suction tip
- Syringe for cuff inflation (Kersten, 1989)
- Water-soluble lubricant

Tracheostomy Tubes

Generally, when mechanical ventilation is initiated, a tracheostomy is not the entry of choice because it is more invasive and takes longer to perform. However, tracheostomy might be performed initially if the patient has received head or neck surgery or has an upper airway obstruction resulting from severe edema (such as burns) or a tumor obstruction. Tracheostomy is more commonly performed on the patient who requires prolonged intubation (over 2 to 3

weeks) because of failure to wean from the ventilator. Many hospitals have established guidelines for limiting the length of time a person is allowed to have an E-T tube in place before receiving a tracheostomy.

Prolonged use of an E-T tube is associated with many complications. Some of these complications can be avoided if a tracheostomy is performed in a timely manner. It should be noted that tracheostomy also is associated with a variety of complications. Currently, there is increasing controversy over when tracheostomy should be performed. (Artificial airway complications are discussed in Section Seven.)

Securing the Artificial Airway

Any type of artificial airway must be secured in place properly to prevent tube displacement and to minimize trauma to mucous membrane. Initially, in an emergency situation, the tube is secured with adhesive tape. Twill tape and a variety of commercially available stabilizers may be used in place of adhesive tape, particularly for prolonged use. Whatever method is used, stabilization of the tube is imperative. Tracheostomy tubes commonly are secured with twill tape or a commercially available tracheostomy band. The tracheostomy tube also may be sutured in place to prevent accidental dislodgement. Once the airway is secured, a chest x-ray should be performed to confirm correct placement.

Supportive Equipment

In addition to the artificial airway and mechanical ventilator, there are other supplies and equipment that must be readily available.

- Two oxygen sources
  One for the ventilator
  One for the resuscitation bag, to provide 100 percent oxygen
- Suction equipment and at least one suction source
- Disposable sterile suction kits or sterile suction catheters, gloves, containers, sterile water
- Oral pharyngeal airway or a bite block if the oral route is used (to prevent closure of the airway if the patient should bite down on the tube)—also facilitates access to the oropharynx for suctioning
- Cuff manometer to check the cuff pressure on a regular basis
- A manual resuscitation bag to provide adequate backup in case of ventilator failure and for suctioning
- If positive end-expiratory pressure (PEEP) is

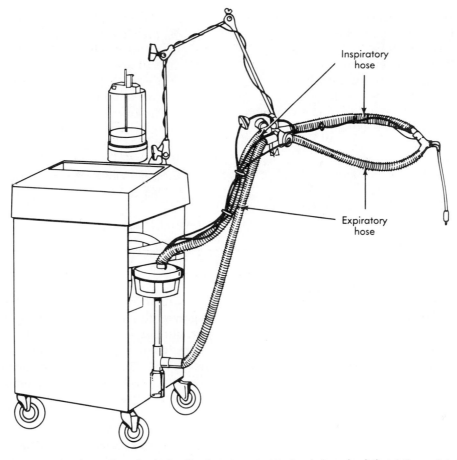

Figure 3-2. Ventilator connected to endotracheal tube. One hose is part of the inspiratory circuit that delivers air to the patient. The other is part of the expiratory circuit. This ventilator is an example of a conventional volume ventilator. (*From* Pulmonary physiology in clinical practice: The essentials for patient care and evaluation, *p. 199, by L. Martin, 1987, St. Louis, MO: C.V. Mosby Co.*)

to be used on the ventilator, a manual resuscitation bag with a PEEP attachment is recommended

In summary, positive pressure mechanical ventilation requires the insertion of an artificial airway, either in the form of an E-T tube, which can be inserted by oral or nasal route, or by performing a tracheostomy. Figure 3–2 shows a volume ventilator attached to an E-T tube. In an emergency, oral intubation using a laryngoscope most commonly is performed because of the speed and accuracy with which it can be placed. Adult artificial airways must have a cuff that is inflated for mechanical ventilation. Neonate and small pediatric E-T tubes do not require cuffs for ventilation. Tracheostomy frequently is performed in those patients requiring prolonged mechanical ventilatory support or long-term assistance with airway clearance.

Section Three Review

1. In the adult, an inflated E-T tube cuff is necessary for mechanical ventilation primarily because
   A. it prevents stomach contents from getting into the lungs
   B. it seals off the nasopharynx from the oropharynx
   C. it prevents air from getting into the stomach
   D. it seals off the lower airway from the upper airway

2. The endotracheal tube size indicated on the tube reflects what measurement?
   A. the length of the tube
   B. the internal diameter of the tube
   C. the circumference size of the tube
   D. the length of the person's airway
3. In an emergency situation, the most common entry route for airway access is
   A. oral intubation
   B. nasal intubation
   C. tracheostomy
   D. oropharyngeal airway
4. Which of the following statements is true about securing the artificial airway?

A. the inflated cuff provides sufficient securing
B. the airway is generally sutured in place
C. a nasotracheal tube does not require securing
D. artificial airways must be secured directly to the patient.

5. When setting up a room for mechanical ventilator use, there must be
   A. one oxygen source
   B. two oxygen sources
   C. clean gloves for suctioning
   D. backup ventilator in room

Answers: 1, D. 2, B. 3, A. 4, D. 5, B.

Section Four: Types of Mechanical Ventilators

At the completion of this section, the learner will be able to describe the types of mechanical ventilators, based on mechanism of force and cycling mechanism.

A common classification of ventilators uses mechanism of force, which is either negative or positive pressure. Figure 3–3 compares the mechanics of spontaneous ventilation, negative pressure ventilation, and positive pressure ventilation.

Negative Pressure Ventilators

Negative pressure ventilators were the first modern ventilators to be developed. The iron lung, a type of negative pressure ventilator, played a crucial role in care of polio victims during the early 1900s. This type of ventilator uses negatively applied pressure to the thorax. Negative pressure ventilatory support does not require use of an artificial airway. Support is delivered by external means. To use a negative pressure ventilator, at least the trunk area of the body is encased in an airtight container. At regular intervals, the air pressure in the tank is reduced in relation to intrapulmonary pressure, causing a lifting of the thorax. The resulting increased thoracic volume decreases intrapulmonary pressure, which, in turn, initiates air flow into the lungs due to the development of a pressure gradient. The amount of negative pressure used is based on the desired tidal volume (V_T)—the higher the desired V_T, the higher the negative pressure required. Patient inaccessibility because of encasement is a major drawback to this form of ventilator support.

With the advent of positive pressure ventilators, negative pressure ventilators rapidly lost favor. Today, although negative pressure ventilators are still in use, positive pressure ventilators are the primary means of ventilatory support. The reader is referred to Blaufuss and Wallace (1987) for further information on negative pressure ventilators.

Positive Pressure Ventilators

Positive pressure ventilators require an artificial airway to deliver ventilatory support. Gases are driven into the lungs through the ventilator's circuitry, which is attached to an artificial airway (E-T or tracheostomy tube). Positive pressure ventilators can be divided into three major types: pressure-cycled, volume-cycled, and time-cycled. The term cycle refers to the mechanism by which the inspiratory phase is stopped and the expiratory phase is started.

Pressure-Cycled Ventilators

Pressure-cycled ventilators deliver a preset pressure of gas to the lungs. The pressure delivered (expressed in centimeters of H_2O) is constant. The volume of air it delivers varies with the lung's compliance and airway resistance. This presents potentially serious support problems, since stiffening lungs, a leak in the system, or a partially obstructed airway can significantly alter the volume of gas delivered. Maintaining an adequate V_T is crucial for normal lung functioning. For this reason, use of pressure-cycled ventilators generally is reserved for short-term use, such as in postanesthesia recovery. Examples of pressure-cycled ventilators include Bennett PR-2 and the Bird-Mark-7.

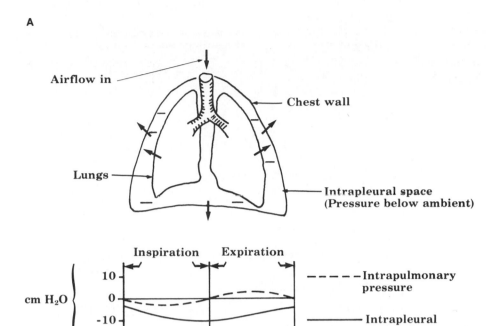

A

Airflow in

Chest wall

Lungs

Intrapleural space
(Pressure below ambient)

Inspiration   Expiration

cm H₂O

10
0
-10

Intrapulmonary
pressure

Intrapleural
pressure

B

Open to
ambient air

Chest
wall

Negative
pressure
ventilator

Below
ambient
pressure

Intrapleural
space

Lung at end exhalation

Lung at end inhalation

Pressure
manometer

cm H₂O

10
0
-10

Intrapulmonary
pressure

Intrapleural
pressure

Figure 3–3. The mechanics of breathing. **A.** The mechanics of spontaneous breathing and the resulting pressure waves. **B.** Negative pressure ventilation and the resulting lung mechanics and pressures. (*From* Mechanical ventilation: Physiological and clinical applications, *pp. 22, 25, 26, by S.P. Pilbeam, 1986, St. Louis: C.V. Mosby Co./Multi-Media Publishing.*) *Continued*

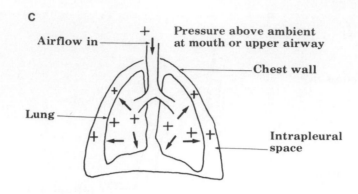

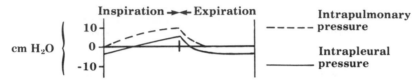

Figure 3–3.   continued   **C.** The mechanics and pressures associated with positive pressure ventilation. Intrapleural pressures are above ambient pressure during end-inspiration.

Volume-Cycled Ventilators

Volume-cycled ventilators are the most common type of ventilators in use today. They are more versatile than the pressure-cycled ventilators. Volume-cycled ventilators deliver a preset volume of gas (measured in milliliters or liters) to the lungs, making volume the constant and pressure the variable. Within a certain preset safety range (pressure limits), the ventilator will deliver the established volume of gas regardless of the amount of pressure it requires. This has the advantage of being able to overcome changes in lung compliance and airway resistance. For example, as lung compliance decreases or airway resistance increases, the pressure at which the gas is delivered to the lungs will increase sufficiently to deliver the desired volume of gas to the lungs. Examples of volume-cycled ventilators include MA-1, MA-2, and Bear-2.

Time-Cycled Ventilators

There are also ventilators that use time as the constant. The length of time allowed for inspiration is controlled, whereas volume and pressure vary.

Time-cycled ventilators frequently are referred to as time-cycled–pressure-limited ventilators, since they also limit the amount of pressure that can be delivered. Time-cycled ventilators have largely replaced volume-cycled ventilators in the management of neonates. Close control of inspiratory time and pressure has been found to better meet the needs of neonates. Some models are used for support of older children and adults, particularly for IMV weaning. Examples of time-cycled ventilators include Babybird, Sechrist IV, Engstrom, and Servo 900.

In summary, negative pressure ventilators require sealing at least the chest of the patient in an airtight tank or shell. They do not require an artificial airway. Negative pressure ventilators are no longer seen commonly in acute care settings. Positive pressure ventilators directly force gases into the lungs using positive pressure. There are various types of positive pressure ventilators available. Pressure-cycled ventilators deliver a set amount of pressure to the lungs. Volume-cycled ventilators deliver a set amount of volume to the lungs and are the most common type of ventilator in use at this time, since it is possible to adjust pressure to meet changes in airway resistance and compliance. Time-cycled ventilators use inspiratory time as their major cycling parameter.

Section Four Review

1. Negative pressure ventilators adjust the tidal volume by
   A. adjusting the amount of negative airflow
   B. adjusting the amount of positive airflow
   C. altering the amount of negative pressure applied
   D. altering the amount of positive pressure applied
2. The term cycle as it applies to mechanical ventilation refers to the mechanism by which
   A. the ventilator turns on and off
   B. inspiration ceases and expiration starts
   C. the concentration of oxygen is controlled
   D. the rate of airflow is maintained
3. Volume-cycled ventilators have an advantage over pressure-cycled ventilators because
   A. they adjust volume as pulmonary pressure changes
   B. they increase airflow as compliance increases
   C. they decrease airflow as airway resistance decreases
   D. they can adjust pressure to changes in lung compliance
4. Pressure-cycled ventilators use which of the following as a constant?
   A. pressure
   B. time
   C. volume
   D. flow rate
5. In adults, time-cycled ventilators are used primarily for which purpose?
   A. initial support
   B. pneumothorax
   C. IMV weaning
   D. adult respiratory distress syndrome

Answers: 1, C. 2, B. 3, D. 4, A. 5, C.

Section Five: Commonly Monitored Ventilator Settings

At the completion of this section, the learner will be able to explain the commonly monitored ventilator settings.

Positive pressure ventilators offer multiple variables that can be manipulated to meet precisely the individual pulmonary needs of the patient. There are certain settings and values related to each variable that must be monitored by anyone taking care of a mechanically ventilated patient whether in a critical care unit or on a general floor. The most commonly monitored settings include tidal volume (V_T), fraction of inspired oxygen (F_{IO_2}), ventilation mode, rate (f), positive end-expiratory pressure (PEEP), continuous positive airway pressure (CPAP), pressure support (PS), peak airway pressure (PAP), and alarms.

Tidal Volume

Tidal volume (TV, V_T) is the amount of air that moves in and out of the lungs in one normal breath. Normal V_T ranges from 7 to 9 mL/kg (or 500 to 800 mL in an adult). If V_T is too low, hypoventilation will occur. If V_T is too high, the patient is at risk for pneumothorax and possible depression of the cardiovascular system. On the mechanical ventilator, V_T commonly is set at 10 to 15 mL/kg to decrease the risk of atelectasis and help stimulate the production of surfactant (Luce et al, 1984). The nurse should note the V_T setting on the control board. On many ventilators, the nurse can monitor the expiratory volume for significant changes that may indicate a change in the patient's pulmonary status, particularly if the patient is on IMV.

Fraction of Inspired Oxygen

F_{IO_2} means the fraction of inspired oxygen. It is always expressed as a decimal. At sea level, the room air that is inhaled into the alveoli is composed of oxygen that is 0.21 of the total concentration of gases in the alveoli. A mechanical ventilator is able to deliver a wide range of F_{IO_2} from 0.21 to 1.0.

Initially, in an emergency situation, F_{IO_2} is commonly set at 0.5 to 1.0 to deliver 50 percent to 100 percent oxygen to the patient. The setting is then increased or decreased based on the patient's Pao_2 and clinical picture. The goal is to maintain the Pao_2 within an acceptable range for the individual, using the lowest level of F_{IO_2}. Prolonged use of F_{IO_2} >0.60 may cause complications associated with oxygen toxicity.

In a semielective situation, the initial F_{IO_2} may

be set at lower levels, based on more individualized oxygenation needs. The patient who has a CO_2-retaining COPD requires special consideration. When maintenance of some degree of patient-initiated breathing is desirable, care must be taken to set the FIO_2 at the lowest level that will deliver an acceptable PaO_2. The use of high concentrations of oxygen on such an individual may obliterate the hypoxic drive to breathe.

Ventilation Mode

The ventilation mode refers to that which initiates the cycling of the ventilator to terminate expiration. The most common modes are assist/control (A/C) and intermittent mandatory ventilation (IMV).

Assist/Control Mode

Many ventilators have an assist mode, a control mode, and an assist/control mode. In assist mode, the ventilator is sensitive to the inspiratory effort of the patient. When the patient begins to inhale, the assist mode triggers the ventilator to deliver a breath at the prescribed settings (called a ventilator or mechanical breath). In the control mode, the ventilator delivers the breaths at a preset rate based on time. It is not sensitive to the patient's own ventilatory effort. Control mode generally is not used alone unless the patient is continuously apneic. A combination of assist and control modes generally is used. Assist/control mode protects the patient in the following manner. The assist part of the mode is sensitive to spontaneous inspiratory effort of the patient, allowing the patient to maintain some control over breathing. At the same time, the control part of the mode acts as a backup should the patient decrease the breathing effort below the preset rate. When A/C mode is used, every breath is a ventilator breath (tidal volume, and so on, as set by the clinician), which differentiates it from IMV. A/C mode commonly is used initially, particularly in patients with acute respiratory failure or respiratory muscle fatigue, because assist/control mode takes over the work of breathing.

Intermittent Mandatory Ventilation

Using the IMV mode, the patient spontaneously breathes through the ventilator circuit, maintaining much of the work of breathing. Interspersed at regular intervals, the ventilator provides a preset ventilator breath. The intervals are based on the IMV rate that is set by the operator. For example, if the IMV is set at 12, the ventilator will deliver a breath approx-

imately every 5 seconds. Between mandatory breaths, the patient's breathing will vary in VT and rate, since it is composed of spontaneous breaths, not ventilator breaths.

Synchronous intermittent mandatory ventilation (SIMV) is a type of IMV. The original IMV mode is not sensitive to the patient's own ventilatory cycle. Thus, an IMV breath can be stacked on top of the patient's own inhalation. SIMV synchronizes a mandatory breath to follow the patient's exhalation. The advantages of SIMV over IMV mode have not been proven, since stacking of breaths has not been shown to be a physiologic hazard. SIMV, however, is more comfortable for the patient because it does not interfere with the normal breathing cycle. IMV/SIMV have certain advantages over the other modes. They decrease the risk of hyperventilation and also provide a better ventilation-perfusion distribution. IMV/SIMV also facilitates the process of ventilator weaning (Kersten, 1989). Figure 3–4 compares the various ventilatory modes.

Rate

Properly setting the ventilator rate (f) is important in establishing adequate minute ventilation $\dot{V}E$. Minute ventilation is the amount of air that moves in and out of the lungs in 1 minute. Tidal volume (VT) and f are the two variables that make up $\dot{V}E$. It can be calculated using the following equation.

$$\dot{V}E = VT \times f$$

These variables are significant because if either one is manipulated, it will affect minute ventilation ($\dot{V}E$). If $\dot{V}E$ becomes too low, hypoventilation will occur, possibly precipitating acute respiratory acidosis. In the CO_2-retaining COPD patient, hyperventilation resulting in decreased CO_2 levels can complicate weaning from the ventilator.

Before being placed on a ventilator, a tachypneic patient should be ventilated manually (using a manual resuscitation bag) to slow respirations to the desired rate. Normal $\dot{V}E$ is 5 to 7 L/minute.

In the A/C mode, initial settings can be several breaths slower than the patient's spontaneous breaths. The rate is then adjusted as the patient's spontaneous rate changes to provide adequate backup. If the patient's breathing pattern is ineffective, the medical team may opt to obliterate the patient's own breathing effort through sedation or use of neuromuscular blocking agents, such as pancuronium. When this is done, the rate on the ventilator will be manipulated with other settings to maintain the arterial blood gases (ABGs) within the acceptable range for the patient.

The IMV rate also is based on providing adequate ventilation for the patient. If the rate is set too slow, hypoventilation may occur, precipitating acute ventilatory failure (respiratory acidosis). If the rate is set too high, it may precipitate respiratory alkalosis by blowing off too much CO_2.

Positive End-Expiratory Pressure

Positive End Expiratory Pressure (PEEP) provides the alveoli with a constant (preset) amount of positive pressure at the end of each expiration. PEEP can be used with a variety of ventilator modes, including A/C and IMV.

Normally, at the end of expiration, alveoli have a tendency to collapse. Providing positive pressure during this phase of the cycle forces the alveoli to remain open, which (1) recruits previously collapsed alveoli, (2) prevents atelectasis, and (3) improves gas exchange (Figure 3–5). As can be seen in Figure 3–6, airway pressure never goes to zero but is always positive.

The amount of PEEP can be monitored on most ventilators by looking at the airway pressure manometer. When no PEEP is being used, the needle on the

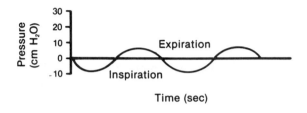

Spontaneous Breathing

Patient has full work of breathing: determining rate, V_T, and rhythm.

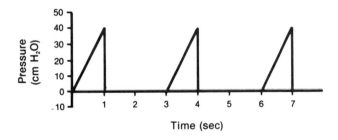

Controlled Ventilation

Patient has no work breathing: ventilator will rhythmically deliver V_T at preset rate.

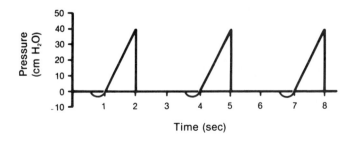

Assist-Control

Patient has minimal work of breathing during initial expansion of chest, then ventilator will deliver preset V_T.

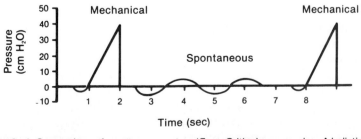

Intermittent Mandatory Ventilation (IMV)

Patient has a variable work of breathing: the mandatory ventilated breaths occur at a preset rate and V_T, but the patient may take spontaneous breaths between the machine-delivered breaths.

Figure 3–4. Comparison of ventilatory modes. (*From* Critical care nursing: A holistic approach, *pp. 352–353, by C.M. Hudak, B.M. Gallo, and J.J. Benz (eds.), 1990, Philadelphia: J.B. Lippincott Co.)*

Continued

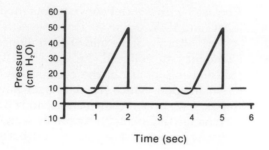

Assist-Control, 10 cm of PEEP

Patient has lessened work breathing as the initial pressure forces are eliminated.

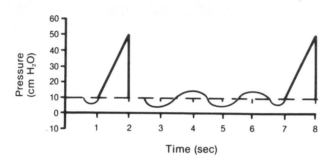

IMV, 10 cm of PEEP

Patient has lessened work of breathing during spontaneous breaths.

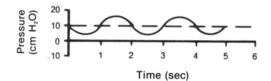

CPAP, Spontaneous Breathing, 10 cm pressure

Patient performing full work of breathing at lower levels of effort due to the elimination of initial pressure forces.

Figure 3–4.   continued

Figure 3–5. Effect of PEEP on oxygenation. During expiration with PEEP, airways that would otherwise collapse are kept open, allowing continued oxygen transfer. In **Example A,** the Pao_2 and Sao_2 improve, and Fio_2 is unchanged. In **Example B,** the Pao_2 is maintained at an acceptable level, whereas the Fio_2 is decreased from 0.70 to 0.50. (*From* Pulmonary physiology in clinical practice: The essentials for patient care and evaluation, *p. 212, by L. Martin, 1987, St. Louis, MO: C.V. Mosby Co.*)

	Inspiration	Expiration	Example A			Example B		
			Fio_2	Pao_2	Sao_2	Fio_2	Pao_2	Sao_2
No PEEP			0.50	40	75	0.70	65	90
PEEP			0.50	54	85	0.50	65	90

pressure manometer should fall back to zero at the end of each breath. When PEEP is present, the needle should fall back only to the level of PEEP. For example, if PEEP is set at 10 cm H_2O, the needle should fall to 10 ± 2 cm H_2O rather than returning to zero.

PEEP has been particularly helpful in treatment of ARDS. Kersten (1989, p. 713) explains.

> By recruiting alveoli and redistributing pulmonary perfusion, PEEP effectively combats refractory hypoxemia and reduced lung compliance,

the hallmarks of ARDS, the disorder routinely requiring PEEP.

PEEP can be adjusted to range from 0 to 45 cm H_2O. It is set at the lowest pressure that will maintain a Pao_2 of ≥60 mm Hg while using ≤ 0.50 Fio_2 and an acceptable cardiac output (Shapiro et al, 1983).

Although PEEP is very helpful in treatment of severe hypoxemia, its use is associated with several significant complications. The risk of complications increases as the amount of PEEP is increased. Com-

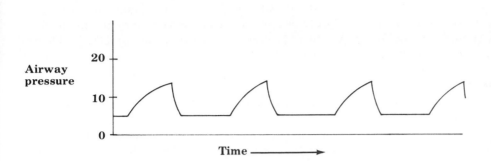

Figure 3–6. Positive end-expiratory pressure (PEEP) airway pressure. Positive end-expiratory pressure (PEEP) during controlled positive pressure ventilation. In this example, there is no spontaneous breathing between machine breaths and no negative deflection of the baseline, which is above the zero point. PEEP may be used with a variety of ventilator modes. (*From* Mechanical ventilation: Physiological and clinical application, *p. 32, by S.P. Pilbeam, 1986, St. Louis: C.V. Mosby Co./Multi-Media Publishing.*)

plications include barotrauma and decreased cardiac output due to decreased venous return to the right side of the heart. The patient on PEEP must be closely monitored for signs and symptoms associated with these two complications.

Criteria for use of PEEP include the following.

- Severe hypoxemia without adequate correction with supplemental O_2 (shunt effect) (e.g., ARDS)
- Acute diffuse lung disease (as opposed to chronic or purely localized processes) (e.g., ARDS, pulmonary edema)
- Restrictive effect (lung volumes reduced, as opposed to increased, as in obstruction) (e.g., Guillain-Barré syndrome, myasthenia gravis) (Luce et al, 1984, p. 221)

Continuous Positive Airway Pressure

Continuous positive airway pressure (CPAP) uses the same principles as PEEP, but it does not require use of a ventilator. CPAP delivers a continuous flow of positive pressure such that airway pressure is never allowed to drop to zero. CPAP can be used with ventilators that have a spontaneous mode, which allows the patient to breathe spontaneously through the ventilator circuitry. The increased resistance associated with spontaneously breathing through a ventilator circuit is thought to increase the work of breathing and thus is a controversial means of delivering CPAP. It is most commonly delivered by a special mask and can be delivered also by a T-piece to an artificial airway.

Pressure Support Ventilation

Pressure support ventilation (PSV), like PEEP, provides positive pressure to the alveoli. However, PSV supports the inspiratory phase, augmenting the patient's tidal volume. The purpose of PSV is to decrease the work of breathing through supporting the

patient's inspiratory efforts. PSV is used primarily as an aid to ventilator weaning. Like PEEP, PSV is adjusted in centimeters of water pressure increments, which commonly range from 5 to 15 cm H_2O (Pilbeam, 1986, p. 296). PSV may be used in conjunction with other modes, particularly IMV. It can be used also as a mode in itself, supporting spontaneous breathing using the ventilator circuitry.

Peak Airway Pressure or Peak Inspiratory Pressure

When using volume-cycled ventilators, the tidal volume is preset to deliver a certain number of milliliters or liters. The pressure it takes to deliver that amount of volume will vary depending primarily on airway resistance and lung compliance. The amount of pressure required to deliver the volume is called the peak airway pressure (PAP) or peak inspiratory pressure (PIP). PIP is measured in centimeters of water pressure and may be visualized on an airway pressure manometer or on a data screen. In the adult, PIPs of <40 cm H_2O are considered desirable. It is known that high PIPs greatly increase the risk of barotrauma and negative effects on other body systems (Section Six). When monitored, PIP should be recorded at regular intervals for trending. Trending refers to taking multiple measurements over an extended period of time to evaluate the parameter for a pattern of change.

Increasing Peak Inspiratory Pressure Trend

This signifies that increasing amounts of pressure are necessary to deliver the preset VT. It is most commonly indicative of increased airway resistance or decreased lung compliance.

Decreasing Peak Inspiratory Pressure Trend

This signifies that less pressure is needed to deliver the VT to the patient. It may indicate an improvement in airway resistance or lung compliance.

Alarms

The patient's life depends on correct functioning of the ventilator and maintenance of a patent airway. To protect the patient, most types of ventilators have been equipped with a system of alarms to alert the caregiver to problems. There are many variables that may be equipped with alarms. Two frequently triggered alarms are the low exhaled volume and high pressure alarms.

The low exhaled volume alarm indicates that there is a loss of tidal volume or a leak in the system. When this alarm goes off, the nurse should focus rapidly on checking to see if the ventilator tubing has become disconnected or if the artificial airway cuff is inadequately filled with air or has a leak. The cuff can be checked by feeling for air leaking out of the nose and mouth. It may be noted also that the patient can suddenly vocalize, which also indicates a leak or insufficiently inflated cuff. A leaking cuff may be checked by deflating and then reinflating the cuff to observe for its ability to attain and then maintain a tracheal seal. If the cuff is ruptured, the nurse needs to notify the medical team immediately and prepare for reintubation.

The high pressure alarm is the most commonly heard alarm. Anything that increases airway resistance can trigger it. Examples of clinical conditions that cause a high pressure alarm include coughing, biting on the tube, secretions in the airway, or water in the tubing. Clearing the airway or tubing most frequently will correct the problem.

If the cause of an alarm is not immediately found or cannot be corrected immediately, the patient should be removed from the ventilator and manually ventilated using a resuscitation bag until the problem is corrected.

Initial Ventilator Settings

When a patient is first placed on the mechanical ventilator, there are certain standard settings that may be used as a guideline. The settings are as follows:

Tidal volume	10–15 mL/kg ideal body weight
Rate	8–12/minute
Mode	Assist/control
FIO_2	0.5–1.0 (less in COPD, if possible)
Peak flow	40–60 L/minute
Inspiratory sensitivity	−1 to −2 cm H_2O

In summary, positive pressure ventilators have many parameters that must be monitored by those persons who work directly with them. This section presents the most commonly monitored mechanical ventilator settings, including V_T, FIO_2, modes (assist/control, IMV/SIMV), rate, PEEP, CPAP, pressure support, PIP, and alarms. Special consideration is given to ventilator setting alterations for management of the patient with CO_2 retaining COPD.

Section Five Review

1. The normal V_T in a spontaneously breathing adult is _____ mL/kg.
   A. 2–5
   B. 5–7
   C. 7–9
   D. 10–15
2. The common V_T setting range on a mechanical ventilator is _____ mL/kg.
   A. 2–5
   B. 5–7
   C. 7–9
   D. 10–15
3. If V_T is set too low on the ventilator, it will cause
   A. hypoventilation
   B. pneumothorax
   C. hypoxemia
   D. hypocapnia

4. A high FIO_2 level (>0.5) is avoided in patients with COPD when possible because
   A. it could cause hyperventilation
   B. it could lead to hypocapnia
   C. it could obliterate the hypoxic drive
   D. it could precipitate metabolic acidosis
5. A major advantage of initial use of A/C mode is that it allows
   A. the diaphragm to exercise
   B. the patient to rest
   C. increased work of breathing
   D. maintenance of some spontaneous breathing
6. SIMV is used primarily for
   A. weaning
   B. full support
   C. acute head injury
   D. acute pulmonary diseases

7. A low minute ventilation ($\dot{V}E$) can cause which of the following?
   A. acute metabolic alkalosis
   B. acute respiratory alkalosis
   C. acute metabolic acidosis
   D. acute respiratory acidosis
8. PEEP affects the alveoli by
   A. increasing alveolar fluid
   B. decreasing their relative size
   C. sealing off nonfunctioning units
   D. maintaining them open at end-expiration
9. PSV is used primarily for what purpose?
   A. to increase PIP
   B. to decrease oxygen need
   C. to decrease work of breathing
   D. to prevent atelectasis
10. An increasing PIP most commonly indicates which of the following?

A. increasing airway resistance and/or decreasing lung compliance
B. decreasing airway resistance and/or decreasing lung compliance
C. increasing airway resistance and increased lung compliance
D. decreasing airway resistance and decreased lung compliance

11. The ventilator low exhaled volume alarm will trigger when
    A. patient is coughing
    B. there is water in the tubing
    C. patient is biting the E-T tube
    D. there is a leak in the system

Answers: 1, B. 2, D. 3, A. 4, C. 5, B. 6, A. 7, D. 8, D. 9, C. 10, A. 11, D.

Section Six: Effects of Mechanical Ventilation on Body Systems

At the completion of this section, the learner will be able to discuss the effects of mechanical ventilation on various body systems.

Positive pressure ventilation (PPV) affects virtually all body systems. Some of the effects can be detrimental to patient outcomes.

Cardiovascular Effects

Spontaneous Breathing

During normal spontaneous inhalation, air is drawn into the lungs due to a drop in intrathoracic pressure. At the same time, the decreased intrathoracic pressure also increases venous return to the heart by drawing blood into the heart and the major thoracic vessels. As blood is moved into the right heart, the right heart chamber enlarges and stretches, enhancing right ventricular preload and stroke volume. During normal exhalation, there is an increase in the flow of blood from the pulmonary circulation to the left heart, increasing left ventricular preload and stroke volume. At the end of spontaneous exhalation, the output of blood decreases in both the right and left heart (Pilbeam, 1986).

Positive Pressure Ventilation

The positive pressure being exerted on the lungs causes a relative increase in intrathoracic pressure, which is then transmitted to all structures in the thorax, including the heart, lungs, and major thoracic vessels. The major vessels become compressed, causing an increase in central venous pressure (CVP). Blood return to the right heart is reduced due to a decreased pressure gradient. The resulting reduction in venous return to the heart causes right preload and stroke volume to decrease. Left ventricular output will fall as a direct result of decreased right ventricular output.

Positive pressure ventilation (PPV) reduces cardiac output by decreasing venous return to the heart in two major ways. First, as described earlier, the presence of positive intrathoracic pressure prevents blood from being pulled into the major thoracic vessels and into the heart. Second, cardiac output is reduced through a squeezing of the heart by the lungs during the inspiratory phase of PPV. Pilbeam (1986, p. 129) clarifies this point:

> The longer the inspiratory phase and the greater the peak pressure, the less the cardiac output. This tamponade effect occurs when reduced venous return to the thorax occurs.

Third, the amount of pressure being exerted on the alveoli is the single most important factor influencing cardiac output when considering pulmonary influences. As the level of pressure is increased, venous return to the heart decreases. The more the heart and pulmonary capillaries are squeezed by the presence of positive pressure, the lower the cardiac output. This helps explain why high levels of PEEP can dramatically reduce cardiac output. Other factors that influence the effects of PPV on the cardiovascular system include lung and thoracic compliance, airway resistance, and the patient's volemic state.

Decreased cardiac output may be manifested as a reduction in arterial blood pressure, particularly if the patient is hypovolemic. However, a normal blood pressure frequently is maintained in PPV patients through the compensatory mechanisms of increased heart rate and increased systemic vascular resistance (SVR) (Pilbeam, 1986).

Pulmonary Effects

PPV alters the relationship of ventilation to perfusion in the lungs. When spontaneously breathing, most inhaled gases flow toward the diaphragm. The distribution of gases to the alveoli normally favors the peripheral and dependent lung areas. Likewise, pulmonary perfusion normally is the greatest in dependent areas, thus matching the lung zones with the most ventilation with the lung zones with the most perfusion.

PPV causes gases to flow through the path of least resistance, which increases ventilation to the nondependent lung areas and large airways. This is largely due to the decreased functioning and stiffening of the diaphragm associated with passive PPV. PPV gas flow will increase ventilation to the healthy lung areas while flow will decrease to the diseased areas, since it meets increased resistance in diseased lung tissue.

When PPV is being used, the positive pressure is transmitted to the pulmonary vessels, pushing the blood to the peripheral lung and to dependent areas. Since perfusion is now the greatest in the periphery and in the dependent lung areas and ventilation is greatest in the nondependent and larger airways, the relationship of ventilation to perfusion is altered— they no longer match well. In areas with the most perfusion, there is decreased ventilation, and in areas with adequate ventilation, perfusion has been reduced. This can create problems with oxygenation that may be reflected in deteriorating arterial blood gases (Pao_2 levels in particular).

Neurovascular Effects

PPV can cause a change in neurovascular status through two major mechanisms. First, intracranial pressure (ICP) can increase, and, second, cerebral perfusion pressure (CPP) can decrease. Patients who have existing intracranial or neurovascular problems are at particular risk when moderate to high ventilation pressures are required. The increased intrathoracic pressure associated with PPV decreases

venous return from the head. The higher the pressure required to ventilate the patient, the greater the effects on the ICP.

Blood flow to the head (cerebral perfusion pressure) may be reduced. If cardiac output drops sufficiently to reduce systolic blood pressure, cerebral perfusion may become compromised. CPP is influenced by two factors: ICP and mean arterial blood pressure (MABP). This relationship is expressed in the statement

$$CPP = ICP - MABP$$

MABP is determined by the systolic and diastolic blood pressures. Therefore, if systolic blood pressure is reduced, so will MABP, thus also reducing CPP. If CPP drops too low, cerebral hypoxia can result (Pilbeam, 1986).

Renal Effects

PPV is associated with a decreased urinary output. The mechanisms for this decrease are multiple, and some are unclear. Two major mechanisms are decreased cardiac output and redistribution of renal blood flow.

Decreased cardiac output is associated with reduced renal perfusion and reduced glomerular filtration rate, which can cause decreased urine output. Pilbeam (1986) states, however, that in patients who are receiving PPV, arterial blood pressure generally is maintained through compensatory mechanisms. It is suggested that when cardiac output has not been reduced significantly, the cause of low urine output may be more associated with a redistribution of intrarenal blood flow that occurs with PPV. This may result from stimulation of the sympathetic nervous system. The redistribution of blood causes kidney function changes. PPV seems to alter renal perfusion in the following manner (Pilbeam, 1986, p. 131).

> Flow to the outer cortex decreases, while flow to the inner cortex and outer medullary tissue (juxta-medullary nephrons) increases. The net result is that urine output decreases by 40%, creatinine clearance decreases by 23% and sodium excretion by 63%.

This redistribution places the most blood in areas of the kidney that reabsorb sodium. If sodium is reabsorbed, water also will be reabsorbed to maintain homeostasis, thus reducing urine output.

Gastrointestinal Effects

PPV can decrease blood flow into the intestinal viscera by increasing visceral vascular resistance. The increased resistance to flow can result in tissue ischemia, which causes increased permeability of the protective mucosal lining. This predisposes the ventilator patient to gastric ulcer formation and gastrointestinal bleeding.

In summary, positive pressure mechanical ventilation affects multiple body systems. *Cardiovascular effects:* cardiac output is reduced due to reduced venous return to the heart. *Pulmonary effects:* gas and blood flow into the lungs is altered, causing a change in distribution of pulmonary blood and gases. Under the influence of positive pressure, gas flow will favor the path of least resistance and will move toward nondependent lung areas and large airways. Pulmonary blood flow (perfusion) will be the greatest in dependent areas and the peripheral lung. *Neurovascular effects:* PPV can increase ICP and CPP because of decreased venous return from the head as well as the change in cardiac output. *Renal effects:* renal perfusion is altered during PPV, causing decreased urinary output. This is believed to be due to decreased cardiac output and the redistribution of renal blood flow, which encourages reabsorption of sodium. *Gastrointestinal effects:* PPV may cause decreased intestinal viscera blood flow, causing tissue ischemia.

Section Six Review

1. PPV affects the cardiovascular system by
   A. increasing cardiac output
   B. decreasing venous return to the heart
   C. increasing arterial blood pressure
   D. increasing venous return to the heart
2. PPV alters the relationship of ventilation to perfusion in what way?
   A. ventilation increases in nondependent lung areas
   B. ventilation increases in the small airways
   C. perfusion increases in the nondependent lung areas
   D. perfusion increases near the large airways
3. PPV influences ICP by
   A. decreasing intrathoracic pressure
   B. increasing cerebral perfusion pressure
   C. decreasing venous drainage from the head
   D. increasing MABP

4. The kidneys are affected by PPV in what way?
   A. decreased sodium retention
   B. redistribution of renal blood flow
   C. renal effects of increased cardiac output
   D. redistribution of urine flow through the kidneys
5. The gastrointestinal system may be adversely affected by PPV due to
   A. increased visceral vascular resistance
   B. increased blood supply to the viscera
   C. increased venous pooling in the viscera
   D. decreased visceral vascular resistance

Answers: 1, B. 2, A. 3, C. 4, B. 5, A.

Section Seven: Major Complications of Mechanical Ventilation

At the completion of this section, the learner will be able to discuss the major complications associated with mechanical ventilation.

Mechanical ventilation is associated with many potential complications. The major complications can be divided into cardiovascular, pulmonary, and gastrointestinal.

Cardiovascular Complications

Positive pressure ventilation (PPV) decreases cardiac output and venous return to the heart by increasing intrathoracic pressure. High levels of PEEP can significantly decrease cardiac output, affecting both preload and afterload of the right ventricle. Clinically, decreased cardiac output results in a decrease in blood pressure, an increased pulse rate, possible arrhythmia development, and decreased urine output.

Hemodynamic monitoring will show a decreased cardiac output, increased pulmonary artery wedge pressure, and increased right atrial pressure (Kersten, 1989).

Pulmonary Complications

Barotrauma

Barotrauma is associated with PPV. Burton and Hogkin (1984) explain that barotrauma probably is initiated by alveolar overdistention through use of pressures or volumes that are excessive. The higher the positive pressure applied, the greater the risk of trauma. Patients who are at the highest risk for development of barotrauma are those requiring high levels of PEEP and high peak airway pressures (PAP) (e.g., end-stage COPD). Barotrauma can manifest itself as pneumothorax, subcutaneous emphysema, or pneumomediastinum. Clinically, barotrauma should be suspected if (1) the patient has a sudden onset of agitation and cough associated with a frequent high pressure alarm, (2) the blood pressure (BP) and ABG rapidly deteriorate, (3) breath sounds suddenly are diminished or absent, or (4) subcutaneous emphysema can be palpated on the anterior neck or chest (Kersten, 1989). If a pneumothorax or pneumomediastinum is diagnosed, insertion of a chest tube should be anticipated and prepared for.

Oxygen Toxicity

Oxygen toxicity is associated with the use of a fraction of inspired oxygen (FIO_2) of ≥ 0.6 for more than 48 hours. The use of FIO_2 of 1.0 can cause pulmonary changes within 6 hours (Pilbeam, 1986). Oxygen toxicity damages the endothelial lining of the lungs and decreases alveolar macrophage activity. It also decreases mucous and surfactant production. If it is allowed to continue for more than 72 hours, the patient may develop a pattern of symptoms similar to ARDS (Pilbeam, 1986). The early signs and symptoms of oxygen toxicity are nonspecific (malaise, fatigue, and substernal discomfort). Because early symptoms are difficult to assess, the nurse should be aware of who is at risk for developing oxygen toxicity on the basis of the length of time that the patient has received an FIO_2 of ≥ 0.6 (or even 0.5). Changes in pulmonary mechanics are the best indicator of oxygen toxicity. A pattern of decreased lung compliance, decreased vital capacity, and increased PIP is noted (Kersten, 1989).

Nosocomial Pulmonary Infection

Nosocomial pulmonary infection is a common major complication of mechanical ventilation. The passing of an E-T tube from the upper airway into the lower airway introduces upper airway contaminants into the lower airway. The presence of an artificial airway bypasses the normal upper airway defense mechanisms. Contamination also occurs as a result of failure to maintain strict aseptic technique during pulmonary suctioning or use of contaminated equipment. These factors, coupled with the physiologically compromised state of most mechanically ventilated patients and tearing of the mucous membranes with tracheal suctioning, places them at high risk for development of a pulmonary infection. Signs and symptoms of a pulmonary infection include development of adventitious breath sounds and changes in sputum color or quantity. Systemically, infection may be evidenced by fever and increased white blood cell (WBC) count. Positive chest x-ray and sputum culture findings are important diagnostic tools.

Gastrointestinal Complications

Gastrointestinal bleeding occurs in approximately 25 percent of patients on mechanical ventilators through development of stress ulcers. Stress ulcers develop as a result of either gastric hyperacidity or, more commonly, from a transient visceral hypoxia episode. In the mechanically ventilated patient, the tissue hypoxia may have occurred related to acute respiratory failure or may be the result of increased resistance to blood flow in the viscera. Stress ulcers, which usually are shallow erosions in the mucosal lining, often cause slow bleeds and may, therefore, frequently not be diagnosed early in their development. For this reason, it is important to check all stools for guaiac.

Symptomatically, the patient will exhibit a decreasing hematocrit and guaiac-positive stools. Stools may be black or dark red. If the ulcer formation is gastric, nasogastric aspirate will be guaiac-positive, and the aspirate will appear bright red to dark red. Preventive interventions include the use of antacids, histamine (H_2) antagonists, or both to maintain a gastric pH of >3.5 (Kersten, 1989).

In summary, there are many potential complications associated with mechanical ventilation. Cardiovascular complications are those associated with a significantly reduced cardiac output. PEEP is especially associated with cardiovascular compromise. Pulmonary complications include barotrauma, associated mostly with higher levels of PEEP, oxygen toxicity, which occurs with high levels of oxygen for a prolonged period of time (oxygen toxicity has been attributed to the development of ARDS), and nosocomial pulmonary infection. Gastrointestinal complications include development of stress ulcers and gastrointestinal bleeding.

Section Seven Review

1. Changes in cardiac output resulting from positive pressure ventilation are associated with which of the following manifestations?
   A. increased arterial blood pressure
   B. increased urinary output
   C. arrhythmia development
   D. decreased pulse rate
2. Which of following are manifestations of pulmonary barotrauma secondary to mechanical ventilation?
   A. onset of increased lethargy
   B. increase in arterial blood pressure
   C. increase in breath sounds over a lung field
   D. increased cough with high pressure alarm triggering
3. Oxygen toxicity affects the pulmonary tissue in which of the following ways?
   A. decreasing macrophage activity
   B. increasing mucous production
   C. increasing surfactant production
   D. decreasing peak inspiratory pressure (PIP)

4. Patients receiving mechanical ventilation are at increased risk of developing a nosocomial pulmonary infection because
   A. the lower airway is defenseless
   B. macrophage activity has been bypassed
   C. normal upper airway defenses are bypassed
   D. normal pulmonary mechanics have been interfered with
5. Gastrointestinal bleeding secondary to mechanical ventilation most frequently manifests itself as
   A. grossly bloody stools
   B. guaiac-positive stools
   C. grossly bloody nasogastric drainage
   D. guaiac-negative nasogastric drainage

Answers: 1, C. 2, D. 3, A. 4, C. 5, B.

Section Eight: Artificial Airway Complications

At the completion of this section, the learner will be able to explain the cause and prevention of artificial airway complications.

Artificial airways have their own set of complications that are primarily pressure damage related.

Nasal Damage

Placing an artificial airway through the nasal passage is associated with trauma to nasal mucous membranes during the passing of the tube. In addition, ischemia and even necrosis of the nares may develop caused by the pressure the tube exerts against the internal nasal wall. Anchoring the tube to the cheeks rather than to the top of the nose will help prevent pressure damage. Choice of the proper size tube also is important in minimizing the risk of damage. Nasotracheal tubes can cause inner ear problems related to their location. The nasotracheal tube can occlude the eustachian tubes, increasing the risk of development of ear pressure problems or inner ear infection.

Cuff Trauma

Although the use of tracheal cuffs is necessary to mechanically ventilate the patient properly, they are associated with potentially severe tracheal and laryngeal injuries. The use of excessive cuff pressures is the major contributing factor in these injuries. Arterial capillary blood flow pressure through the trachea is low (<30 mm Hg). A high pressure force, such as is delivered by an overinflated cuff, exerts a pressure that is higher than capillary pressure, causing circulation in the cuffed area to be compromised. Decreased or obliterated blood flow to an area of tissue causes ischemia, which, if allowed to continue for an extended period of time, can produce necrosis. Necrosis of the trachea, larynx, or both is associated with the development of fistulas, fibrosis, and ulceration.

Proper monitoring and control of cuff pressures decreases the risk of complications significantly. Cuff pressures need to be monitored at least once every shift. Safe cuff pressure ranges between 20 and 25 mm Hg (27 to 34 cm H_2O). If a cuff manometer is not available, it is simple to make one using a three-way or four-way stopcock, a 10 mL syringe, and a sphygmomanometer (Figure 3–7).

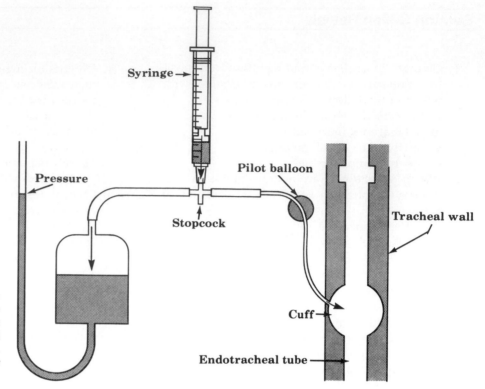

Figure 3–7. The use of syringe, mercury manometer, and three-way stopcock for measuring cuff pressure. (*From Mechanical ventilation: Physiological and clinical applications, p. 307, by S.P. Pilbeam, 1986, St. Louis: C.V. Mosby Co./Multi-Media Publishing.*)

A minimum occluding pressure technique may also be used to reduce the risk of pressure-related cuff damage. Using this technique, the cuff is inflated only to the point at which it seals the airway during the mechanical ventilation. Cuff pressure should be regularly checked using this technique and should not exceed 20 to 25 mm Hg.

Artificial airways can damage one or both vocal cords as a result of traumatic introduction of the tube or damage related to pressure of the tube against the cords. Fistula formation is also a major concern. Should tracheal injury from a cuff cause a fistula to form between the trachea and esophagus, gastric secretions can be aspirated into the lungs. Tracheoesophageal (T-E) fistulas should be suspected if tube feeding or food is aspirated during tracheal suctioning. The patient can be tested for a T-E fistula by placing food dye in food products, such as liquid drinks or tube feedings. During E-T suctioning, the secretions are monitored for the presence of the food dye, which if present, is indicative of esophageal contents in the lower airway. Proper cuff technique and use of correct tube size can minimize cuff-related complications.

In summary, the patient who requires an artificial airway is at risk for developing a complication related to its use. Artificial airway complications are primarily due to the effects of pressure on delicate mucous membranes. Nasal damage may occur during passage of the tube or may be caused by the pressure of the tube against the nares or nasal passage. Cuff trauma is caused by excessive pressure being exerted against the trachea, compromising blood flow to the surrounding mucosa. Cuff pressures should be measured on a regular basis and should be maintained at 20 to 25 mm Hg (27 to 34 cm H_2O). The use of a minimum occluding pressure technique also can be used to reduce the chances of damage to the trachea. The presence of an artificial airway can damage one or both vocal cords. The formation of a T-E fistula is a potentially serious complication that can cause aspiration of esophageal or stomach contents into the lower airways. Placing food dye in oral or tube feedings can test for the presence of a T-E fistula.

Section Eight Review

1. The presence of a nasotracheal tube can affect the ears because it can
   A. occlude the eustachian tubes
   B. exert direct pressure on the inner ears
   C. cause inner ear ischemia
   D. directly damage the eustachian tubes
2. High endotracheal tube cuff pressures can damage the trachea when cuff pressure is
   A. increased during coughing
   B. reduced due to a leak
   C. lower than surrounding capillary pressure
   D. higher than surrounding capillary pressure
3. Normal tracheal capillary pressure is about ____ mm Hg.
   A. <10
   B. <20
   C. <30
   D. <40
4. Safe tracheal cuff pressure ranges are ____ mm Hg.
   A. 10–15
   B. 15–20
   C. 20–25
   D. 25–30
5. T-E fistula formation secondary to tracheal cuff complications can cause
   A. sepsis
   B. aspiration pneumonia
   C. gastric ulcerations
   D. esophageal varices

Answers: 1, A. 2, D. 3, C. 4, C. 5, B.

Section Nine: Innovations in Mechanical Ventilation

At the completion of this section, the learner will be able to discuss three innovations in mechanical ventilation.

Several important innovations in mechanical ventilation have received increased attention over the past several years. These include microprocessor ventilators, high frequency jet ventilators, and independent lung ventilation.

Microprocessor Ventilators

Microprocessor-controlled ventilators (MPV), such as the Bennett 7200, the Bear V, and Infant Star, are gaining popularity in acute care settings. Microprocessor-controlled means that the ventilator functions by computer commands. MPVs essentially perform the same functions as other sophisticated non-microprocessor ventilators, but often more rapidly. They, however, have several potential advantages that the noncomputerized ventilators do not possess. They can be hooked up to a printer and to a central control module at the nursing station. MPVs also have the capability of automatic ventilator setting changes based on computer-analyzed arterial blood gases (ABGs). Since they use computer software, the MPVs can be updated easily by obtaining updated software rather than purchasing a new ventilator. The control board on the MPV looks very different from that of the conventional ventilators. Rather than the usual dials, switches, buttons, and needles that are present on the conventional control boards, MPVs have, primarily, pressure-sensitive boards with digital readouts.

High-Frequency Jet Ventilation

High-frequency jet ventilation (HFJV) was described originally in 1977 by Klain and Smith (Pilbeam, 1986). HFJV requires a special ventilator and a modified E-T tube. A regular E-T tube can be modified satisfactorily for HFJV use if the special tube (the Hi-Lo Jet Tube) is not available. The Hi-Lo Jet Tube looks like a conventional E-T tube except that it also has a jet catheter and pressure monitor line built into it. Pilbeam (1986, p. 301) provides a good synopsis of how HFJV works.

> HFJV uses a high pressure gas source that can be regulated to produce short, rapid jets of gas through a small bore cannula into the airway above the carina. Air from a second gas source can be entrained by the jet stream. HFJV has a frequency range of about 100 to 400 cycles per minute (1.7 to 6.7 Hz) although rates may go higher than this. Tidal volumes are about the same or slightly larger than deadspace volumes.

Uses for HFJV are still being developed and researched. At present, this technique is used for treatment of severe respiratory failure, idiopathic pulmonary fibrosis secondary to ARDS (Smith, 1988), patient conditions in which conventional PPV is either not effective or is contraindicated, and for use during certain types of chest surgery.

Independent Lung Ventilation

Independent lung ventilation (ILV) is the delivery of PPV to each lung independent of the other, using a special double-lumen artificial airway.

At this time, ILV is used most commonly for treatment of respiratory failure associated with asymmetrical lung pathology (e.g., unilateral chest trauma, unilateral ARDS). When the lungs are injured asymmetrically, $\dot{V}/\dot{Q}$ mismatch between the two lungs develops (Siegel et al, 1985). This means that the injured or diseased lung will have volume and pressure needs that are different from the needs of the uninjured lung. By using ILV, the differing requirements of each lung can be individually addressed simultaneously. Ideally, the use of ILV significantly enhances gas exchange, reduces barotrauma, and is able to reverse some of the more fixed changes associated with ARDS (Siegel et al, 1985).

ILV frequently is synchronized to decrease the risk of cardiac complications. When synchronization is used (called SILV, synchronized independent lung ventilation), both lungs inhale and exhale (cycle) at the same time. SILV requires the use of two ventilators that are connected by a cable to make them capable of coordinating their cycles. If regular ILV is used, the ventilators are not connected to each other. The Servo 900 ventilators have this capability and are used frequently for SILV.

In summary, there are a variety of innovations in mechanical ventilation available in a rapidly changing market. Microprocessor-controlled ventilators perform many of the same functions as older generation ventilators. They, however, offer more versatility in mode choice and can monitor and make adjustments using computer speed and accuracy. They also offer updating through software packages. High-frequency jet ventilation is a very different concept in mechanical ventilation, using short, very rapid blasts of gas at 100 to 400 cycles per minute. Independent lung ventilation requires a special artificial airway that can allow ventilation of each lung independently. This innovative form of mechanical ventilation allows the clinician more freedom to meet the needs of each lung independently. At this time, independent lung ventilation is being tested primarily in cases of respiratory failure that is asymmetrical in nature (involving one lung but not the other).

Section Nine Review

1. Which of the following statements is true regarding MPVs?
   A. the ventilator functions by computer commands
   B. the ventilator does not have its own control panel
   C. the control board looks identical to non-microprocessor ventilators
   D. the ventilator has many more functions than a nonmicroprocessor ventilator
2. The HFJV is used primarily for which of the following problems?

   A. pneumothorax
   B. viral pneumonia
   C. unilateral chest trauma
   D. severe respiratory failure
3. At this time, ILV primarily is used on
   A. severe bilateral pneumonia
   B. severe diffuse respiratory failure
   C. asymmetrical respiratory failure
   D. COPD

Answers: 1, A. 2, D. 3, C.

Posttest

The following Posttest is constructed in a case study format. A patient is presented. Questions are asked based on available data. New data are presented as the case study progresses.

Mary R., 55 years of age, has a 20-year history of smoking. She has been treated medically for emphysema for several years. Mary weighs 115 pounds. She is admitted to the hospital with a diagnosis of acute respiratory failure.

1. If Mary's tidal volume was 300 mL, her alveolar ventilation would be ____ mL.
   A. 8.4
   B. 50
   C. 185
   D. 300
2. To be clinically called acute ventilatory failure, which of the following arterial blood gas results must be present?
   A. pH <7.35
   B. $Paco_2$ >50 mm Hg
   C. Pao_2 <60 mm Hg
   D. HCO_3 <18 mm Hg
3. Mary has a low ventilation-perfusion ratio due to pulmonary shunting. Shunting refers to
   A. blood that does not go through the heart
   B. normal alveolar ventilation with poor perfusion
   C. diminished pulmonary ventilation and perfusion
   D. normal perfusion past unventilated alveoli

Mary is showing evidence of ventilatory fatigue. It is decided that she will require intubation and mechanical ventilation.

4. Mary's intubation is a semielective one. For increased comfort, she may have which type of artificial airway inserted?
   A. oral endotracheal tube
   B. nasotracheal tube
   C. tracheostomy tube
   D. oral pharyngeal airway

Mary is placed on a Bear-2, a volume-cycled ventilator.

5. The primary advantage of using a volume-cycled ventilator is that this type of ventilator
   A. overcomes changes in airway resistance
   B. does not require a cuffed artificial airway
   C. automatically alters volume as pressure changes

D. delivers higher levels of oxygen than other ventilators
6. Mary's tidal volume is set at 700 mL. A large tidal volume is set on a mechanical ventilator for which of the following reasons?
   A. to decrease peak airway pressure
   B. to decrease pneumothorax occurrence
   C. to decrease ventilator breaths
   D. to decrease atelectasis occurrence

Mary's minute ventilation is 5.6 L/minute. Her Bear-2 settings are currently as follows: VT 700 mL, f 8/minute. Her $Paco_2$ has increased from 45 mm Hg in the last hour to the latest level of 55 mm Hg.

7. Assuming that the tidal volume cannot be manipulated further, how can the rate be manipulated to increase the minute ventilation to 7 L/minute?
   A. decrease the rate to 6/minute
   B. increase the rate to 10/minute
   C. increase the rate to 12/minute
   D. increase the rate to 14/minute
8. If Mary was placed on PEEP, the level of PEEP could be monitored by the nurse in which manner?
   A. the PIP should increase by 10 cm H_2O during inspiration
   B. the PIP should decrease by 10 cm H_2O during inspiration
   C. the airway pressure manometer needle should fall only to 10 cm H_2O during expiration
   D. the airway pressure manometer should fall to negative 10 cm H_2O during expiration

Mary has improved, and weaning from the ventilator has begun. The decision is made to place Mary on synchronous intermittent mandatory ventilation (SIMV) of 12/minute with pressure support of 10 cm H_2O.

9. Pressure support ventilation is used for which of the following reasons?
   A. it makes inspiration easier
   B. it makes expiration easier
   C. it keeps alveoli open through the breathing cycle
   D. it increases PIP during inspiration

10. Mary's PIP has increased steadily for the past 3 hours. This trend may indicate
    A. increased lung compliance
    B. decreased airway resistance
    C. decreased lung compliance
    D. increased lung ventilatory capacity
11. Mary's low exhaled volume alarm keeps triggering. The problem is not found immediately. The nurse should
    A. call the physician
    B. manually ventilate
    C. check connections again
    D. put more air in the tracheal cuff
12. When Mary was on PEEP, the nurse would expect which of the following trends secondary to changes in cardiac output?
    A. decreased blood pressure, increased pulse
    B. increased blood pressure, increased pulse
    C. decreased blood pressure, decreased pulse
    D. increased blood pressure, decreased pulse
13. If Mary developed a right lower lobe (RLL) pneumonia while receiving mechanical ventilation, how would airflow be affected?
    A. ventilation would not be effected
    B. ventilation to RLL would increase
    C. ventilation to all right lung fields would decrease
    D. ventilation to RLL would decrease
14. Mary's urine output before mechanical ventilation was approximately 100 mL/hour over a 24-hour period. Once mechanical ventilation was initiated, the nurse should expect which trend for urine output?
    A. decrease
    B. increase slightly
    C. increase significantly
    D. remain approximately the same
15. While Mary is on the mechanical ventilator, the nurse will need to monitor her closely for development of a stress ulcer related to
    A. visceral tissue ischemia
    B. increased visceral blood flow
    C. increased visceral venous return
    D. decreased visceral vascular resistance
16. The nurse will need to monitor Mary for development of a nosocomial pulmonary infection. Assessments that would support this problem include
    A. sputum is green
    B. lung sounds are clear
    C. large quantity of sputum
    D. increased serum white blood cell count
17. To prevent complications associated with endotracheal trauma, the nurse should maintain the cuff pressure within what range?
    A. 10–15 mm Hg
    B. 15–20 mm Hg
    C. 20–25 mm Hg
    D. 25–30 mm Hg

Posttest Answers

Question	Answer	Section	Question	Answer	Section
1	C	One	10	C	Five
2	B	Two	11	B	Five
3	D	Two	12	A	Five
4	B	Three	13	D	Six
5	A	Four	14	A	Six
6	D	Five	15	A	Six
7	B	Five	16	A	Seven
8	C	Five	17	C	Eight
9	A	Five			

REFERENCES

Burton, G.C., and Hodgkins, J.E. (1984). *Respiratory care: A guide to clinical practice*, 2nd ed. Philadelphia: J.B. Lippincott Co.

Blaufuss, J.A., and Wallace, C.J. (1987). Negative pressure ventilation. *Crit. Care Nursing.* 9:14–30.

Hudak, C.M., Gallo, B.M., and Benz, J.J. (1990). *Critical care nursing: A holistic approach*. Philadelphia: J.B. Lippincott Co.

Kersten, L. (1989). *Comprehensive respiratory nursing: A decision making approach.* Philadelphia: W.B. Saunders Co.

Luce, J.M., Tyler, M.L., and Pierson, D.J. (1984). *Intensive respiratory care.* Philadelphia: W.B. Saunders Co.

Martin, L. (1987). *Pulmonary physiology in clinical practice: The essentials for patient care and evaluation.* St. Louis: C.V. Mosby Co.

Pilbeam, S.P. (1986). *Mechanical ventilation: Physiological and clinical applications.* St. Louis: C.V. Mosby/Multi-Media Publishing.

Shapiro, B., Cane, R., and Harrison, R. (1983). Positive end-expiratory pressure in acute lung disease. *Chest.* 83:558–563.

Shapiro, B.A., Kacmarek, R.M., Cane, R.D., Peruzzi, W.T., and Hauptman, D. (1991). *Clinical application of respiratory care,* 4th ed. St. Louis: Mosby Year Book.

Siegel, J.H., Stoklosa, J.C., Borg, U., et al. (1985). Quantification of asymmetric lung pathophysiology as a guide to the use of simultaneous independent lung ventilation in posttraumatic and septic adult respiratory distress syndrome. *Ann. Surg.* 202:425–438.

Smith, S. (1988). High-frequency ventilation in the treatment of idiopathic pulmonary fibrosis complicating ARDS: A nursing challenge. *Crit. Care Nurse Q.* 11:29–35.

ADDITIONAL READING

Barnes, T.A. (1988). *Respiratory care practice.* Chicago: Year Book Medical Publishers.

Vasbinder-Dillon, D. (1988). Understanding mechanical ventilation. *Crit. Care Nursing* 8:42–56.

Nursing Care of the Patient with Altered Respiratory Function

Kathleen Dorman Wagner

The module, *Nursing Care of the Patient with Altered Respiratory Function,* is designed to integrate the major points discussed in the modules, *Respiratory Process, Gas Exchange and Blood Gas Analysis,* and *Mechanical Ventilation.* This module summarizes relationships between key concepts and assists the learner in clustering information to facilitate clinical application. The module is divided into three parts. The first part discusses assessment data frequently used in deriving appropriate nursing diagnoses for a patient with a respiratory problem. The second part

is divided into two sections. It applies the content in an interactive learning style. Using a case study format, the learner is encouraged to identify nursing actions based on the assessment of a patient with a restrictive pulmonary disease in Section One and a patient with an obstructive pulmonary disease in Section Two. Consequences of selecting a particular action are discussed. Rationale for all answers is presented. The last part presents the nursing management of a patient requiring mechanical ventilation. The module ends with a brief summary of its major points.

Objectives

At the completion of the module, *Nursing Care of Patients with Altered Respiratory Function,* the learner will be able to

1. Describe an appropriate database for a patient with a pulmonary disorder

2. Explain the assessment of the patient with a restrictive pulmonary disorder

3. Discuss development of nursing diagnoses appropriate to patients with restrictive pulmonary disorders

4. Explain the development of a plan of care for the patient with a restrictive pulmonary disorder

5. Describe the assessment of the patient with an obstructive pulmonary disorder

6. Discuss development of nursing diagnoses appropriate to patients with obstructive pulmonary disorders

7. Explain the development of the plan of care for the patient with an obstructive pulmonary disorder

8. Describe the nursing management of the physiologic needs of the patient requiring mechanical ventilation

9. Discuss the nursing management of the psychosocial needs of the patient requiring mechanical ventilation

10. Explain weaning of the patient from the mechanical ventilator

Glossary

Accessory muscles. Muscles not normally used during quiet breathing that are available for assisting either inspiration or expiration during times of increased work of breathing

Albumin. A simple nonmuscle protein primarily found in blood plasma

Assist/control mode. A mechanical ventilation mode that combines two single modes: assist, a patient-sensitive mode, and control, a time-triggered mode; considered a supportive breathing mode

Chronic obstructive pulmonary disease (COPD). A group of pulmonary diseases that cause obstruction to expiratory airflow

Circumoral. The area around the mouth, as in circumoral cyanosis

Cor pulmonale. Right heart hypertrophy and enlargement secondary to pulmonary disease

Crackles (rales). Adventitious breath sound associated with fluid or secretions or both in small airways or alveoli

Dyspnea. Difficulty breathing

Emphysema. A chronic obstructive pulmonary disease (COPD); a destructive pulmonary process characterized by enlargement of alveoli and destruction of lung tissue

Extubation. Removal of an endotracheal or tracheostomy tube from the patient's airway

Hemoptysis. Blood secretions from the lower airway

Hypokalemia. Serum potassium level that is below normal

Intermittent mandatory ventilation (IMV). A mechanical ventilator mode that allows the patient to breathe spontaneously through ventilator circuitry while interspersing mandatory mechanical breaths at even intervals via a preset rate; generally considered a weaning mode

Intubation. Placement of an endotracheal or tracheostomy tube into the patient's airway

Mucociliary escalator. The body's natural mechanism of clearing the airway of unwanted foreign matter and secretions through use of mucus and ciliated epithelium

NANDA. North American Nursing Diagnosis Association

Negative inspiratory force (NIF). The amount of negative pressure a person can exert

Pa_{CO_2}. The partial pressure of carbon dioxide as it exists in the arterial blood

Pa_{O_2}. The partial pressure of oxygen as it exists in the arterial blood

Parenchyma. The body of an organ; organ tissue

Parietal pleura. The moist membrane that adheres to the thoracic walls, diaphragm, and mediastinum

Paroxysmal nocturnal dyspena (PND). A form of transient mild pulmonary edema that occurs at night; it is associated with cardiac disease

Pleurisy (pleuritis). Pain caused by inflammation of the parietal pleura

Positive end-expiratory pressure (PEEP). An expiratory support device that requires a mechanical ventilator; PEEP maintains above ambient alveolar pressures at end-expiration, enhancing diffusion and recruiting collapsed alveoli

Respiratory insufficiency. A state of pulmonary compensation in which normal blood gases are maintained only at the expense of the cardiopulmonary system

Restrictive disease. Pulmonary disorders associated with a decrease in lung volumes

Synchronous intermittent mandatory ventilation (SIMV). A form of intermittent mandatory ventilation (IMV) mode in which the mandatory breaths are synchronized to the patient's own during inspiration

Tidal volume. The volume of air moved in and out of the lungs during normal breathing

Ventilatory failure. A condition caused by alveolar hypoventilation; clinically it is called acute respiratory acidosis

Visceral pleura. The moist membrane that adheres to the lung parenchyma and is adjacent to the parietal pleura

Weaning. The process by which a patient becomes independent of mechanical ventilator assistance

Wheeze. Adventitious breath sound caused by air passing through constricted airways

RESPIRATORY ASSESSMENT

Nursing History

When a patient is admitted to the hospital in acute distress, the nurse initially assesses airway, breathing, and circulation (ABCs) and immediately takes appropriate action based on those assessments. As soon as is feasible, information regarding the immediate events leading to admission should be obtained. A recent history gives important clues as to the etiology and chain of events related to the current problem.

The presence of severe respiratory distress limits the amount of health history information a patient is able to relate. Minimize questions directed to the patient to reduce the stress on breathing, stating all inquires in such a way that they require very brief answers.

Historical data of particular importance to assess in the patient with pulmonary problems include the following.

Social History

Assess tobacco and alcohol use. Tobacco use is associated with many pulmonary diseases, and current use may aggravate further acute pulmonary problems. Alcohol use in association with prescribed drug therapy may adversely affect the patient's respiratory condition. Problems with alcohol withdrawal can complicate the cardiopulmonary status should delirium tremens develop.

Nutritional History

The nutritional state of a pulmonary patient is crucial to assess because malnutrition is contributory to the development of respiratory failure. There are several ways in which this can happen. First, a protein–calorie deficit weakens muscles, including the respiratory muscles. Second, malnutrition is associated with a weakened immune system, which increases susceptibility to infection and makes it harder to fight against existing infections. The increased stress associated with an acute infection can precipitate acute respiratory failure. Third, a high-carbohydrate diet increases the overall carbon dioxide load in the body. This may lead to ventilatory complications in certain patients (Farzan, 1985).

Cardiopulmonary History

The lungs, heart, and blood vessels comprise a common circuit. For this reason, factors that alter any part of the circuit can cause a subsequent alteration in other parts. It is often difficult to differentiate a problem of pulmonary or cardiovascular etiology. Because of this, obtaining sufficient data regarding the cardiovascular system will be invaluable in planning the management of the patient. Of particular importance is to collect data concerning preexisting cardiovascular or pulmonary problems and prehospitalization activity tolerance levels.

Elimination History

Urinary elimination is not directly affected by pulmonary function. It can, however, be indirectly affected when the patient experiences a severe hypoxic episode. If the kidneys sustain an acute hypoperfusion/hypoxic episode, acute tubular necrosis and acute renal failure could result.

Bowel elimination can negatively affect pulmonary status when constipation occurs. A full, extended bowel can push abdominal contents against the diaphragm, restricting expansion of the lungs. Oxygen consumption also can be increased when the patient strains to evacuate a hard stool, further compromising oxygen levels in patients with marginal or poor arterial blood gases. Patients with pulmonary disorders often experience constipation related to decreased activity levels and decreased intake of fluids and appropriate foods.

Sleep–Rest History

Pulmonary problems frequently interfere with sleep and rest. There are a variety of reasons for this. If the respiratory problem is severe enough to cause hypoxia, the patient often exhibits restlessness associated with inadequate oxygenation of the brain. Pulmonary disorders often increase the work of breathing, which can interfere with rest and sleep. Patients in respiratory distress may sleep poorly because they fear that they will cease to breathe when they are unaware. Others cannot sleep because of their level of general discomfort. Dyspnea and air hunger are very frightening and threatening experiences for pulmonary patients.

Common Complaints Associated with Pulmonary Disorders

If a respiratory problem is suspected, the nurse should focus on eliciting information concerning the most common respiratory complaints: dyspnea, chest pain, cough, sputum, and hemoptysis.

Dyspnea

Dyspnea is a subjective (patient-based) symptom. It refers to the feeling of difficult breathing or shortness of breath. Physiologically, dyspnea is associated with increased work of breathing, a supply and demand imbalance. Increased work of breathing occurs when ventilatory demands go beyond the body's ability to respond. Progressive dyspnea is noted commonly in both restrictive and obstructive pulmonary disorders (Kersten, 1989).

Orthopnea is a type of dyspnea closely associated with cardiac problems or severe pulmonary disease. It refers to a state in which the patient assumes a head-up position to relieve dyspnea. Orthopnea may be mild (the patient may require several pillows to sleep comfortably in bed), or it may be severe (the patient may require sitting upright in a chair or in bed).

One type of dyspnea is of particular interest in differentiating cardiac from pulmonary disorders. Paroxysmal nocturnal dyspnea (PND) is associated with left heart failure. The typical patient report is that of waking during the night, after being asleep for several hours, with a sudden onset of severe dyspnea. On sitting up or getting out of bed, the dyspnea is relieved, and the patient is able to resume sleep. PND is a form of transient, mild pulmonary edema. It is believed that fluids that have been congested in the lower extremities during the day due to gravity drainage shift to the heart and lungs, causing a fluid volume overload when the person becomes horizontal (as in sleep) for several hours.

Chest Pain

The type of chest pain the patient describes can be helpful in differentiating cardiogenic (originating from the heart) from pleuritic (originating from the pleura) pain. Cardiogenic pain generally is described as dull, pressurelike discomfort often radiating to the jaw, back, or left arm. If asked to point to the painful area, the patient often uses the palm of the hand, indicating a somewhat general area. Cardiogenic pain is unaffected by breathing. (Cardiogenic pain is discussed further in Module 9, *Nursing Care of the Patient with Altered Tissue Perfusion*.)

Pleuritic pain frequently is described as sharp and knifelike, and the patient is able to point to the pain focal area with one finger. When the patient is between breaths or the breath is held, pain decreases or ceases. The pain increases with deep breathing. A pleural friction rub may sometimes be auscultated at the focal pain point and can be described as sounding like leather being rubbed together.

Most pulmonary disorders affecting only the lung parenchyma (lung tissue) are not associated with chest pain as an early symptom because the parenchyma is insensitive to pain. For example, lung cancer frequently goes undetected until a routine chest x-ray is taken or the tumor impinges on innervated thoracic structures, causing deep pain. Like lung tissue, the attached visceral pleura is insensitive. The parietal pleura, however, is well innervated, and when inflammation (called pleurisy, pleuritis) occurs, it can trigger the sharp pain as previously described (Figure 4–1).

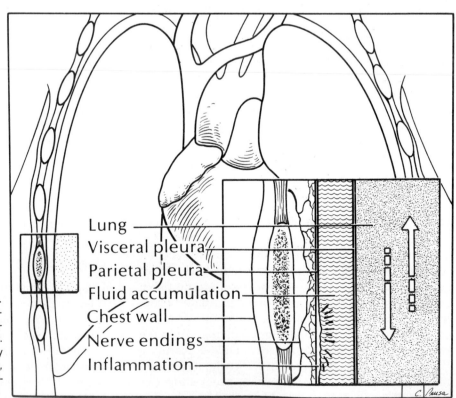

Lung
Visceral pleura
Parietal pleura
Fluid accumulation
Chest wall
Nerve endings
Inflammation

Figure 4–1. The source of pleural pain. When the parietal pleura is irritated and inflamed, the nerve endings located in the parietal pleura send pain signals to the brain. (*From* Clinical manifestations of respiratory disease, 2nd ed., p. 71, by T.R. Des Jardins, 1990, Chicago: Year Book Medical Publisher, Inc.)

Cough

Coughing is an important reflex activity that assists the mucociliary escalator in removing secretions and foreign particles from the lower airway. It is triggered by irritation, the presence of foreign particles, or obstruction of the airway. The patient should be asked to provide the following information about cough: frequency, character, duration, triggers, and pattern of occurrence.

Sputum

A description of sputum production is important to assess in a pulmonary patient. If the patient has a disease that is associated with chronic production of sputum, he or she should be asked to describe the usual quantity, characteristics, and color. It is important to get the patient to describe any changes in sputum associated with the current pulmonary problem.

If a sputum specimen is ordered for laboratory studies, it is best to obtain the specimen in the early morning on awakening because secretions pool during sleep. To assure that the specimen is not composed of upper airway secretions, instruct the patient to take several large breaths and then cough forcefully from the diaphragm. If the patient's cough is weak and nonproductive, deep tracheal suctioning may be necessary, collecting the specimen in a special suction trap device, such as the Luken tube. The sputum specimen should precede initiation of antibiotic therapy.

Hemoptysis

Hemoptysis refers to bloody secretions coughed up from the lower airway. Hemoptysis should be differentiated from blood that is spit out of the mouth from other sources, for example, nose, mouth, or gastrointestinal bleeding. Hemoptysis may result from cardiovascular or pulmonary problems.

Common causes of cardiovascular-related hemoptysis include pulmonary embolism and cardiogenic pulmonary edema secondary to left heart failure. The most common source of hemoptysis, however, is lung disease, particularly as a result of infection and neoplasms. Lung diseases associated with hemoptysis include bronchitis, bronchiectasis, pneumonia, tuberculosis, fungal and parasitic infections, and lung tumors (Farzan, 1985; Dolan, 1991). Information to obtain concerning hemoptysis includes color, consistency and quantity, and frequency and duration.

Components of the Respiratory Assessment

The initial general nursing assessment focuses on all body systems in detail. Once the initial assessment is completed and baseline data are documented, the nurse conducts more specific shift assessments. These frequent bedside assessments often are focused on organ systems (or functional patterns) that have the potential for changing rapidly, indicating a status change in actual or potential patient problems.

Assessing Common Respiratory Symptoms

Regular assessment of the common respiratory symptoms of dyspnea, chest pain, cough, hemoptysis, and sputum are important in monitoring the patient for acute changes in respiratory status.

Dyspnea

Objectively, the nurse may note tachypnea, nasal flaring, use of accessory muscles, or abnormal arterial blood gases. The patient may voluntarily assume a high Fowler sitting position secondary to orthopnea. Severe tachypnea, a respiratory rate of over 30 breaths per minute, significantly increases the work of breathing. If allowed to continue for a prolonged period of time, respiratory muscle fatigue can occur, which may ultimately cause acute respiratory failure.

Chest Pain

Objective data the nurse may note include splinting, shallow respirations, tachypnea, facial changes associated with pain, and increased blood pressure and pulse.

Cough and Sputum

Objectively, the nurse can observe the strength, character, and frequency of the cough. Sputum may consist of a variety of substances, such as mucus, pus, bacteria, or blood. Sputum should be monitored on a regular basis for quantity, characteristics (thin, thick, tenacious), color, and odor. Careful attention to sputum changes should be noted and documented, since they may reflect a change in the patient's pulmonary status. Normal secretions are thin and clear. Sputum color varies depending on the underlying problem (Table 4–1).

TABLE 4–1. SPUTUM COLOR AND CONSISTENCY AND UNDERLYING PROBLEMS

Color and Consistency	Underlying Problem
Yellow-green	Bacterial infection
White, tenacious, mucoid	Acute asthma
Rust colored/blood-tinged	Trauma of coughing, pneumonia, pulmonary infarction
Frothy, pink-tinged	Pulmonary edema

Hemoptysis

When hemoptysis is noted, it should be assessed for color, consistency, and quantity. The frequency and duration also should be noted and documented.

Respiratory Physical Assessment

Vital Signs

Vital signs give important baseline data. They should include at least arterial blood pressure, pulse, respirations, and temperature. They also may include invasive hemodynamic monitoring assessments, such as central venous pressure (CVP), intraarterial pressure, pulmonary artery pressure, and cardiac output. Hemodynamic monitoring generally is initiated when cardiac involvement is suspected or fluid status is questioned. If the patient's condition is purely pulmonary in nature, data collected from hemodynamic monitoring may be of insufficient use to warrant such an invasive procedure. The presence of pulmonary hypertension can alter hemodynamic measurements.

Inspection and Palpation

Skin coloring should be inspected closely for cyanosis. Observe the lips, earlobes, and beneath the tongue for central cyanosis, which may indicate prolonged hypoxia. Cyanosis is not a very reliable indicator of hypoxia, since it is dependent on the amount of reduced hemoglobin present. Its value, therefore, is as supportive rather than diagnostic data. Observe chest movement for symmetry of expansion and the rate, depth, and pattern of breathing. If the patient has sustained chest trauma or has chest tubes in place, the chest should be observed for changes in appearance and palpated for subcutaneous emphysema and areas of tenderness.

Percussion

Percussion is an assessment skill that often is not used on a regular shift-by-shift basis in the acute care setting. It can be used to detect the presence of air, fluid, or consolidation under the area being percussed.

Auscultation

Auscultation is one of the most important pulmonary assessments. The diaphragm of the stethoscope is best for hearing most breath sounds, auscultating in a pattern that allows comparison of one lung to the other. One must first be able to recognize normal breath sounds to be able to recognize and differentiate abnormal sounds.

Normal Breath Sounds. These are divided into three types: vesicular, bronchial (tubular), and bronchovesicular. Table 4–2 differentiates the various normal sounds as summarized from Brunner and Suddarth (1988) and Hudak et al (1990).

Abnormal Breath Sounds. The chest should be auscultated routinely for diminished or absent sounds in any field. The presence of abnormal breath sounds is associated with a change in lung status, such as partial or complete obstruction of a part of the airway by secretions or fluid.

TABLE 4–2. NORMAL BREATH SOUNDS

Breath Sound	Normal Location	Description
Vesicular	Peripheral lung fields	Whispery rustling quality; quiet and low pitched; inspiratory phase is longer than expiratory phase; no distinct pause between inspiration and expiration
Bronchial (tubular)	Over the trachea	High-pitched, loud sound; pause heard between inspiratory and expiratory phases; expiration phase is longer than inspiration (abnormal if heard in peripheral lung; may indicate a consolidation, such as pneumonia)
Bronchovesicular	In all lobes near major airways	Sound is between vesicular and bronchial

Adventitious breath sounds are the lung sounds that are heard on top of other breath sounds. They are never considered normal. Adventitious sounds may be caused by fluid or secretions in the airways or alveoli, by alveoli opening or collapsing, or by bronchoconstriction. Adventitious sounds are classified as crackles, wheeze, and rub. The older terms, rales and rhonchi, have been included in parentheses to clarify where they fit into the newer recommended terminology.

Crackles (previously called rales) are heard as relatively discrete, delicate popping sounds of short duration. They are associated with either fluid or secretions in the small airways or alveoli, or opening of alveoli from a collapsed state. Crackles are heard most commonly during inspiration. Crackles may be described as fine or coarse. Fine crackles are very delicate and high pitched and are of very short duration. Such conditions as atelectasis or pneumonia are associated with fine crackles. Coarse or loud crackles are louder, lower-pitched sounds of longer duration than fine crackles. They are heard in such conditions as bronchitis and pulmonary edema.

Wheeze (previously divided into rhonchi and wheeze) is caused by air passing through constricted airways. The constriction may be caused by bronchospasm, fluid, secretions, edema obstructing the airway, or the presence of an obstructing tumor or foreign body. Wheeze has a musical quality that may be high pitched or low pitched. It may be heard on inspiration or expiration and is of long duration.

Pleural rub is caused by an inflammation of the pleural linings (membranes). When inflammation occurs, the linings become resistant to free movement. The characteristic sound is heard during breathing and has been described as sounding like leather rubbing together or creaking.

Focused Respiratory Assessment

The onset of acute respiratory distress can be rapid and severe. The nurse should be alert to changes from previously assessed baseline data. Rapid respiratory assessment should focus on the following cluster of data that strongly suggest an acute alteration in respiratory function.

- Suddenly increased restlessness and agitation (hypoxia)
- Suddenly decreased responsiveness, increased lethargy (hypercapnia)
- Significant change in pattern of breathing
    Respiratory rate <10 or >30/minute
    Shallow or erratic breathing

- Increased cyanosis or duskiness
- Increased use of accessory muscles
- Increased dyspnea or orthopnea
- Increase in adventitious breath sounds or development of abnormal breath sounds
- Changing trends noted in vital signs (blood pressure, pulse, respirations)
    Increasing trends indicate that compensation is occurring
    Decreasing trends indicate that decompensation is occurring
- Presence of pain

NURSING PROCESS

Section One: Restrictive Disease

CASE STUDY 1. MARY R, A PATIENT WITH RESTRICTIVE DISEASE

You are the nurse assigned to admit Mary R, 38 years old, who is a direct admission from a family practice clinic. No other information is available. You have just been informed that Mary has been brought to the floor and has been assisted into bed.

Initial Appraisal

On walking into her room for the first time, you quickly note the following.
General Appearance. Mary is a black female of small stature. She appears well nourished and tidy in appearance. She is still fully clothed except for her shoes. She is wearing glasses.
Signs of Distress. Mary's respirations are rapid and shallow. She is moving restlessly in the bed. A frequent, harsh cough is heard, and secretions are audible during coughing. Perspiration is noted on Mary's face.
Other. You do not note any intravenous lines or oxygen in use. A man of approximately the same age is in the room with Mary, talking quietly to her. He identifies himself as James, her husband.

Focused Respiratory Assessment

Mary's clothing is exchanged quickly for a hospital gown to make assessment easier and make her more comfortable. Because Mary appears to be in acute respiratory distress, you immediately perform a rapid assessment focusing first on her pulmonary status. The results are as follows.

Mary is restless and oriented to person, place, and time. Her respiratory rate is 32/minute, shallow and regular. Her mucous membranes are dusky. Her respirations are labored. She is using accessory muscles on her neck during inspiration. Crackles and wheezes are auscultated in the right middle and right lower lobes of her lungs. A pleural friction rub is auscultated at the right anterior axillary line, fifth intercostal space. Her current blood pressure is 140/88 (baseline, according to her husband, is 130/76), pulse is 120/minute, and temperature is 102F (orally). She is complaining of increased short-ness of breath that does not improve when the head of the bed is raised. Though her cough is weak, she is expectorating a small amount of thick, green sputum.

After this initial assessment, you call her admitting physician. The physician gives the following stat. phone orders.

- Arterial blood gas (ABG)
- Complete blood cell count (CBC)
- Electrolytes
- Portable chest x-ray
- Sputum for culture and gram stain

QUESTION

Considering Mary's symptoms and assuming that the tests cannot all be performed at the same time, which test should you order to be done first?
1. Electrolytes
2. Portable chest x-ray
3. ABG
4. CBC

ANSWER

3 is correct. Since Mary appears to be in acute respiratory distress, priority tests would be, first, the ABG, which is a rapid, accurate method of measuring oxygenation and acid-base status. *Discussion of incorrect options:* The second priority is the chest x-ray, a rapidly performed diagnostic test that helps locate and differentiate the pulmonary problem. The CBC and electrolytes, although important, do not have a direct impact on Mary's respiratory status. The sputum specimen should be obtained as soon as possible. Results of the culture will not be available for several days.

Stat. Test Results
Arterial blood gases (on room air)
pH = 7.37, $Paco_2$ = 42 mm Hg, Pao_2 = 68 mm Hg, HCO_3 = 26 mEq/L, Sao_2 = 78%
CBC (Normal ranges from Jennings, 1991, and Stark, 1991.)

WBC = 15,000   (Normal range 3500–11,000/μL)
RBC = 4.8   (Normal range 3.8–5.2 × 10^6/μL in females)
Hg = 14   (Normal range 11.7–15.7 g/dL in females)
Hct = 42%   (Normal range 34.9–46.9% in females)

Electrolytes (Normal ranges are from Jennings, 1991, and Stark, 1991.)

Sodium (Na) = 142   (Normal range 136–145 mEq/L)
Potassium (K) = 4.5   (Normal range 3.5–5.5 mEq/L)
Chloride (Cl) = 104   (Normal range 96–106 mEq/L)
Calcium (Ca) = 9.2   (Normal range 8.5–10.5 mg/dL)

Portable chest x-ray results
    Right middle lobe (RML) and right lower lobe (RLL) infiltrates are consistent with pneumonia
Sputum for culture and gram stain
    Results pending on culture
    Gram stain: gram-positive clustered cocci

QUESTION

Which of the following statements is true regarding the laboratory or x-ray data?
1. The ABG shows evidence of acid-base balance with mild hypoxemia
2. The electrolytes show evidence of possible overhydration
3. The CBC does not show evidence of an infectious process
4. The gram stain is consistent with a viral infection

ANSWER

1 is correct. The ABG shows acid-base balance with mild hypoxemia. *Discussion of incorrect options:* The electrolytes show evidence of possible dehydration in high normal sodium and chloride levels. The increased white blood cell count on the CBC is consistent with the presence of an infectious process. The high normal hematocrit may suggest dehydration when considered with the high normal sodium and chloride levels. The chest x-ray confirms pneumonia as a diagnosis. The presence of gram-positive clustered cocci in the sputum gram stain is consistent with staphylococci. The gram stain helps differentiate the causative agent before confirmation by the sputum culture results, which take several days.

The results of the ABG are called to the physician immediately, and oxygen is initiated at 4 L/minute per nasal cannula. The physician states that she will be at the hospital to see Mary shortly.

Focused Nursing History

Since Mary is in too much distress to be interviewed directly, you decide to talk with her husband to obtain the most important critical historical data that may have an impact on Mary's present situation. The complete nursing database will be completed within the first 24 hours postadmission. Her husband gives the following history.

Mary began exhibiting common cold symptoms approximately 10 days ago. About 4 days ago, Mary's fever began to increase, accompanied by severe chilling. Her cough became productive, with green sputum. The cough has prevented Mary from sleeping very much for the past several nights. She has been complaining of a pattern of increasingly severe shortness of breath. Mary is not currently taking any prescription drugs. She has been taking several over-the-counter medications to relieve her symptoms: a nonnarcotic cough preparation and acetaminophen. For the past several days, she has been complaining of a transient sharp pain in her lower right chest that increases with breathing. Mary is allergic to penicillin. She has a 20-year history of smoking 1/2 to 1 pack of cigarettes per day but has not been able to smoke for several days because of shortness of breath. She rarely drinks any alcoholic beverages.

Systematic Bedside Assessment

Before the physician's arrival, you initiate a head-to-toe assessment.

Head and Neck. Mary's overall skin coloring is difficult to assess because it is dark. Therefore, her mucous membranes are assessed, and they are dusky in color. Mary continues to be completely oriented but remains restless. Slight nasal flaring is noted. She has nasal cannula oxygen delivering 4 L/minute. She does not have jugular vein distention. No other abnormalities of the head or neck are noted.

Chest. Pulmonary status is as previously noted in the Focused Respiratory Assessment.

Cardiac status is as follows. Pulmonary adventitious sounds make it somewhat difficult to clearly discriminate sounds. S_1 and S_2 and no murmur are auscultated. Sounds are regular, with a rate of 122/minute.

Abdomen. The abdomen is flat. Positive bowel sounds are auscultated in all quadrants. Mary denies any abdominal tenderness. It is soft to palpation.

Pelvis. Mary voided 125 mL of clear, dark amber urine, with a specific gravity of 1.030.

Extremities. There is poor skin turgor. The skin is hot and diaphoretic. No peripheral edema is noted. The nailbeds are difficult to assess due to dark pigmentation. Peripheral pulses are palpable in all four distal extremities.

Posterior. No skin breakdown is noted, and there is no sacral edema. Posterior breath sounds are crackles and wheezes present on the right side to midlung field.

Development of Nursing Diagnoses

Clustering Data. You have just completed your head-to-toe assessment and are now ready to develop a problem list based on the subjective and objective data that you have collected thus far. To cluster your data, you look for abnormalities found during the assessment. Mary's major symptom at this particular time is her labored, rapid, shallow respirations. Thus, these primary symptoms can initiate your first cluster of critical cues (abnormal data that help define a problem). (Carpenito, 1987; Kersten, 1989).

CLUSTER 1 (from previous history and physical assessment data).

Subjective data: Patient complaining of dyspnea unaffected by position changes. Cold symptoms for 10 days. Increasing pattern of shortness of breath that does not seem to be affected by changing height of head of the bed. Cough with green sputum is noted. Chills and fever that have worsened over several days. Is complaining of a transient sharp pain in her lower right chest that increases with breathing. Has had difficulty sleeping due to frequent coughing.

Objective data: Labored, shallow respirations. Respiratory rate is 28/minute. Accessory muscles are in use. Crackles and wheezes heard in RML and RLL in anterior fields and to midchest in posterior right field. Pleural friction rub is auscultated at right anterior axillary line, fifth intercostal space. ABG shows that mild hypoxemia is present. Chest x-ray indicates an RML/RLL infiltrate. Gram stain shows gram-positive clustered cocci. Her cough is weak. Secretions, which are very thick and green, are difficult for her to expectorate. Fever and chills are present.

QUESTION

Based on these data, which of the following nursing diagnoses would you select as being appropriate in planning Mary's care?
1. Impaired gas exchange
2. Ineffective airway clearance
3. Ineffective breathing pattern
4. All of the above

ANSWER

4 is correct. Mary's pulmonary problem is a complex one that requires a wide variety of medical and nursing interventions. NANDA has approved all three of the three presented pulmonary-related nursing diagnoses as individual diagnoses. However, because complex patients, such as Mary, often have all three of the pulmonary-related nursing diagnoses, Carpenito (1987) offers an alternative that joins all three NANDA diagnoses, **Alteration in respiratory function**

- **Ineffective breathing pattern:** hypoventilation related to weakness, pleural pain, fatigue
- **Impaired gas exchange** related to alveolar consolidation, pooling of secretions
- **Ineffective airway clearance** related to thick secretions associated with pulmonary infection and dehydration, pleural pain, ineffective cough

The use of the **Alteration in respiratory function** option may be useful in facilities that do not require strict adherence to the NANDA-approved diagnoses.

Expected patient outcomes (evaluative criteria) for Mary would include

1. Normal respiratory rate, depth, and rhythm
2. Improved or clear breath sounds
3. No dyspnea
4. Usual mental status
5. Mucous membranes are usual color
6. ABGs within normal limits for patient (Ulrich et al 1986)

For the purposes of Mary's case study, only the pulmonary related nursing diagnoses are developed further. However, in a true clinical situation, as the nurse creating Mary's plan of care, you would continue to develop other clusters based on primary critical cues and supporting cues from the data already collected. If data is insufficient, you should follow through on collecting the necessary data to confirm or refute your hypotheses.

Based on the preliminary data collected on Mary, there is sufficient support to state the following nursing diagnoses.

- **Alteration in comfort:** pleural pain
- **Alteration in fluid volume:** deficit
- **Self-care deficit**
- **Sleep pattern disturbance**
- **Potential injury:** physiologic related to development of complications
  1. Delayed resolution of pneumonia
  2. Superinfection
  3. Exudative pleural effusion
  4. Atelectasis
  5. Acute respiratory failure (Ulrich et al, 1986)

Developing the Plan of Care

Mary's pneumonia is a restrictive pulmonary disease process. She has many signs and symptoms consistent with restrictive diseases. Table 4–3 presents common signs and symptoms of restrictive diseases as summarized from Kersten (1989).

Treatment goals based on the restrictive nature of her disease include (1) optimizing her oxygenation status, (2) promoting airway clearance, and (3) maintaining functional alveoli. These general goals are reflected in the nursing diagnoses and expected patient outcomes (EPOs) on the nursing care plan. For example, optimizing oxygenation status is addressed in the nursing diagnoses, impaired gas exchange and ineffective airway clearance. Accomplish-

TABLE 4–3. SIGNS AND SYMPTOMS OF RESTRICTIVE DISEASE

Increased respiratory rate
Decreased tidal volume
Normal to decreased Pao_2
Shortness of breath
Cough
Chest pain or discomfort
Fatigue
History of weight loss

ment of the goal is measured in such criteria as ABG within normal limits for patient, usual skin color, usual mental status, and improved lung sounds.

Nursing interventions are based on activities to help Mary meet her EPOs. They consist of collaborative interventions, which are activities ordered by the physician but require some actions by the nurse, and independent interventions, activities that are within the nursing scope of practice to write and carry out as nursing orders.

Collaborative Interventions Related to Pulmonary Status. The physician's orders may include the following.

1. *Pulmonary drug therapy.* Mary will be receiving several drugs while hospitalized. Oxygen therapy has been ordered to treat Mary's mild hypoxemia. The minimal goal of oxygen therapy is to increase the Pao_2 to at least 60 mm Hg. Other types of drug therapy that probably will be ordered for Mary include antibiotics for treatment of pneumonia and analgesics for treatment of pleuritic pain. She may not receive a cough suppressant in this stage of her pneumonia because a productive cough is a protective reflex to help rid the lungs of unwanted secretions. If necessary, she also may receive drug therapy through hand-held nebulization or metered dose inhaler. Drugs that commonly are inhaled include bronchodilators and steroids.
2. *Laboratory and x-ray testing.* These may be ordered intermittently. Of particular interest will be the ABG, CBC, and chest x-ray to follow progress of the therapeutic plan.
3. *Percussion and postural drainage.* P and PD may be ordered to facilitate airway clearance. In many hospitals, this is

performed by respiratory therapy. P and PD also can be done by the nurse if she is properly trained as ordered by the physician, or it may be an independent nursing action, depending on hospital policy.

4. *Intravenous fluids.* These may be ordered to promote hydration, which is crucial in loosening secretions for improved airway clearance. An IV access site also is necessary for IV antibiotic therapy, if ordered.

Independent Nursing Interventions

1. Assess for decreased respiratory function (report abnormal)
   - Respirations <8/minute or >30/minute
   - Increasingly shallow, labored breathing
   - Increasing dyspnea or central cyanosis
   - Change in mental status
     Increased restlessness
     Increased lethargy
   - Increasingly abnormal ABGs
   - Increasingly abnormal breath sounds, adventitious sounds
   - Change in sputum
   - Accessory muscle use
2. Turn every 2 hours
3. Cough and deep breathe every 1 to 2 hours
4. Incentive spirometry every 1 to 2 hours
5. Encourage fluids to 2 to $2\frac{1}{2}$ L/24 hours or 600 to 800 ml/8 hour shift
6. Tracheal suction if needed
7. Position of comfort, with head of bed elevated >30 degrees
8. Monitor effects of drug therapy
9. Monitor test results (report abnormal)
10. Instruct patient or family about condition, procedures, medications, treatment
11. Encourage self-care as tolerated

Plan Evaluation and Revision

Mary's pulmonary plan of care is now developed and ready to execute. Her progress is monitored at regular intervals to evaluate the effects of the various therapeutic actions. If progress is not being noted toward attainment of Mary's various expected patient outcomes, her plan may need revisions, examining alternative interventions that may be more effective.

Mary's plan of care is effective, and she responds rapidly to her antibiotic therapy and her pulmonary hygiene program. Because she does not have underlying pulmonary disease, her recovery is uncomplicated. Before discharge, she will need to receive teaching concerning continuing her antibiotic therapy as prescribed, increasing her activities slowly at home, smoking cessation, and pulmonary hygiene.

Section Two: Obstructive Pulmonary Disease

——— CASE STUDY 2. PETER M, A PATIENT WITH OBSTRUCTIVE PULMONARY DISEASE ———

You are a registered nurse working on a general surgical floor in a 300-bed community hospital. You have, as part of your assignment, Mr. Peter M, a 68-year-old status post-transurethral resection (TUR) of 3 days. You have just heard the shift report, in which you received the following information about Peter.

At 2:00 PM, vital signs are BP 150/90 (baseline is 130/84), pulse 100/minute and slightly irregular, rate 38/minute, temperature 98.6F (oral). He has 2 L of oxygen ordered per nasal cannula. His lungs sound a little more congested, and breathing seems more labored. He has been on bedrest since surgery. He has a history of emphysema. His post-TUR status is stable. His urinary status has been uneventful since surgery. Urine is clear, and a 3-way Foley catheter is in place. It will probably be discontinued today. His appetite has been poor. He has an IV of 5% dextrose in 0.45% normal saline in a right peripheral line. The nurse reporting off suggests that you watch Peter closely this evening, stating that he seems weaker today. He has been fully alert and awake throughout the day. The nurse also reports that Peter has gained 4 pounds over the past several days.

Significant History

Peter is a retired teacher. He has a smoking history of $1\frac{1}{2}$ to 2 packs per day for over 40 years. He currently smokes, although he states that he has reduced his smoking to about $\frac{1}{2}$ packs per day for the past 2 years. He was diagnosed with pulmonary emphysema approximately 10 years ago and congestive heart failure approximately 2 years ago. He states that he drinks an occasional glass of beer or wine but not on a regular basis. He has a prescribed low sodium diet that his wife cooks for him. Over the past year, he has had increasing difficulty passing urine. Tests showed benign prostatic hypertrophy. His TUR was an elective procedure. He has no known allergies. His appetite has been poor for the past several days due to complaints of nausea, though he has not been vomiting. His medications taken at home include theophylline (Theodur), digoxin, oxygen, furosemide (Lasix), and prednisone. He indicates that he has a hard time keeping up with all his medications and forgets some of them at times. He has been maintained on these medications during hospitalization. He usually sleeps, using two large pillows to help him breathe better. He is able to attend to his own needs at home but becomes increasingly short of breath with climbing the 15 steps to the second story of his home to go to his bedroom.

Initial Appraisal

It is now 3:30 PM, and you are making your patient rounds with initial appraisals. On approaching Peter's bed, you note the following.

General Appearance. Peter M is an elderly Caucasian male. He is barrel chested and poorly nourished in appearance, with little body fat noted. He is in bed sitting upright, leaning forward with his arms stretched out to his knees.

Signs of Distress. Respirations are rapid, with a prolonged expiratory phase. His breathing is noisy, with an expiratory wheeze heard while you are standing at the foot of the bed. You note pulling of his neck muscles during inspiration. Coloring appears dusky.

Other. There is approximately 50 mL of urine in his Foley bag. You note a 3-way Foley catheter in place. Urine is clear and yellow. A bladder irrigant bag is hanging but is not running. The IV fluid is infusing at the correct rate. He has oxygen running at 2 L/minute per nasal cannula. He is oriented to his name and the year but cannot tell you where he is. No one else is in the room with him.

Focused Respiratory Assessment

Because your initial appraisal of Peter included abnormal assessments that are overtly respiratory, you rapidly focus in on a more complete respiratory assessment. You do this, however, with the understanding that pulmonary signs and symptoms can be of pulmonary or cardiac origin. Your assessment is as follows.

His vital signs currently are respiratory rate 32/minute and labored. Pulse 115/minute; S_1 and S_2 are present though the sounds are hard to distinguish because of his loud adventitious breath sounds. BP is 156/92. You auscultate loud coarse rhonchi on both inspiration and expiration, and expiratory wheeze is heard bilaterally. Breath sounds can be heard distantly in apices but are progressively diminished from mid to low lung fields bilaterally. He has a full rolling cough, but he is unable to clear the secretions from his lungs. His bedside chart shows an intake > output balance of 1500 mL over the past 24 hours.

Following respiratory data collection and based on Peter's history, you decide that his signs and symptoms may not be completely of pulmonary origin. You, therefore, quickly assess his cardiovascular status.

Cardiovascular Status. You note positive jugular vein distention. Peter has 3+ pitting edema of his lower legs. You cannot distinguish heart sounds sufficiently to assess for S_3 and S_4 reliably. His current urine output is 50 mL in a 2-hour period. Breath sounds are too diminished to clearly assess for presence of crackles in the bases.

Following your focused assessment, you call your report to the physician, who orders the following stat. orders.

- Portable chest x-ray
- ABG
- Furosemide 40 mg IV now
- Aminophylline drip at 35 mg/hour
- Serum electrolytes
- Digoxin and theophylline levels
- ECG

QUESTION

Considering Peter's present condition and assuming that the orders cannot all be carried out at the same time, which stat. physician order should you do first?
1. IV furosemide
2. ABG

3. Digoxin and theophylline levels
4. Chest x-ray

ANSWER

2 is correct. Obtaining the ABG first is a rapid and accurate method of measuring his oxygenation and acid-base status. *Discussion of incorrect options:* The IV furosemide would be next in priority to help relieve fluid volume excess problems. The nurse should be aware, however, that Peter has been on long-standing Digoxin therapy. It will be very important to check his electrolyte level at the earliest opportunity for possible hypokalemia problems, particularly since he is receiving furosemide, a potent loop diuretic that is very potassium depleting. Low serum potassium associated with Digoxin therapy can precipitate Digoxin toxicity. The portable chest x-ray and ECG also can be ordered rapidly, but there often is a delay before these procedures are actually performed.

Stat. Test Results
Portable chest x-ray
Right heart enlargement consistent with cor pulmonale. Hyperlucency is present, with flattening of the diaphragm. Increased anteroposterior (A/P) diameter is present. Bullous lesions are noted.
Arterial blood gases
pH = 7.32, $Paco_2$ = 75 mm Hg, Pao_2 = 70 mm Hg, HCO_3 = 36 mEq/L, Sao_2 = 84%
Electrolytes
    Na = 138 mEq/L, K = 4.0 mEq/L, Cl = 102 mEq/L, Ca = 9.2 mg/dL

Digoxin level
    0.22 ng/mL (Normal range 0.8–1.8 ng/mL)
Theophylline level
    15 μg/mL (Toxic level >20 μg/mL)
ECG
Right ventricular leads show changes consistent with cor pulmonale. Changes also are noted consistent with digitalis effects. Unifocal premature ventricular contractions are present.

QUESTION

Which of the following statements is correct regarding the significance of laboratory and other test data?
1. The ABG shows metabolic acidosis with mild hypoxemia
2. The electrolytes are all within acceptable limits
3. The chest x-ray finding of cor pulmonale is an uncommon finding in COPD
4. The premature ventricular contractions are of concern because of the patient's digoxin level

ANSWER

2 is correct. Peter's electrolytes levels are not significant at this time. However, they continue to be monitored carefully while he is receiving diuretics because of the potential for electrolyte depletion complications. *Discussion of incorrect options:* His portable chest x-ray showed evidence of cor pulmonale, right heart enlargement, and hypertrophy of pulmonary etiology. It is associated frequently with some degree of right heart failure. The lung fields are consistent with emphysematous changes. His ABG showed acute respiratory acidosis with mild hypoxemia. Patients with chronic obstructive diseases frequently undergo progressive ABG alterations. Normal ABG values are relative numbers in

patients with COPD. Over time, $Paco_2$ increases due to the progressive pulmonary dysfunction that interferes with elimination of carbon dioxide from the body. The body is very intolerant to changes in pH. Therefore, as $Paco_2$ progressively increases, bicarbonate (HCO_3) is increasingly retained by the kidneys to maintain the pH within physiologically acceptable limits.

If Peter has very severe emphysema, he may breathe normally on a hypoxic drive. He, like many COPD patients, may be tolerant of relatively low Pao_2 levels and high $Paco_2$ levels. His current pH is below the normal range, however, which tells you that at this time, he for some reason has moved from a state of chronic insufficiency to acute respiratory failure. (For review, see Modules on *Respiratory Process* and *Gas Exchange and Blood Gas Analysis*.)

Peter's digoxin level is toxic. This is not uncommon in older patients receiving chronic digoxin therapy. Digoxin toxicity is potentially dangerous. As the nurse, you would hold the drug and inform the physician of the test results. Digoxin generally is held until levels return to therapeutic levels. His theophylline level is within the therapeutic range at this time. Patients on chronic theophylline therapy often become toxic, however, developing symptoms of nausea and vomiting, increased heart rate, dysrhythmias, insomnia, headache, and increased irritability (McKenry and Salerno, 1989).

Peter's ECG shows evidence of his chronic drug therapy and his cor pulmonale. The presence of premature ventricular contractions is significant because of his Digoxin toxic state, which can precipitate many arrhythmias and conduction problems.

Systematic Bedside Assessment

Once you have completed the various stat. activities on Peter, you begin your head-to-toe assessment.

Head and Neck. Circumoral and earlobe duskiness is noted. Oxygen is in place at 2 L/minute. Responsiveness level: He is oriented to name and month but not to place, although he has been reminded recently. His speech is breathless, and he is able to talk in one to two word phrases only. Purse-lipped breathing is noted. Positive jugular vein distention is noted at 45 degrees.

Chest. The chest is as previously assessed in the pulmonary and cardiac assessment.

Abdomen. His abdomen is distended and tight. He complains of tenderness in his right upper quadrant. Bowel sounds are auscultated in all four quadrants but are hypoactive.

Pelvis. A 3-way Foley catheter is present. He denies pain at this time. Urine output in the bag is 50 mL for a 2-hour period. The urine color is clear and amber. No drainage is noted around the catheter at the meatus.

Extremities. Mild digital clubbing is noted. His nailbeds are dusky, and capillary refill is <3 seconds. His skin is warm and flaky dry. He has a peripheral IV in his right forearm. The site is negative for edema, redness, or heat; 1+ edema is noted in both hands, and 3+ edema is noted in the lower legs. He has positive peripheral pulses. When he is on his feet, you are able to palpate his dorsalis pedis pulses but not his posterior tibial pulses.

Posterior. No skin breakdown is noted at this time, but redness is noted in several areas along the spinous processes of the vertebrae and on the coccyx. Scattered rhonchi are auscultated throughout the posterior fields, and sounds are diminished.

Development of Nursing Diagnoses

Clustering Data. Following your systematic bedside assessment, there are sufficient data to develop nursing diagnoses. The first step is to cluster data based on major abnormal cues.

CLUSTER 1.

Subjective data: Peter has a long history of pulmonary emphysema. He continues to smoke, although he has decreased his intake to 1/2 pack per day. His at-home pulmonary medications include Theo-Dur, oxygen, and prednisone.

Objective data: Peter's respiratory rate is 32/minute and labored. Pursed-lip breathing is noted. He is sitting upright in bed, leaning forward. His expiratory phase is noticeably longer than his inspiratory phase. He is using his accessory muscles to breathe. Loud rhonchi and wheezes are present. A full rolling cough is noted, but he is unable to cough up and expectorate the secretions. His pulse is 115/minute, and blood pressure is 156/92. His theophylline level is within normal limits. His latest ABG showed acute respiratory acidosis with mild hypoxia. He has oxygen per nasal cannula running at 2 L/minute. Circumoral and earlobe duskiness is noted.

QUESTION

Based on these data, which of the following nursing diagnoses would you select as being appropriate in planning Peter's care?
1. **Impaired gas exchange**
2. **Ineffective airway clearance**
3. **Ineffective breathing pattern**
4. All of the above

ANSWER

4 is correct. Peter's critical cues show evidence of all three respiratory relation nursing diagnoses.

- **Ineffective airway clearance** related to excessive secretions, ineffective cough, and pooling of secretions
- **Impaired gas exchange** related to ineffective airway clearance, ineffective breathing pattern, and decrease in functional lung surface area
- **Ineffective breathing pattern** related to anxiety and dysfunction of the muscles of respirations

Expected patient outcomes (evaluative criteria) for Peter would include

1. Normal respiratory rate, depth, and rhythm
2. Decreased dyspnea
3. Usual or improved breath sounds
4. Usual mental status
5. ABGs within normal limits for patient (Ulrich et al, 1986)

If Peter's emphysema is severe, his blood gases may never attain the usual normals. ABG normal values often are altered in patients with chronic obstructive diseases. His acceptable ranges might be

- pH 7.35–7.45 (remains unchanged with disease)
- $Paco_2$ <50 mm Hg (increases with obstructive disease)
- Pao_2 >50 mm Hg (decreases with obstructive disease)
- Sao_2 ≥85% (decreases with obstructive disease)

Peter's age of 68 also influences his acceptable Pao_2 range. It is known that normal aging decreases the number of functioning alveoli. For this reason, Pao_2 has a normal tendency to decrease with age.

CLUSTER 2. Peter's assessment had sufficient evidence to develop a picture consistent with a pulmonary-related problem and a possible cardiovascular problem. Because the pulmonary and cardiovascular systems actually exist as a single cardiopulmonary circuit, the possible cardiovascular problem is briefly explored.

Subjective data: Peter has a 2-year history of congestive heart failure. At-home cardiac-related medications include Digoxin and furosemide. He usually sleeps on two pillows.

Objective data: Jugular vein distention is present, and 3+ edema is noted in his lower legs. His current urine output is 50 mL in a 2-hour period. Chest x-ray shows evidence of cor pulmonale. Digoxin level is >2.0 (toxic). ECG results were consistent with cor pulmonale and showed premature ventricular contractions. He has experienced a 4-pound weight gain over the past several days.

Based on these data, a nursing diagnosis of **Alteration in cardiac output: decreased,** related to ineffective right heart pumping associated with right heart hypertrophy, is noted. Appropriate patient outcomes would need to be decided on and interventions performed to address this problem. This second cluster of data was included to exemplify the common cardiac complications associated with chronic respiratory disease. Nursing management of the patient with cardiovascular problems is addressed in Module 9, *Nursing Care of the Patient with Altered Tissue Perfusion.*

Other nursing diagnoses supported by the existing data include

- **Activity intolerance**
- **Alteration in comfort: nausea**
- **Alteration in nutrition: less than body requirements**
- **Anxiety**
- **Knowledge deficit**
- **Self-care deficit**
- **Potential alteration in skin integrity**

Developing the Plan of Care

Peter's emphysema is an obstructive pulmonary disease. He has many of the signs and symptoms that are typical of obstructive diseases (Table 4–4).

Patients with chronic obstructive pulmonary disease often are admitted to hospitals for reasons unrelated to their pulmonary disorder, such as was the case of Peter with his genitourinary problem. When a patient with COPD is admitted to the hospital for any reason, the health care team must incorporate management of the chronic problem with management of the acute problem if complications are to be avoided.

Many patients with COPD exist in a day-to-day state of chronic respiratory insufficiency; that is, they are able to maintain a relatively normal (balanced supply and demand) acid-base and oxygenation state only at the expense of the other body systems. For example, to compensate, the cardiovascular system increases blood pressure and pulse, the renal system increases retention of bicarbonate, the lungs increase the respiratory rate, and the hematopoietic system increases red blood cell production. This is accomplished through compensatory mechanisms. These mechanisms, however, are finite in their abilities to compensate and vary in the length of time they take to respond to new de-

mands. When a person, like Peter, is placed under an acute physiologic or psychologic stress (i.e., surgery, hospitalization, trauma, acute illness), the sudden increase in physiologic demand may go beyond the ability of the body to supply the necessary oxygen and eliminate the increased carbon dioxide. From the time of hospital admission, Peter was under increased stress and thus was at increased risk for developing some complication.

Overall goals in planning Peter's pulmonary care are consistent with his obstructive pulmonary disease needs and include (1) optimizing ventilation and (2) maintaining adequate oxygenation. A plan using both collaborative and independent interventions will be developed to accomplish these goals.

Collaborative Interventions Related to Peter's Pulmonary Status. The physician's orders may include the following.

1. *Pulmonary drug therapy.* Peter, like many patients with COPD, is on long-term bronchodilator and steroid therapy. Bronchodilators dilate the smooth muscle of the bronchi, decreasing airway obstruction. There are two major groups of bronchodilators, the methyl xanthines (e.g., aminophylline, theophylline) and the sympathomimetic bronchodilators (e.g., isoetharine, albuterol, terbutaline, metaprotenol). His bronchodilators may be administered orally, IV, by hand-held nebulizer, or by metered-dose inhaler. Corticosteroids sometimes are ordered for treatment of restrictive diseases but are used more commonly as treatment of obstructive diseases. This group of drugs reduces inflammation, promotes bronchodilation, and inhibits bronchoconstriction (McKenry and Salerno, 1989). In the presence of acute infection, corticosteroid therapy may be contraindicated because of its immunosuppressant activity. Prolonged use of corticosteroids is associated with many adverse effects, and thus their use is closely weighed in terms of benefits and risks before initiation of long-term therapy. Corticosteroids may be administered orally or by aerosol. Examples of commonly used drugs include prednisone, methylprednisone, and prednisolone (McKenry and Salerno, 1989).

   Oxygen therapy will be ordered carefully. If Peter is a carbon dioxide re-

---

TABLE 4–4. SIGNS AND SYMPTOMS OF OBSTRUCTIVE DISEASE

Increased anterior posterior chest diameter

Increased expiration time

Increased $Paco_2$

Shortness of breath

Cough

Excessive mucoid secretions (emphysema associated with chronic bronchitis)

Malnourished appearance (emphysema)

Activity intolerance

Tripod sitting position (emphysema)

tainer, his respiratory center is driven by a hypoxic drive. Moderate to high oxygen concentrations may turn off his drive to breathe. Peter's oxygen concentration most likely will be maintained at 2 to 3 L/nasal cannula, or 28 percent Venti-Mask. Analgesic therapy may be ordered to control Peter's postsurgical pain. His respiratory status needs to be monitored closely for signs and symptoms of respiratory depression, such as slowing respiratory rate or increasingly shallow respirations. Many analgesics are associated with respiratory depression, increasing the risk of acute ventilatory failure. This is of particular concern in patients with severe pulmonary problems.

3. *Laboratory and x-ray tests.* These may be ordered intermittently if significant clinical changes are noted in Peter's status. They will, most likely, not be ordered on a regular basis. Of particular interest would be ABG, electrolytes, and CBC. A serum albumin may be ordered if the physician is concerned about possible malnutrition.

4. *Pulmonary function tests.* Pulmonary function tests may be ordered if the physician wants to either (1) obtain baseline data concerning Peter's current pulmonary function status or (2) compare his current status with previously documented pulmonary function data.

5. *Diet.* A special diet may be ordered that is low carbohydrate, high protein, and high fat. Patients with chronic respiratory diseases frequently experience a loss of appetite from coughing, shortness of breath, general fatigue, excessive mucous production, and the side effects of drug therapy. Hypoxia, associated with advanced pulmonary disease, decreases the endurance of the respiratory muscles and increases energy consumption due to an increased work of breathing. The combination of anorexia and hypoxia causes the chronic respiratory patient to lose weight. Ultimately, there is a decreased supply associated with an ever increasing demand.

Chronic respiratory patients may need to control carbohydrate intake. Normally, carbohydrates comprise the majority of dietary intake. Carbohydrate me-tabolism causes CO_2 production that is higher than what is produced by fat or protein. A high carbohydrate diet may precipitate acute respiratory failure in the acutely ill respiratory patient because the malnourished state weakens the respiratory muscles, resulting in a decreased tidal volume. A decrease in tidal volume can result in alveolar hypoventilation. The combination of increased carbon dioxide in the alveoli and decreased alveolar ventilation causes increasing $Paco_2$ levels, which ultimately can cause acute respiratory acidosis.

The malnourished respiratory patient has a lower than normal protein level. Protein is vital to proper body function. Serum albumin (normal ≥ 3.5 g/dL) determination is a frequently used laboratory test to measure nonmuscle protein. Albumin is one of the best malnutrition predictors. Approximately 55 percent of plasma in the blood is albumin. A serum albumin level of <2.5 g/dL is considered critically low, decreasing the patient's chance of survival through an acute illness (Dougherty, 1988).

Independent Nursing Interventions. Nursing management of Peter, a patient with obstructive pulmonary disease, is essentially the same as management of the patient with restrictive pulmonary disease (refer to Case Study 1, Independent Nursing Interventions). Emphasis is placed on airway clearance and pulmonary hygiene. His nutritional status needs to be improved and monitored closely. His oxygenation status and therapy will require close assessment for therapeutic and nontherapeutic effects to prevent loss of his hypoxic drive to breathe if he is a CO_2 retainer. Encouraging him to maintain activities, such as getting up into a chair, walking in the room or hall, all help maintain or strengthen activity tolerance and reduce the risk of immobility complications.

Plan Evaluation and Revision

Peter's plan of care should be evaluated at regular intervals. Evaluation will be based on the status of specific expected patient outcomes. If evaluation shows lack of forward progress toward attaining or maintaining goals, the plan needs to be revised, seeking alternatives to care that will be more successful.

PATIENT REQUIRING MECHANICAL VENTILATION

In Case Studies 1 and 2, Mary R and Peter M were successful in meeting their outcome criteria and were subsequently discharged home without further complications. In Part III, we are going to assume that Peter developed a complication of bedrest—pneumonia—and his condition has deteriorated. He has demonstrated increasing respiratory distress and has been transferred to the critical care unit for close observation. Stat. ABGs are drawn and show acute respiratory failure. The decision is made to intubate and initiate mechanical ventilation.

Many patients, like Peter, with chronic obstructive or chronic restrictive pulmonary diseases eventually develop acute respiratory failure secondary to infection, severe lung tissue destruction, airway obstruction, or respiratory muscle failure, particularly at the end-stage of the disease. When experiencing an acute respiratory disease superimposed on chronic pulmonary insufficiency, the compensatory mechanisms may not be able to respond adequately to treatment, precipitating the onset of failure.

Other patients develop acute respiratory failure as the result of a sudden life-threatening event of a nonrespiratory nature, such as multiple trauma, cardiac arrest, or severe head injury. Any person who is not able to adequately maintain oxygenation or ventilation is a candidate for initiation of mechanical ventilation. Criteria for mechanical ventilation are presented in Module 3, *Mechanical Ventilation.*

Patient Care Goals

The general goals and outcome criteria appropriate to the management of Peter while receiving mechanical ventilation may be divided into two major groupings: support of his physiologic needs and support of his psychosocial needs.

Support of Physiologic Needs

Support of Peter's physiologic needs is accomplished through interventions that promote optimal oxygenation, provide adequate ventilation, protect the airway, support tissue perfusion, and provide adequate nutrition.

Support of Psychosocial Needs

Support of Peter's psychosocial needs centers around interventions to reduce anxiety, provide a balance of sleep and activity, promote communication, and support the family.

Nursing Management of Physiologic Needs

Peter's nursing management will be planned around interventions to attain the previously stated goals. The first three goals, promote optimal oxygenation, provide adequate ventilation, and protect the patient's airway, are all addressed through implementation of the three pulmonary related nursing diagnoses as follows.

Ineffective Airway Clearance

Since Peter is now requiring positive pressure ventilation, he will have an endotracheal (E-T) tube inserted to directly access and seal off his lower airway. The length and relatively small internal diameter of artificial airways will make it difficult, if not impossible, for Peter to clear his own airway. The problem of airway clearance is compounded by general weakness and fatigue or diminished responsiveness level, any of which also hinders airway clearance.

Airway clearance is a top priority nursing goal in management of the patient with an artificial airway. If airway patency is not maintained, Peter's breathing and cardiovascular status eventually will fail due to hypoxia or hypercarbia.

> Remember to apply the ABCs—*Airway, Breathing, Circulation*—in that order.

The primary reason that airway patency becomes compromised is airway obstruction caused by excessive, thick, or pooled secretions. Each of these situations must be managed properly by the nurse.

Excessive Secretions

Excessive secretions are removed by suctioning Peter's artificial airway on an as necessary basis, which may be every few minutes during initial intubation to several times a shift in chronic intubation. His breath sounds should be assessed every 1 to 2 hours for the presence of secretions. If adventitious breath sounds are auscultated in the large airways, suctioning should be performed. Coughing, whether or not it sets off the ventilator's high pressure alarm, may indicate a need for suctioning. The nurse often can hear the secretions without the use of a stethoscope, particularly during coughing. Coughing, however, can occur due to tracheal irritation or bronchospasm or because the tip of the airway is touching the carina. The last two situations can precipitate severe coughing spasms. Because coughing may occur without the presence of secretions in the large airways, the nurse should assess the situation first. Unnecessary suctioning causes needless trauma to the delicate mucous membranes in the trachea and also depletes oxygen levels.

Good rules to apply are

- Always assess before suctioning
- Do not suction unnecessarily
- Follow approved protocols for suctioning
- Monitor the patient closely for adverse effects of suctioning, such as arrhythmias and hypoxia

In most circumstances, the nurse will maintain Pao_2 levels during suctioning if the following common protocol is maintained.

Step 1. Hyperoxygenate/hyperventilate. Deliver 100 percent oxygen accompanied by manually ventilating the patient with a resuscitation (Ambu) bag for four to five breaths (two-handed ventilating will give significantly larger breaths than one-handed ventilating).
Step 2. Suction. Use moderate, not high, suction pressure. If secretions are too thick to be aspirated, instill approximately 3 mL of sterile saline down the airway during hyperventilation. Apply suction only on withdrawal, rotating the catheter while using intermittent suction and withdrawing the catheter within 10 seconds.
Repeat Steps 1 and 2 until the airway is cleared.
Step 3. Return the patient to the ventilator.

There are many variations to suctioning protocols. Some hospitals only hyperoxygenate by temporarily increasing the ventilator's oxygen concentration (Fio_2) to 100 percent (for 1 to 5 minutes). Hyperventilation may be part of such a policy. Hyperventilation can be accomplished through a SIGH or other intermittent large inhaled volume mechanism on the ventilator that, when manually triggered, will deliver a breath that is 1.5 to ≥2 times the patient's set tidal volume. In patients with acute neurologic injury, protocol may call for initial hyperoxygenation/hyperventilation for 1 or more minutes before initiation of the suctioning protocol.

Suction catheters may be divided into two major groups: open and closed systems. Both systems are used for suctioning artificial airways, but only open systems are used without an artificial airway in place. Each type of system has its own suctioning protocol. Closed system catheters are self-contained within a sheath attached directly to the artificial airway. A closed catheter system remains in the artificial airway system between suctioning, allowing it to be used multiple times. Open systems generally are single-use catheters and require introduction of the catheter into the artificial airway from outside the artificial airway system. Further discussion of suctioning systems is beyond the scope of this module.

If Peter needs to be placed on positive end-expiratory pressure (PEEP), a different suctioning protocol may be required. Patients on PEEP often do not tolerate being detached from the ventilator for any reason. Loss of PEEP can precipitate oxygen desaturation and may make the patient hemodynamically unstable. Several approaches may be used: (1) the usual suctioning protocol, (2) the usual suctioning protocol using a manual resuscitation bag that has a special PEEP attachment, set at the prescribed PEEP level, or (3) suctioning without removing the patient from the ventilator by either an inline closed suction system or introducing a suction catheter into the closed system through a special port on top of the ventilator adaptor nozzle. Research is continuing on which type of suctioning system and protocol is best in specific situations. All types of suctioning have associated problems, including infection, hypoxia, trauma, arrhythmias, trauma to mucous membranes, and others.

Thick Secretions

These may well be a major problem in preventing airway clearance. Properly hydrating Peter is the most important means of thinning his secretions, since secretions are composed primarily of water. Mechanically ventilated patients receive warmed, humidified gases that facilitate liquefication of secretions. Instillation of sterile normal saline down the airway is a common method of thinning secretions, as previously described.

Pooled Secretions

Pooled secretions can cause obstruction of major airways or can plug the tip of the artificial airway. Proper suctioning, liquefying secretions, and turning Peter every 1 to 2 hours all help prevent obstruction by pooling.

Impaired Gas Exchange

Treatment of impaired gas exchange is the major reason for placing patients, like Peter, on a mechanical ventilator (i.e., impending ventilatory failure or acute respiratory failure). Ventilators can manipulate carbon dioxide levels directly by causing alveolar hyperventilation or hypoventilation.

Alveolar hyperventilation is associated with decreasing carbon dioxide levels and respiratory alkalosis. It can be patient induced if Peter is on the assist/control (A/C) mode and is hyperventilating for any reason (e.g., anxiety, pain, head injury), since he can blow off too much carbon dioxide. It also can be induced mechanically by setting the rate and tidal volume too high on the ventilator. Sometimes, as in patients with increased intracranial pressure, mild respiratory alkalosis is induced intentionally to facilitate cerebral vasoconstriction through low carbon dioxide levels.

Alveolar hypoventilation is associated with increasing carbon dioxide levels and respiratory acidosis. Hypoventilation may be patient induced, for example, in the patient on synchronous intermittent mandatory ventilation (SIMV) mode (or other spontaneous breathing mode) whose breathing is very shallow. It also can be induced mechanically by setting the rate and tidal volume too low on the ventilator.

A changing arterial blood gas trend may indicate a change in Peter's respiratory or metabolic status, reflecting an improvement or deterioration in his condition. The cause of the imbalance needs to be found and treated to correct the imbalance. It is the nurse's responsibility to monitor the ABG trends, observe Peter's condition, notify the physician of increasing abnormalities, follow up on orders received, and monitor the ventilator settings at established intervals. The nurse also can facilitate gas exchange by taking actions to maintain airway clearance and effective breathing patterns. (Ventilator settings to be monitored are discussed in the *Mechanical Ventilation* module.)

Ineffective Breathing Patterns

Patients may be placed on the mechanical ventilator because of ineffective breathing patterns, consisting of any significant changes in the breathing rate, rhythm, or depth from the patient's baseline normals (e.g., tachypnea, bradypnea, apnea, hypoventilation, hyperventilation). Changes in breathing patterns can affect oxygenation and acid-base status, as previously described.

Peter is triggering the ventilator at 30 times per minute. Breathing patterns that remain too rapid may need to be controlled once the patient is placed on the ventilator to prevent hyperventilation problems. A variety of analgesics (e.g., IV morphine) or sedatives (e.g., benzodiazepines, such as Valium and Ativan) may be ordered. In some patients, a neuromuscular blocking agent (e.g., curare or Pavulon) may be ordered if the breathing pattern is adversely affecting Peter's progress and cannot be controlled using analgesics or sedatives. The nurse should assess for possible causes of the rapid pattern and take steps to relieve the problem when possible. Rapid breathing patterns may stem from fear, anxiety, pain, or such physiologic problems as acid-base imbalance or head injury.

Protection of the Airway

Protecting the airway is a major goal in Peter's care while he is on the ventilator. Any artificial airway can be fairly easily dislodged, either partially or completely. Because of this, the nurse must always take steps to minimize the possibility of dislodgment, which could precipitate respiratory compromise. During bedside care, dislodgment is at the highest risk while moving the patient from side to side in bed or in transferring in or out of bed. Certain nursing actions minimize this risk, such as (1) maintaining sufficient slack on the ventilator tubing to minimize tension on the airway during moving, (2) disconnecting the patient from the ventilator and manually ventilating during transfer in and out of bed, and (3) adequately securing the airway through correct taping or other stabilizing device. Tracheostomy tubes often are sutured in place as well as being tied around the neck. Securing an E-T tube using twill tape may not stabilize the tube sufficiently to prevent accidental dislodgment.

If Peter is not fully oriented or is uncooperative, he may pull the airway out. To prevent accidental or intentional dislodgment by the patient, many hospitals have a standard policy of applying soft wrist restraints at all times to patients on a mechanical ventilator. When restraints are in use, neurovascular checks should be performed routinely distal to the restraints. The purpose of the restraints needs to be explained and intermittently reinforced to both Peter and his family, emphasizing that they are in place for protection of the airway. Patients and families frequently view restraints as a punishment or unnecessary restriction of freedom.

Alteration in Cardiac Output

The general goal, support tissue perfusion, can be addressed using the nursing diagnosis: **Alteration in**

cardiac output: decreased. Positive pressure ventilation profoundly affects the normal hemodynamics of the body by increasing intrathoracic pressures and decreasing venous return to the heart, which decreases cardiac output. The use of PEEP further compromises cardiac output by further decreasing venous return. These effects are described in detail in Module 3, *Mechanical Ventilation.*

Hemodynamic Effects of Mechanical Ventilation

Peter, while on the mechanical ventilation, may have a pulmonary artery flow-directed catheter inserted to closely monitor his hemodynamics status, particularly since he has a history of cardiovascular problems. Table 4–5 shows the hemodynamic trends associated with mechanical ventilation, as summarized from Daily and Schroeder (1989).

If he does not have a pulmonary artery catheter inserted, the nurse can assess for the clinical manifestations of decreased cardiac output, such as confusion, restlessness, decreased urine output, flattened neck veins, and clammy, cool skin (Daily and Schroeder, 1989). Management of the patient with decreased cardiac output is described in detail in Module 9, *Nursing Care of the Patient with Altered Tissue Perfusion.*

Ulrich et al (1986) suggest the following major nursing interventions in planning care of the patient with decreased cardiac output.

- Monitor for and report signs and symptoms of decreased cardiac output
- Implement measures to improve cardiac output
  1. Perform actions to reduce cardiac workload
  2. Monitor for therapeutic and nontherapeutic effects of the following if administered
     a. Positive inotropic agents
     b. Beta-adrenergic blocking agents
     c. Antiarrhythmics
     d. Intravenous infusions
  3. Prepare client for invasive measures
- Consult physician if signs and symptoms of decreased cardiac output persist or worsen

Alteration in Nutrition

Before Peter's current respiratory crisis, his nutritional state was poor. Now, having been placed on a mechanical ventilator, he will have additional nutritional problems needing to be addressed. Peter has an **Alteration in nutrition: less than body requirements.** During the acute phase of his illness, he will

TABLE 4–5. HEMODYNAMIC EFFECTS OF MECHANICAL VENTILATION

Measured Pulmonary Artery Catheter Parameter	Trend
Right atrial pressure	Increased
Pulmonary artery pressure	Increased
Pulmonary artery wedge pressure	Usually increased
Left arterial pressure	Usually increased
Peripheral arterial pressure	Unchanged or decreased
Cardiac output	Decreased

maintain a nothing-by-mouth status. The presence of an E-T tube, even with a properly inflated cuff, places him at risk for aspiration of microparticles that can leak around the endotracheal cuff and contaminate the lower airway. This can precipitate complications associated with aspiration. Avoiding food and fluids by oral route and maintaining excellent oral hygiene, which includes frequent oral suctioning, reduce the risk of microaspiration problems.

The importance of maintaining or improving nutritional integrity in the respiratory compromised patient was discussed earlier, in Case Study 2. Maintaining a malnourished state with its negative nitrogen balance will significantly decrease Peter's chances of successful weaning from the mechanical ventilator because of respiratory muscle atrophy and weakness. Regaining nutritional integrity is a crucial aspect of care management because it has a direct impact on Peter's ability to improve his condition.

While on mechanical ventilation, Peter has a small-bore feeding tube inserted, either nasogastric or nasoenteric. Feedings ideally are initiated within 3 days of artificial airway placement to prevent gastrointestinal complications and to initiate early nutritional support. As described in Case Study 2, pulmonary patients may require special consideration of carbohydrate loading because of the high carbon dioxide by-product produced, which can further complicate Peter's acid-base balance. Management of the patient with alterations in nutrition is detailed in Module 20, *Nursing Care of Patients with Altered Metabolism.*

Nursing Management of Psychosocial Needs

Anxiety

Peter is experiencing a high level of anxiety associated with the insertion of the E-T tube, the mechanical ventilator, and the critical care environment. Anxiety is a common complaint of patients, such as Peter, who have chronic respiratory problems. Many chronic pulmonary diseases are progressive in nature. Thus a pattern of increasing disability is experienced.

Nett and Petty (1985, p 413) summarize many of the anxiety-producing questions commonly voiced by chronic obstructive disease patients.

- Can I live?
- Can I hope?
- Can I work?
- Can I love?
- Can I thrive?

As many chronic pulmonary diseases progress, patients experience an increasing pattern of hospital admissions for complications of their disease. Ultimately, at end-stage disease, these patients most commonly die of complications of their disease, such as severe respiratory failure or cor pulmonale.

When patients are experiencing acute respiratory distress, they often are anxious. Severe dyspnea often is associated with fear of suffocation or dying. All energy is focused toward breathing when acute distress exists. Being placed on a mechanical ventilator may be received by the patient either with relief or with an increased state of anxiety. The nursing diagnosis to deal with this problem is: **Anxiety,** which is frequently associated with the unfamiliar environment, unfamiliar invasive breathing assist device, loss of control, painful procedures, lack of understanding of procedures, and fear of dying.

Management of Peter's anxiety while he is on the mechanical ventilator combines collaborative and independent nursing interventions. Sedation commonly is ordered to decrease anxiety levels, which, in turn, helps him breathe with the ventilator. The sedation may be in the form of narcotics or sedatives. A high anxiety state must be brought under control if Peter is to decrease his work of breathing and oxygen consumption. Narcotics are particularly useful if the breathing pattern needs to be subdued because they have respiratory depressant side effect. This is sometimes the case in patients who have uncontrolled tachypnea. When oxygen consumption is very high, it may be decided to use a neuromuscular blocking agent to paralyze the respiratory muscles, producing rapid apnea and total skeletal muscle paralysis. Neuromuscular blocking agents do not alter the responsiveness level of the patient. Therefore, while in the paralyzed state, this group of patients should receive intermittent IV sedation at regular intervals to reduce anxiety and to enhance mental rest.

Nursing interventions regarding anxiety will include

- Monitoring for anxiety status

- Implementing measures to reduce anxiety
- Maintaining a restful environment
- Explaining all procedures and diagnostic tests
- Assessing for therapeutic and nontherapeutic effects of sedation

Sleep Pattern Disturbance

While on the ventilator, Peter experiences interruptions throughout the 24-hour day. Airway clearance and other maintenance nursing interventions frequently require disturbing a resting or sleeping high acuity patient. The nursing diagnosis addressing this problem is **Sleep pattern disturbance.**

Management of this problem often is a matter of careful planning on the part of the nurse. Clustering activities to allow for prolonged periods of undisturbed rest, particularly during the night hours, is a nursing goal. Minimizing interruptions at night for suctioning and turning and other high priority interventions requires coordination and good communication among the entire nursing team.

Communication and Sensation

The presence of an artificial airway prevents Peter from verbally communicating. This alteration is addressed in the nursing diagnosis: **Impaired verbal communication.** Peter may require frequent reminders that he will be able to talk once the tube is removed, with a brief explanation of why he cannot talk at this time. Peter, who is fully responsive, may become very frustrated when he cannot make his needs understood. There are alternative communication methods available. To evaluate appropriate types of communication alternatives, the nurse will need to evaluate Peter's visual status. If he cannot see well or his glasses are not available, communication alternatives are reduced significantly.

The nurse has a variety of communication alternatives from which to experiment for effectiveness, for example, an alphabet or picture board for the patient to point to. Alphabet boards are not very satisfactory for many patients because they cannot concentrate sufficiently or do not have the strength to point to multiple letters for writing a message. Some facilities have a talking board, on which the patient touches the appropriate picture and the board verbally states the particular need. Use of any type of picture board depends on the patient's ability to see the pictures. Some patients are able to write on a board with paper and pencil or other type of writing board, such as magic slates or small chalk board.

Patience on the part of the nurse is a major component of successful communication with a mechanically ventilated patient. Simple needs often can be expressed through lip reading or hand signals. It is easier to lip read with a patient who has a nasotracheal tube rather than an orally placed tube.

Family Support

The psychosocial needs of Peter's family cannot be forgotten while he is being managed on the ventilator. Families vary on how they perceive the ventilator. Peter's family may express relief that his breathing status is now protected. This is particularly true of families of patients who have had several past intubations. Peter's family initially may find the presence of the artificial airway and mechanical ventilator a frightening experience. The frequent alarms and his inability to communicate verbally are the basis of many of the questions asked of the nurse. Family members need to be oriented to the equipment in direct simple terms. Frequent updates should be given on Peter's status in terms they can understand. It also is appropriate to remind the family, as necessary, that Peter will be able to talk once the tube is removed if a temporary tracheostomy or E-T tube is in place. The nurse may have to translate communications from Peter to his family.

Weaning the Patient from the Mechanical Ventilator

Peter's pneumonia is now resolved, and it is believed that he is ready for removal from the mechanical ventilator. Just as criteria are used in making the decision to place a patient on a mechanical ventilator, essentially the same criteria are used in deciding if the patient is ready to begin the weaning process. Ventilator weaning refers to the activities involved in attaining total independence from the mechanical ventilator. Weaning can be a rapid process or a very slow process. A variety of factors are involved in the speed at which weaning is done.

Rapid Weaning (Short-Term)

Sometimes a patient with no significant lung disease requires short-term mechanical ventilation (e.g., surgery, drug overdose). Once the underlying problem is corrected (i.e., reversal of anesthesia effects), the patient is evaluated for ventilator weaning, using special criteria. Nett et al (1987) suggest the following weaning routine: If the criteria are met, the patient is removed from the ventilator and placed on a T-piece at 40 percent moist oxygen for 30 minutes. During the trial period, the patient is monitored for comfort, ECG status, and ABG status. If these criteria remain within acceptable limits (Pao_2 remaining stable, and $Paco_2$ remaining at ≤ 5 mm Hg of the level present while on the ventilator), the patient is suctioned, rested for a short period on the ventilator, and extubated.

Slow Weaning (Long-Term)

Patients, like Peter, who have underlying chronic lung disease (i.e., emphysema or pulmonary fibrosis) that is complicated by some acute problem (i.e., pneumonia) frequently will not be weaned as rapidly as patients with normal lungs. Long-term weaning is performed on patients who are resistant to weaning for a variety of reasons. Problems that may cause a failure to wean include excessive respiratory muscle work of breathing, respiratory muscle fatigue, anemia or malnutrition, excessive secretions, infection, unstable hemodynamic state, fear and anxiety, and others (Norton and Neureuter, 1989). This group of patients often is in a poorer state of general health than the fast weaning group. Their ability to readjust to negative pressure normal breathing from long-term positive pressure breathing often is slow and requires retraining and restrengthening of the respiratory muscles. Systematic correction of problems before initiating the weaning process significantly increases the chances for successful weaning.

Indications for Initiation of Weaning

Weaning Peter from the ventilator should not be considered until the original problem that caused the need for mechanical ventilation has been resolved. Peter's general condition should be at least stabilized if not improved. His ABGs should be within acceptable limits for him. PEEP should no longer be in use. His nitrogen balance should be relatively normal, with a serum albumin of >2.5 g/dL. Vital signs should be within normal limits for Peter, with a respiratory rate of less than 30/minute. His pulmonary mechanics should show a spontaneous tidal volume of >4 to 5 mL/kg, a minute volume of <10 L/minute, and a negative inspiratory force (NIF) of greater than -25. These mechanics are easy to measure and can be performed by anyone with the proper training. Peter must be willing to be weaned, particularly if manual weaning is to be used. Lack of cooperation frequently will lead to failure no matter how well the other criteria are being met.

Methods of Weaning

Manual Weaning

Manual weaning was the original method of removing a patient from a ventilator, and it is still commonly used. Manual weaning is accomplished through following a schedule of removal from the mechanical ventilator for increasing periods of time. If this method were used on Peter, he would be taken off the ventilator and his artificial airway would be attached to a humidified oxygen source. The nurse would then closely monitor Peter for signs of weaning intolerance, such as respiratory rate >30/minute, a significant increase in blood pressure and pulse, a minute ventilation of over 10 L/minute, development of cyanosis, or a decrease in oxygen saturation on pulse oximetry to below his acceptable level.

Manual weaning requires close patient contact throughout the weaning period, since the nurse plays a crucial part in monitoring him and coaching correct breathing rate and depth for the trial period. The nurse's calm reassurance will be instrumental in assisting Peter past the period of anxiety often associated with removal from the mechanical ventilator. Manual weaning is performed on an increasing schedule either throughout the 24-hour period or throughout the day and evening. The amount of time Peter is kept off the ventilator may start at 5 minutes and increase to the entire day, except at night, before full independence. Manual weaning must be individually designed, based on Peter's changing status from day to day.

Manual weaning is a strengthening exercise for the respiratory muscles. Complete removal from the ventilator forces the respiratory muscles to take over complete work of breathing, without any assistance from the ventilator for increasing blocks of time. Muscle strength is increased through use of the weaning procedure and good nutrition and hydration. There are several disadvantages to manual weaning. First, it may be a frightening experience to Peter, who is more accustomed to positive pressure breathing. Abrupt removal from the ventilator may precipitate high anxiety, which will hinder the weaning process. Second, manual weaning is time consuming for the nurse. During the period that Peter is off the ventilator, particularly in the early stages of weaning, the nurse generally is needed directly at the bedside, coaching, monitoring, and encouraging him.

Ventilator Weaning

This is a newer weaning method than manual weaning. The most common type of ventilator weaning at this time is the SIMV mode. Using this ventilator mode, Peter is given mandatory mechanical (ventilator) breaths at preset intervals every minute. Between the mechanical breaths, Peter is able to exercise his respiratory muscles spontaneously. The SIMV rate initially may be set fairly high, near Peter's own respiratory rate. The rate of mandatory breaths is then decreased by two-breath increments one to two times per day (as tolerated by him) until the SIMV rate is down to four breaths per minute. Once the mandatory rate is at four breaths per minute, a spontaneous mode (such as CPAP) or a T-piece trial is attempted for a minimum of 30 minutes. If Peter tolerates the weaning procedure and all parameters remain within acceptable boundaries, he can be extubated. Kearney et al (1990, pp 13–14) suggest the following extubation and postextubation protocol.

- Have cool humidified oxygen set up at the bedside
- Suction out the patient's E-T tube and mouth
- Deflate the endotracheal tube cuff
- Remove the tube at end-inspiration
- Encourage cough and deep breathing
- Apply humidified oxygen

Following extubation, particular attention must be given to excellent pulmonary hygiene, including a routine of coughing, deep breathing, and incentive spirometry. Various aerosol therapies, percussion, and postural drainage may be ordered to prevent or treat complications, if necessary. Peter will need to be monitored closely for signs and symptoms of respiratory distress after extubation.

SIMV weaning is an endurance exercise for the respiratory muscles. The muscles work continuously over the entire day except when the SIMV breath triggers a positive pressure breath, which allows a single breath rest. Ventilator weaning generally is thought to be less traumatic to the patient because it does not involve removal from the ventilator. It also is often less time consuming for the nurse to monitor the patient who is having the SIMV rate slowly manipulated.

Mechanical weaning, just as manual weaning, requires careful monitoring of Peter's status. Some patients do not tolerate decreasing SIMV rates. This tolerance may change on a day to day basis. Weaning often is not a smooth undertaking. In patients with underlying disease, changing status can require temporary cessation of weaning. This is particularly true if Peter should develop another pneumonia. Such a status change may first manifest itself in a sudden intolerance to weaning. During active weaning, schedules need to be followed carefully. Long-term weaning often is a challenge for the nurse, the patient, and the family.

Peter's plan of care is successful, and he is finally weaned 35 days after being placed on the ventilator. After another week of observation, he is discharged home with a home health referral. Peter was fortunate in this admission because he was able to be weaned from the ventilator. As his pulmonary disease progresses, weaning may become increasingly difficult, possibly leading to eventual ventilator dependence. Superior teaching will be necessary for Peter concerning health maintenance and avoidance of infection. Taking excellent care of himself hopefully will help him avoid another episode of respiratory failure that could significantly decrease his quality of life should he again require mechanical ventilation.

Conclusion

Nursing management of the patient with restrictive or obstructive pulmonary disease focuses on optimizing ventilation and oxygenation. This module has presented subjective and objective data relevant to pulmonary diseases, including differentiating pulmonary from cardiogenic symptoms. There are three primary respiratory nursing diagnoses: **Impaired gas exchange, ineffective breathing pattern,** and **ineffective airway clearance.** Each of these diagnoses has been described in detail using the case studies of Mary R, a patient with restrictive pulmonary disease, and Peter M, a patient with obstructive pulmonary disease. Each case study was presented using the nursing process framework. Collaborative as well as independent nursing interventions were discussed. An important part of high acuity pulmonary care is care of the patient requiring mechanical ventilation. To facilitate exploration of this, the case study of Peter was further expanded, placing him in acute respiratory failure. Mechanical ventilation was then discussed, following Peter from the placement of the artificial airway through weaning him from the ventilator.

REFERENCES

Brunner, L.S., and Suddarth, D.S. (1988). *Textbook of medical-surgical nursing,* 6th ed. Philadelphia: J.B. Lippincott Co.

Carpenito, L.J. (1987). *Nursing diagnosis: Application to clinical practice,* 2nd ed., pp. 481–498. Philadelphia: J.B. Lippincott.

Daily, E.K., Schroeder, J.S. (1989). *Techniques in bedside hemodynamic monitoring,* 4th ed., pp. 341–357. St. Louis: C.V. Mosby Co.

Des Jardins, T.R. (1990). *Clinical manifestations of respiratory disease,* 2nd ed. Chicago: Year Book Medical Publisher, Inc.

Dolan, J.T. (1991). *Critical care nursing: Clinical management through the nursing process,* pp. 551–715. Philadelphia, F.A. Davis Co.

Dougherty, S. (1988). The malnourished respiratory patient. *Crit. Care Nurse.* 8(4):13–22.

Farzan, S. (1985). *A concise handbook of respiratory diseases,* 2nd ed. Reston, VA: Reston Publishing Co., Inc.

Hudak, C.M., Gallo, B.M., and Lohr, T. (1990). *Critical care nursing: A holistic approach,* 5th ed. Philadelphia: J.B. Lippincott Co.

Jennings, B.M. (1991). The hematologic system. In J.G. Alspach (Ed.) *Core curriculum for critical care nursing,* pp. 675–747. Philadelphia: W.B. Saunders.

Kearney, P. A., Hale, G., Medin, D., and Sublett, D. (1990). *Mechanical ventilation: University of Kentucky Medical Center.* Lexington, KY: University of Kentucky.

Kersten, L.D. (1989). *Comprehensive respiratory nursing: A decision-making approach.* Philadelphia: W.B. Saunders Co.

McKenry, L.M., Salerno, E. (1989). *Mosby's pharmacology in nursing,* 17th ed., pp. 617–666. St. Louis: C.V. Mosby Co.

Nett, L.M., and Petty, T.L. (1985). *Chronic obstructive pulmonary disease,* 2nd ed. New York: Marcell Dekker, Inc.

Nett, L.M., Morganroth, M.L., and Petty, T.L. (1987). Weaning from the ventilator: Protocols that work. *Am. J. Nursing.* 91(9):1174–1177.

Norton, L.C., and Neureuter, A. (1989). Weaning the long-term ventilator-dependent patient. Common problems and management. *Crit. Care Nurse.* 9(1):42–52.

Stark, J.L. (1991). The renal system. In J.G. Alspach (Ed.) *Core curriculum for critical care nursing,* pp. 472–608. Philadelphia: W.B. Saunders.

Ulrich, S.P., Canale, S.W., and Wendell, S.A. (1986). *Nursing care planning guides: A nursing diagnosis approach.* Philadelphia: W.B. Saunders Co.

PART II

Perfusion

Perfusion

James P. McGraw

This self-study module is intended for the novice nurse caring for the acutely ill patient. The focus of this module is the physiologic concepts that influence the performance of the cardiovascular system, with particular focus on the heart. An understanding of these concepts will allow the nurse to apply them to a variety of clinical situations in order to understand and predict cardiovascular performance.

The module is subdivided into sections that define terms and normal values, describe key relationships between variables, identify common clinical conditions that influence these variables, and present the clinical assessments that can be made of these variables.

Each module builds on the previous ones. You are urged to complete each of them and their posttests sequentially.

Objectives

At the completion of this module, *Perfusion,* you will be able to

1. Define and state adult normal values for cardiac output, heart rate, and stroke volume
2. Define preload, contractility, and afterload
3. Describe the effect of the Frank-Starling law on cardiac output
4. Describe the relationship among pressure, flow, and resistance
5. State some of the conditions that affect heart rate, preload, contractility, and afterload
6. Identify the common clinical assessments made to evaluate the heart rate, preload, contractility, and afterload

---

Pretest

1. The stroke volume multiplied by the heart rate equals the
   A. cardiac output
   B. cardiac index
   C. pulse pressure product
   D. left ventricular stroke work index
2. The normal cardiac output for an adult at rest is approximately
   A. 1.2 L/minute
   B. 3.4 L/minute
   C. 5.0 L/minute
   D. 7.0 L/minute
3. The resistance against which the heart must pump blood is known as the
   A. preload
   B. afterload
   C. upload
   D. download
4. The Frank-Starling law states that within physiologic limits, the heart will
   A. beat no faster than the body's demand for oxygen dictates
   B. pump all of the blood delivered to it
   C. completely empty of blood with each beat
   D. extract only the amount of oxygen needed from its blood supply
5. Pressure is the mathematical product of
   A. flow and volume
   B. flow and resistance
   C. viscosity and resistance
   D. viscosity and volume

6. Which of the following will depress myocardial contractility?
   A. epinephrine
   B. digitalis
   C. sympathetic nervous system activity
   D. hypoxia
7. Profound hemorrhage initially would result in
   A. decreased afterload
   B. decreased preload
   C. increased preload
   D. increased pulse pressure
8. The number of heartbeats too weak to be transmitted to the periphery can be measured by
   A. pulse pressure
   B. brachiopopliteal gradient
   C. electrocardiogram
   D. apical–radial pulse deficit
9. Heart rate may be slowed by
   A. straining to move bowels
   B. sympathetic nervous system stimulation
   C. physical exertion
   D. loss of 20 percent of circulating blood volume
10. Which of the following is consistent with diminished preload to the right ventricle?
    A. ascites
    B. jugular venous distention
    C. hepatic engorgement
    D. poor skin turgor

Pretest answers: 1, A. SV × HR = CO. 2, C. 3, B. 4, B. 5, B. 6, D. 7, B. 8, D. 9, A. 10, D.

Glossary

Afterload. The resistance against which the heart pumps blood

Aldosteronism. A disorder caused by increased secretion of an adrenal hormone, aldosterone, which results in retention of sodium and water and loss of potassium and hydrogen ions by the kidneys

Anaphylaxis. An abrupt, transient, allergic reaction with contraction of the smooth muscle and dilation of the capillaries

Aortic valve. The valve between the left ventricle and the aorta

Apical–radial pulse deficit. The difference between the apical and radial pulse rates, which reflects the number of heartbeats too weak to be transmitted to the periphery

Arteriole. A terminal artery that has a muscular wall that feeds directly into the capillaries

Arteriosclerosis. Degeneration, hardening, or thickening of the arterial walls

Ascites. An accumulation of serous fluid in the peritoneal cavity

Body surface area. A measure of overall body size using both height and weight in its calculation

Cardiac index. Cardiac output divided by body surface area

Cardiac output. The amount of blood pumped by the heart each minute

Cardiomyopathy. Disease of the myocardium

Compliance. The change in volume resulting from an incremental increase in pressure within a structure

Contractility. The ability of a muscle to shorten when stimulated; in particular, the force of myocardial contraction

Dyspnea. A subjective sensation of shortness of breath

Ejection fraction. The portion of ventricular end-diastolic volume that is pumped from the ventricle in one beat

Flow. The volume of blood passing a point per unit of time, specifically, cardiac output

Frank-Starling law. The principle that states that within physiologic limits, the heart will pump as much blood as is delivered to it

Hypoxia. Subnormal levels of oxygen in blood or tissue

Mitral valve. The valve between the left atrium and left ventricle

Myocarditis. Inflammation of the myocardium

Nomogram. A series of scales arranged so that calculations can be performed graphically

Orthostatic hypotension. Subnormal blood pressure caused by a change in body position, such as rising from supine to standing

Parasympathetic nervous system. The part of the autonomic nervous system that tends to increase secretions, increase tone in smooth muscle, and dilate blood vessels; in particular, it slows the heart rate

Preload. The degree of stretch in myocardial fibers at the end of diastole

Pulmonic valve. The valve between the right ventricle and the pulmonary artery

Septic shock. Shock resulting from an acute infection, associated with dilation of the peripheral vasculature

Stenosis. A narrowing of a passage, particularly narrowing of the orifice of a cardiac valve

Stroke volume. The volume of blood pumped with each heartbeat

Sympathetic nervous system. The part of the autonomic nervous system that tends to decrease secretions, decrease smooth muscle tone, and contract blood vessels; in particular, it increases the rate and strength of myocardial contraction

Tricuspid valve. The valve between the right atrium and right ventricle

Turgor. Fullness; skin turgor refers to the fullness of the peripheral interstitial space, which is assessed by pinching the skin and noting the speed of recoil to its original shape

Abbreviations

bpm. Beats per minute

BSA. Body surface area

CI. Cardiac index

CO. Cardiac output

HR. Heart rate

S_3. Third heart sound, which is commonly found in normal youths and frequently is associated with congestive heart failure in later life

S_4. Fourth heart sound, which frequently is associated with congestive heart failure, myocardial infarction, and hypertension

SV. Stroke volume

Section One: Cardiac Output

At the completion of this section, you will be able to define and state adult normal values for cardiac output, heart rate, and stroke volume. These definitions and values will be applied to the content of later sections.

Cardiac output (CO) is the amount of blood

pumped by the heart each minute. CO is a critical aspect of cardiovascular performance in both health and illness. Understanding how CO changes in response to changing conditions in the body will allow you to predict how the body will respond to different effects of injury or disease.

The normal CO is approximately 4.5 to 6.0 L/minute (Guyton, 1986). The normal CO for individuals can vary significantly depending on body size. A tall, heavy person will need more CO to feed all of his or her cells than will a short light person. Because of this, when CO is measured, it usually is corrected to account for body size. The correction is calculated by dividing the CO by the body surface area (BSA) and is called the cardiac index (CI). The normal CI is 3.5 to 4.5 L/minute/m² (Guyton, 1986). The BSA is calculated via the use of nomograms or computer programs from the patient's height and weight. For example, if two patients each have a CO of 5.0 L/minute but one has a BSA of 1.0 m² and the other has a BSA of 2.0 m², their CIs (5.0 L/m² and 2.5 L/m², respectively) illustrate that the perfusion of tissue is quite different despite their equal COs.

The heart pumps blood one burst at a time, with each heartbeat. The volume of blood pumped with each heartbeat is called the stroke volume (SV). The CO is the volume of each beat (SV) times the heart rate (HR).

$$SV \times HR = CO$$

Given a normal heart rate of approximately 72 bpm (range 60–100) and CO of approximately 5 L/minute, it is possible using this equation to determine that the usual stroke volume for an adult is approximately 70 mL.

$$\frac{5000 \text{ mL/minute}}{72 \text{ bpm}} = 69 \text{ mL/beat}$$

Changes in either the HR or SV will alter the CO. Fortunately, the body uses the interrelationship between these two factors to keep the CO at the level needed. For example, if the SV should fall, the body would immediately increase the HR to compensate and keep the CO unchanged. Conversely, if the HR should drop, the SV will increase and may allow the CO to remain unchanged. Of course, there is a limit to the capacity of the body to use these compensatory efforts to maintain CO.

In summary, the CO is the product of SV and HR. Both SV and HR can be modified to ensure that the CO is adequate to meet the body's needs.

Section One Review

---

1. The volume of blood pumped by the heart each minute is the
   A. stroke volume
   B. cardiac output
   C. cardiac index
   D. ejection fraction
2. A normal cardiac output for an adult at rest is approximately
   A. 1.2 L/minute
   B. 3.4 L/minute
   C. 5.0 L/minute
   D. 7.0 L/minute

3. The normal adult stroke volume is approximately
   A. 7 mL
   B. 17 mL
   C. 70 mL
   D. 700 mL
4. A patient has a stroke volume of 60 mL and a heart rate of 70 bpm. What is his cardiac output?
   A. 420 mL/minute
   B. 1.1 mL/minute
   C. 4.2 mL/minute
   D. 150 mL/minute

Answers: 1, B. 2, C. 3, C. 4, C. SV × HR = CO

$$\frac{70 \text{ mL}}{\text{beat}} \times \frac{60 \text{ beats}}{\text{minute}} = \frac{4200 \text{ mL}}{\text{minute}}$$

Section Two: Preload, Afterload, and Contractility

At the completion of this section, you will be able to define preload, contractility, and afterload.

There are a great number of factors that affect the CO. If you understand how the four determinants of CO affect CO, you will understand easily how each of the multitude of factors in injury and disease affects CO.

The four determinants of CO are

- Heart rate (HR)
- Preload
- Contractility
- Afterload

"Where" you may ask, "Is stroke volume?" Stroke volume (SV) is determined by the interplay of preload, contractility, and afterload.

$$HR \times SV = CO$$

Preload
Contractility
Afterload

Heart Rate

If the SV is held constant, any change in the HR will result in an immediate change in the CO. For example, if the SV is 70 mL and the HR drops from 70 bpm to 50 bpm, the CO will drop from 4.9 L/minute to 3.5 L/minute. If the pulse should rise from 70 bpm to 100 bpm and the SV should stay at 70 mL, the CO would rise from 4.9 L/minute to 7.0 L/minute.

Although the most effective way to manipulate CO is through HR, this manipulation has limits. If the pulse rises too high (approximately >150 bpm), the SV will begin to drop because the heart has too little time during diastole to fill with blood properly.

Preload

Preload is the amount of stretch in the myocardial fibers at the end of diastole (just before the onset of systole) (Guyton, 1986). Usually this is thought of as the volume of blood in the ventricle at end-diastole. The greater the volume of blood in the ventricle, the greater the amount of stretch that the fibers experience. Preload is greatly affected by the volume of blood delivered to the heart by the venous system. If the venous system brings a large volume of blood to the ventricle, there will be much stretch and high preload. If the venous system brings a small volume of blood to the ventricle, there will be less stretch and less preload.

Injury or illness of the myocardium can make the myocardial cells less stretchable. If this should occur, increased volume within the ventricle may be re-

quired to stretch the myocardial cells to the same degree. This situation is known as diminished myocardial compliance (Guyton, 1986).

In addition, if the heart should fail to eject the usual volume from the ventricle, excess will remain in the ventricle at the end of systole. When the usual amount of venous blood rushes in during diastole, it will be added to the remainder from the previous beat. This will result in an unusually large volume being in the ventricle at the end of diastole, resulting in increased preload.

Contractility

Contractility is the force with which the heart pumps blood. If the heart contracts forcefully, it will push out much of the blood in the ventricle. If the heart is pumping poorly, the result will be a drop in the SV. Many variables affect the force with which the heart muscle contracts. Contractility is the result of the contractile activity of the myocardial cells. Anything that enhances or diminishes the ability of these cells to contract vigorously will affect contractility.

Even when working perfectly, the ventricle does not eject all of the blood it contains. Usually, the ventricle ejects only 60 percent of the blood that it contains at the end of diastole. This measure of the portion of blood ejected is known as the ejection fraction and is a commonly measured index of myocardial function.

Afterload

Afterload is the resistance against which the ventricle must pump blood (Guyton, 1986). There is an optimal amount of resistance necessary for the system to work properly. The major influence on afterload is the mechanical resistance to flow offered by the arterial system. Other variables include the pulmonic and aortic valves, which may become stenotic and unable to fully open during systole.

Summary

HR affects CO directly if the SV does not change. SV has a direct effect on CO. SV is determined by preload, contractility, and afterload. An increase in the HR to compensate for diminished SV is common.

Section Two Review

1. The degree of stretch of myocardial cells at the end of diastole is known as
   A. preload
   B. contractility
   C. compliance
   D. distensibility

2. The vigor of myocardial cell's muscular activity is known as
   A. automaticity
   B. conduction
   C. contractility
   D. afterload

3. The resistance against which the ventricle pumps blood is known as
   A. preload
   B. blood pressure
   C. compliance
   D. afterload

Answers: 1, A. 2, C. 3, D.

Section Three: The Frank-Starling Law

At the completion of this section you will be able to describe the effect of the Frank-Starling law on CO. All of the four factors mentioned earlier are related to CO. However, there is a particular relationship between preload and SV that is so important it deserves special attention.

Within limits, the heart will pump the amount of blood delivered to it each beat. This is known as the Frank-Starling law of the heart. In other words, as preload increases, so does SV, and as preload decreases, SV falls (Figure 5–1A). Unfortunately, this law only applies within a range of normal.

You will note that until a critical point is reached, as preload increases, so does SV. As you can see,

there is an optimal preload for the heart to have maximal SV. If the patient's cardiovascular system is too far to the right past the optimal point, we can improve SV by lowering preload. Conversely, if the patient is on the far left part of the curve, we can improve SV by increasing preload.

It is important to realize that the Frank-Starling curve can change depending on the condition of the myocardium.

Note that with poor contractility shown in Figure 5–1B, the curve has moved down so that SV is less than normal at each point along the curve.

In summary, under normal conditions, SV increases and decreases as preload increases and decreases. Injury or disease can alter the response of the myocardium to changes in preload.

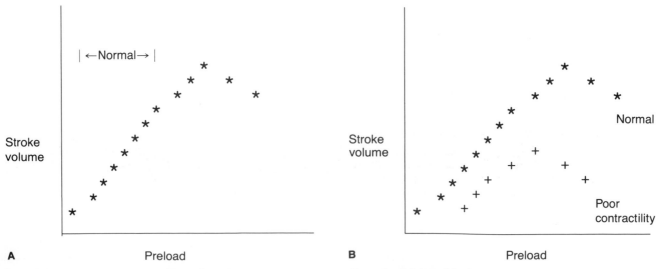

Figure 5–1. Graphs demonstrating the Frank-Starling law of the heart.

Section Three Review

1. The Frank-Starling law states that within physiologic limits the heart
   A. pumps as fast as it receives more blood
   B. pumps as much blood as it receives
   C. pumps less blood as it receives more blood
   D. pumps an unchanging amount of blood regardless of how much it receives

2. Disease may decrease the contractility of the myocardium. This means that if the preload decreases, the SV will
   A. increase
   B. decrease
   C. stay the same
   D. it cannot be determined from this information

Answers: 1, B. 2, B.

Section Four: Pressure, Flow, and Resistance

At the completion of this section, you will be able to describe the relationship among pressure, flow, and resistance. This relationship will help you to understand how cardiac output and vascular resistance relate to blood pressure. These are relationships that often are manipulated in acutely ill patients.

Many aspects of cardiovascular physiology are similar to the plumbing that we use every day. One critical concept of hemodynamics that can be thought of in this way is the relationship among flow, pressure, and resistance.

Imagine a system with a pump, a rigid tube, and a valve some distance from the pump as shown in Figure 5–2. If the valve is half closed, the pressure in the tube will increase as the rate of the liquid pumped is increased. If the pump were to run very fast with the valve partially closed, the pressure in the pipe would become great. If, on the other hand, the pump output remained constant and the valve were opened completely, there would be little pressure in the tube. This relationship among flow, resistance, and pressure can be mathematically expressed as

$$\text{Flow} \times \text{resistance} = \text{pressure}$$

In other words, just as SV and HR could compensate for each other to keep CO unchanged, flow and resistance can be adjusted to keep pressure steady. The flow in the cardiovascular system is the CO, the resistance is the afterload (the vascular resistance usually is the major component of this), and the pressure is the blood pressure.

In summary, blood pressure is the product of CO and vascular resistance. Blood pressure can be changed by adjustments in both CO and vascular resistance.

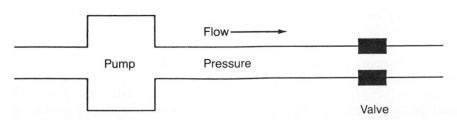

Figure 5–2. Diagram demonstrating the hemodynamic concept of the relationship among flow, pressure, and resistance.

Flow ⟶

Pump   Pressure

Valve

Section Four Review

1. The mathematical relationship among flow, resistance, and pressure is

    A. flow $= \dfrac{\text{resistance}}{\text{pressure}}$

    B. resistance $= \dfrac{\text{flow}}{\text{pressure}}$

    C. pressure $\times$ flow $=$ resistance
    D. flow $\times$ resistance $=$ pressure
2. What is the flow in the cardiovascular system?
    A. cardiac output
    B. heart rate
    C. stroke volume
    D. blood pressure
3. What is the resistance in the cardiovascular system?
    A. preload
    B. afterload
    C. contractility
    D. compliance
4. If pressure drops and flow remains unchanged, resistance must be
    A. increased
    B. decreased
    C. unchanged
    D. cannot be determined

Answers: 1, D. 2, A. 3, B. 4, B.

Section Five: Conditions That Affect Cardiac Output

At the end of this section, you will be able to state some of the conditions that affect HR, preload, contractility, and afterload. This information will allow you to apply these concepts in clinical situations.

Heart Rate

HR is controlled predominantly by the heart's pacemaker sites, which are influenced by the interplay of the sympathetic and parasympathetic nervous systems. The sympathetic nervous system causes the fight-or-flight reaction, where the body's resources are mobilized to counteract a real or perceived threat. The cardiovascular effects of sympathetic nervous system stimulation include increased HR, increased contractility, and vasoconstriction. The parasympathetic system causes generally the opposite effects, with a slowing and retarding of cardiovascular performance.

Any stresses that cause the activation of the sympathetic nervous system will cause an increased HR. The stressors that can be responsible for this include anything that is perceived as a threat, ranging from speaking in front of large groups to fleeing a burning house. In the hospital environment, stimuli that activate the sympathetic nervous system include pain, anxiety, and sensory overstimulation, in addition to the physiologic causes. On a physiologic level, anything that causes a drop in SV is likely to cause an increase in HR in an effort to compensate and hold

CO constant. In addition, there are numerous other causes of increased HR, including cardiac conduction system dysfunction, drug effects, and hormone imbalances.

HR is slowed most commonly by increased activity of the parasympathetic nervous system. There are numerous causes of this, ranging from drug effects and poisoning to straining hard to have a bowel movement. Other sources of a low HR include impaired impulse generation or conduction in the heart.

Preload

As you learned earlier, preload is the amount of stretch of myocardial fibers at the end of diastole, and preload can be thought of as being the amount of blood in the ventricle at end-diastole. Thus, preload can be altered by changing the amount of blood delivered to the heart by the venous system.

Loss of blood volume from hemorrhage, dehydration, diuretic use, or movement of fluid out of the vascular space into the extravascular compartment will result in a drop in preload. Diminished preload also can be caused by failure of the atrioventricular valve (either tricuspid or mitral) to allow free flow of blood into the ventricle. Loss of tone in the venous system can cause the venous vessels to dilate and hold more blood, which will result in less blood being delivered to the ventricle and a drop in preload. In addition, very fast HRs can so shorten diastole that there is insufficient time for the ventricle to fill adequately, resulting in diminished preload.

Increased blood volume will result in increased preload. Conditions that can cause increased blood volume are renal failure, fluid overload from IV therapy, aldosteronism (with retention of sodium and water), and excess sodium in the diet. Increased preload also occurs when the heart is unable to pump out the amount of blood received from the venous system. When this occurs, the remaining blood is still in the ventricle when the new flood of venous blood arrives to be pumped. As a result, the end-diastolic volume rises. One can imagine that if the heart continued to fail to pump the amount of blood delivered to it, there would be increasing congestion as the venous blood returned to the heart but was not promptly ejected into the arteries. This is precisely what happens in congestive heart failure: the heart pumps less blood than is delivered to it, and there is congestion in the venous system that drains into the affected ventricle. If the left ventricle fails, this congestion occurs in the pulmonary vascular bed. If the right ventricle fails, the congestion occurs in the systemic venous system.

Contractility

Contractility is the force with which the heart pumps blood. Contractility is much like HR in that it is heavily influenced by the autonomic nervous system. Sympathetic stimulation of the heart results in increased contractility, and conversely, parasympathetic stimulation causes decreased contractility. Other major determinants of contractility include oxygenation (hypoxia or ischemia decrease contractility), myocardial disease (myocarditis, cardiomyopathy),

and drug effects (many narcotics and anesthetic agents are direct myocardial depressants). Drugs that increase myocardial contractility include digitalis, epinephrine, and dopamine.

Afterload

Afterload is the resistance against which the heart must pump blood. The major determinant of afterload is the resistance to flow caused by the arterial system. Most of the arterial resistance is at the arterioles and is due to the tone in the muscles of their walls. Anything that causes changes in the arteriolar vascular tone can cause changes in afterload. For example, stimulation of the sympathetic nervous system will cause constriction of the arterioles and increase afterload. Drugs can relax or constrict the arterioles and cause a prompt drop or rise in afterload. The arterioles can be dilated by septic shock, spinal cord injury, or anaphylaxis.

Further resistance to flow can be caused by failure of the pulmonic or aortic valve to allow free flow of blood from the ventricle to the artery. In this case, the stenosed valve would cause an increase in afterload.

Summary

Each determinant of CO can be affected by numerous clinical conditions. Thus, clinical conditions can have an impact on CO by their influence on preload, afterload, contractility, and HR.

Section Five Review

1. Decreased HR can be caused by
   A. decreased SV
   B. anxiety
   C. parasympathetic stimulation
   D. pain
2. Increased preload can be caused by
   A. mitral stenosis
   B. loss of venous vascular tone
   C. very fast HRs
   D. congestive heart failure
3. Increased contractility can be caused by
   A. ischemia
   B. hypoxia
   C. cardiomyopathy
   D. sympathetic stimulation

4. Increased afterload can be caused by
   A. sympathetic stimulation
   B. septic shock
   C. anaphylaxis
   D. spinal cord injury

Answers: 1, C. 2, D. 3, D. 4, A.

Section Six: Assessments of Cardiac Output

At the completion of this section, you will be able to identify the common clinical assessments made to evaluate the determinants of CO discussed in previous sections.

Heart Rate

Evaluating the HR is relatively easy. A simple count of the radial pulse is useful for determining the number of heartbeats that are strong enough to reach the periphery. A count of the apical HR is useful to determine the total HR. Usually, these two rates are equal, but there may be a deficit between the apical rate and the radial rate caused by irregular heart rhythms that result in SV varying from beat to beat, which results in some beats being too weak to be felt at the radial artery (this is called the apical–radial pulse deficit). Electronic monitoring of the ECG is a useful but incomplete assessment of HR, for one cannot determine the character of the pulse from the ECG.

Preload, like contractility and afterload, is infrequently measured directly at the bedside. Usually, we must rely on indirect measures that allow us to estimate or infer the preload, contractility, or afterload. The methods of directly measuring these factors that require invasive tests and equipment are not discussed here. You will note that the right ventricular contractility, right ventricular afterload, and left ventricular preload are difficult to assess at the bedside because the cardiovascular structures where these exist are embedded deeply in the chest and are unavailable for examination.

Preload

Preload for the right ventricle is assessed by looking at the systemic venous system. The assessment items include the following (Bates, 1987).

Increased Right Heart Preload

- Jugular venous distention (JVD) (immediate sign)
- Ascites
- Hepatic engorgement
- Peripheral edema

(require several hours to days to appear)

Decreased Right Heart Preload

- Poor skin turgor
- Dry mucous membranes
- Orthostatic hypotension

Preload for the left heart is assessed by looking at the pulmonary venous system. These assessment items include the following.

Increased Left Heart Preload

- Dyspnea
- Cough
- Third heart sound (S_3)
- Fourth heart sound (S_4)

Decreased Left Heart Preload

Unfortunately, there are no noninvasive assessments that indicate specifically diminished left ventricular preload. Usually, if the left heart has insufficient preload, the right heart has the same situation, and we can rely on signs of diminished right ventricular preload.

Contractility

Assessing the force of myocardial contraction is done by looking at the quality of the heartbeat when isolated from HR.

Pulse

The character of the pulse is noted at the radial artery. Increased contractility will demonstrate a bounding, vigorous pulse, whereas diminished contractility will demonstrate a weak, thready pulse. It is important to note that contractility is difficult to measure indirectly by physical signs, since so many other factors may alter the character of the pulse. Decreased contractility usually is determined by exclusion of other causes of poor cardiac output.

Pulse Pressure

The pulse pressure is the difference between diastolic and systolic blood pressures. The pulse pressure reflects how much the heart is able to raise the pressure in the arterial system with each beat. The normal pulse pressure is approximately 40 mm Hg (Guyton, 1986). Within the restrictions noted, the pulse pressure can be a useful, objective, noninvasive indicator of myocardial contractility.

Afterload

As was mentioned previously, indirect assessment of right ventricle afterload is difficult because of the location of the pulmonary arterial system deep in the chest. However, it is possible for us to assess the systemic arterial system for signs of increased or decreased afterload. Even though we may find signs of altered afterload in some patients, they will not be present in all patients with altered afterload. It is necessary to remember once again that all of these determinants of CO are interrelated, and it can be difficult to isolate individual factors at the bedside without invasive tests.

Increased Systemic Afterload

Cool, clammy extremities may indicate that the arterioles to the skin have been constricted.

Systemic hypertension may indicate that the heart is pushing blood out against great resistance.

Nonhealing wounds on the extremities and thick brittle nails are indicators of chronic poor perfusion of the extremities, which may imply high vascular resistance (Bates, 1987).

Decreased Systemic Afterload

Warm, flushed extremities may indicate that the arterioles have relaxed and are offering little resistance to blood flow.

Summary

The status of preload, afterload, contractility, and HR can be assessed partially by clinical examination. Comprehensive assessment of these determinants can assist the clinician to identify the cause of altered CO.

Section Six Review

1. The total number of heartbeats is reflected in the pulse counted at the
   A. femoral artery
   B. cardiac apex
   C. carotid artery
   D. radial artery
2. Signs of increased preload for the right ventricle include
   A. jugular venous distention
   B. cool clammy skin
   C. bounding pulse
   D. dry mucous membranes

3. Signs of decreased contractility include
   A. bounding pulse
   B. diminished pulse pressure
   C. ascites
   D. poor skin turgor
4. Signs of increased afterload for the left ventricle include
   A. cool, moist skin
   B. thin, flexible toenails
   C. liver engorgement
   D. peripheral edema

Answers: 1, B. 2, A. 3, B. 4, A.

Posttest

Do not refer back to the text to answer these questions.

1. What is the relationship among stroke volume, cardiac output, and heart rate?
   A. $SV \times CO = HR$
   B. $SV \times HR = CO$
   C. $CO \times HR = SV$
   D. $CO = \dfrac{HR}{SV}$

2. The degree of stretch in the myocardial fibers at the end of diastole is called
   A. preload
   B. contractility
   C. afterload
   D. compliance

3. In the healthy heart, the response to an increase in preload is for SV to
   A. increase
   B. decrease
   C. stay the same
   D. cannot be determined from the available data

4. If afterload increases and CO remains the same, what will happen to blood pressure?
   A. increase
   B. decrease
   C. stay the same
   D. cannot be determined from the available data

5. Myocardial ischemia will most directly influence
   A. preload
   B. afterload
   C. contractility
   D. vascular tone

6. Physical examination reveals jugular vein distention, ascites, and liver engorgement. These suggest
   A. increased left ventricular preload
   B. decreased left ventricular preload
   C. increased right ventricular preload
   D. decreased right ventricular preload

7. Sudden physiologic stress, such as escaping a burning building, will result in
   A. increased heart rate and increased afterload
   B. increased heart rate and decreased afterload
   C. decreased heart rate and increased afterload
   D. decreased heart rate and decreased afterload

8. Extremely rapid heart rate can decrease CO because there is inadequate time in each cycle for
   A. systolic ejection
   B. diastolic filling
   C. valve closure
   D. intraventricular conduction

9. If an adult patient has a blood pressure of 80/60 mm Hg, the pulse pressure is
   A. increased
   B. decreased
   C. normal
   D. unknown from these limited data

10. Following hemorrhage, cool, clammy skin most suggests
    A. increased contractility
    B. decreased contractility
    C. increased afterload
    D. decreased afterload

Posttest Answers

Question	Answer	Section	Question	Answer	Section
1	B	One	6	C	Six
2	A	Two	7	A	Five
3	A	Three	8	B	Five
4	A	Four	9	B	Six
5	C	Five	10	C	Six

REFERENCES

Bates, B. (1987). *A guide to physical examination and history taking,* 4th ed. Philadelphia: J.B. Lippincott.

Guyton, A. (1986). *Textbook of medical physiology,* 7th ed. Philadelphia: W.B. Saunders.

Hemodynamic Monitoring

Paula Hogsten

The critically ill patient has complex nursing needs. This module focuses on the integration of hemodynamic concepts and physical findings in the nursing assessment of the critically ill patient. The underlying physiologic principles of pulmonary artery monitoring will be linked to the information generated by a pulmonary artery catheter. This information combined with astute observation and assessment skills can guide the nursing management of an acutely ill patient.

A 10-question pretest is provided to assess baseline knowledge of the concepts presented in this module.

Objectives

On completion of the module, *Hemodynamic Monitoring,* the learner will be able to

1. Describe the purpose and functional components of a basic pulmonary artery catheter
2. Understand the concept of thermodilution cardiac output determination
3. Recognize the normal right atrial waveform pattern
4. Relate right ventricular preload to the right atrial pressure
5. Identify common physical findings and appropriate nursing interventions related to abnormal right atrial pressure
6. Recognize the normal right ventricular waveform pattern
7. State normal right ventricular pressure
8. Identify appropriate nursing interventions related to right ventricular waveforms

9. Recognize the normal pulmonary artery waveform pattern
10. State normal pulmonary artery pressure
11. Identify common physical findings and appropriate nursing interventions related to abnormal pulmonary artery pressures
12. Recognize the normal pulmonary artery wedge pattern
13. State normal pulmonary artery wedge pressure
14. Relate left ventricular preload to pulmonary artery wedge pressure
15. Identify common physical findings and appropriate nursing interventions related to abnormal wedge pressures
16. Understand the physiology underlying the arterial waveform
17. Identify the components of a normal arterial waveform

18. Understand the implications of selected derived hemodynamic parameters

19. Calculate mean arterial pressure, cardiac index, and systemic vascular resistance

---

Pretest

1. Filling pressure of the right ventricle (right ventricular preload) is measured through the pulmonary artery catheter port opening into the
   A. superior vena cava
   B. right atrium
   C. right ventricle
   D. pulmonary artery

2. The greatest potential for dysrhythmias occurs when the pulmonary artery catheter passes through the
   A. superior vena cava
   B. right atrium
   C. right ventricle
   D. pulmonary artery

3. The BEST definition of preload is
   A. the ejection fraction
   B. the volume of blood returning to the heart
   C. stretch exerted on the ventricular walls at end-diastole
   D. the resistance the ventricle must overcome to eject its contents

4. Preload of the left ventricle is measured INDI-RECTLY by
   A. cardiac output
   B. pulmonary artery systolic pressure
   C. pulmonary artery diastolic pressure
   D. pulmonary artery wedge pressure (PAWP)

5. Afterload is estimated by determining the
   A. pulmonary artery wedge pressure
   B. right atrial pressure (RAP)
   C. cardiac index (CI)
   D. systemic vascular resistance (SVR)

6. Which of the following pulmonary artery pressures (PAP) fall within the normal range?
   A. PAP = 40/22, PAWP = 18
   B. PAP = 26/12, PAWP = 10
   C. PAP = 18/7, PAWP = 3
   D. PAP = 34/26, PAWP = 23

7. Normal range for cardiac output is
   A. 2–6 L/minute
   B. 4–8 L/minute
   C. 6–10 L/minute
   D. 8–12 L/minute

8. The dicrotic notch on the pulmonary artery waveform represents
   A. atrial contraction
   B. closure of the pulmonic valve
   C. closure of the aortic valve
   D. the beginning of ventricular systole

9. The right atrial waveform and the _____ waveform are similar in appearance.
   A. the pulmonary artery wedge
   B. the right ventricular
   C. the pulmonary artery
   D. systemic arterial

10. The dicrotic notch on the arterial waveform represents
    A. atrial contraction
    B. closure of the pulmonic valve
    C. closure of the aortic valve
    D. the beginning of ventricular systole

Pretest answers: 1, B. 2, C. 3, C. 4, D. 5, D. 6, B. 7, B. 8, B. 9, A. 10, C.

Glossary

Afterload. Resistance to ventricular systole, i.e., the pressure the ventricle has to overcome to eject the stroke volume; afterload is calculated as the systemic vascular resistance (SVR) for the left ventricle, and as pulmonary vascular resistance (PVR) for the right ventricle

Cardiac index (CI). Cardiac output (CO) individualized to body size (2.4 to 4.0 L/minute/m²)

Cardiac output (CO). The amount of blood ejected from the heart each minute (4–8 L/minute)

Frank-Starling law of the heart. The more myocardial fibers are stretched during diastole, the more they will shorten (contract) during systole and the greater will be the force of contraction until a physiologic limit has been reached

Mean arterial pressure (MAP). Directly measured by arterial line or calculated from systolic and diastolic cuff readings (normal 70–90 mm/Hg)

Preload. The pressure (stretch) exerted on the walls of the ventricle by the volume of blood filling the heart at end-diastole; left ventricular preload is measured indirectly by the pulmonary artery wedge pressure (PAWP); right ventricular preload is measured directly by the right atrial pressure (RAP)

Pulmonary artery diastolic pressure (PAD). Reflects diastolic filling pressure in left ventricle (normal 8–15 mm/Hg)

- The pulmonary artery diastolic pressure (PAD) approximates the left ventricular end-diastolic pressure; normally, PAD is 2–5 mm/Hg higher than pulmonary artery wedge pressure (PAWP)

Pulmonary artery systolic pressure (PAS). Pressure generated by the right ventricle during systole (normal ~ 20–30 mm/Hg)

Pulmonary artery wedge pressure (PAWP). Pressure obtained when the inflated balloon wedges in a small branch of the pulmonary artery reflecting pressures from left heart (normal 4–12 mm/Hg)

- PAWP reflects the preload status of the left ventricle; a high PAWP suggests a relative or actual hypervolemia (a high filling pressure), and a low PAWP suggests hypovolemia (a low filling pressure)

Pulmonary vascular resistance (PVR). The afterload of the right ventricle; the resistance the right ventricle must overcome to eject blood into the pulmonary artery (37–250 dynes/second/cm⁻⁵); adjusting for body size provides the index of this parameter (PVRI = 255–285 dynes/second/cm⁻⁵m²)

Right atrial pressure (RAP or CVP). A measure of the pressure in the right ventricle at end-diastole; this is right ventricular preload (normal ~ 2–8 mm/Hg)

Stroke volume (SV). The amount of blood ejected from the heart into systemic circulation with each contraction (normal 60–130 mL/beat); adjusting for body size provides the index (SVI = 33–47 mL/beat/m²)

Systemic vascular resistance (SVR). Afterload of left ventricle; the resistance the left ventricle must overcome to open the aortic valve and eject the stroke volume into the aorta (800–1200 dynes/second/cm⁻⁵); adjusting for body size provides the index of this parameter (SVRI = 1970–2390 dynes/second/cm⁻⁵m²)

Normal values from Alspach (1985), Darovic (1987) and Shoemaker (1988).

Cardiac Pressures

RA mean	2–6 mm/Hg
RV	20–30 mm/Hg
PAS	20–30 mm/Hg
PAD	8–15 mm/Hg
PAWP	4–12 mm/Hg

Common Formulas

Co	$SV \times HR$
CI	$\dfrac{CO}{BSA}$
MAP	$\dfrac{SBP + 2\ (DBP)}{3}$
SVR	$\dfrac{[(MAP\text{-}RAP) \times 80]}{CO}$
PVR	$\dfrac{[(PA\text{-}PAWP) \times 80]}{CO}$

Normal Values

CO	4–8 L/minute		SVR	800–1200 dynes/second/cm⁻⁵
CI	2.4–4.0 L/minute/m²		SVRI	1970–2390 dynes/second/cm⁻⁵
SV	60–100 mL/beat		PVR	37–250 dynes/second/cm⁻⁵
SVI	33–47 mL/beat/m²		PVRI	255/285 dynes/second/cm⁻⁵

Abbreviations

AOEDP. Aortic end-diastolic pressure

BSA. Body surface area

CI. Cardiac index

CO. Cardiac output

CVP. Central venous pressure

DBP. Diastolic blood pressure

HR. Heart rate

LA. Left atrium

LV. Left ventricle

LVEDP. Left ventricular end-diastolic pressure

MAP. Mean arterial pressure

PA. Pulmonary artery

PAD. Pulmonary artery diastolic

PAP. Pulmonary artery pressure

PAS. Pulmonary artery systolic

PAWP. Pulmonary artery wedge pressure

PVR. Pulmonary vascular resistance

RA. Right atrium

RV. Right ventricle

RAP. Right atrial pressure (also known as central venous pressure, CVP)

RVEDP. Right ventricular end-diastolic pressure

SBP. Systolic blood pressure

SV. Stroke volume

SVR. Systemic vascular resistance

SVRI. Systemic vascular resistance index

Various terms are used by health care professionals to refer to a pulmonary artery catheter, including right heart catheter, Swan or Swan-Ganz catheter, flow-directed thermodilution catheter, and pulmonary artery catheter. This module uses the term pulmonary artery catheter.

Section One: The PA Catheter

At the completion of this section, the learner will describe the purpose and functional components of a basic pulmonary artery catheter.

Purpose

The pulmonary artery catheter is an invasive diagnostic tool that can be used at the bedside for the following purposes.

1. Determination of the pressures within the right heart and pulmonary artery and indirect measurement of left heart pressures
2. Determination of cardiac output (CO)
3. Sampling mixed venous blood from the pulmonary artery ($S\bar{v}o_2$)
4. Infusion of fluids

A special pulmonary artery catheter is available with a fiberoptic filament that terminates in the pulmonary artery. In addition to allowing all the basic functions listed above, the fiberoptic filament in this catheter allows for continuous monitoring of the oxygen saturation of the blood in the pulmonary artery. This is known as the mixed venous oxygen saturation, or $S\bar{v}o_2$. Continuous monitoring of this parameter provides more information than intermittent or spot sampling. Knowledge of the $S\bar{v}o_2$ is used to assess the adequacy of oxygen delivery to the tissues.

Basic Construction

The pulmonary artery catheter is constructed of a radiopaque polyvinylchloride. Several sizes and various options are available to meet the needs of an adult or pediatric population. Options include such items as a heparin coating to reduce the risk of

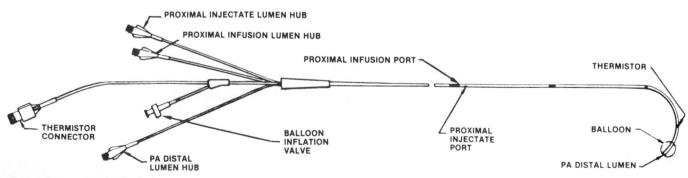

Swan-Ganz VIP™ Catheter

Figure 6–1. A five lumen pulmonary artery catheter. (*Reprinted with permission © 1991, Baxter Healthcare Corporation. Swan-Ganz^R is a registered trademark of Baxter Healthcare Corporation, Inc.*)

thrombus formation, an extra lumen for IV infusions, and pacing capacity. The catheter is marked at 10 cm intervals to facilitate insertion. Color-coded extrusions or ports on the proximal end provide access to the catheter lumens. A typical or basic five-lumen pulmonary artery catheter is illustrated in Figure 6–1.

Components and Pertinent Points

Proximal Injectate Lumen/Hub

This port terminates in the right atrium and is labeled proximal. It monitors right atrial pressure (RAP) when connected to a transducer. The injectate for CO is pushed through this lumen, and IV fluids can be infused through this port. (To avoid an inadvertent bolus of potent medications, do not infuse vasoactive drips through the port selected for cardiac output determinations.)

Proximal Infusion Lumen/Hub

When present, this optional lumen terminates in the right atrium and is labeled infusion. It is used typically as a central access site for IV fluid infusions. It can be used for CO determination if the proximal injectate lumen occludes.

Distal Lumen/Hub

This port terminates in the pulmonary artery and is labeled distal. It is attached to a transducer for continuous monitoring of pulmonary artery pressure (PAP) waveform. Pulmonary artery wedge pressure (PAWP) is obtained through this port, and mixed venous blood is obtained or sampled from this port. Maintaining 300 mm Hg pressure on the flush solution promotes patency. Medications are not infused through this port.

Thermistor Connector

The proximal end attaches to the CO computer cable. It terminates near the tip of the catheter in the pulmonary artery, and it detects changes in blood temperature for CO determination.

The pulmonary artery catheter is a fluid-filled line with a thermistor wire terminating near the distal end. If the thermistor hub must be disconnected from the CO computer, cover it with the original cap or a finger cot to protect the patient from microshock.

Balloon Inflation Valve

This valve is contiguous with the small balloon at the distal end of the catheter. A gate valve mechanism on the hub locks the port in an open or closed position. The maximum recommended inflation volume should not be exceeded. Inflation is stopped as soon as the waveform changes to a PAWP pattern. Deflation is passive, since manual deflation may damage the balloon integrity. Never leave the balloon in the inflated position.

In most hospitals, the nurse is responsible for preparing the patient, the equipment, and all necessary supplies. Before insertion of a PA catheter, the integrity of the catheter balloon is verified, the equipment is calibrated for accuracy, and the cables are attached correctly to the monitor. The proximal and distal ports of the catheter are attached to one or more transducers. Simply stated, a transducer senses the pressure changes in the heart and great vessels. These pressure fluctuations are changed to an electrical signal and relayed to the monitor, which converts the signal into a waveform and corresponding digital readout.

The insertion of a PA catheter is always a sterile procedure. Along with the physician, the nurse is responsible for careful observation and monitoring of the patient during the insertion process. Once the catheter is inserted by the physician, the nurse assumes responsibility for patient safety, comfort, and system maintenance. It is the responsibility of the nurse to be aware of unit specific policies and procedures related to hemodynamic monitoring.

The PA catheter is a complex tool that has enhanced the care of acutely ill patients. An understanding of the functional components of a PA catheter along with knowledge of where each lumen exits into the heart and pulmonary artery are important. This information is expanded on in each section of this module. Collecting data is not the end-point of hemodynamic monitoring. Careful clinical assessment integrated with the data collected from a PA catheter can be used to provide information about the capacity of the heart to function as a pump. This knowledge can be used to plan nursing interventions and provide for more precise manipulation of fluids and medications that can improve cardiac function and patient outcome. Proper use of a PA catheter can enable health care providers to intervene proactively rather than reactively.

Section One Review

1. Which port of the pulmonary artery catheter is used to obtain a right atrial pressure (RAP)?
   A. proximal port
   B. distal port
   C. thermistor wire port
   D. balloon inflation port
2. Which lumen is used for obtaining cardiac output (CO) determinations?
   A. proximal port lumen
   B. distal port lumen
   C. thermistor wire lumen
   D. balloon inflation port lumen
3. The purpose of protecting the thermistor hub whenever it must be disconnected from the CO computer cable is to
   A. prevent IV fluid leaks
   B. decrease the potential for an air embolism to occur
   C. avoid inaccurate CO readings
   D. provide for the electrical safety of the patient
4. The pressure reading from the _____ lumen is always continuously monitored.
   A. proximal lumen
   B. distal lumen
   C. thermistor wire lumen
   D. balloon port lumen

5. Why should vasoactive drugs never be infused through the port used for CO determinations?
   A. the size of the lumen is too small
   B. a bolus injection of a potent drug will occur every time CO is obtained
   C. CO readings will be less accurate
   D. some vasoactive drugs are not compatible with the catheter material
6. What is the best way to deflate the balloon on the PA catheter?
   A. slowly pull back on the syringe plunger
   B. quickly pull back on the plunger to limit inflation time
   C. allow the balloon to deflate passively
   D. remove the syringe from the hub directly after inflation
7. Which lumen is used to monitor PAP?
   A. proximal port lumen
   B. distal port lumen
   C. thermistor wire lumen
   D. balloon inflation port lumen

Answers: 1, A. 2, A. 3, D. 4, B. 5, B. 6, C. 7, B.

Section Two: Cardiac Output

At the completion of this section, the learner will understand the concept of thermodilution cardiac output determination.

Cardiac output (CO) is the amount of blood ejected from the heart into the systemic circulation each minute. It is the product of the heart rate (HR) times the stroke volume (SV). The SV is determined by the effects of preload, afterload, and contractility on the ventricle. It is important to understand what these terms mean because they will be expanded on throughout this module. Preload is the pressure or stretch exerted on the walls of the ventricle by the volume of blood filling the heart at end-diastole. Afterload is the resistance to ventricular systole, i.e., the pressure the ventricle has to overcome to open the aortic valve and push blood out into the systemic circulation. Contractility is the capacity of the heart to shorten its muscle fibers to squeeze or contract. These three things interact to determine the CO (Fig-

ure 6–2). This is true for both the right and left ventricles, but primary emphasis is placed on the left ventricle because it is the capacity of the left ventricle to function as a pump that determines patient outcome.

The normal range for CO is 4 to 8 L/minute. CO is a generic parameter that allows health care providers to place the patient's CO inside or outside of the normal range. Keep in mind that this very important parameter does not address the effect body size has on CO requirements. The cardiac index (CI), which references CO to body size, is discussed in Section Eight.

Although there are various methods for deter-

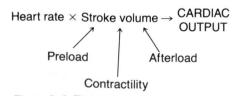

Figure 6–2. The determinants of cardiac output.

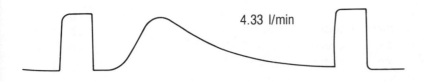

4.33 l/min

Figure 6–3. A normal cardiac output curve. (*Reprinted with permission © 1991, Baxter Healthcare Corporation.*)

mining CO, the thermodilution method is the one most commonly used and is the focus of this section. The thermodilution method uses the theory of temperature change to calculate CO. The proximal end of the thermistor lumen of the PA catheter is connected to a CO computer by a special cable. The distal end of the thermistor wire terminates about 1.6 inches (4 cm) before the tip of the catheter. This thermistor bead is exposed to the blood flowing through the PA. It is through this thermistor wire that the CO computer can sense temperature changes of the blood.

To determine CO by thermodilution, a bolus of fluid is injected into the right atrium through the proximal injectate port of the PA catheter. For accuracy, this injection must be smooth, rapid, and timed to occur within 4 seconds. This fluid bolus, or injectate, mixes with the blood and is pumped through the right ventricle into the PA. The fluid bolus transiently drops the blood temperature in the PA. As blood continues to be pumped into the PA, the blood temperature warms to prebolus level. The blood temperature change and the duration of the change are sensed by the CO computer.

The duration of the change in blood temperature caused by the fluid bolus is analyzed by the CO computer and a time/temperature CO curve is formed (Figure 6–3). The area under the curve represents the cardiac output. This area is calculated by the computer and displayed digitally in liters/minute. There is an inverse relationship between the size of the curve and the CO. A small curve indicates a rapid return of the blood to its baseline temperature and, therefore, a high CO. A large curve indicates a slow return to baseline temperature and, therefore, a low CO. A notched or uneven curve indicates poor injection technique, and the value obtained should not be accepted.

Obtaining valid CO determinations is an important nursing responsibility. There is a variety of CO systems in use, and each one requires the input of specific data. These data are loaded into the system before obtaining the first CO. Most systems require input of some or all of the following data before use.

- French size and length of the catheter (the catheter model)
- Temperature of the injectate used (iced or room temperature)
- How the injectate temperature is measured, i.e., an inline temperature probe or a bath probe
- The injectate volume selected (5 mL or 10 mL)

Some free-standing CO computers require only a single numerical constant to be dialed in before use. This constant is obtained from the package insert provided with the PA catheter. The constant is selected from a chart that considers the catheter model, the bath temperature, and the injectate volume selected.

It is important that the correct information be provided to the system before obtaining COs. If the volume or temperature of the injectate is changed during the course of hemodynamic monitoring, this information must be provided to the system, or the CO determinations will be inaccurate.

General Considerations

The volume and temperature of the injectate used to determine CO will vary according to hospital policy and patient condition. A common practice is for three sequential CO determinations to be performed using 10 mL of saline or dextrose for each determination. If one of the results varies more than 10 percent, it is rejected. The average of at least two similar values is accepted for the CO.

Selection of either room temperature or iced injectate generally is considered acceptable (according to unit policy) as long as the proper constant is used. Although there remains some controversy, research suggests that there is no significant difference between iced injectate and room temperature injectate unless the patient is hypothermic. In hypothermia, there may not be a wide enough temperature difference between the injectate and the patient's temperature to ensure accuracy.

Room temperature injectate frequently is used for the initial CO determination to allow quick evaluation. However, once the choice is made to use either iced or room temperature injectate, it should stay consistent with that patient.

Additionally, there has been debate on the importance of patient positioning and the timing of the bolus injection on the accuracy of CO results. The literature suggests that there is no significant difference in measurements as long as the transducer is at the level of the phlebostatic axis and elevation of the backrest is 45 degrees or less in the patient with normal hemodynamics and 20 degrees or less in the patient with unstable hemodynamics.

The timing of the bolus injection should coincide with the end-expiration phase of the patient's breathing cycle. This is thought to provide more consistency in the results.

For more information on injectate temperature, patient position, and timing of the bolus injection, the reader is referred to the reference list.

Section Two Review

1. The normal cardiac output is
   A. 1–4 L/minute
   B. 2–6 L/minute
   C. 4–8 L/minute
   D. 6–10 L/minute
2. The thermodilution method of CO determination is based on
   A. a blood temperature change over time
   B. the length of time it takes for dye to be circulated
   C. the temperature of the injectate
   D. the volume of the injectate

3. To increase the accuracy of CO determinations, which of the following techniques of injecting the fluid bolus is considered best?
   A. inject slowly and smoothly over 1 minute
   B. inject smoothly within a 4-second interval
   C. inject rapidly over 8 seconds
   D. intermittently inject the volume over 30 seconds
4. Failure to provide the computer with a correct computation constant will
   A. not significantly alter the CO result
   B. result in inaccurate CO determinations
   C. be compensated for by throwing out grossly abnormal values
   D. not be a problem because the computer will not work without a constant

Answers: 1, C. 2, A. 3, B. 4, B.

Section Three: Right Atrial Pressure

At the completion of this section, the learner will relate right ventricular preload to the mean right atrial pressure, recognize the normal pressure/morphology of a right atrial waveform, and identify common physical findings and nursing interventions related to abnormal right atrial pressures.

Right atrial pressure (RAP) is synonymous with central venous pressure (CVP). It is obtained from the proximal port of the PA catheter, which opens into the right atrium. The RAP is always read as a mean pressure, and the normal range is 2 to 8 mm Hg.

The importance of RAP is its use as an estimate of right ventricular preload, i.e., the volume status of the right heart. Recall from Section Two that preload

is the stretch exerted on the walls of the ventricle by the volume of blood filling the ventricle at the end of diastole. Although the blood volume in the right ventricle at the end of diastole cannot be measured, the pressure exerted by that volume can be measured. RAP then reflects the pressure in the right ventricle at the end of diastole. Also known as right ventricular end-diastolic pressure, it is abbreviated RVEDP. Measurement of the RVEDP is possible because the tricuspid valve remains open until the end of right ventricular diastole, allowing right ventricular pressure to be transmitted to the right atrium. This is why the RAP can be used to evaluate right heart preload. It is not a reliable indicator of left heart preload.

The right atrial waveform has a characteristic undulating pattern that is a result of: atrial contraction (produces the *a* wave), the bulging of the tricuspid

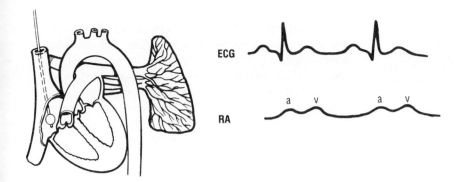

ECG

RA   a   v   a   v

Figure 6–4. A right atrial waveform (RA) with the *a* and *v* wave components identified. (*Reprinted with permission © 1991, Baxter Healthcare Corporation.*)

valve into the atria during ventricular contraction (produces the *v* wave), and passive atrial filling during ventricular systole (Figure 6–4).

The RAP and waveform can be monitored by attaching a transducer to the proximal port of the PA catheter. Simply stated, a transducer converts the pressure transmitted through the catheter into a waveform and digital readout, which can be displayed on the monitor. The RAP will be used later in the hemodynamic calculations addressed in another section of this module.

Conditions Leading to an Elevated Right Atrial Pressure

Fluid overload increases intravascular volume, and, therefore, the preload. In right heart failure, decreased contractility increases preload by causing a relative hypervolemia. The failing right ventricle just cannot empty itself well. Pulmonic stenosis, pulmonary hypertension from any cause, including chronic lung disease or pulmonary embolism, all increase the pressure the right heart has to overcome to eject blood into the PA (increased afterload). When less blood is ejected from the right ventricle into the PA, it is reflected in an increased RAP, i.e., increased right heart preload. Chronic or severe left heart failure (inadequate cardiac output) can lead to elevated RAP.

Clinical Findings

Clinical findings associated with an increased RAP vary according to the cause and duration. Signs and symptoms may include all or some of the following: distended neck veins, tachycardia, a right ventricular gallop (S3, S4, or both), right upper quadrant tenderness from liver engorgement, dependent or generalized edema.

When elevated RAP is a result of left heart failure, signs and symptoms of left ventricular failure

also will be found. These are discussed in Section Five of this module.

Intervention

Intervention for an elevated RAP is determined by the cause. In general, care is directed toward decreasing venous return to the right heart (optimizing preload), increasing right ventricular contractility, and decreasing the workload of the heart. Preload can be reduced by fluid and sodium restrictions and administration of diuretics or vasodilating medications. Contractility is enhanced with inotropic medications, such as digoxin. Nursing orders include careful and frequent assessment of the response to interventions, meticulous intake and output, daily weights, and implementation of a plan of care designed to decrease patient energy requirements. Information on special diet restrictions and medications should be provided to the patient and family.

Conditions Leading to a Low Right Atrial Pressure

A low right atrial pressure (low preload) is a result of hypovolemia or poor venous return to the heart for any reason.

Clinical Findings

Clinical findings accompanying low right heart filling pressures depend on the severity of the condition. Typical findings include tachycardia, hypotension, diminished pulse amplitude, flat neck veins, poor skin turgor, dry oral mucosa, and decreased urine output.

If right heart preload (volume) is severely reduced, the signs and symptoms of shock also will be present.

Intervention

Intervention is directed toward enhancing the pre-load status of the right ventricle. General nursing care includes continuous evaluation of the response to fluid replacement by frequent nursing assess-ments, careful intake and output measurements, and daily weights.

The RAP is an indicator of right heart preload. It is obtained from the proximal port of the PA catheter, and the normal range is 2 to 8 mm Hg. Treatment of either low or high RAP is guided by an ongoing eval-uation of the hemodynamic response to interven-tions. Nursing care consists of both collaborative and independent nursing actions. The provision of infor-mation and emotional support to the patient and family is an important nursing function.

Section Three Review

1. Right atrial pressure (RAP) is measured through which port of the PA catheter?
   A. proximal port
   B. distal port
   C. thermistor wire port
   D. balloon inflation port
2. RAP is a reflection of
   A. the pulmonary artery wedge pressure (PAWP)
   B. preload of the right heart
   C. afterload of the right heart
   D. left heart function
3. Normal mean RAP is
   A. less than 4 mm Hg
   B. 2–8 mm Hg
   C. 6–12 mm Hg
   D. 14–20 mm Hg

4. Right heart failure would result with an RAP that was
   A. lower than normal
   B. above normal
   C. within normal range
   D. unchanged
5. Hypovolemia would result with an RAP that was
   A. lower than normal
   B. above normal
   C. within normal range
   D. unchanged
6. With chronic lung disease, one would expect to find an RAP that was
   A. lower than normal
   B. above normal
   C. within normal range
   D. unchanged

Answers: 1, A. 2, B. 3, B. 4, B. 5, A. 6, B.

Section Four: Right Ventricular Pressure

At the completion of this section, the learner will recognize the normal right ventricular waveform pat-tern, state normal right ventricular pressure, and identify appropriate nursing interventions related to right ventricular waveforms.

Right ventricular (RV) pressure is obtained as a systolic/diastolic reading. The normal RV systolic pressure is 20 to 30 mm Hg. This represents the pres-sure necessary to exceed the pressure in the PA (RV afterload), open the pulmonary valve, and eject blood into the pulmonary circulation. RV diastolic pressure range is 2 to 8 mm Hg. This end-diastolic pressure directly reflects the preload status of the RV

and should approximate the right atrial pressure (RAP).

The RV waveform has a characteristic pattern. It consists of a steep upstroke and a sharp downstroke (Figure 6–5). Compare this waveform to the right atrial waveform in Figure 6–4. Although there is a marked increase in systolic pressure, the RV diastolic pressure remains essentially the same as the RAP.

The RV waveform typically is seen by the nurse on only two occasions.

1. During insertion as it is floated through the RV
2. If the catheter tip retreats from its proper position in the PA into the RV

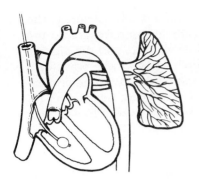

ECG

RV

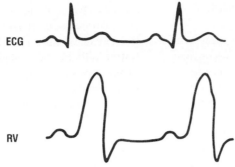

Figure 6–5. Right ventricular (RV) waveform. (*Reprinted with permission © 1991, Baxter Healthcare Corporation.*)

Irritation of the RV endothelium by the catheter tip may result in premature ventricular contractions (PVCs) or other dysrhythmias. For this reason, it is important to recognize the RV waveform and its corresponding pressures.

The cardiac rhythm and waveforms should be monitored by the nurse as the catheter is floated into the PA. Once the catheter has been properly positioned in the PA, a change to an RV waveform should be reported immediately to the physician to expedite repositioning of the catheter. Some hospitals or units have specific nursing interventions to follow when a PA catheter retreats into the RV. It is the responsibility of the nurse to be aware of unit policy related to this event. In addition to observing for dysrhythmias and notifying the physician for repositioning, some policies may instruct the RN to:

1. Pull the catheter back into the right atrium
   or

2. Inflate the balloon to foster flotation of the catheter tip back into the PA

Close observation of the cardiac rhythm is indicated whenever the catheter tip is in the RV. Once the catheter has been inserted, the exposed portion of the catheter is considered contaminated and should not be advanced unless a sterile sleeve was placed over the catheter before insertion. Use of these optional sleeves allows repositioning of the catheter without increasing the risk of infection.

RV waveforms should be seen only during insertion and removal of the catheter. The presence of the RV waveform at any other time suggests improper positioning and implies an increased risk for the development of dysrhythmias. Careful observation of the patient and the cardiac rhythm is indicated when the catheter is in the RV. The nurse is responsible for being aware of and following specific unit policy related to this situation.

Section Four Review

1. The normal range for right ventricular (RV) systolic pressure is
   A. 10–20 mm Hg
   B. 20–30 mm Hg
   C. 30–40 mm Hg
   D. 40–50 mm Hg
2. The normal range for RV diastolic pressure is
   A. 2–8 mm Hg
   B. 4–10 mm Hg
   C. 6–12 mm Hg
   D. 8–14 mm Hg

3. Select the best description of an RV waveform.
   A. soft undulating pattern
   B. steep upstroke followed by a sharp downstroke
   C. sharply notched with a slow downstroke
   D. almost flat
4. The greatest potential for dysrhythmias occurs when the PA catheter is in the
   A. superior vena cava
   B. right atrium
   C. right ventricle
   D. pulmonary artery

Answers: 1, B. 2, A. 3, B. 4, C.

Section Five: Pulmonary Artery Pressure

At the completion of this section, the learner will state normal pulmonary artery pressure, recognize the typical morphology of a pulmonary artery waveform, and identify common physical findings and nursing interventions related to abnormal pulmonary artery pressures.

Pulmonary artery pressure (PAP) is read as a systolic and diastolic pressure. It is obtained from the distal port of the PA catheter. Under normal conditions, the PAP is considered to reflect both right and left heart pressures.

The PA systolic (PAS) pressure reflects the highest pressure generated by the right ventricle during systole. The normal range is 20 to 30 mm Hg. In the absence of COPD, pulmonary embolism, mitral stenosis, and heart rates greater than 125, the PA diastolic (PAD) pressure can be used to estimate the left ventricular preload status. This is possible because there are no valves to impede the transmission of left atrial pressure to the PA. The normal range for PAD pressure is 8 to 15 mm Hg. Once the PAD pressure has been demonstrated to correlate with the pulmonary artery diastolic wedge pressure (PAWP), it can be used to follow the left ventricular preload status.

The PA waveform is always monitored continuously by a transducer attached to the distal port of the catheter. The transducer converts the pressure transmitted from the PA into an electrical signal, which is converted into waveform and digital readout that can be displayed on the monitor. The PA waveform has a characteristic pattern (Figure 6–6). It consists of a steep upstroke and a downstroke that is distinguished by a dicrotic notch formed by the closure of the pulmonic valve.

Review the RV waveform (Figure 6–5) and compare it to the PA waveform in Figure 6–6. The systolic peaks of the RV and PA waveforms are approximately equal. However, in the PA waveform, notice that the diastolic pressure (bottom of the waveform) raises, and a dicrotic notch is present on the downstroke. The dicrotic notch is formed by closure of the pulmonic valve. If the catheter tip retreats into the RV, the diastolic pressure will drop, and the dicrotic notch will be lost. Knowledge of these waveform properties allows the nurse to identify catheter position correctly. This is important because catheter retreat into the RV could result in dysrhythmias (Section Four).

Elevated Pulmonary Artery Systolic Pressure

Any condition that elevates RV systolic pressure will be reflected in an elevated PAS pressure. Examples include RV infarction and failure, pulmonary hypertension, cardiac tamponade, and chronic or severe LV failure.

Clinical Findings

Clinical findings associated with an elevated PAS pressure vary according to the cause, severity, and duration of the elevated pressure. Signs and symptoms may include all or some of the following: distended neck veins, RV gallop (S3 or S4), liver engorgement and right upper quadrant (RUQ) tenderness, and dependent or generalized edema.

Elevated Pulmonary Artery Diastolic Pressure

Conditions that affect the left heart such as angina or myocardial infarction, fluid overload, mitral stenosis, and hemodynamically significant tachycardia, are associated with a high PAD pressure.

Clinical Findings

Clinical findings associated with left heart failure may result in some or all of the following signs and

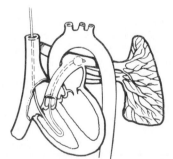

Figure 6–6. Pulmonary artery (PA) waveform. (*Reprinted with permission © 1991, Baxter Healthcare Corporation.*)

symptoms: dyspnea, tachycardia, LV gallop (S3 or S4), and bilateral crackles (rales) in the lungs. An elevated PAD pressure can result also from conditions that cause pulmonary hypertension. Validate the PAD pressure by comparing it with the PAWP before using it to follow LV function.

Intervention

Intervention for an elevated PAS or PAD pressure is determined by the cause. In general, care is directed toward reducing preload by administering diuretics and imposing fluid and sodium restrictions. When these fail, vasodilating drugs, such as nitroglycerin (Tridil) and nitroprusside (Nipride), are used. Cardiac contractility may be improved by the use of inotropic medications, such as digoxin, dobutamine, dopamine, and amrinone. Nursing care includes intake and output measurements, daily weights, positioning for comfort, and alterations in the plan of care based on an ongoing assessment of the patient's response to interventions. Care is directed also toward reducing the workload of the heart by planning activities to allow rest periods. The educational needs of the patient and family related to care, diet, medications, and activity should be incorporated into the plan of care.

Low Pulmonary Artery Diastolic Pressure

Low PAD pressure typically indicates an actual or relative hypovolemia, i.e., a low preload state related to inadequate venous return to the left heart.

Clinical Findings

Clinical findings associated with low preload states include tachycardia, flat neck veins, clear lungs, dry oral mucosa, poor skin turgor, hypotension, and decreased urine output. If severe, the signs and symptoms of advanced shock, such as cool and clammy skin, also may be seen.

Intervention

Intervention is directed toward improving LV preload through volume replacement. Nursing care includes managing fluid replacement through an ongoing assessment of the patient's hydration status and hemodynamic parameters. Daily weights and accurate intake and output records are important.

Under normal conditions, the PAS and PAD pressures provide a means for assessing both right and left heart function. Knowledge of the typical PA waveform assists the nurse to recognize incorrect catheter placement. Normal hemodynamics must be understood before abnormal ones can be explored. Integrating hemodynamic parameters with careful physical assessment findings allows the nurse to plan interventions to improve patient outcome.

Section Five Review

1. The normal range for pulmonary artery systolic (PAS) pressure is
   A. 10–20 mm Hg
   B. 20–30 mm Hg
   C. 30–40 mm Hg
   D. 40–50 mm Hg
2. The normal range for pulmonary artery diastolic (PAD) pressure is
   A. 2–8 mm Hg
   B. 4–10 mm Hg
   C. 6–12 mm Hg
   D. 8–15 mm Hg
3. Select the best description of a pulmonary artery (PA) waveform.
   A. soft undulating pattern
   B. steep upstroke followed by a sharp downstroke
   C. sharply notched upstroke with a steep downstroke
   D. steep upstroke and a downstroke distinguished by a dicrotic notch
4. Under normal conditions, a high PAD pressure suggests
   A. hypovolemia (low preload)
   B. hypervolemia (high preload)
   C. good left heart function
   D. right heart failure

5. The nurse should expect primary interventions for a PAD pressure of 2 mm Hg to be
   A. administering diuretics and implementing fluid restrictions
   B. managing and assessing the effects of volume replacement
   C. administering medications to increase contractility
   D. no intervention because 2 mm Hg is acceptable

Answers: 1, B. 2, D. 3, D. 4, B. 5, B.

Section Six: Pulmonary Artery Wedge Pressure

At the completion of this section, the learner will recognize the normal pulmonary artery wedge pattern, state normal pulmonary artery wedge pressure, relate left ventricular preload to pulmonary artery wedge pressure, and identify common physical findings and appropriate nursing interventions related to abnormal wedge pressures.

Preload is defined as the pressure or stretch exerted on the wall of the ventricle by the volume of blood filling it at end-diastole. Frank-Starling law of the heart states that the more myocardial fibers are stretched during diastole, the more they will shorten (contract) during systole and the greater will be the force of contraction until a physiologic limit has been reached. The way myocardial fibers are stretched is through preload or volume.

This concept of preload applies to both the right and left ventricle, but emphasis is placed on the left ventricle (LV) because it is the capacity of the LV to function as a pump that determines patient outcome. LV preload can be measured directly only during a cardiac catheterization. However, the pulmonary artery wedge pressure (PAWP) provides an indirect estimate of LV preload. It is obtained through the distal port of the PA catheter. The normal range is 4 to 12 mm Hg. Like the right atrial pressure (RAP), the PAWP is always read as a mean pressure.

The pulmonary artery wedge waveform (Figure 6–7) is similar in appearance to the right atrial waveform (Figure 6–4). It is an undulating waveform caused by: left atrial contraction (produces the *a* wave), bulging of the mitral valve into the left atrium during ventricular contraction (produces the *v* wave), and passive atrial filling during ventricular systole.

To obtain a wedge pressure, the catheter balloon is inflated slowly, allowing the catheter to float and wedge in a small branch of the PA. Inflation is stopped as soon as the characteristic PAWP pattern is observed (Figure 6–7). The inflated balloon stops the forward flow of blood through that vessel. The catheter tip senses the pressure in front of the balloon. Since there are no valves in the pulmonary circulation, the catheter can sense the pressure in the left atrium. Further, the mitral valve remains open until the end of diastole. This allows the left atrium and ventricle to function as one chamber until the mitral valve closes at the end of diastole. In this way, the PAWP reflects the left ventricular end-diastolic pressure (LVEDP). In the absence of mitral valve disease, the PAWP is considered an accurate estimate of left ventricular preload.

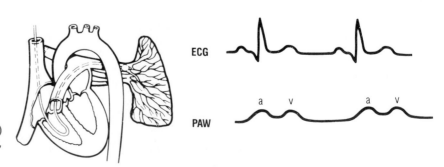

Figure 6–7. Pulmonary artery wedge (PAW) waveform. (*Reprinted with permission © 1991, Baxter Healthcare Corporation.*)

Key Points To Follow When Obtaining Pulmonary Artery Wedge Pressure

- Observe the waveform constantly during inflation, and stop inflation as soon as the PAWP is identified.
- Use the smallest inflation volume possible, and do not exceed the maximum recommended volume to reduce the risk of balloon rupture (typically ≤1.5 mL).
- Maintain inflation only long enough to obtain a stable reading.
- Allow the balloon to deflate passively to avoid damaging the balloon.

Elevated Pulmonary Artery Wedge Pressure

Any condition that increases the left ventricular end-diastolic blood volume will result in an elevated PAWP. This can occur with

- An actual fluid overload, i.e., an increased preload from hypervolemia
- A relative fluid overload, i.e., an increased preload caused by inadequate emptying of the ventricle related to poor contractility
- A stenotic aortic valve, which can impede the emptying of the ventricle (high afterload)
- A stenotic mitral valve, which creates a high left atrial pressure that is then reflected back into the pulmonary vasculature
- High systemic blood pressure, which can impede the ejection of blood from the left ventricle into the systemic circulation (high afterload)

The PAWP can be used to evaluate ventricular compliance. An elevated PAWP waveform suggests a stiff, noncompliant left ventricle that is poorly contractile.

Clinical Findings

Clinical findings related to an elevated PAWP will vary according to the degree of elevation but typically include tachycardia, exertional dyspnea, paroxysmal nocturnal dyspnea (PND), crackles (rales) in the lung fields, and an S3 or S4 gallop at the apex. Untreated, a failing left ventricle can deteriorate until the symptoms of profound cardiogenic shock are seen.

Intervention

Interventions are directed toward optimizing preload by administration of diuretics and vasodilators along with sodium and fluid restrictions. Control of dysrhythmias will help the heart to pump more effectively. Afterload, the resistance that the heart has to overcome to open the aortic valve and eject the stroke volume, is reduced by administration of vasodilators, such as nitroprusside (Nipride) and prazosin (Minipress). By dilating the peripheral vessels, these drugs reduce afterload, promote emptying of the ventricle, and effectively reduce cardiac work. Contractility is enhanced by careful titration of inotropic medications, such as digoxin, dobutamine (Dobutrex), and amrinone (Inocor). Frequent nursing assessments, meticulous intake and output records, and daily weights are crucial to follow the response to treatment. Activities should be paced to the tolerance of the patient.

Low Pulmonary Artery Wedge Pressure (Low Preload)

A low PAWP typically is related to inadequate circulating blood volume.

Clinical Findings

Clinical findings include flat neck veins, clear lungs, low pulse pressure, decreased urine output, hypotension, tachycardia, and likely complaints of thirst.

Intervention

Interventions include careful replacement of fluid or blood products by correlating the PAWP with an ongoing assessment of the patient's response to treatment. Hourly urine output, careful intake and output records, and daily weights are indicated.

Section Six Review

1. What is the normal range of the pulmonary artery wedge pressure (PAWP)?
   A. 2–10 mm Hg
   B. 4–12 mm Hg
   C. 8–16 mm Hg
   D. 10–18 mm Hg
2. Select the best description of a PAWP waveform.
   A. soft undulating pattern
   B. steep upstroke followed by a sharp downstroke
   C. sharply notched with a slow downstroke
   D. a sawtooth pattern
3. In hypovolemic states, the PAWP would be
   A. well within the normal range
   B. low normal or below normal range
   C. high normal or above the normal range
   D. high or low

4. In congestive heart failure, the PAWP would be
   A. well within the normal range
   B. low normal or below normal range
   C. high normal or above the normal range
   D. high or low
5. Which waveform most closely resembles the PAWP waveform?
   A. right atrial waveform
   B. right ventricular waveform
   C. pulmonary artery waveform
   D. systemic arterial waveform

Answers: 1, B. 2, A. 3, B. 4, C. 5, A.

Section Seven: Systemic Arterial Pressure

At the completion of this section, the learner will understand the physiology underlying the arterial waveform and identify the components of a normal arterial waveform.

Blood pressure is a function of blood flow (cardiac output) and the elasticity of the blood vessels. Systolic blood pressure normally ranges between 100 and 140 mm Hg. Systolic pressure reflects the highest pressure exerted by the left ventricle as it ejects the stroke volume into the aorta. Diastolic blood pressure normally ranges between 60 and 80 mm Hg. The mean arterial pressure (MAP) normally ranges between 70 and 90 mm Hg (Section Eight). The basic concept of blood pressure and the physiology related to an arterial waveform are the focus of this section.

Advantages of direct (invasive) blood pressure monitoring in the critically ill patient include

- Knowledge of minute to minute changes in blood pressure
- Increased accuracy of measurement in the hypotensive patient
- More precise titration of medications and fluids
- The capacity to obtain arterial blood gases and blood samples without pain and discomfort to the patient

The arterial waveform has a characteristic morphology that is related to the cardiac cycle (Figure 6–8). When the aortic valve opens, blood is ejected into the aorta. This forms a steep upstroke on the arterial waveform, called the anacrotic limb. The top of this limb represents the peak, or highest systolic pressure, which appears digitally on the monitor as the systolic pressure. After this peak pressure, the waveform descends. This descent forms the dicrotic limb and represents systolic ejection of blood that is continuing at a reduced force. The descending, or dicrotic, limb is disrupted by the dicrotic notch, which is an important point on the waveform. The dicrotic notch represents closure of the aortic valve and the beginning of ventricular diastole. The lowest portion of the waveform (baseline) represents the diastolic pressure and is reflected digitally on the monitor.

Arterial monitoring is a frequent occurrence in critical care units. The nurse typically is responsible for setting up the equipment for an arterial insertion, calibrating the equipment to ensure accurate readings, and assisting the physician with the procedure. The two most common sites for arterial monitoring are the radial artery and the femoral artery.

Once the arterial catheter is placed, the nurse is responsible for patient safety and comfort and the maintenance of the system. Securing the pressure tubing to prevent dislodgment and possible exsanguination is an important nursing responsibility. To overcome the arterial pressure and prevent the blood from backing up into the pressure tubing, a pressure bag is placed around the flush solution bag and inflated to about 300 mm Hg. Depending on hospital policy, the flush solution may or may not contain an anticoagulant, heparin or sodium citrate.

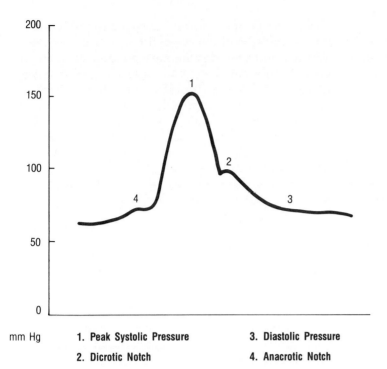

200

150

100

50

0

mm Hg

1. **Peak Systolic Pressure**   3. **Diastolic Pressure**
2. **Dicrotic Notch**   4. **Anacrotic Notch**

Figure 6–8. Components of the arterial waveform. (*Reprinted with permission © 1991, Baxter Healthcare Corporation.*)

Monitoring circulation distal to the insertion site is another important nursing function. The skin color and temperature distal to the insertion site should be assessed and documented along with the pulse at regular intervals. Any alteration in circulation should be brought to the attention of the physician promptly. The site should be observed frequently for signs of infection: redness, warmth, edema, and drainage. Specific responsibilities related to arterial monitoring usually are delineated in unit policy and procedure manuals.

Arterial monitoring provides the capacity to follow the patient's blood pressure on an almost continuous basis. Depending on specific monitor characteristics, digital blood pressure readings usually are updated at 4- to 6-second intervals. This allows the nurse to monitor the patient's response to interventions without having to disturb the patient to take a manual reading. Additionally, arterial blood gases and blood samples can be drawn without pain or discomfort to the patient.

Section Seven Review

1. The dicrotic notch on the descending limb of the arterial waveform represents
   A. opening of the aortic valve
   B. closure of the aortic valve
   C. the beginning of ventricular systole
   D. the diastolic pressure
2. The highest point on the arterial waveform denotes the
   A. anacrotic limb
   B. peak systolic pressure
   C. mean arterial pressure
   D. diastolic pressure
3. The lowest point on the arterial waveform represents the
   A. anacrotic limb
   B. peak systolic pressure
   C. mean arterial pressure
   D. diastolic pressure
4. The indentation on the descending limb of the arterial waveform is called the
   A. anacrotic limb
   B. dicrotic notch
   C. peak systolic pressure
   D. dicrotic limb

Answers: 1, B. 2, B. 3, D. 4, B.

Section Eight: Derived Parameters

At the completion of this section, the learner will understand the use and implications of selected derived hemodynamic parameters and calculate mean cardiac index, arterial pressure, and systemic vascular resistance.

Cardiac Index

As discussed in Section Two, cardiac output (CO) is the amount of blood ejected from the heart in 1 minute. The normal range is 4 to 8 L/minute. As a generic or raw value, the CO does not take the size of the patient into account. The cardiac index (CI) individualizes the CO to the patient by taking body size into consideration. Knowledge of the CO and body surface area (BSA) is all that is necessary to determine the CI. The formula is

$$CI = \frac{CO}{BSA}$$

The normal CI is 2.4 to 4.0 L/minute/m².

The BSA is simply a function of height and weight. Most monitors will calculate the BSA when the patient's height and weight have been entered. This method provides the most accurate estimate of BSA. An alternative method for obtaining the BSA is to use the DuBois body surface area chart (Figure 6–9). This chart is comprised of three columns, one listing weight, one listing height, and one with the BSA estimate. A ruler placed across the three-column chart in a manner that connects the patient's height and weight will intersect the BSA of the patient.

The following example demonstrates the importance of calculating the cardiac index.

	Patient A	Patient B
Height	6'0"	5'0"
Weight	216 lb	118 lb
BSA	2.22 m²	1.50 m²
CO	4.0 L/minute	4.0 L/minute
CI	1.89 L/minute/m²	2.4 L/minute/m²

Both patients have a CO of 4.0 L/minute, which falls within the normal range, but the CI of Patient A is well below normal and suggests a shock state. Using the CO alone would not have indicated the gravity of the patient's hemodynamic status. The CI provides meaning to the CO.

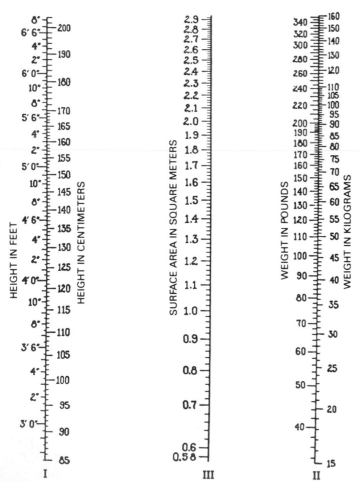

Figure 6–9. Dubois body surface chart. (By Boothby and Sandiford of the Mayo Clinic; with permission of the Mayo Foundation.)

Mean Arterial Pressure

The mean arterial pressure (MAP) is an approximation of the average pressure in the systemic circulation throughout the cardiac cycle. Normal range is 70 to 90 mm Hg. MAP is a function of CO and the resistance of the blood vessels. The MAP is provided as a digital readout when an arterial line or automatic blood pressure equipment is in use. The MAP obtained from an arterial line is the most accurate because the mean actually is measured.

When direct arterial monitoring is not available, the MAP must be calculated. Keep in mind that MAPs calculated from cuff pressures (automatic or manual) have a potential for error because of extraneous factors, such as: the wrong size cuff, differences in hearing or sensitivity of the instrument, and patient movement.

The formula for MAP reflects the components of the cardiac cycle. In normal heart rates, systole accounts for one third of the cycle and diastole comprises two thirds of the cycle.

$$MAP = \frac{(SBP + 2\ DBP)}{3}$$

Normal MAP is 70 to 90 mm Hg.

Systemic Vascular Resistance

Systemic vascular resistance (SVR) is an estimate of left ventricular afterload. Recall from Section Two that afterload is the resistance the left ventricle must overcome to open the aortic valve and eject the stroke volume into the systemic circulation. Afterload, then, is one of the primary determinants of myocardial oxygen demand. The harder the heart must work to pump blood out of the ventricle, the higher the oxygen requirements become. This is an important aspect to consider during regulation of potent vasoactive medications.

Although afterload generally is considered to be the resistance provided by the systemic vascular bed, anything that impedes ejection from the ventricle, including a stenotic aortic valve, constitutes afterload. Afterload can only be measured directly during cardiac catheterization as the aortic end-diastolic pressure (AOEDP). At the bedside, SVR is used to estimate afterload.

Most monitors will calculate the SVR. If this capacity is not available, the following formula is used for manual calculation.

$$SVR = \frac{(MAP - RAP) \times 80}{CO}$$

The SVR is expressed in dynes/second/cm^{-5}, and the normal range is 800 to 1,200 dynes/second/cm^{-5}. Like the CO, the SVR is a generic, or raw, value. To individualize it to the patient, the CI is substituted for the CO in the formula. The formula for the SVR index (SVRI) is as follows.

$$SVRI = \frac{(MAP - RAP) \times 80}{CI}$$

The normal range for the SVRI is 1,970 to 2,390 dynes/second/$cm^{-5}m^2$. The indices of CI and SVRI are far better indicators of the patient's hemodynamic status than the CO and SVR alone because the indices are referenced to body size.

Elevated Systemic Vascular Resistance

A high SVR is typically manifested by cool, pale skin resulting from constriction of the peripheral vascular bed. Intervention is determined by the cause. In hypothermia, peripheral vasoconstriction occurs as a compensatory mechanism intended to keep the central core warm. In this circumstance, warming the patient may be the only intervention necessary to dilate the constricted peripheral vasculature, normalize the SVR, and improve the CO.

Hypovolemia also results in an elevated SVR. Inadequate circulating blood volume induces several compensatory mechanisms, one of which is to induce the peripheral vascular beds to constrict. This mechanism results in the shunting of as much peripheral blood volume as possible back to the vital organs (heart, lung, and brain) to keep the patient alive. The increased SVR raises the blood pressure. Fluid or blood volume replacement should normalize the SVR.

In cardiac failure, low blood pressure initiates similar compensatory mechanisms. The peripheral vascular beds constrict in an attempt to increase the blood return to the heart and thereby increase the blood pressure. However, the increase in afterload caused by the constriction in the vascular beds makes it even more difficult for a heart that is already failing to overcome the pressure in the aorta, open the aortic valve, and eject the SV. Primary intervention for this condition is careful titration of a vasodilator medication, such as nitroprusside (Nipride) or amrinone (Inocor), which has the added effect of improving myocardial contractility in addition to reducing afterload. Careful dilatation of the vascular beds reduces the cardiac work required to overcome aortic pressure and open the aortic valve. Reducing an elevated afterload makes it easier for the heart to eject the SV, lessens cardiac work, and can improve the CO.

Low Systemic Vascular Resistance

Low SVR frequently is manifested by warm skin that may appear flushed. Conditions that generate a low SVR include septic, neurologic, and anaphylactic shock. In these conditions, mechanisms occur that initiate dilatation of the peripheral vasculature, lowering the SVR and resulting in a low blood pressure. Intervention is directed toward increasing the SVR. Norepinephrine (Levophed) and moderate to high doses of dopamine hydrochloride are two medications that can induce vasoconstriction and thereby raise the blood pressure.

The derived parameters of MAP, CI, and SVR provide important information about the cardiac sta-tus. Recall from Section Two that CO is determined by preload, afterload, and contractility. The PAWP is a preload indicator, and the SVR is an afterload in-dicator. The calculations for estimating contractility are beyond the scope of this module. Correlating he-modynamic parameters with physical assessment can assist the nurse in clinical decision making at the bedside. Integration of this knowledge can enable the nurse to provide both independent and col-laborative nursing interventions. These are the de-rived hemodynamic parameters used most com-monly. The reader is referred to a cardiac hemodynamics text for more indepth information on these and other derived parameters.

Section Eight Review

1. Normal range for the mean arterial pressure (MAP) is
   A. 60–80 mm Hg
   B. 70–90 mm Hg
   C. 80–100 mm Hg
   D. 90–110 mm Hg
2. Using the DuBois chart (Figure 6–9), determine the body surface area (BSA) for a patient who is 5'0" tall and weighs 140 pounds.
   A. 1.60
   B. 1.80
   C. 2.40
   D. 1.82
3. Using the following hemodynamic parameters: mean arterial pressure (MAP) = 90 mm Hg, right arterial pressure (RAP) = 6 mm Hg, cardiac output (CO) = 6.2 L/minute, body sur-face area (BSA) = 1.8 m², calculate the cardiac index (CI).
   A. 2.00
   B. 3.44
   C. 4.50
   D. 2.96

4. Using the hemodynamic parameters in ques-tion 3, calculate the systemic vascular resistance (SVR).
   A. 1,832 dynes/second/cm^{-5}
   B. 622 dynes/second/cm^{-5}
   C. 1,083 dynes/second/cm^{-5}
   D. 1,274 dynes/second/cm^{-5}
5. What would be the systemic vascular resistance index (SVRI)?
   A. 3,200 dynes/second/cm^{-5}m²
   B. 1,020 dynes/second/cm^{-5}m²
   C. 2,195 dynes/second/cm^{-5}m²
   D. 1,953 dynes/second/cm^{-5}m²

Answers: 1, B. 2, A. 3, B. 4, C. 5, D.

Posttest

Do not refer to the text to answer these questions.

1. In viewing a cardiac output (CO) curve, a large curve indicates
   A. a normal CO
   B. a high CO
   C. a low CO
   D. an error in technique
2. The hemodynamic measurement for right heart preload is the
   A. pulmonary artery wedge pressure
   B. pulmonary artery systolic pressure
   C. right atrial pressure
   D. cardiac output
3. It is important to recognize a right ventricular waveform because
   A. a catheter in the right ventricle can induce dysrhythmias
   B. this pattern is the one that should be monitored constantly
   C. this is the best indicator of hemodynamic status
   D. the catheter tip should be in the right ventricle at all times
4. A normal pulmonary artery pressure waveform will demonstrate the following characteristics.
   A. soft undulating pattern
   B. steep upstroke followed by a sharp downstroke
   C. sharply notched upstroke with a steep downstroke
   D. steep upstroke and a downstroke distinguished by a dicrotic notch
5. Afterload is best defined as the
   A. volume filling the ventricle at end-diastole
   B. blood ejected from the heart in 1 minute
   C. resistance to ventricular ejection
   D. ability of the cardiac muscle to contract

6. Pulmonary artery wedge pressure is the hemodynamic measurement for
   A. right ventricular preload
   B. right ventricular contractility
   C. left ventricular preload
   D. left ventricular afterload
7. The nurse would expect primary intervention for a symptomatic patient with a pulmonary artery wedge pressure of 3 mm Hg to be
   A. fluid restriction
   B. decreasing preload
   C. volume replacement
   D. decreasing afterload
8. Cardiac index (CI) is more specific than CO because
   A. CI is a direct measurement instead of an estimate
   B. CI takes the size of the patient into consideration
   C. CO can be affected by afterload
   D. CO is dependent on patient position
9. To assess the afterload status of the left ventricle, one should
   A. calculate the pulmonary vascular resistance
   B. calculate the systemic vascular resistance
   C. determine the mean arterial pressure
   D. determine the cardiac index
10. Which is the most important parameter to follow when titrating inotropic drugs on a patient with poor left ventricular function?
   A. cardiac output
   B. cardiac index
   C. mean arterial pressure
   D. right atrial pressure

Posttest Answers

Question	Answer	Section	Question	Answer	Section
1	C	Two	6	C	Six
2	C	Three	7	C	Six
3	A	Four	8	B	Eight
4	D	Five	9	B	Eight
5	C	Two	10	B	Eight
5	C	Eight			

REFERENCES

Alspach, J.G., and Williams, S.M. (1985). *Core curriculum for critical care nursing*, 3rd ed. Philadelphia: W.B. Saunders Co.

Darovic, G.O. (1987). *Hemodynamic monitoring*. Philadelphia: W.B. Saunders Co.

Shoemaker, W. (1988). *The textbook of critical care medicine*, 2nd ed. Philadelphia: W.B. Saunders Co.

ADDITIONAL READING

Cason, C.L., and Lambert, C.W. (1987). Backrest position and reference level in pulmonary artery pressure measurement. *Clin. Nurse Specialist*. 1 (4):159–165.

Chulay, M., and Miller, T. (1984). The effect of backrest elevation on pulmonary artery and pulmonary capillary wedge pressures in patients after cardiac surgery. *Heart Lung*, 13 (2):138–140.

Guyton, A.C. (1986). *Textbook of medical physiology*, 7th ed. Philadelphia: W.B. Saunders Co.

Kern, L.S. (1988). *Cardiac critical care nursing*. Rockville, Maryland: Aspen Publishers, Inc.

Laurent-Bopp, D., and Gardner, P.E. (1988). Clinical nursing research in cardiac care. In L.S. Kern (ed). *Cardiac critical care nursing*, pp. 475–476. Rockville, Maryland: Aspen Publishers, Inc.

Nemens, E.J., and Woods, S.L. (1982). Normal fluctuations in PA and PCW pressures in acutely ill patients. *Heart Lung*. 11 (5):393–398.

Quail, S.J. (1984). *Comprehensive intra-aortic balloon pumping*. St. Louis: C.V. Mosby Company.

Reidinger, M.S., and Shellock, F.G. (1984). Technical aspects of thermodilution method for measuring CO. *Heart Lung*. 13 (3):215–221.

Schermer, L. (1988). Physiologic and technical variables affecting hemodynamic measurements. *Crit. Care Nurse*. 8 (2):33–42.

Tilkian, A.G., and Daily, E.K. (1986). *Cardiovascular procedures: Diagnostic techniques and therapeutic procedures*. St. Louis: C.V. Mosby Company.

Urban, N. (1986). Integrating hemodynamic parameters with clinical decision-making. *Crit. Care Nurse*. 6 (2):33–42.

Woods, S.L., Grose, B.L., and Laurent-Bopp, D. (1982). Effect of backrest position on pulmonary artery pressures in critically ill patients. *Cardiovasc. Nurs*. 18 (4):19–24.

Module 7

Cardiac Monitoring and Related Interventions

Pamela Stinson Kidd

This module, *Cardiac Monitoring and Related Interventions,* is written at the core knowledge level for individuals who provide nursing care for acutely ill patients. It provides a basic review of common dysrhythmias. The module translates the cardiac cycle in order to promote understanding of the implications of dysrhythmias. Guidelines for electrocardiogram (ECG) interpretation are included. The module does not attempt to discuss every potential dysrhythmia a nurse may encounter in the clinical setting. Instead, it provides a systematic approach to understanding automaticity and conduction that can then be applied to practical situations. The learner must go to outside sources for additional experience in ECG interpretation. Section One discusses auto-maticity. Sections Two and Three include guidelines for interpretating ECG patterns and normal sinus rhythmn. Section Four addresses who is at risk for dysrhythmias. Section Five through Eleven cover basic dysrhythmias. Section Twelve provides a review of thrombolytic therapy. Basic pharmacology and mechanical treatment of common dysrhythmias are addressed in Sections Thirteen and Fourteen, respectively. The module ends with a summary of nursing actions for the patient requiring cardiac monitoring (Section Fifteen). It is suggested that the learner review those concepts that have been missed in the review questions before proceeding to the next section.

Objectives

Following completion of the module, *Cardiac Monitoring and Related Interventions*, the learner will be able to

1. Describe the membrane permeability changes of cardiac cells
2. Discuss the relationship between membrane permeability and serum electrolyte levels
3. Describe the normal cardiac conduction system
4. Identify common ECG patterns reflecting abnormal cardiac automaticity (sinus, atrial junctional, and ventricular origin)
5. Identify common ECG patterns reflecting abnormal cardiac conduction

6. Describe ECG patterns commonly associated with myocardial infarction
7. Discuss indications for thrombolytic therapy
8. Identify nursing responsibilities in thrombolytic therapy
9. Discuss medications frequently used in treating cardiac disturbances
10. Identify nursing responsibilities associated with cardiac pacing
11. Identify nursing responsibilities when caring for a patient being cardiac monitored

---

Pretest

1. The isoelectric line on the ECG pattern represents
   A. depolarization of cardiac cells
   B. an ectopic pacemaker
   C. the resting membrane potential
   D. cellular influx of potassium

2. Which of the following statements reflects events during the relative refractory period?
   A. there is a temporary decrease in excitability
   B. the cell can respond to a stimulus of greater intensity than normal
   C. depolarization occurs
   D. a flux of negatively charged ions out of the cell occurs

3. Failure to sense means that an artificial pacing device is
   A. not producing depolarization
   B. competing with the patient's own rhythm
   C. allowing ectopic beats to occur
   D. producing conduction delays

4. Digitalis glycosides may do all of the following EXCEPT
   A. increase the heart's sensitivity to electrical shock
   B. slow impulse conduction
   C. decrease automaticity
   D. block the effect of catecholamines

5. P waves in sinus rhythms
   A. are always positively deflected
   B. should precede the QRS complex
   C. are 0.08 seconds in length
   D. are followed immediately by a T wave

6. Hyperkalemia produces
   A. tall, peaked T waves
   B. absent T waves
   C. flat T waves
   D. inverted T waves

7. Junctional rhythms commonly occur
   A. as a protective mechanism in SA node abnormalities
   B. in response to ventricular escape beats
   C. as an indication of reperfusion in thrombolytic therapy
   D. when a pacing device fails to capture

8. In a fast-paced rhythm (greater than 100 beats per minute), which of the following is the most plausible?
   A. parasympathetic nervous system is stimulated
   B. AV node is pacing the heart
   C. ventricular conduction is slowed
   D. decreased cardiac output may occur

9. Sinus dysrhythmias are usually
   A. warning signs of impending heart failure
   B. life threatening
   C. harmless
   D. related to chronic coronary problems

10. The main difference between ventricular tachycardia and ventricular fibrillation is
    A. absence of P waves
    B. regularity of R to R interval
    C. widening of the QRS complex
    D. lengthening of the PR interval

11. Supraventricular tachycardia is
    A. produced by a ventricular pacemaker
    B. the result of delayed atrioventricular conduction
    C. produced by a pacemaker above the ventricles
    D. associated with sympathetic response to pain

12. The ventricular rate in atrial flutter is
    A. greater than 250 beats per minute
    B. dependent on the number of impulses that pass through the AV node
    C. regular
    D. greater than the atrial rate

13. In ventricular tachycardia, the
    A. P waves are inverted
    B. QRS complexes are less than 0.12 seconds
    C. R to R interval is irregular
    D. P waves are buried in the QRS complexes

14. The difference between type I and type II second degree heart block is
    A. dropping of a QRS complex
    B. rate of the rhythm
    C. progressive lengthening of the PR interval
    D. widening of the QRS complex

15. Premature ventricular contractions (PVCs) may be treated in all of the following circumstances EXCEPT when
    A. the patient is asymptomatic
    B. they occur in a couplet only
    C. they occur from multiple sites
    D. they occur in a bigeminy pattern

16. Complete heart block is characterized by
    A. lengthening of the PR interval
    B. dropping of the QRS complex
    C. regular P to P and R to R intervals
    D. QRS complexes greater than 0.12 seconds

17. Which of the following individuals would be eligible for thrombolytic therapy?
    A. 90-year-old with chest pain of 3 hours duration
    B. 65-year-old with chest pain relieved by three nitroglycerin tablets
    C. 60-year-old with chest pain of 2 hours duration
    D. 80-year-old with ST elevation in two contiguous leads
18. An elevated ST segment suggests
    A. ventricular irritability
    B. impaired ventricular depolarization
    C. impaired atrial depolarization
    D. impaired ventricular repolarization

19. Which of the following ECG changes usually are present in myocardial infarction?
    A. T wave and ST segment changes
    B. P wave changes
    C. lengthening of the PR and ST segments
    D. premature ventricular contractions (PVCs)
20. Tissue plasminogen activator (TPA) may produce which of the following complications?
    A. anaphylaxis
    B. hives
    C. hematuria
    D. vomiting

Pretest answers: 1, C. 2, B. 3, B. 4, D. 5, B. 6, A. 7, A. 8, D. 9, C. 10, B. 11, C. 12, B. 13, D. 14, C. 15, A. 16, C. 17, C. 18, D. 19, A. 20, C.

Glossary

Absolute refractory period. The period after an action potential when a stimulus cannot produce a second action potential no matter how strong the stimulus is

Action potential. Signal produced from rapid change in membrane permeability that is transmitted from one part of the nerve or muscle cell to another

Automaticity. Ability to initiate an impulse

Bigeminy. A cardiac rhythm of one SA node-generated beat followed by one premature ventricular contraction

Cardioversion. A synchronized direct current electrical countershock that depolarizes all the cells simultaneously, allowing the SA node to resume the pacemaker role

Compensatory pause. A pause produced by suppression of the SA node by a premature beat (In a compensatory pause, the next P wave following the premature beat occurs on time as if it was not affected by the premature beat. If the suppression is for a prolonged period, the next P wave will be delayed (noncompensatory pause). Thus, the P to P interval between the premature beat and the normal beat is longer than the P to P interval between two normal beats.)

Conductivity. The ability of a cell to carry or transport an impulse

Contractility. The ability of a muscle to shorten when stimulated, in particular, the force of myocardial contraction

Defibrillation. An unsynchronized direct current electrical countershock that depolarizes all the cells simultaneously, allowing the SA node to resume the pacemaker role

Depolarization. A state where the membrane potential is less negative than the resting membrane potential

Ectopic. Extra heartbeat initiated by a focus other than the SA node

Excitability. Ability to respond to an impulse

Excitation–contraction coupling. Linking of the electrical and mechanical events in the heart; each individual myocardial cell is stimulated to contract sequentially so that contraction of the atria is followed by contraction of the ventricles

Fast response action potential. Action potential of a myocardial working cell. Created by a more negative resting membrane potential, which encourages the rapid entry of sodium into the cell

Isoelectric. Occurs when the muscle is completely polarized or depolarized; no potential is recorded on the ECG

Plateau phase. Part of the repolarization when the calcium channels open to allow movement of calcium into the cell to help maintain the cell in a depolarized state

Relative refractory period. The period after an action potential when a stimulus can produce a second action potential if the stimulus is greater than threshold level

Repolarization. Return of the cellular membrane to its resting membrane potential

Resting membrane potential. Point at the end of repolarization when the membrane is relatively permeable to potassium but is almost impermeable to sodium; thus, intracellular concentration of potassium is greater than extracellular concentration

Sarcolemma. Cell membrane of a muscle fiber

Slow response action potential. Action potential of a pacemaker cell characterized by the slow movement of sodium into the cell because the sarcolemma is permeable to sodium ions

Supranormal period. The period after an action potential during which a stimulus that is slightly less than normal can precipitate another action potential

Trigeminy. A cardiac rhythm of two SA node-generated beats followed by one premature ventricular contraction

---

Abbreviations

AV node. Atrioventricular node

APSAC. Anisoylated plasminogen streptokinase activator complex

CPK. Creatine phosphokinase

ECG. Electrocardiogram

mV. Millivolts

PAC. Premature atrial contraction

PTCA. Percutaneous transluminal coronary angioplasty

PVC. Premature ventricular contraction

SA node. Sinoatrial node

TPA. Tissue plasminogen activator

Section One: Membrane Permeability

At the completion of this section, the learner will be able to briefly explain membrane permeability changes in cardiac cells.

The resting membrane potential of cardiac cells is represented by an isoelectric line on the ECG pattern. There is no deflection, since there is no movement of ions across the sarcolemma. Normally, the intracellular concentration of potassium is greater than the extracellular concentration (Kemp and Dolan, 1991). The concentration of sodium ions is greater extracellularly. The intracellular potential becomes increasingly negative because potassium diffuses externally. In addition, proteins and phosphates remain internally, and they are negatively charged. Polarization occurs when enough potassium has diffused to create a cell net charge of −90 mV (Guyton, 1986).

There are five phases of an action potential: depolarization (phase 0), early repolarization (phase 1), plateau phase (phase 2), repolarization (phase 3), and resting membrane potential (phase 4). During depolarization, the cell is almost impermeable to sodium unless a stimulus occurs. This stimulus may be electrical in origin, such as the firing of the sinoatrial (SA) node or defibrillation. Chemical changes also may precipitate depolarization. Hypoxia and its ac-

companying respiratory acidosis as well as pharmaceutical agents (i.e., sodium bicarbonate) may serve as chemical stimuli. In depolarization, more sodium moves into the cell through the fast sodium channels and creates a fast response action potential. The inside of the cell becomes positively charged.

The process of repolarization takes place over phases 1, 2, and 3. In early repolarization, sodium channels close. During the plateau phase, calcium channels open. These channels are slow in relation to the preceding sodium channels. The influx of calcium helps to maintain the positive charge (depolarization) a little longer. Chemical blockage of the channels may be used to treat cardiac abnormalities (Section Thirteen). In phase 3, repolarization, potassium moves back into the cell to create the original electrochemical gradient.

During the resting membrane potential phase (phase 4), repolarization is completed, and the original electrochemical gradient is in place. The cell is ready to be depolarized again. The absolute refractory period begins in phase 0 and lasts until the midpoint of phase 3. During this period, the cell cannot respond to another stimulus regardless of the strength of the stimulus. The relative refractory period begins at the midpoint of phase 3 and lasts until the beginning of phase 4. A stronger than normal stimulus may produce depolarization. During

TABLE 7–1. PHASES OF AN ACTION POTENTIAL

Phase 0	Depolarization	Movement of sodium into cell (fast channels open)
Phase 1	Early repolarization	Closure of fast sodium channels
Phase 2	Plateau	Calcium moves into cell (slow channels open)
Phase 3	Repolarization	Potassium moves into cell
Phase 4	Resting membrane potential	Electrochemical gradient returned to normal Sarcolemma almost impermeable to sodium

the supranormal period (phase 4), a weaker than normal stimulus can produce depolarization. A common example of a stimulus producing depolarization during the supranormal or relative refractory period is premature atrial and ventricular beats. These are discussed later in the module. Table 7–1 summarizes the phases of the action potential.

In summary, it is helpful to remember that sodium, calcium, and potassium always are located both intracellularly and extracellularly. The total of these electrolytes remains the same. The action potential changes where the total is distributed, at the location of the ions. Figure 7–1 depicts the ion changes throughout the action potential.

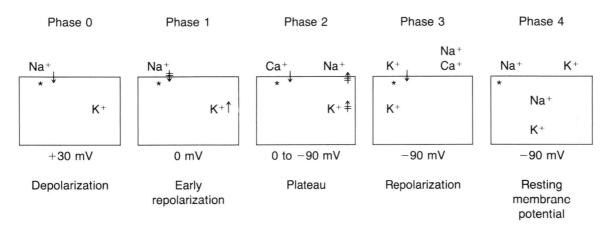

Figure 7–1. Membrane permeability changes. Cell membrane permeability changes throughout depolarization and repolarization. * = protein⁻, phosphate⁻; ↑ ↓ = rapid; ⧺ ⧻ = slow.

Section One Review

1. Depolarization may occur in direct response to all of the following EXCEPT
   A. chemical stimuli
   B. acidosis
   C. defibrillation
   D. hyperglycemia
2. Potassium is located primarily
   A. intracellularly
   B. in skeletal muscle
   C. extracellularly
   D. in cardiac muscle
3. During the relative refractory period
   A. a larger than normal stimulus occurs
   B. the SA node fires
   C. depolarization may occur
   D. the cardiac cell is not able to be stimulated

4. The three major electrolytes associated with automaticity are
   A. sodium, potassium, and calcium
   B. potassium, glucose, and sodium
   C. calcium, phosphate, and proteins
   D. potassium, calcium, and phosphate
5. The movement of calcium into the cell promotes
   A. depolarization
   B. repolarization
   C. the refractory period
   D. closure of the slow channels

Answers: 1, D. 2, A. 3, C. 4, A. 5, A.

Section Two: Cardiac Conduction

At the completion of this section, the learner will be able to describe the cardiac conduction system and the normal ECG complex.

There are two types of myocardial cells, working cells and pacemaker cells. Pacemaker cells have a slow response action potential. The resting membrane potential of pacemaker cells is unstable, and the cell membrane is somewhat permeable to sodium. The slow diffusion of sodium into the cell precipitates depolarization without a preceding impulse. Only pacemaker cells possess automaticity or the ability to initiate an impulse. Conversely, the working cells have a stable resting membrane potential. In order for depolarization to occur, a stimulus must be present. Working cells are responsible for contractility. Both working and pacemaker cells have the ability to respond to stimuli (excitability) and regularity (rhythmicity) and to conduct impulses (Toledo and Dolan, 1991).

The sinoatrial (SA) node is considered to be the pacemaker of the heart, since it controls the heart rate normally between 60 and 100 beats per minute (bpm). When abnormalities occur with the firing of the SA node, another cardiac cell will discharge. An ectopic pacemaker is a new site of impulse formation within the heart (Meltzer et al, 1983). The impulse is transmitted from the atria to the ventricles along a cardiac conduction pathway (Figure 7–2). Myocardial contraction occurs when the ventricular muscle is stimulated. The combined events of depolarization and repolarization comprise the electrical phases of the cardiac cycle.

The normal ECG complex consists of several components. The P wave indicates atrial depolarization, firing of the SA node. The PR interval depicts atrial conduction of the impulse, through the AV node to the ventricles. The normal length of the PR interval is 0.12 to 0.20 second. A longer PR interval suggests a conduction delay usually in the area of the AV node.

The QRS complex reflects ventricular depolarization and atrial repolarization. The atrial repolarization is overpowered by the ventricular depolarization because the ventricular muscle mass is larger than that of the atria. Therefore, atrial repolarization is not seen on the ECG. QRS complexes may be of various sizes and configurations. Figure 7–3 illustrates common QRS configurations. The QRS segment is less than 0.12 second in length. A prolonged QRS complex indicates abnormal impulse conduction through the ventricles.

The ST segment demonstrates ventricular conduction. It represents the completion of ventricular depolarization and the beginning of ventricular re-

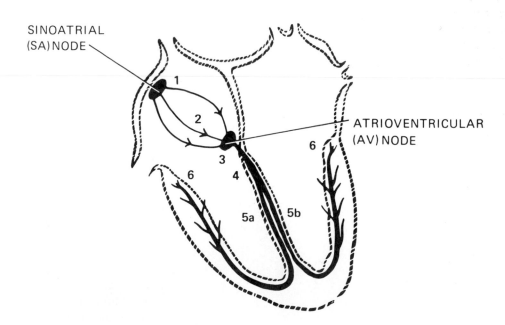

Figure 7–2. Conduction system of the heart. The impulse originates in the SA node (1). It spreads through the atrial muscles along three bands of tissue known as the internodal tracts (2), causing atrial contraction. It reaches the AV node (3), where it is momentarily slowed before passing on to the bundle of His (4). The impulse descends through the bundle of His and down the right and left bundle branches (5a, 5b). Reaching the terminal Purkinje fibers (6), the impulse stimulates the ventricular myocardial cells at the Purkinje–myocardial junction. Ventricular contraction then occurs. (*From* Intensive coronary care: A manual for nurses, *p. 116, by L. Meltzer et al, 1983, Bowie, MD: Brady Co.*)

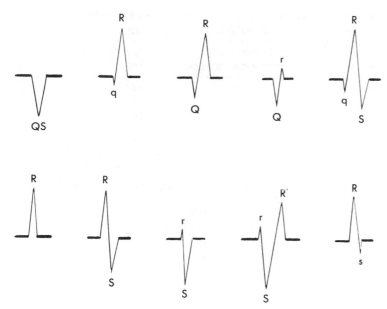

Figure 7–3. Common QRS complex configurations. (*From Clinical electrocardiography: A simplified approach, ed. 3, by A. L. Goldberger and E. Goldberg, 1986, St. Louis: CV Mosby.*)

polarization. The segment should be isoelectric, with no deflections present, because positive and negative charges are balanced. Deflections in the ST segment usually indicate ventricular muscle injury. The T wave depicts ventricular repolarization. T waves also are affected by ventricular muscle injury because of interference with repolarization. An example of a clinical condition with potential ventricular muscle injury is acute myocardial infarction.

The QT interval represents ventricular depolarization and repolarization. It is measured from the beginning of the QRS complex to the end of the T wave. The QT interval is usually less than 0.40 second in length, depending on heart rate. As heart rate increases, the QT interval will shorten. If the heart rate decreases, the QT interval will lengthen.

Electrical transmission can be connected with mechanical events of the heart. Diastole occurs during atrial depolarization and at the end of ventricular repolarization. This is depicted by the end of the T wave to the R wave on the ECG. Systole begins at the peak of the QRS complex (ventricular depolarization) and continues to the end of the T wave (ventricular repolarization). This relationship helps to explain why cardiac output is affected when a dysrhythmia occurs. Figure 7–4 illustrates the relationship between the ECG and the cardiac cycle.

To summarize, the ECG reflects the cardiac conduction pathway. Abnormalities in conduction will appear on the ECG. The cardiac cycle depends on proper electrical transmission and conduction in order to maintain an adequate cardiac output. The nor-

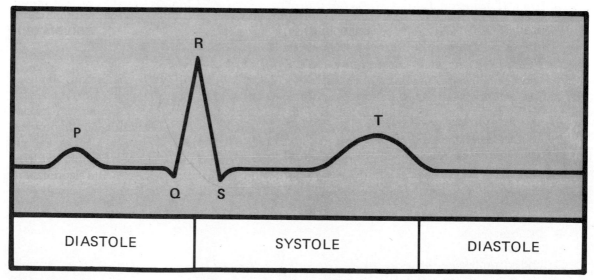

Figure 7–4. Relationship between ECG and cardiac cycle. Relationship of electrocardiogram to diastole and systole. (*From Intensive coronary care: A manual for nurses, p. 124, by L. Meltzer et al, 1983, Bowie, MD: Brady Co.*)

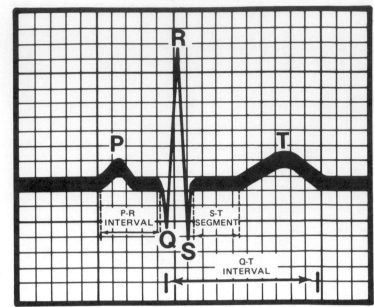

Figure 7–5. Normal electrocardiogram. (*From* Intensive Coronary Care: A Manual for Nurses, *p. 123, by L. Meltzer et al, 1983, Bowie, MD: Brady Co.*)

mal ECG (normal sinus rhythm) has a rate between 60 and 100 bpm. The SA node paces the rhythmn (P wave), and the impulse is transmitted to the ventricles within 0.20 second (PR interval). The ventricles depolarize, representing contraction or systole, within 0.12 second. The complete sequence of ventricular events occur within 0.40 second (QT interval). Figure 7–5 is a diagram of a normal ECG.

Section Two Review

1. Abnormalities in the firing of the SA node usually
   A. result in cardiac arrest
   B. result in the discharging of another pacemaker cell
   C. produce tachydysrhythmias
   D. result in heart blocks
2. A PR interval greater than 0.20 second
   A. is normal
   B. indicates a pacemaker other than the SA node is firing
   C. indicates a delay in conduction
   D. is too fast to maintain adequate cardiac output
3. Atrial repolarization is reflected in the
   A. P wave
   B. PR interval
   C. T wave
   D. QRS complex

4. The QT interval indicates all of the following EXCEPT
   A. atrial recovery
   B. ventricular depolarization
   C. ventricular recovery
   D. atrial depolarization
5. Systole is associated with
   A. ventricular depolarization
   B. atrial depolarization
   C. AV nodal conduction
   D. P wave on the ECG

Answers: 1, B. 2, C. 3, D. 4, D. 5, A.

Section Three: Interpretation Guidelines

At the completion of this section, the learner will be able to identify a system for interpreting ECG patterns.

The ECG is printed on graph paper. Each small block of the graph paper is equal to 1 mm, or 0.04 second on the horizontal axis. The horizontal axis of the graph paper represents time. The vertical axis of the graph paper represents contractility. Each small block is equivalent to 1 mV on the vertical axis. For the purposes of basic ECG interpretation, time is the most important factor to consider. Since each small block equals 0.04 second, a large block, comprised of five small blocks equals 0.20 second. Five large blocks comprise 1 second.

There are six steps to follow in interpreting an ECG.

1. Measure the rate
2. Examine the R to R interval
3. Examine the P wave
4. Measure the PR interval
5. Check to see if P waves are followed by a QRS complex
6. Examine the QRS complex

There are three ways the rate can be calculated. The first two methods discussed can be used only when the rate is regular. The number of 0.04-second boxes can be counted between two R waves and divided into 1,500. The number of 0.20-second boxes can be counted between two R waves and divided into 300. The last method is based on a 6-second cardiac strip. ECG paper is marked at the top margin in 3-second intervals. The number of R waves in a 6-second strip (30 large blocks, 150 small blocks) is multiplied by 10 to get the heart rate by minute (6 × 10 = 60 seconds). Figure 7–6 demonstrates all three methods of rate calculation.

Next, the R waves should be examined. If the R waves appear in regular intervals (are constant), the rhythm is described as a regular rhythm. If the R waves do not occur in a regular pattern, a dysrhythmia is present.

Normally, P waves precede each QRS complex. If P waves are absent, one of two things may be occurring. If the atria are firing fast and chaotically, the P waves are replaced by irregular, rapid oscillations. This condition is known as atrial fibrillation (Section Six). If the SA node is not serving as pacemaker and another cell below the SA node is serving as the pacemaker, P waves are absent. Cardiac cells in the area of the AV node can pace the heart at a rate of 40 to 60 bpm. Pacemaker cells in the Purkinje fibers and ventricles pace at a rate less than 40 bpm. Generally, if the atria are discharging chaotically, the rate will be greater than 60 bpm. If the atria are not discharging and the pacer is outside the SA node, the rate will be less than 60 bpm.

The next step in ECG interpretation is to measure the PR interval. If it is greater than 0.20 second in length, a delay in conduction is present. For example, first degree heart block (Section Ten) is a condition in which the PR interval is prolonged but of constant length. QRS complexes are always present.

Next, check to see if P waves are followed by a QRS complex. If P waves are present but they are not followed consistently by a QRS complex, a second or third degree heart block (Section Ten) may be present.

The final step is examination of the QRS complexes. The complex should be less than 0.12 second in length unless there is a delay in the impulse reaching the ventricles. A widening of the QRS complex encourages spontaneous firing of ventricular ectopic pacemakers (premature ventricular complexes) (Section Nine) as an inefficient compensation to maintain systole and thus cardiac output.

Figure 7–7 illustrates the application of the principles discussed in this section. Each ECG tracing is like a fingerprint. No two are alike, but the system for analyzing the tracing is the same. The system outlined in this section should provide a consistent and comprehensive approach to ECG interpretation.

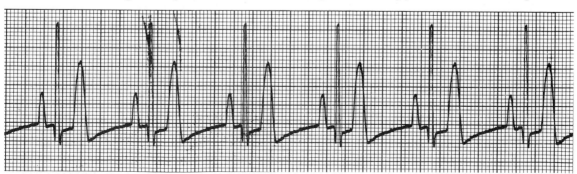

Figure 7–6. Calculation of heart rate. Method one: Using 0.04-second boxes between R waves: 24 (0.04) boxes: 1,500 divided by 24 = 63 bpm. Method two: Using 0.20-second boxes between R waves: 4.5 (0.20) boxes: 300 divided by 4.5 = 66 bpm. Method three: Number of R waves in a 6-second strip = 6: 6 times 10 = 60 bpm.

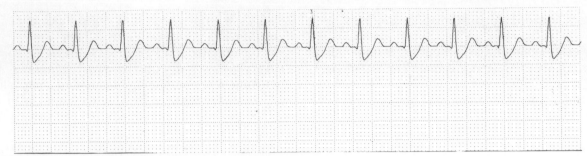

Figure 7–7. Interpretation of ECG using six-step process.

1. Measure the rate. There are 12 R waves in the 6-second strip:

$12 \times 10 = 120$. There are 12 small boxes (0.04) between two R waves: $\dfrac{1500}{12} = 125$

There are approximately 2.5 large boxes (0.20) between two R waves: $\dfrac{300}{2.5} = 120$

2. Examine the R to R interval. The interval is regular; therefore, the rhythm is regular.
3. Examine the P wave. The P waves are the same configuration.
4. Measure the PR interval. The interval is constant and measures 4 small boxes (0.4) or 16 seconds.
5. Check to see if the P waves are followed by a QRS complex. P waves are followed by QRS complex.
6. Examine the QRS complex. The complexes are the same configuration and measures 2 small boxes (0.04) or 8 seconds.

Section Three Review

1. Using the small block method (0.04 second), the heart rate in the ECG in Figure 7–8 would be
   A. 76
   B. 85
   C. 80
   D. 72
2. Using the large block method (0.20 second), the heart rate in the ECG in Figure 7–9 would be
   A. 35
   B. 30
   C. 40
   D. 45

3. Using the number of R waves in a 6-second strip method, the heart rate in the ECG in Figure 7–10 would be
   A. 120
   B. 140
   C. 130
   D. 70
4. The QRS complex should
   A. be greater than 0.12 second
   B. precede the P wave
   C. differ in configuration
   D. precede the T wave

Answers: 1, A. 2, B. 3, A. 4, D.

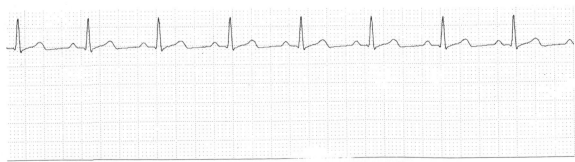

Figure 7–8. Normal sinus rhythm rate equals 1500 divided by 19×0.04-second boxes = 76.

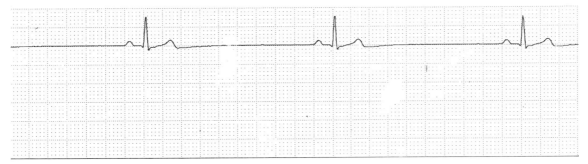

Figure 7–9. Sinus bradycardia rate equals 300 divided by 10 × 0.20-second boxes = 30.

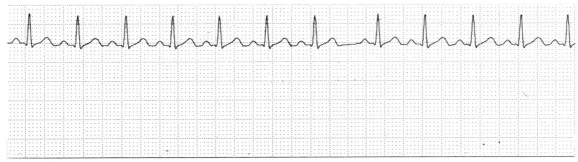

Figure 7–10. The sinus tachycardia rate equals 12 R waves × 10 = 120.

Section Four: At Risk Factors

At the completion of this section, the learner should be able to identify factors that place a person at risk for developing dysrhythmias.

Anyone who has an alteration in tissue perfusion is at risk for a dysrhythmia. The alteration may be peripheral in nature, as in chronic hypertension. The increased afterload or resistance the heart must pump against in order to maintain an adequate cardiac output (CO) eventually produces ventricular enlargement and decreased contractility (Starling's law). The heart rate will try to increase as a way of maintaining CO, since the stroke volume (SV) is diminished. An alteration in cardiac perfusion due to coronary artery disease predisposes to dysrhythmias because of potential myocardial ischemia. The ventricles will not be able to depolarize as effectively (QRS complex), and repolarization may be inefficient (T wave). Thus, abnormal ventricular beats or blocks in conduction may occur.

A fluid volume deficit encourages the appearance of tachydysrhythmias. The heart rate increases again in response to a diminished CO. Fluid volume overload eventually will result in ventricular enlargement and decreased contractility. Premature beats, cardiac conduction blocks, and abnormalities in heart rate may appear in response to the excess fluid volume.

Electrolyte abnormalities place a person at risk for dysrhythmias. Hypokalemia decreases the amount of positive ions available to produce depolarization. Depolarization becomes more difficult and repolarization is extended. Therefore, the PR interval may be longer, and the T wave may be flat. An extra wave may follow the T wave (U wave). Bradydysrhythmias and conduction blocks are common. Premature ventricular contractions (PVCs) may occur if the heart rate is too slow. Hyperkalemia produces easier depolarization and short repolarization. Tall, peaked T waves are present. Eventually the cell becomes too positive to respond and depolarize, and asystole occurs. Before asystole, the PR interval lengthens, and the QRS complex widens.

Calcium works in combination with sodium. Hypocalcemia allows more sodium to enter the cell, since a positive intracellular charge must be obtained for depolarization to occur. The sodium enters the cell in an uncontrolled fashion, producing tetany or spontaneous and continuous depolarization. Tachydysrhythmias occur, leading to cardiac arrest as a result of cellular exhaustion. Hypercalcemia repels sodium. Both ions tend to remain extracellularly, decreasing neuromuscular excitability. Depolarization is delayed because the cell remains negatively charged. Bradydysrhythmias and conduction blocks occur.

Magnesium is required for intracellular enzyme reactions. A deficit of magnesium will increase the irritability of the nervous system and can produce dysrhythmias (Guyton, 1986). Hypermagnesemia is associated with renal failure. Central nervous system depression results. The ECG may demonstrate a prolonged PR interval, wide QRS complexes, and bradycardia (Thelan et al, 1990).

In summary, a person may be at risk for developing cardiac dysrhythmias if an alteration in tissue perfusion, fluid volume, or electrolyte values is present.

Section Four Review

1. Increased afterload increases the risk for dysrhythmias because
   A. it increases automaticity
   B. increasing pressure stimulates ectopic pacemakers
   C. it delays cardiac conduction
   D. it produces an influx of potassium ions
2. Excess fluid volume increases the risk for dysrhythmias because
   A. it increases automaticity
   B. it decreases contractility
   C. it increases cardiac conduction
   D. it produces an influx of sodium ions
3. Hypokalemia results in
   A. delayed conduction
   B. increased automaticity
   C. widened QRS complexes
   D. inverted P waves

4. Hypocalcemia results in
   A. decreased sodium influx into the cell
   B. delayed repolarization
   C. spontaneous depolarization
   D. spontaneous conduction
5. Hypermagnesemia may produce
   A. tachydysrhythmias
   B. bradycardia
   C. shortened PR intervals
   D. ST segment depression

Answers: 1, A. 2, B. 3, A. 4, C. 5, B.

Section Five: Sinus Dysrhythmias

At the completion of this section, the learner will be able to describe common dysrhythmias arising from the SA node and their treatment.

Sinus bradycardia is described as less than 60 bpm and originating from the SA node, as evidenced by a regular P wave preceding each QRS complex. The only abnormality noted in this rhythm is the rate. This rhythm may be present in athletes because they have improved their cardiac muscle and thus their stroke volume (SV). The heart rate can decrease and still maintain an efficient CO. Sinus bradycardia may not be treated unless the person experiences symptoms of decreased CO, such as syncope, hypotension, and angina. If the rate drops too low, the chance of ectopic pacemakers firing increases. Lethal ventricular dysrhythmias may result. Sinus bradycardia is treated by administering atropine because it blocks the parasympathetic innervation to the SA node, allowing normal sympathetic innervation to gain control and increase SA node firing. Figure 7–11 illustrates sinus bradycardia.

Sinus tachycardia has a rapid rate ranging from 100 to 150 bpm. There are no other abnormal characteristics associated with this rhythm. The rapid rate results from sympathetic nervous stimulation. This stimulation may be in response to fear, increased activity, hypermetabolic states (such as fever), pain, and decreased CO due to hypovolemia or ventricular failure. Sinus tachycardia may produce angina if the CO decreases to the point of decreasing coronary circulation if myocardial oxygen demand is increased without an increase in coronary circulation. Treatment is aimed at relieving the cause of increased sympathetic stimulation. Nursing measures, such as

TABLE 7–2. SUMMARY OF DIFFERENCES IN SINUS DYSRHYTHMIAS

Rhythm	Characteristics	Treatment Strategies
Sinus bradycardia	Rate less than 60 bpm	Atropine
Sinus tachycardia	Rate greater than 100 bpm	Antianxiety measures Pain relief measures Antipyretics Oxygen Digitalis

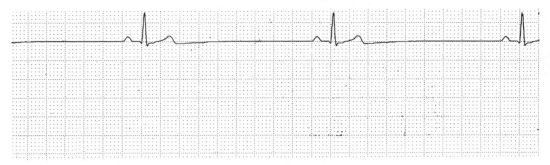

Figure 7–11. Interpretation of sinus bradycardia using the six-step process.
1. Rate = 30
2. R to R interval regular
3. P wave has same configuration
4. PR interval = 0.20
5. P wave precedes QRS: yes
6. QRS complex = 0.04

imagery, distraction, and promoting a calm environment, as well as drug therapy may be necessary. Sedatives, tranquilizers, antianxiety agents, analgesics, and antipyretics may be used. Figure 7–12 is an ECG tracing of sinus tachycardia.

In summary, sinus dysrhythmias are characterized by regular rates. They usually are harmless unless CO becomes compromised. The nurse should assess the patient for signs of decreasing level of consciousness, hypotension, and angina. When these symptoms occur, the dysrhythmia is treated. Table 7–2 compares sinus dysrhythmias.

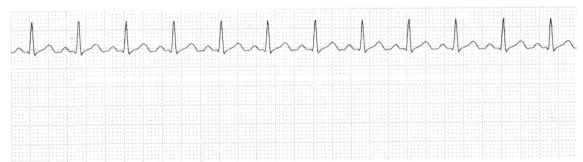

Figure 7–12. Interpretation of sinus tachycardia using the six-step process.
1. Rate = 120
2. R to R interval regular
3. P wave has same configuration
4. PR interval = 0.12
5. P wave precedes QRS: yes
6. QRS complex = 0.04

Section Five Review

1. Sinus bradycardia originates from
   A. delayed AV conduction
   B. AV nodal area
   C. Purkinje fibers
   D. SA node

2. Atropine is used to treat sinus bradycardia because it
   A. inhibits the AV node
   B. stimulates the sympathetic nervous system
   C. blocks the parasympathetic nervous system
   D. enhances ventricular conduction

3. Sinus tachycardia may result from all the following EXCEPT
   A. parasympathetic stimulation
   B. anxiety
   C. pain
   D. fever

4. Decreasing level of consciousness associated with sinus tachycardia indicates
   A. decreased ventricular contractility
   B. decreased cardiac output
   C. increased atrial filling
   D. decreased AV conduction

Answers: 1, D. 2, C. 3, A. 4, B.

Section Six: Atrial Dysrhythmias

At the completion of Section Six, the learner will be able to identify basic atrial dysrhythmias.

Common atrial dysrhythmias are supraventricular tachycardia, atrial flutter, and atrial fibrillation. Each of these dysrhythmias is characterized by a rapid rate. Most patients describe a fluttering sensation in the chest, dyspnea, lightheadedness, or angina when experiencing these dysrhythmias. The rapid heart rate decreases ventricular filling time and CO.

Supraventricular tachycardia has a rate between 150 and 250 bpm. The rhythm is regular, but P waves are not distinguishable, since they are buried in the preceding T wave. The QRS complex appears normal because ventricular conduction is not affected. Normal QRS complexes indicate that the ectopic pacemaker is located above the ventricles. The exact location may not be distinguishable without having a 12-lead ECG available. Treatment remains the same regardless of pacemaker origin. If the patient is not experiencing symptoms, drug therapy is initiated to slow the rate. Calcium blocking agents are used to prevent the influx of calcium, thus positive charges, into the cell, discouraging depolariza-

tion. Verapamil commonly is administered. Digitalis preparations, propranolol, or quinidine also may be used. In cases where the patient is experiencing distress or is unresponsive to drug therapy, cardioversion is used to rapidly correct the dysrhythmia. Figure 7–13 is an example of supraventricular tachycardia.

Atrial flutter has a faster rate than supraventricular tachycardia. The atrial rate will be greater than 250 bpm. The ventricular rate depends on the number of impulses that pass through the AV node. The ventricular rate may be irregular if some of the impulses are blocked. The atrial oscillations appear as sawtooth waves. A fast ventricular rate decreases CO in the absence of digitalis toxicity. Cardioversion is the preferred method of treating this dysrhythmia. Calcium channel blockers, beta-blocking agents, and digitalis preparations may be used (Section Thirteen). Atrial flutter is described by the number of atrial oscillations between each QRS complex (Figure 7–14).

Atrial fibrillation is a condition in which the atria are contracting so fast that they are unable to refill before ejection. Therefore, the ventricles are filled inadequately and CO is diminished. The atria are not

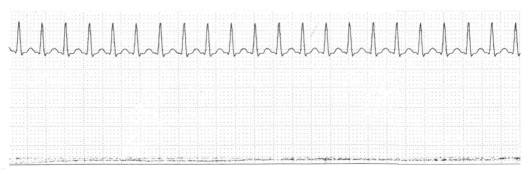

Figure 7–13. Interpretation of supraventricular tachycardia using the six-step process. (*Note:* This is not a 6-second strip.)
1. Rate = 250
2. R to R interval regular
3. P wave: difficult to distinguish
4. PR interval: cannot calculate
5. P wave precedes each QRS: cannot identify
6. QRS complex = 0.04

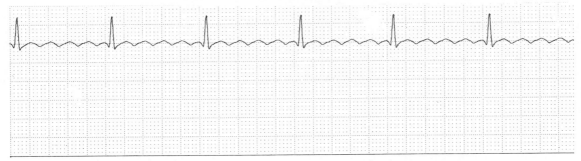

Figure 7–14. Interpretation of atrial flutter with 5.1 conduction using the six-step process.
1. Rate: atrial: unable to calculate
   ventricular = 60
2. R to R interval regular
3. P wave: cannot distinguish, flutter wave present

4. PR interval: cannot calculate
5. P wave precedes each QRS: cannot identify
6. QRS complex = 0.06

able to empty completely because of the fast rate of depolarization. Blood that remains in the atria is prone to forming clots, predisposing the person to cerebrovascular attacks.

Atrial fibrillation has an irregular ventricular response. The QRS complexes are normal in appearance but occur at irregular intervals. This is manifested clinically as a difference between the apical heart rate and the peripheral pulse rate because the SV may be inadequate with some beats to produce a peripheral pulse. The atria may be discharging at a rate greater than 400 bpm. Absent P waves and irregular QRS intervals are characteristic of this dysrhythmia. Verapamil or digitalis preparations are used to treat this disorder. Cardioversion also may be used. Atrial fibrillation may not be treated if it is of long-standing duration and does not produce symptoms. Figure 7–15 is an example of atrial fibrillation.

In summary, atrial dysrhythmias have a rapid atrial response and are characterized by absent P waves. A complication of these dysrhythmias may be decreased CO if the ventricular response also is rapid, resulting in inadequate ventricular filling. Table 7–3 compares atrial dysrhythmias.

TABLE 7–3. SUMMARY OF DIFFERENCES IN ATRIAL DYSRHYTHMIAS

Rhythm	Characteristics	Treatment Strategies
Superventricular tachycardia	R to R interval regular Atrial rate 150 to 250 bpm	Beta-blocking agents (propranolol) Calcium channel blocking agents (verapamil) Digitalis Cardioversion Overdrive pacing
Atrial flutter	R to R interval may be regular or irregular Atrial rate may be up to 350 bpm Sawtoothed waves	Cardioversion Digitalis
Atrial fibrillation	Irregular R to R interval Atrial rate greater than 350 bpm	Digitalis Cardioversion Calcium channel blocking agents (verapamil)

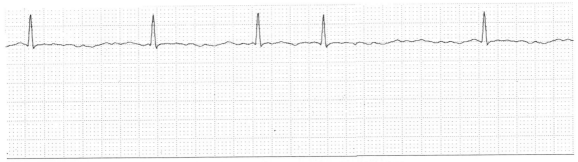

Figure 7–15. Interpretation of atrial fibrillation using the six-step process.
1. Rate: atrial: unable to calculate
   ventricular = 50
2. R to R interval irregular
3. P wave: undistinguishable

4. PR interval: cannot calculate
5. P wave precedes each QRS: cannot identify
6. QRS complex = 0.06

Section Six Review

1. Atrial dysrhythmias produce symptoms of lightheadedness or angina because
   A. cardiac output is decreased
   B. ventricular conduction is delayed
   C. SA node is competing for pacemaker status
   D. coronary vasodilation occurs
2. Verapamil may be used to treat supraventricular tachycardia because it
   A. increases AV conduction
   B. prevents influx of calcium into the cell
   C. prolongs repolarization
   D. blocks potassium movement extracellularly

3. Atrial fibrillation predisposes a person to a cerebrovascular attack because it produces
   A. cardiac fatigue
   B. inadequate emptying of the atria
   C. ventricular exhaustion
   D. decreased cerebral circulation

Answers: 1, A. 2, B. 3, B.

Section Seven: Junctional Dysrhythmias

At the completion of Section Seven, the learner will be able to identify common junctional dysrhythmias.

Junctional dysrhythmias occur because the SA node fails to fire. They have a protective function. The junctional area is located around the AV node. Pacemaker cells in this area have an intrinsic rate of 40 to 60 bpm. Once the pacemaker cell discharges, it spreads upward to depolarize the atria and downward to depolarize the ventricles. Since the ventricles usually are depolarized in a downward fashion, the QRS complex will appear normal. The atria are depolarized in an abnormal manner. Therefore, the P

wave will be inverted (in lead II). The timing of the P wave is abnormal. It may precede the QRS complex, but the PR interval is shorter. The P wave may be buried in the QRS complex and be indistinguishable. It is possible that the P wave follows the QRS complex.

The term *junctional tachycardia* refers to a junctional rhythm with a rate greater than 100 bpm. If the rate of the rhythm is between 60 and 100 bpm, it is called an accelerated junctional rhythm. Figure 7–16 shows an accelerated junctional rhythm pattern.

Digitalis increases the automaticity of the AV node. Therefore, digitalis toxicity may precipitate junctional rhythms. The dysrhythmia is treated by

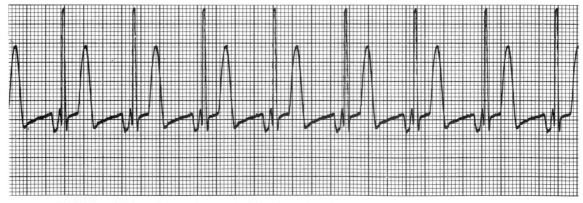

Figure 7–16. Interpretation of accelerated junction rhythm using the six-step process.
1. Rate = 80
2. R to R interval regular
3. P wave: same configuration, inverted
4. PR interval = 0.04
5. P wave precedes QRS: yes
6. QRS complex = 0.08

withholding the medication. Usually the patient can tolerate junctional rhythms. However, if the patient experiences symptoms of decreased CO because the rate is too slow, atropine may be administered. A pacemaker may be inserted as a protective measure in case the junction fails or if the patient is symptomatic. Table 7–4 compares junctional rhythms.

In summary, junctional rhythms are a protective mechanism when the SA node fails to discharge appropriately. Depolarization of the atria is abnormal. Therefore, the P wave may fall before, during, or after the QRS complex.

TABLE 7–4. SUMMARY OF DIFFERENCES IN JUNCTIONAL DYSRHYTHMIAS

Rhythm	Characteristics	Treatment Strategies
Junctional rhythm	Rate 40–60 bpm Inverted or absent P waves	May not be treated if patient is asymptomatic Atropine Pacemaker insertion
Junctional tachycardia	Rate greater than 100 bpm Inverted or absent P waves	May not be treated if patient is asymptomatic Pacemaker insertion Associated with digitalis toxicity (withhold digitalis if appropriate)

Section Seven Review

1. Junctional rhythms are
   A. precursors to ventricular dysrhythmias
   B. a protective mechanism
   C. generated by the SA node
   D. considered an atrial dysrhythmia
2. Junctional tachycardia is classified as a junctional rhythm with a rate
   A. greater than 40 bpm
   B. greater than 60 bpm
   C. greater than 100 bpm
   D. between 60 and 100 bpm
3. The P wave in a junctional rhythm
   A. is bizarre in configuration
   B. is always abnormal in location
   C. can appear anywhere in relation to the QRS complex
   D. is flat

Answers: 1, B. 2, C. 3, C.

Section Eight: Ventricular Dysrhythmias

At the completion of this section, the learner will be able to identify common ventricular dysrhythmias.

Ventricular dysrhythmias are considered the most lethal. Inadequate ventricular ejection produces inadequate CO. Coronary and peripheral ischemia results, producing necrosis and cell death. Two common ventricular dysrhythmias are ventricular tachycardia and ventricular fibrillation.

Ventricular tachycardia may follow premature ventricular contractions (PVCs) (Section Nine). It is classified as three or more consecutive PVCs occurring at a rapid rate, usually greater than 140 bpm. Although the SA node continues to fire, ectopic pacemakers in the ventricles fire spontaneously and bear no relationship to the SA node-initiated impulse. P

waves are not identifiable because they are buried in the QRS complexes. The R to R interval may be regular. The QRS complex is greater than 0.12 second. Short runs of ventricular tachycardia can be tolerated. A danger of ventricular tachycardia is that it may develop into ventricular fibrillation. Patients may be alert while experiencing ventricular tachycardia, and a carotid pulse may still be present. As CO diminishes, loss of consciousness ensues. Witnessed ventricular tachycardia is treated with a precordial thump over the sternum. Cardioversion may be used. Lidocaine is the drug of choice in decreasing ventricular irritability. Figure 7–17 is an example of ventricular tachycardia.

Ventricular fibrillation is the most common cause of sudden death. The patient will be unresponsive and without a pulse and requires emergency

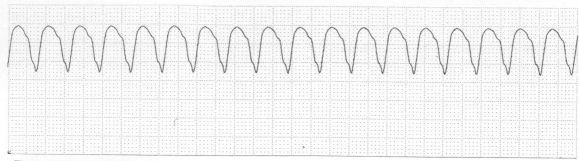

Figure 7–17. Interpretation of ventricular tachycardia using the six-step process.
1. Rate: atrial: unable to calculate
       ventricular = 180
2. R to R interval regular
3. P wave: undistinguishable
4. PR interval: unable to calculate
5. P wave precedes each QRS: no
6. QRS complex = 0.28

treatment. Cardiopulmonary resuscitation is initiated. Defibrillation is the treatment of choice and is used beginning with 200 J and progressing up to 360 for a total of three times (American Heart Association, 1987). A bolus of epinephrine is administered. If the patient remains pulseless, an IV lidocaine bolus is administered. Once the patient has converted from ventricular fibrillation and has a pulse, a continuous infusion of lidocaine is initiated. Myocardial infarction and premature ventricular beats may precede the development of ventricular fibrillation. The ECG pattern is chaotic. It is impossible to identify any PQRST waves, and the rhythm is grossly irregular. Figure 7–18 is an example of ventricular fibrillation.

To summarize, ventricular dysrhythmias are more life threatening than other dysrhythmias and require immediate treatment. They are recognizable by absent P waves, and regular, wide QRS complexes or, in the case of ventricular fibrillation, chaotic wave forms. Table 7–5 compares ventricular dysrhythmias.

TABLE 7–5. SUMMARY OF DIFFERENCES IN VENTRICULAR DYSRHYTHMIAS

Rhythm	Characteristics	Treatment Strategies
Ventricular tachycardia	R to R interval regular Absent P wave Wide QRS but somewhat uniform Rate greater than 150 bpm	Lidocaine Cardioversion
Ventricular fibrillation	R to R interval irregular Absent P wave Wide QRS, no uniformity Rate undeterminable	CPR Defibrillation Epinephrine Lidocaine

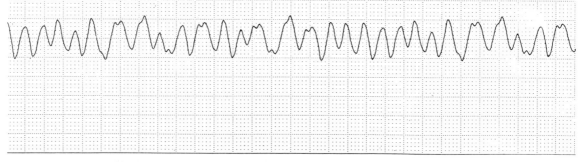

Figure 7–18. Interpretation of ventricular fibrillation using the six-step process.
1. Rate: atrial: unable to calculate
       ventricular = unable to calculate
2. R to R interval irregular
3. P wave: undistinguishable
4. PR interval: unable to calculate
5. P wave precedes each QRS: no
6. QRS complex: no uniformity, unable to calculate

Section Eight Review

1. Ventricular tachycardia
   A. may be harmless
   B. follows premature ventricular contractions (PVCs)
   C. results from SA node fatigue
   D. produces ventricular rates less than 100 bpm
2. In ventricular fibrillation, the ECG pattern
   A. is chaotic
   B. has recognizable QRS complexes
   C. has inverted T waves
   D. has a regular atrial rate

3. The treatment of choice in ventricular fibrillation is
   A. lidocaine
   B. epinephrine
   C. cardioversion
   D. defibrillation

Answers: 1, B. 2, A. 3, D.

Section Nine: Premature Contractions

At the completion of Section Nine, the learner will be able to distinguish premature beats and identify their origin.

Premature beats may originate in the atria, junctional area (AV node), or ventricles. Since premature junctional beats are treated in the same manner as premature atrial beats (PACs), discussion is limited to PACs and premature ventricular beats (PVCs).

In PACs, the P wave is abnormal in shape, since a focus other than the SA node is initiating the impulse. Therefore, there will be differences in the P wave configurations. The rhythmn is irregular because there is a slight pause after the premature beat to allow for the SA node to get ready to initiate a beat after it responded to the premature stimulus.

The remaining components of the ECG are normal. PACs do not pose a serious threat unless they occur at a rate greater than six per minute. This rate suggests the future development of atrial tachycardia or atrial fibrillation. Digitalis preparations usually are used to treat multiple PACs. Figure 7–19 is an example of a PAC.

PVCs originate in the ventricles and do not stimulate the atria retrospectively. Thus, P waves are absent in a PVC. The rhythmn is irregular because of the compensatory pause before the next stimulus arrives to initiate a normal ventricular beat. The QRS complex is wide, greater than 0.12 second in length, and distorted. PVCs may originate from one irritable cell in the ventricles. Unifocal PVCs originate from the same location, and thus they appear the same in configuration. Multifocal PVCs originate from

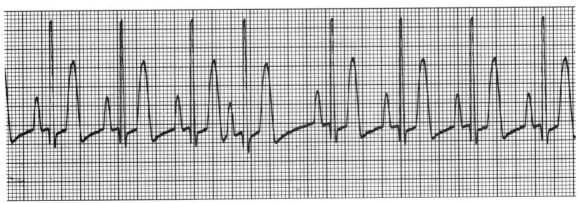

Figure 7–19. Interpretation of sinus rhythm with premature atrial contraction using the six-step process.
1. Rate = 80
2. R to R interval irregular
3. P wave: same configuration
4. PR interval = 0.16
5. P wave precedes QRS: yes
6. QRS complex = 0.08

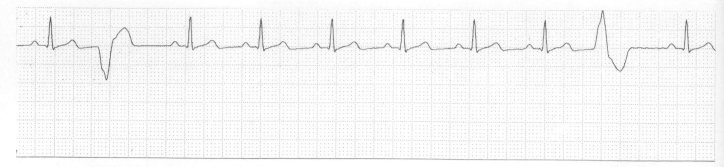

Figure 7–20. Interpretation of sinus rhythm with multifocal PVCs using the six-step process. (*Note:* Strip is longer than 6 seconds = 37 (0.20) boxes.)
1. Rate = 70
2. R to R interval irregular
3. P wave: same configuration
4. PR interval = 0.16
5. P wave precedes each QRS: no
6. QRS complex varies, 0.06 to 0.32

multiple irritable ventricular cells. Therefore, they have various shapes. Thus, all of the premature beats have wide and chaotic QRS complexes, but they are not identical to one another unless they arise from the same site.

PVCs may appear in healthy individuals. Caffeine, alcohol intake, and stress may produce ventricular irritability. A major responsibility of the nurse is determining factors contributing to their occurrence. Ischemia is the most dangerous cause of PVCs. Hypoxia, acidosis, hypokalemia, and digitalis toxicity also are associated with PVCs. It is important to remember that not all PVCs are treated. This is especially true in cases where PVCs originate because the underlying cardiac rhythm is too slow. Treating the PVCs may decrease CO further.

There are certain circumstances that warrant close observation of PVCs because they are associated with future development of ventricular tachy-

cardia and ventricular fibrillation (Thelan et al, 1990, p. 203). In the situations listed, lidocaine may be administered prophylactically if the patient has underlying cardiac disease.

1. Greater than 6 PVCs per minute
2. PVCs occurring together (couplet)
3. Multifocal PVCs
4. A run of ventricular tachycardia (more than 3 PVCs in a row)

Procainamide, followed by bretylium, may be administered if the PVCs are refractory to lidocaine. Figure 7–20 is an example of sinus rhythm with multifocal PVCs.

The patient's underlying cardiac rhythm and the type of PVC (unifocal vs multifocal) should be described. The timing of the PVCs can be described if they occur in a repeatable pattern. For example, bigeminy is a pattern of one normal SA node-

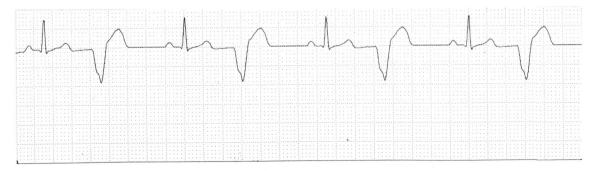

Figure 7–21. Interpretation of ventricular bigeming using the six-step process.
1. Rate = 40
2. R to R interval regular
3. P wave: same configuration
4. PR interval = 0.16
5. P wave precedes each QRS: no
6. QRS complex varies, 0.08 to 0.36

initiated beat followed by one PVC. Trigeminy is a pattern of two normal beats followed by one PVC. Figure 7–21 is an example of ventricular bigeminy.

In summary, PACs usually are harmless and are not treated unless they are present at a rate of six or greater a minute. PVCs may be more life threatening, since they indicate ventricular irritability. Multiple PVCs, multifocal PVCs, a couplet of PVCs, and a run of ventricular tachycardia may be treated with lidocaine if the patient has underlying cardiac disease, since they may predispose to life-threatening dysrhythmias. Table 7–6 compares premature contractions.

TABLE 7–6. SUMMARY OF DIFFERENCES IN PREMATURE CONTRACTIONS

Contraction	Characteristics	Treatment Strategies
Premature atrial contraction	PR interval may be normal or prolonged QRS may be absent after P wave	Reduce caffeine intake May not be treated if patient is asymptomatic Beta-blocking agents (propranolol)
Premature ventricular contraction	PR interval absent in premature beat QRS greater than 0.12	May not be treated if patient is asymptomatic Reduce caffeine intake Decrease stress Lidocaine

Section Nine Review

1. Which of the following statements best describes premature beats?
   A. they originate anywhere along the cardiac conduction pathway
   B. they originate in the atria
   C. they originate in the ventricles
   D. they originate in the junctional (AV nodal) area
2. Premature atrial contractions (PACs) should be treated when
   A. they occur as a pair
   B. they originate from different sites
   C. they occur greater than six per minute
   D. they occur in a repeatable pattern

3. Premature ventricular contractions (PVCs) may be associated with
   A. hyponatremia
   B. hypocalcemia
   C. hypoglycemia
   D. hypokalemia
4. In PVCs, the QRS complex is
   A. greater than 0.12 second
   B. negatively deflected
   C. isoelectric
   D. preceded by a T wave

Answers: 1, A. 2, C. 3, D. 4, A.

Section Ten: Conduction Abnormalities

At the completion of this section, the learner will be able to distinguish the three most common and life-threatening conduction abnormalities.

Conduction can be inhibited anywhere along the cardiac conduction pathway. Normally, conduction of the impulse will be blocked in its transmission from the SA node to the ventricles. Delays may occur at the AV nodal area. Ischemia to the AV node, digitalis, antiarrhythmic agents, and increased parasympathetic activity can produce blocks in conduction.

A first degree heart block is denoted by a prolonged PR interval (greater than 0.20 second.) There is a delay in conduction through the AV node. The rest of the ECG is normal. If the patient is asymptomatic and the PR interval is less than 0.28 second, no treatment usually is necessary. If the PR interval is greater than 0.28 second, the patient will be at risk for premature beats, complete heart block (discussed later in this section), and asystole. Atropine may be administered, or a temporary pacing catheter may be placed. Figure 7–22 is an example of first degree heart block.

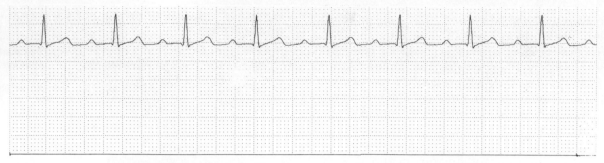

Figure 7–22. Interpretation of first degree heart block using the six-step process.
1. Rate = 80
2. R to R interval regular
3. P wave: same configuration
4. PR interval = 0.24
5. P wave precedes QRS: yes
6. QRS complex = 0.06

In second degree heart block, an impulse is not transmitted to the ventricles because it is completely blocked in the AV nodal area. Therefore, a P wave will be present, but a QRS complex will not follow. The rhythmn is irregular because of the missing QRS complexes. In some cases, the PR interval will lengthen progressively before the dropping of the QRS complex (Wenckebach or type I second degree heart block). In type II second degree heart block, the PR intervals are of constant duration before the blocking of the P wave. This type of heart block is less common but is considered more serious, since it is associated with third degree heart block and asystole (Meltzer et al, 1983). The nurse should determine the ventricular rate (number of QRS complexes) of the rhythmn and the frequency of dropped beats. Angina, light headedness, and dyspnea may occur because of decreased cardiac output. In the case of type I second degree heart block, if the rate is below 60 bpm and the patient is asymptomatic, no treat-ment may be initiated. The patient is observed. A patient with type II second degree heart block, whether symptomatic or asymptomatic, usually will receive a transvenous pacemaker. The point at which the pacemaker is inserted may vary, since symptoms are managed with medications initially. Regardless of the type of second degree block, if the patient experiences symptoms, atropine is administered, followed by isoproterenol, or an external pacemaker may be used. Eventually, a transvenous pacemaker may need to be inserted for symptomatic patients with type I second degree heart block (American Heart Association, 1987). Figure 7–23 is an example of type I second degree heart block, and Figure 7–24 is an example of type II second degree heart block.

Complete heart block requires emergency treatment because the atria and ventricles are contracting independently. Thus, the CO is greatly diminished because of inadequate filling of the ventricles. Impulses are not conducted through the AV node. The

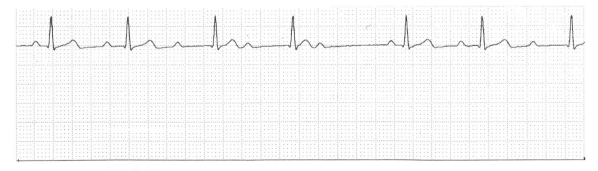

Figure 7–23. Interpretation of type I second degree heart block using the six-step process.
1. Rate: ventricular: 70
   atrial: 80
2. R to R interval irregular
3. P wave: same configuration
4. PR interval varies, 0.20 to 0.48
5. P wave precedes QRS: yes, but QRS does not always follow P wave
6. QRS complex = 0.06

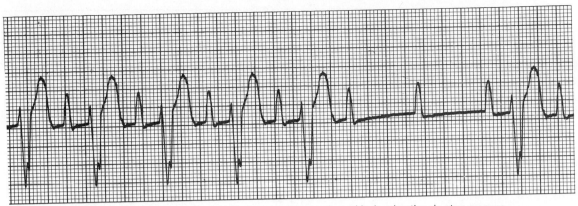

Figure 7–24. Interpretation of type II second degree heart block using the six-step process.
1. Rate: ventricular: 60
       atrial: 80
2. R to R interval irregular
3. P wave: same configuration
4. PR interval = 0.28
5. P waves are not followed by QRS complex in 2 places
6. QRS complex = 0.12

atria and ventricles may fire at a regular rate, but they do not function as a single unit. The P to P wave interval will be regular, as will the R to R wave interval, but the PR interval will vary. There is no relationship between the P wave and the QRS complex, since the atria and the ventricles are being paced by a separate pacemaker. The QRS complex is wide and chaotic due to the ventricular origin of the stimulus. Complete heart block usually is associated with myocardial infarction. In rare cases, the ventricular rate is fast enough to maintain CO, and symptoms may be less severe. Usually, the patient experiences confusion and syncope. Complete heart block may progress to ventricular fibrillation. Treatment of complete heart block is the same as that for type II second degree heart block. If symptomatic, the patient is administered atropine, followed by isoproterenol, ex-

ternal pacing, and transvenous pacing. Figure 7–25 is an example of complete heart block.

In summary, abnormalities can occur along the cardiac conduction pathway that interfere with transmission of the impulse from the atria to the ventricles. The least severe of these abnormalities is first degree heart block. The impulse is transmitted to the ventricles, but there is a delay at the AV nodal area. Impulses from the atria to the ventricles are periodically blocked in second degree heart block. In type I, the PR interval progressively lengthens before the blocked impulse. In type II, the PR interval remains constant. Complete heart block is a medical emergency. It is treated with the placement of a temporary cardiac pacemaker, since the atria and ventricles are contracting independently, decreasing CO. Table 7–7 compares atrioventricular blocks.

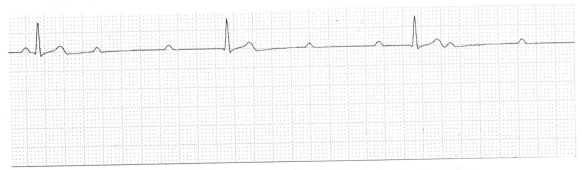

Figure 7–25. Interpretation of complete heart block using the six-step process.
1. Rate: ventricular: 30
       atrial: 70
2. R to R interval regular
3. P wave: same configuration
4. PR interval varies
5. P wave precedes each QRS: no
6. QRS complex = 0.06

Section Ten Review

1. Which of the following may produce blocks in impulse conduction?
   A. ischemia
   B. sympathetic stimulation
   C. fever
   D. antipyretic agents
2. The difference between type I and type II second degree heart block is
   A. dropping of the QRS complex
   B. regularity of the rhythm
   C. length of the PR interval
   D. P wave configuration
3. Complete heart block is characterized by
   A. constant PR interval
   B. heart rate less than 50 bpm
   C. QRS complexes less than 0.12 second
   D. regular P to P and R to R intervals
4. First degree heart block should be treated if
   A. the PR interval is irregular
   B. the PR interval is greater than 0.28 second
   C. the PR interval is isoelectric
   D. the PR interval is negatively deflected

Answers: 1, A. 2, C. 3, D. 4, B.

TABLE 7–7. SUMMARY OF DIFFERENCES IN ATRIOVENTRICULAR (AV) BLOCKS

Block	Characteristics	Treatment Strategies
First degree	PR interval greater than 0.20 R to R interval is regular	May not be treated if patient is asymptomatic Atropine
Second degree, Mobitz type I	Atrial rate is greater than ventricular rate R to R interval is irregular	Commonly associated with digitalis toxicity (withhold digitalis if appropriate)
	PR interval gradually lengthens until a P wave is blocked (no QRS follows the P wave)	Atropine Pacemaker insertion
Second degree, Mobitz type II	Atrial rate is greater than ventricular rate There is no consistent pattern to the blocking of the P wave R to R interval irregular	Atropine Pacemaker insertion
Third degree, complete	PR interval may be normal or prolonged, but it is consistent	
	PR interval varies R to R interval regular QRS may be widened	Pacemaker insertion

Section Eleven: Myocardial Infarction

At the completion of this section, the learner will be able to describe ECG changes in lead II associated with myocardial infarction.

The heart is supplied by three coronary arteries: anterior descending, circumflex, and right coronary artery. The anterior descending artery supplies the anterior left and right ventricle. The circumflex artery supplies the left atria and left lateral and posterior ventricle. The right coronary artery supplies the right atria and ventricle. There are four basic areas where an infarction can occur: anterior, inferior, lateral, or posterior aspect of the heart. Although this module does not discuss 12-lead ECG interpretation, certain leads have changes depending on the location of the infarct. For example, an anterior myocardial infarction will demonstrate changes in leads I, AVL, V_2, and V_3.

Ischemic changes may be visible in a single monitored lead, but it is not possible to confirm the presence and location of an infarction. Ischemia may impair repolarization. Thus, the T wave may be changed, since it corresponds with ventricular repolarization. The T wave may be inverted. As ischemia progresses into injury, repolarization is impaired even further. The ST segment may demonstrate changes. It may be either elevated or depressed depending on the lead that the cardiac monitor is displaying. Diagnosis of infarction requires a 12-lead ECG. Figure 7–26 is an example of ischemic changes in lead II.

As injury progresses into infarction, the area becomes necrotic and is without electrical activity. The

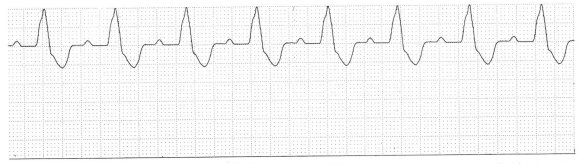

Figure 7–26. Characteristics of ischemia in lead II. Note the severe ST depression. Interpretation using the six-step process.
1. Rate = 80
2. R to R interval regular
3. P wave: same configuration
4. PR interval = 0.20
5. P wave precedes QRS: yes
6. QRS complex = 0.12 to 0.16

Q wave may be deep and wide, since the area over the infarcted site is unable to exhibit electrical activity. The ECG pattern depicted is produced by the area opposite the infarcted site. The infarcted site serves as a window through which the electrical activity of the opposite side is transmitted. The electrical activity moves away from the necrotic zone, producing a deep, wide, negatively deflected Q wave.

The treatment for myocardial infarction is focused on decreasing myocardial demands and increasing myocardial oxygen supply. Oxygen should be administered. Angina should be relieved through the use of narcotics and coronary vasodilators. Thrombolytic therapy using streptokinase (Streptase), anisoylated plasminogen streptokinase activator (Eminase), or tissue plasminogen activator (TPA, Alteplase) may be initiated.

In summary, any of the ECG changes discussed in this section indicate myocardial circulatory compromise. Prompt intervention may stop or reverse the sequence of events. The nurse should alert the physician to the occurrence of T wave and ST segment changes, since these may indicate impending or actual myocardial infarction.

Section Eleven Review

1. Ischemia produces changes in
   A. ventricular depolarization
   B. atrial depolarization
   C. ventricular repolarization
   D. AV conduction
2. Ischemia may be reflected by
   A. wide QRS complexes
   B. T wave changes
   C. isoelectric ST segment
   D. pathologic Q waves
3. A wide, deep Q wave may represent
   A. lack of electrical activity over a necrotic area
   B. slowed ventricular conduction
   C. impaired atrial repolarization
   D. ventricular irritability
4. A myocardial infarction usually will produce
   A. changes in the P and T wave configurations
   B. changes in the QRS complex
   C. T wave and ST segment changes
   D. lengthening of the PR and QT intervals

Answers: 1, C. 2, B. 3, A. 4, C.

Section Twelve: Thrombolytic Therapy

At the completion of this section, the learner will be able to identify selection criteria for thrombolytic therapy and nursing responsibilities associated with thrombolytic therapy.

Thrombolytic therapy has been used to lyse a clot in the coronary artery in order to prevent necrosis of the cardiac muscle. Reperfusion rates of 75 percent have been attained in some clinical trials (Brewer-Senerchia, 1989). The goals of thrombolytic therapy are to maintain patency of the coronary artery, assess and prevent bleeding, avoid myocardial ischemia, prevent reocclusion, preserve left ventricular function, and reduce mortality (Martin et al, 1990). There are three types of thromboblytic agents on the market: synthetic proteins (urokinase for intracoronary administration only, streptokinase), tissue plasminogen activator (TPA) (produced by gene cloning techniques), and anisoylated plasminogen streptokinase activator complex (derived from human plasma).

Streptokinase is a synthetic protein derived from group C beta-hemolytic streptococci. This agent lyses clots by activating plasminogen at the clot site and in the circulation. It is a nonspecific drug, since it has no affinity for plasminogen bound at the thrombus site. Individuals may be allergic to streptokinase if they have experienced streptococcal infections or previously received streptokinase and have developed antibodies. The typical dosage is 1.5 million units.

Anisoylated plasminogen streptokinase activator complex (APSAC) is the newest thromobolytic agent. It binds with fibrin before activation. Therefore, long-term infusions are contraindicated. It is administered as an IV bolus of 30 units over 5 minutes. It requires less nursing administration time. Antibody formation may occur with the use of this agent.

TPA has an affinity for plasminogen that has been incorporated into a clot, and it does not affect circulating plasminogen except with higher doses. Therefore, hemorrhage is less of a possibility. The typical dosage is 80 mg IV. TPA has been shown to be a more effective thrombolytic agent than streptokinase, but survival rates are not statistically greater (Brewer-Senerchia, 1989). One advantage is the ability to re-treat a patient who reoccludes, since there is no chance of antibody formation.

Additional medications may be used in conjunction with thrombolytics. Antiplatelet agents may be administered. The administration of asprin in combination with a hemolytic agent has produced decreased mortality as compared to administering the hemolytic agent alone (Brewer-Senerchia, 1989). Di-

TABLE 7–8. ELIGIBILITY CRITERIA FOR THROMBOLYTIC THERAPY

Chest pain of longer than 30 minutes and less than 6 hours duration, unrelieved with nitroglycerin
ST segment elevation of at least 1 mm in two contiguous leads
Age less than 75 years

pyridamole may be used at the end of infusion of the hemolytic agent. Lidocaine may be given to prevent ventricular dysrhythmias. Heparin may be administered to prevent additional thrombi. Initially, a 5,000 unit IV bolus usually is administered. This is followed by a 800 to 1,000 units/hour continuous IV drip. Heparin therapy is not recommended for 4 hours after the use of APSAC because of increased risk of bleeding (Grigg and Stromberg, 1990).

Eligibility criteria to determine which patients are suitable for thrombolytic therapy are being validated through research. Table 7–8 summarizes the eligibility criteria currently being used. Age has been documented as a factor, but recent research has demonstrated successful reperfusion in people up to 93 years of age (Grigg and Stromberg, 1990). The rate of complications does not appear to be different based on age (Bennett and Grines, 1990). Patients with chest pain but a normal ECG or just the presence of ST depression do not appear to benefit from thrombolytic therapy (Bennet and Grines, 1990). Persons with chest pain of longer than 6 hours duration may benefit from treatment, even though some necrosis may already exist. Collateral circulation and electrical stability of the myocardium may be improved by late treatment. Contraindications generally are categorized as absolute or relative based on the degree of risk of bleeding. Table 7–9 summarizes contraindications for thrombolytic therapy. The learner should be aware that the literature is not conclusive for contraindications or the classification of contraindications as absolute or relative. Table 7–9 serves as a summary of the literature. Physician preference and patient stability also are factors to be considered.

Nursing responsibilities include identifying which patients are suitable for thrombolytic therapy. Prophylactic pressure dressings may need to be applied to wounds and arterial and venous puncture sites. The nurse must assess for signs of bleeding. Neurologic checks should be performed routinely to detect signs of intracranial bleeding. All drainage should be tested for blood. Monitoring vital signs and laboratory tests is another responsibility. A drop in the hematocrit may indicate the need for a transfusion. Partial thromboplastin time and prothrombin time should be monitored, and anticoagulant therapy should be discontinued if these are elevated greater than 2.5 times normal values. Packed red

TABLE 7–9. CONTRAINDICATIONS TO THROMBOLYTIC THERAPY

Absolute	Relative
Active internal bleeding	Recent biopsy, delivery
Recent surgery or noncompressible artery puncture	Genitourinary or gastrointestinal bleeding within last 10 days
CPR greater than 1 minute	Pregnancy
Previous cerebrovascular accident	Pericarditis, bacterial endocarditis
Intracranial/intraspinal surgery or trauma within 2 months	Liver dysfunction
Severe hypertension (SBP 180 mm Hg or greater, DBP 110 mm Hg or greater)	Likelihood of left heart thrombus
	Prior anticoagulation (when using streptokinase)

blood cells, cryoprecipitate or plasma may be administered. Protamine sulfate may be administered to counteract anticoagulant therapy. The patient may need computerized tomography scanning to detect bleeding sources. Patients who develop an allergic reaction may need IV antihistamines and steroids.

Nursing responsibility also includes assessing for reperfusion. There are several signs of reperfusion. The patient experiences pain relief. Vital signs may change, with bradycardia and hypotension occurring. The ST segment on the ECG may return to baseline. The patient may have PVCs. Creatinine phosphokinase (CPK) levels may peak rapidly, since the artery is reopened, and the enzyme that is released from the necrotic tissue is able to flow into the general circulation.

Long-term treatment includes beta-blockers and calcium channel blockers, nitrates, asprin, and anticoagulants. The patient may not understand why treatment is long term, since he or she may have been told that the damage was stopped or the infarction was prevented.

In summary, thrombolytic therapy when initiated within 6 hours of the onset of myocardial infarction helps to prevent necrosis of cardiac muscle. Three thrombolytic agents currently are being used: streptokinase, ASPAC, and TPA. Nursing responsibilities focus on identifying suitable patients, administering thrombolytic agents, monitoring for bleeding complications, and assessing the degree of reperfusion.

Section Twelve Review

1. Which of the following patients would be most eligible for thrombolytic therapy?
   A. 45-year-old patient with chest pain relieved by three nitroglycerin tablets
   B. 70-year-old patient with chest pain of 15 minutes duration
   C. 50-year-old patient with ST elevation in two contiguous leads
   D. 60-year-old patient with ST depression in lead II
2. Nursing interventions for a patient receiving thrombolytic therapy should include
   A. urinary catheter care
   B. neurologic checks
   C. vigorous mouth care
   D. preparing IV sites with a straight razor
3. A complication NOT associated with TPA is
   A. bleeding from IV sites
   B. antibody reaction
   C. cerebrovascular attack
   D. hematuria

4. Which of the following patients is contraindicated for thrombolytic therapy with streptokinase?
   A. 20-year-old patient with history of gastrointestinal bleeding 15 days ago
   B. 55-year-old patient with history of bleeding gums
   C. 65-year-old who received streptokinase 3 months ago
   D. 30-year-old patient who was pulseless and received CPR for less than a minute
5. Reperfusion is indicated by which of the following symptoms?
   A. hypotension
   B. decrease in CPK level
   C. chest pain does not radiate to jaw
   D. tachycardia

Answers: 1, C. 2, B. 3, B. 4, C. 5, A.

Section Thirteen: Pharmacologic Interventions and Nursing Implications

At the completion of this section, the learner will be able to identify common drug classifications used in treating cardiac disturbances. The learner is referred to a pharmacology text to get specific information on dosage and administration. Nursing implications associated with administration of these agents are addressed briefly. Cardioversion and defibrillation are discussed because of the relationship between drug therapy and electric shock with some agents.

Antiarrhythmic agents are used in treating cardiac disturbances. The antiarrhythmics have several subcategories, class I through class IV. Additionally, class I has three subcategories, A, B, and C. Each of these drugs is capable of producing new dysrhythmias or worsening current dysrhythmias. Therefore, constant ECG monitoring is required as these medications are initiated.

Class IA drugs reduce automaticity and prolong the refractory period of the heart. They are indicated in the treatment of atrial dysrhythmias and PVCs. Class IB drugs decrease refractory periods but do not affect automaticity to a great extent. These drugs are used chiefly in the treatment of ventricular dysrhythmias. Class IC agents decrease spontaneous depolarization. They are also used in treating ventricular dysrhythmias.

Class II agents block the defects of the catecholamines (i.e., epinephrine). They decrease automaticity and slow down conduction. Their exact effects depend on which catecholamine receptor they block. Catecholamines may affect four different receptors: alpha$_1$ vasoconstriction, alpha$_2$ norepinephrine release, beta$_1$ cardiac stimulation, and beta$_2$ vasodilation and bronchodilation. For example,

phentolamine (Regitine) is an alpha-blocking agent. Therefore, it produces vasodilation. However, most of the agents used to treat dysrhythmias in this category are beta-blocking agents. Thus, they decrease cardiac stimulation and may produce vasoconstriction and bronchoconstriction. Drugs in this category are used in treating tachydysrhythmias. These drugs may not be used in patients with congestive heart failure, severe bradycardia, and second degree or higher heart block because of decreased cardiac stimulation. They may be contraindicated in asthma due to bronchoconstriction. Since class II drugs decrease the heart rate, the heart rate may be unable to increase to maintain CO in some situations, such as exercise. In cases of cardiac arrest, the heart may be less sensitive to sympathomimetic drugs (i.e., epinephrine) because of the beta-blocking effect.

Class III agents prolong refractory periods, the direct opposite effect of class IB drugs. They increase the fibrillation threshold (making the cell more resistant) of the cells. Thus, they are indicated in the treatment of ventricular dysrhythmias.

Class IV agents are calcium channel blockers. These drugs block the entry of calcium through the cell membranes, thereby decreasing depolarization. Verapamil is the most commonly used calcium channel blocker for dysrhythmias. Nifedipine is another drug in this category that is used to treat hypertension.

Digitalis glycosides may be used to treat decreased contractility seen in congestive heart failure. These drugs also slow impulse conduction through the AV node. They may be used in the treatment of atrial or supraventricular dysrhythmias before using class II or IV agents. Digitalis increases the heart's sensitivity to electric shock and may precipitate ven-

TABLE 7–10. COMPARISON OF ANTIARRHYTHMIC AGENTS

Category	Examples	Effect	Indications
Class IA	Quinidine (Cardioquin) Procainamide (Pronestyl) Disopyramide (Norpace)	Reduce automaticity Prolong refractory period	PVCs Atrial fibrillation and flutter
Class IB	Lidocaine (Xylocaine) Mexiletine (Mexitil) Tocainide (Tonocard)	Decrease refractory period	PVCs Ventricular tachycardia or fibrillation
Class IC	Encainide (Enkaid) Flecainide (Tambocor)	Decrease spontaneous depolarization	PVCs Ventricular tachycardia
Class II	Propranolol (Inderal) Esmolol (Brevibloc)	Decrease automaticity Decrease conduction	Atrial/supraventricular dysrhythmias
Class III	Amiodarone (Cordarone) Bretylium (Bretylol)	Prolong refractory period	Ventricular tachycardia or fibrillation
Class IV	Verapamil (Calan)	Decrease conduction	Supraventricular dysrhythmias
Digitalis glycosides	Digoxin (Lanoxin)	Decrease conduction through AV node	Congestive heart failure Atrial dysrhythmias

tricular fibrillation (Shlafer and Marieb, 1989). Thus, cardioversion should be attempted before administering digitalis. Table 7–10 summarizes antiarrhythmic agents.

Cardioversion is used to treat supraventricular tachycardia that is resistant to medication and ventricular tachycardia in an unstable patient. The unstable patient may be hypotensive, dyspneic, experiencing chest pain, or have evidence of congestive heart failure, myocardial infarction, or ischemia (AHA, 1987). Analgesia may be provided before the electric shock. A synchronizer knob is pushed on the defibrillator machine, which allows the machine to discharge during firing of the ectopic impulse. Low voltages are tried initially (50 J to 100 J depending on the size of the patient). Cardioversion can be repeated using larger voltages if it is unsuccessful. Defibrillation is used to treat ventricular tachycardia in an unresponsive patient and ventricular fibrillation. Defibrillation is an unsynchronized electric shock that usually administers a larger number of joules than cardioversion (200 J up to 360 J). Defibrillation may be repeated.

Nursing responsibilities in drug therapy focus on monitoring the ECG pattern to determine the response to drug therapy. Drug serum levels should be examined before administering the drug to prevent toxicity. The patient's pulse must be assessed for 1 minute before administering each dose, since many of these agents decrease the heart rate. If the heart rate is too slow (i.e., below 60 bpm), the physician should be notified, since the medication may need to be withheld. The nurse must teach patients how to obtain their heart rate and to determine regularity by assessing their pulse for 1 minute. The need to take the medications as prescribed and to report cardiac-related symptoms, such as palpitations, chest pain, wheezing, fatigue, and syncope, must be stressed.

In summary, antiarrhythmic agents are classified in four large categories. They usually act by decreasing automaticity or by affecting the refractory period. Impulse conduction may be delayed. They may help correct or worsen a dysrhythmia. Thus, nursing responsibilities include careful monitoring of the patient's ECG pattern and clinical response.

Section Thirteen Review

1. Beta-blockers (class II agents) may produce which of the following side effects?
   A. weight gain
   B. hypokalemia
   C. wheezing
   D. hives
2. Cardioversion should not be attempted in a digitalized patient because
   A. digitalis increases the heart's sensitivity to electric shock·
   B. digitalis prevents electric stimulation of the heart
   C. extra voltage is required to produce the desired effect
   D. defibrillation is indicated
3. A patient on a beta-blocking agent may not respond to sympathomimetic agents in cardiac arrest because
   A. it competes with the sympathomimetic agent for the beta receptor site
   B. they inhibit the effect of catecholamines
   C. alpha receptors are also blocked
   D. the sympathomimetic agent is administered too late in the arrest

4. The difference between cardioversion and defibrillation is
   A. defibrillation uses a lower amount of joules
   B. cardioversion is synchronized
   C. defibrillation cannot be repeated
   D. cardioversion is used only to treat atrial dysrhythmias
5. Nursing responsibilities in administering antiarrhythmic agents include
   A. administering all agents by IV route
   B. obtaining a 12-lead ECG before each administration
   C. Monitoring the patient's pulse for 30 seconds before administration
   D. checking drug serum levels

Answers: 1, C. 2, A. 3, B. 4, B. 5, D.

Section Fourteen: Pacemaker Therapy

At the completion of this section, the learner will be able to identify indications for pacemaker therapy, types of pacemakers, and nursing implications for the patient being mechanically paced.

Pacemakers may be inserted in addition to drug therapy. An artificial pacemaker is indicated when one of three conditions exists: failure of the conduction system, failure to initiate an impulse spontaneously, and failure to maintain primary pacing control (spontaneous impulses may occur, but they are not synchronized). There are three commonly used pacing mechanisms: external, epicardial, and endocardial.

External pacing can be used in the same circumstances as an internal pacing device. The major difference is that it is always a temporary measure. The external pacer can be set for continuous or demand pacing. It delivers electric impulses to the myocardium transthoracically through two electrode pads placed on the chest. An endocardial pacer is placed later. Epicardial pacing is inserted during open heart surgery by placing electrodes directly on the surface of the heart. Endocardial pacers usually are inserted through the subclavian, jugular, or femoral veins into the right ventricle, where it is lodged.

Pacemakers can be programmed to pace different areas of the heart at specific time intervals and to respond to a level of stimulation. Most pacemakers are designed to pace the ventricles. In this case, a spike will occur before the QRS complex. This method of pacing may be used when transmission of impulses from the atria is being blocked (i.e., complete heart block, Section Ten). The atria also may be paced. A spike will appear before the P wave. This method of pacing may be used with sinus node disease. AV sequential pacing may be used to synchronize heart depolarization in order to maintain CO. In this type of pacing, both the atria and the ventricles are paced. Spikes appear before the P wave and the QRS complex.

The number of times the pacemaker will fire is determined by the sensitivity setting of the pacemaker. If the sensitivity is low, the pacemaker basically ignores the patient's ventricles and will pace more frequently. If the sensitivity is high, the patient's ventricles will be allowed to discharge. Most pacemakers are set on demand, with a high sensitivity setting. A paced beat only occurs when the patient's atria or ventricles fail to discharge. If the pacemaker competes with the patient's own impulse generation, the term *failure to sense* is used. This is a potentially dangerous situation, since the pacemaker may discharge an impulse during the relative refrac-

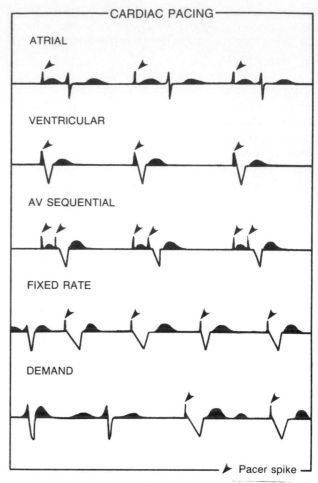

Figure 7–27. ECG examples of artificial cardiac pacing (see text for discussion). Arrow indicates pacer spike. (*From E. McErlean and G. Whitman, 1991, p. 859. Therapeutic modalities in the treatment of the patient with cardiovascular dysfunction. In J. Dolan, ed.* Critical care nursing: Clinical management through the nursing process. *Philadelphia: F.A. Davis.*)

tory or supranormal periods of ventricular repolarization, precipitating ventricular fibrillation. The term *failure to capture* is used to describe the situation in which the pacemaker initiates an impulse, but the stimulus is not strong enough to produce depolarization. A pacing spike may be present, but P waves or QRS complexes or both are absent. Figure 7–27 is an example of artificially paced ECG patterns.

An automatic internal defibrillator may be implanted in patients who chronically experience runs of symptomatic ventricular tachycardia. The device will discharge to override the ectopic ventricular pacemaker. An automatic external defibrillator may be used by some medical and nursing service personnel and laypersons to treat ventricular tachycardia and ventricular fibrillation. The ECG pattern is detected through pads placed on the patient's chest. If a lethal dysrhythmia is detected, the paddles will discharge to defibrillate the patient.

Nursing care includes preparing the patient for insertion of an endocardial pacemaker or applying an external pacing device correctly. The ECG pattern must be monitored to determine that the pacemaker is pacing at the correct rate (demand vs fixed), capturing with each impulse, and sensing the patient's own rhythm. Additionally, the nurse assesses the threshold (minimal amount of output required to initiate depolarization) of the pacemaker. The learner is referred to the literature associated with each artificial

pacing device to determine the correct method of checking the threshold for that device.

In summary, there are three forms of artificial pacing: external, epicardial, and endocardial. The atria or the ventricles may be paced. The rate may be set on demand or continuous setting. The pacing device may fail to sense and compete with the patient's own rhythm. The device may fail to capture by initiating an impulse that is not sufficient to depolarize myocardial cells. Nursing care focuses on assisting with insertion or application and monitoring threshold, capture, and sensitivity of the device.

Section Fourteen Review

1. An external pacing device
   A. is used only to treat supraventricular dysrhythmias
   B. is a temporary measure
   C. requires the patient to be alert in order to function
   D. can be set only in continuous mode
2. An epicardial pacing device
   A. is placed through the subclavian vein
   B. is applied to the chest wall
   C. is inserted in open heart surgery
   D. is used exclusively for AV sequential pacing

3. Failure to sense means
   A. the pacing device is turned off
   B. depolarization is not occurring
   C. the patient is tachycardic
   D. the pacing device is competing with the patient's own rhythm
4. Failure to capture means
   A. depolarization does not occur after a pacer-generated impulse
   B. atria and ventricles are not contracting in a synchronous manner
   C. the pacing device needs to be replaced
   D. the patient will require cardioversion

Answers: 1, B. 2, C. 3, D. 4, A.

Section Fifteen: Nursing Care of the Patient Being Cardiac Monitored

At the completion of this section, the learner will be able to discuss nursing interventions appropriate for the patient who is being cardiac monitored.

There are several nursing actions for a patient requiring cardiac monitoring. The chest wall should be shaved and treated with an adhesive (i.e., tincture of benzoin, skin preparation) before placement of the electrodes, especially for individuals who are sweating profusely. This will help to ensure a good connection. Sites may be rotated every 24 hours to prevent skin breakdown. The sensitivity knob of the cardiac monitor may need to be adjusted in order to view complexes. Alarms on the monitor should be set and

left on and be audible to the nurse. An ECG strip should be recorded and placed on the nursing assessment record on a regular basis.

The patient should have explained to him or her why cardiac monitoring is required. Patients may need to be reassured that they are protected from electric shocks from the equipment. They may need to know that the alarms may sound as a result of patient movement and other factors in addition to cardiac abnormalities.

To summarize, a patient experiencing cardiac dysrhythmias may be observed only or treated using drugs, a pacemaker, or electric shock. The nursing care for a patient being cardiac monitored includes decreasing the patient's fear and increasing his or her knowledge regarding the procedure. A patient who is experiencing a dysrhythmia may be in pain and anxious. The nurse must prioritize care by identifying and treating the dysrhythmia per physician orders. However, interventions can be conducted in a humanistic manner, thereby decreasing anxiety and myocardial oxygen demands through all available routes.

Section Fifteen Review

1. Which of the following patients may need the skin prepared in order to obtain a good connection for the monitoring electrode?
   A. dyspneic patient
   B. diaphoretic patient
   C. obese patient
   D. elderly patient
2. Alarms on the cardiac monitor
   A. may be left off if the patient is in normal sinus rhythm
   B. should be kept low to prevent patient disturbance
   C. should be audible and left on
   D. may be set to the patient's highest heart rate demonstrated
3. Which of the following knobs may need to be turned if the complex is too small to view on the screen?
   A. capture knob
   B. volume knob
   C. alarm knob
   D. sensitivity knob

Answers: 1, B. 2, C. 3, D.

Posttest

1. Fluid volume deficit primarily produces
   A. tachydysrhythmias
   B. cardiac conduction blocks
   C. bradysrhythmias
   D. wide QRS complexes
2. Hypercalcemia results in
   A. increased automaticity
   B. premature atrial contractions (PACs)
   C. bradysrhythmias
   D. tall, peaked T waves
3. When the SA node is pacing the heart, the heart rate will be
   A. irregular
   B. less than 50 bpm
   C. less than 100 bpm
   D. regular
4. The ST segment should be
   A. less than 0.20 second
   B. isoelectric
   C. positively deflected
   D. peaked
5. Time is represented by
   A. vertical axis of the ECG paper
   B. color of ink on the ECG paper
   C. horizontal axis on the ECG paper
   D. asterisk at the bottom of the ECG paper
6. The length of the QT interval may vary in relation to
   A. blood pressure
   B. age
   C. heart rate
   D. sex
7. Depolarization is precipitated by
   A. potassium moving into the cell
   B. calcium moving out of the cell
   C. sodium moving into the cell
   D. sodium moving out of the cell
8. QRS complexes should be
   A. preceded by a T wave
   B. isoelectric
   C. positively deflected
   D. less than 0.12 second

9. Sinus bradycardia may be normal in
   A. athletes
   B. persons experiencing stressful situations
   C. elderly patients
   D. persons with hypertension

10. The major difference between cardioversion and defibrillation is
    A. the number of times each can be repeated
    B. one method is synchronized to discharge with an ectopic impulse
    C. one method is used to treat delays in cardiac conduction
    D. one method requires the patient to be alert

11. Atrial fibrillation is characterized by
    A. sawtoothed P waves
    B. regular QRS intervals
    C. absent P waves
    D. atrial rate less than 250 bpm

12. Verapamil may be used to treat
    A. sinus dysrhythmias
    B. conduction blocks
    C. ventricular dysrhythmias
    D. atrial dysrhythmias

13. Junctional tachycardia is differentiated from an accelerated junctional rhythm by
    A. presence of P wave
    B. length of PR interval
    C. rate of the rhythm
    D. QRS configuration

14. Premature atrial contractions (PACs) are usually
    A. preceded by a hypoxic episode
    B. a signal of ventricular irritability
    C. harmless
    D. associated with digitalis toxicity

15. Streptokinase may produce which of the following side effects?
    A. anaphylaxis
    B. thrombophlebitis
    C. pulmonary emboli
    D. vomiting

16. Failure to capture means the artificial pacing device
    A. is competing with the patient's own rhythm
    B. is not producing depolarization
    C. needs new batteries
    D. is causing PVCs

17. Type II second degree heart block
    A. is associated with ventricular irritability
    B. is more omnious than type I second degree heart block
    C. is less than 50 bpm
    D. requires treatment with verapamil

18. Which of the following patients, based on their history, would NOT be suitable for thrombolytic therapy?
    A. motor vehicle crash 6 months ago
    B. reperfusion by TPA 1 year ago
    C. right cerebrovascular attack 2 months ago
    D. delivered 6-pound daughter 6 months ago

19. ST segment depression is characteristic of
    A. impaired ventricular repolarization
    B. hypokalemia
    C. digitalis toxicity
    D. atrial irritability

20. Drugs that block beta-receptors (i.e., propranolol, esmolol, and nadolol) will
    A. decrease automaticity
    B. increase contractility
    C. increase conduction
    D. stimulate the AV node

Posttest Answers

Question	Answer	Section	Question	Answer	Section
1	A	Four	11	C	Six
2	C	Four	12	D	Six
3	C	Two	13	C	Seven
4	B	Two	14	C	Nine
5	C	Three	15	A	Twelve
6	C	Two	16	B	Fourteen
7	C	One	17	B	Ten
8	D	Two	18	C	Twelve
9	A	Five	19	A	Eleven
10	B	Thirteen	20	A	Thirteen

REFERENCES

American Heart Association. (1987). *Textbook of advanced cardiac life support.* Dallas, Texas: American Heart Association.

Bennet, K., and Grines, C. (1990). Current controversies in patient selection for thrombolytic therapy. *J. Emergency Nursing.* 16:191–194.

Brewer-Senerchia, C. (1989). Thrombolytic therapy: A review of the literature on streptokinase and tissue plasminogen activator with implications for practice. *Crit. Care Nursing Clin. of North Am.* 1:359–371.

Grigg, J., and Stromberg, R. (1990). Immediate emergency department intervention in myocardial infarction. *Topics Emergency Med.* 12 (4):19–28.

Guyton, A. (1986). *Textbook of medical physiology,* 7th ed. Philadelphia: W.B. Saunders Co.

Kemp, D., and Dolan, J. (1991). Anatomy and physiology of the cardiovascular system. In J. Dolan (ed.) *Critical care nursing: Clinical management through the nursing process,* pp. 719–750. Philadelphia: F.A. Davis.

Martin, S., Chesnick, P., and Young, J. (1990). Invasive cardiac procedures after myocardial infarction: Which procedure when and its relationship to thrombolysis. *J. Emergency Nursing.* 16:202–207.

Meltzer, L., Pinneo, R., and Kitchell, J. (1983). *Intensive coronary care.* Bowie, Maryland: Brady Co.

Shlafer, M., and Marieb, E. (1989). *The nurse, pharmacology, and drug therapy.* Redwood City, California: Addison-Wesley.

Thelan, L, Davie, J., and Urden, L. (1990). *Textbook of critical care nursing: Diagnosis and management.* St. Louis: C.V. Mosby Co.

Toledo, L., and Dolan, J. (1991). Electrocardiography: An overview. In J. Dolan (ed.), *Critical care nursing: Clinical management through the nursing process,* pp. 789–827. Philadelphia: F.A. Davis.

Shock States

Karen L. Johnson

The major function of the cardiovascular system is to deliver blood, oxygen, and nutrients to the cells, tissues, and organs of the body and to remove metabolic wastes. When this fails to occur, a state of shock occurs.

Defining shock is more difficult than defining other disease entities. No one seems to agree on one concise definition because shock is a syndrome, a complex of signs and symptoms that describe a sequence of changes that occur when the circulation fails to meet its major objective. One of the best definitions of shock, primarily because it is nonspecific, was offered by Samuel Gross over 100 years ago. He characterized shock as a "rude unhinging of the machinery of life." Continuing research has improved the understanding of the basic concepts of shock. There seems to be a growing consensus that shock occurs when delivery of oxygen to organs is insufficient to meet metabolic demands and remove metabolic wastes (Greenburg, 1988). Buran (1987, p. 19) describes shock as the "inability of oxygen delivery to support metabolic demands of the tissues." Because of an imbalance between oxygen supply and demand

in shock, a functional impairment develops in cells, tissues, and eventually body systems (Rice, 1991a). The relationship between oxygen supply (delivery) and oxygen demand (consumption) serves as the conceptual framework for shock in this module.

This self-study module is composed of six sections. Sections One and Two review the principles of oxygen delivery and consumption. Section Three describes the pathologic mechanisms of impaired oxygen delivery and consumption for shock states. In Sections Four and Five, information is given to assist the learner in understanding compensatory mechanisms and clinical manifestations that occur with shock. The final section describes medical and nursing interventions that optimize oxygen delivery and decrease oxygen consumption. Each section includes review questions to help the reader evaluate understanding of section content before moving on to the next section. All section reviews and the Pretest and Posttest in the module include answers. It is suggested that the learner review those concepts that have been missed in the review questions before proceeding to the next section.

Objectives

At the completion of this module, the learner will be able to

1. Identify factors that control oxygen delivery
2. Identify conditions that alter oxygen consumption

3. Describe the pathologic mechanisms of impaired oxygen delivery and oxygen consumption for each of the four functional classifications of shock states
4. Describe the physiologic compensatory mecha-

nisms that occur to correct the imbalance of oxygen delivery and consumption in shock

5. List the clinical manifestations and hemodynamics for each of the four functional shock states

6. State the medical and nursing interventions that optimize oxygen delivery and decrease oxygen consumption

Pretest

1. Oxygen delivery is
   A. the product of cardiac output and the amount of hemoglobin in the blood
   B. the product of cardiac output and arterial oxygen content
   C. dependent on the amount of oxygen in the blood and size of the vessels
   D. dependent on the amount of blood passing pulmonary capillaries
2. Oxygen delivery in response to tissue needs occurs as a result of
   A. autoregulation
   B. inotropic activity
   C. chronotropic activity
   D. dopaminergic stimulation
3. Oxygen consumption is
   A. dependent on oxygen delivery
   B. dependent on the amount of blood extracted by the tissues
   C. the amount of oxygen used by the body
   D. dependent on the size of the blood vessels
4. Neuromuscular blocking agents
   A. increase oxygen consumption
   B. decrease oxygen consumption
   C. increase oxygen delivery
   D. decrease oxygen delivery
5. Common to all shock states is
   A. blood pressure of 90 mm Hg, heart rate greater than 100 bpm
   B. loss of blood volume
   C. decreased oxygen delivery with decreased oxygen consumption
   D. impaired oxygen delivery with increased oxygen consumption
6. Which of the following shock states have similar pathologic mechanisms?
   A. neurogenic and septic shocks
   B. anaphylactic and cardiogenic shocks
   C. left-sided cardiogenic shock and right-sided cardiogenic shock
   D. carbon monoxide poisoning and cardiac tamponade

7. Which of the following is NOT one of the sympathetic nervous system's fight-or-flight responses?
   A. increased heart rate
   B. dilation of pupils
   C. increased respiratory rate
   D. increased intestinal peristalasis
8. Which of the following is a potent vasoconstrictor?
   A. renin
   B. aldosterone
   C. angiotensin II
   D. ADH
9. In neurogenic shock, signs and symptoms are related to
   A. loss of spinal fluid
   B. damaged parasympathetic cells
   C. loss of hypothalamic control
   D. loss of sympathetic innervation
10. Shock states
   A. increase oxygen consumption
   B. decrease oxygen consumption
   C. increase oxygen delivery
   D. do not affect oxygen delivery and consumption
11. Which of the following decreases oxygen consumption?
   A. hyperventilation
   B. hyperthyroid
   C. sedation
   D. hyperthermia

Pretest answers: 1, B. 2, A. 3, C. 4, B. 5, D. 6, A. 7, D. 8, C. 9, D. 10, A. 11, C.

Glossary

Autologous blood. Blood lost from the patient, which is diverted via a collection tube to a collection chamber, mixed with an anticoagulant, and reinfused back into the same patient

Military antishock trousers (MAST). Trouserlike suit that encloses the legs, thighs, and trunk and exerts a variable degree of compression on the underlying tissues; theoretically, this garment empties the veins in these portions of the body and returns more blood to the systemic circulation; also called pneumatic antishock garment (PASG)

Oxygen consumption. The amount of oxygen used by the body; described as a product of cardiac output and the difference between arterial oxygen content and venous oxygen content

Oxygen delivery. The product of cardiac output and arterial oxygen content

Pneumatic antishock garment. *See* Military antishock trousers (MAST)

Abbreviations

ACTH. Adrenocorticotropic hormone

ADH. Antidiuretic hormone

ATP. Adenosine triphosphate

Cao_2. Oxygen content of arterial blood

CI. Cardiac index

CO. Cardiac output

CVP. Central venous pressure

Do_2. Oxygen delivery

GI. Gastrointestinal

Hct. Hematocrit

Hg. Hemoglobin

HR. Heart rate

IABP. Intraaortic balloon counterpulsation

MAP. Mean arterial pressure

MDF. Myocardial depressant factor

MSO_4. Morphine sulfate

MSOF. Multisystem organ failure

O_2. Oxygen

$Paco_2$. Partial pressure of dissolved gas in the plasma of arterial blood due to carbon dioxide

Pao_2. Partial pressure of dissolved gas in the plasma of arterial blood due to oxygen

PAP. Pulmonary artery pressure

PAWP. Pulmonary artery wedge pressure

RAP. Right atrial pressure

SVR. Systemic vascular resistance

Vo_2. Oxygen consumption

Section One: Oxygen Delivery

At the completion of this section, the learner will be able to identify factors that control oxygen delivery.

The major function of the circulatory system is to deliver oxygen to tissues (Demling, 1988). Cells require oxygen for efficient adenosine triphosphate (ATP) production. ATP provides the cells with energy needed to maintain their specific cell function. Since oxygen cannot be stored, ATP synthesis requires a continuous supply of oxygen. Oxygen delivery is dependent on the amount of blood ejected from the left ventricle and the amount of oxygen carried in that blood. Oxygen delivery (Do_2) is described as the product of cardiac output (CO) and arterial oxygen content (Cao_2) in the equation

$$Do_2 = Cao_2 \times CO$$

The amount of oxygen delivered to the tissues each minute is 900 to 1,100 mL/minute (Mims, 1989). Assessment of CO, hemoglobin, and arterial oxygen content can be used to evaluate the adequacy of oxygen delivery in critically ill patients (Mims, 1989). Factors that control oxygen delivery include (1) the heart's pumping ability, (2) local tissues autoregulation, and (3) autonomic nervous system regulation.

Under normal circumstances, the volume of blood ejected by the left ventricle is proportional to the body's demands. The amount of blood pumped by the heart depends on the heart rate and stroke volume. When tissues require more oxygen, the heart rate will increase in an attempt to augment CO to deliver more oxygenated blood. Tissues have the ability to regulate their own blood supply by dilating or constricting local blood vessels through the mechanism of autoregulation. Tissues have varying energy requirements and have this autoregulation ability to meet their metabolic needs. Autoregulation serves to protect tissues by controlling the blood flow and oxygen delivery in response to individual tissue needs.

The autonomic nervous system exerts partial control of oxygen delivery through excitatory or inhibitory effects on the heart, lungs, and blood vessels. Autonomic signals are transmitted through two subdivisions, the sympathetic and parasympathetic systems. The sympathetic nervous system mediators control oxygen delivery by affecting the heart's inotropic and chronotropic activity. Specific cell mediators (catecholamines) present in the cardiovascular and respiratory systems, when stimulated, result in a specific cell response. The types of cell receptors that respond to the catecholamines are alpha$_1$ and alpha$_2$, beta$_1$ and beta$_2$, and dopaminergic receptors. Stimulation and physiologic response of these receptors are listed in Table 8–1.

In summary, the major function of the cardiovascular system is oxygen delivery to tissues.

TABLE 8–1. ALPHA, BETA, AND DOPAMINERGIC RECEPTOR STIMULATION AND PHYSIOLOGIC RESPONSE

Receptor	Stimulation	Physiologic Response
Alpha$_1$	Vasoconstriction Intestinal relaxation	Increased vascular resistance Increased pressure and afterload
Alpha$_2$	Suppression of norepinephrine	Controls excess catecholamine release
Beta$_1$	Increased myocardial rate and contractility	Increased cardiac output Increased myocardial oxygen consumption
Beta$_2$	Bronchodilation Vasodilation	Decreased airway resistance Decreased vascular resistance
Dopaminergic	Renal vasodilation Mesenteric vasodilation	Increased renal blood flow Increased mesenteric blood flow

Oxygen delivery is determined by the amount of oxygen in arterial blood and CO. Oxygen delivery is controlled in proportion to tissue metabolic demands for oxygen. Factors that control oxygen delivery include the heart's ability to function as a pump, vasodilation and vasoconstriction, which are influenced by local tissue autoregulation, and the mediators of the sympathetic and parasympathetic nervous systems.

The delivery of oxygen to tissues must be adequate to meet the oxygen demands. Oxygen consumption is discussed in the next section.

Section One Review

1. Which of the following factors do not control oxygen delivery?
   A. local tissue regulation
   B. the heart's pumping ability
   C. autonomic nervous system regulation
   D. the amount of oxygen saturated with hemoglobin
2. A continuous supply of oxygen is
   A. not necessary, since oxygen is stored in the cells
   B. required for ATP synthesis
   C. dependent on the amount of blood ejected from the left ventricle
   D. dependent on adequate supplies of hemoglobin

3. Which of the following occurs to deliver more oxygenated blood with increased demands for oxygen?
   A. release of oxygen from hemoglobin
   B. vasoconstriction
   C. increase in cardiac output (CO)
   D. bronchoconstriction
4. Administration of a drug that stimulates dopaminergic receptors would
   A. decrease pressure
   B. increase CO
   C. increase renal blood flow
   D. decrease afterload

5. Stimulation of an alpha$_1$-receptor produces
   A. vasoconstriction
   B. vasodilation
   C. increased heart rate
   D. bronchodilation

Section Two: Oxygen Consumption

At the completion of this section, the learner will be able to define oxygen consumption and identify conditions that alter oxygen consumption.

Adequacy of tissue perfusion is determined by a balance between oxygen supply (delivery) and oxygen demand (consumption). When tissues have increased energy demands, they extract more oxygen from the blood. Different organs have different oxygen demands to perform their functions and, therefore, extract different amounts of oxygen from hemoglobin. The heart extracts about 11.5 percent, the brain extracts about 6.2 percent, and the kidneys extract about 1.5 percent (Demling, 1988).

Oxygen consumption (Vo_2) is a measurement of the amount of oxygen used by the body. Oxygen consumption is described as the product of CO and the difference between arterial oxygen content and venous oxygen content in the equation

$$Vo_2 = CO \times c(a - v)o_2$$

Oxygen consumption is depicted in Figure 8–1.

Conditions may exist that can alter tissue demands for oxygen. These conditions are summarized in Table 8–2. Oxygen consumption varies in proportion to body temperature. There is a 10 to 13 percent increase in oxygen consumption for every degree (C) in temperature above normal (Buran, 1987). Like-

TABLE 8–2. CONDITIONS THAT ALTER OXYGEN CONSUMPTION

Increase O$_2$ consumption	Hyperventilation, hyperthermia, trauma, sepsis, anxiety, stress, hyperthyroidism, increased muscle activity
Decrease O$_2$ consumption	Hypoventilation, hypothermia, sedation, neuromuscular blocking agents, anesthesia, hypothyroidism, inactivity

wise, hypothermia decreases metabolic rates and, therefore, decreases oxygen consumption. Skeletal injuries can increase oxygen consumption by 10 to 30 percent, severe infections can increase oxygen consumption by 60 percent, and major burns can increase oxygen consumption by 100 percent (Buran, 1987). Injured tissue requires more oxygen for repair and also stimulates the development of a hypermetabolic state. Neuromuscular blocking agents (e.g., pancuronium, vecuronium) may be administered to decrease resting muscle tone so little energy and thus oxygen are consumed.

Increased CO usually is the first compensatory mechanism initiated to meet an increased tissue oxygen demand or a decreased oxygen supply to the tissues (Von Rueden, 1989). When increased oxygen demands cannot be compensated by an increased CO, the tissues increase the amount of oxygen they

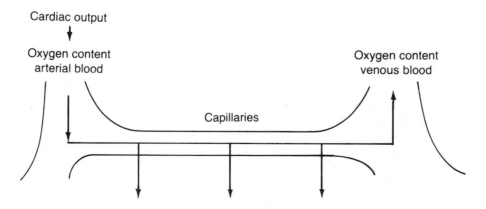

Tissues extract from hgb the amount
of oxygen needed to perform their function

Figure 8–1. Oxygen consumption.

extract from the blood. When these compensatory mechanisms fail and cellular oxygen demands exceed supply, ATP production is altered, anaerobic metabolism ensues, and lactic acid is produced (Shoemaker, 1987).

Ongoing assessment of oxygen delivery and consumption can be made in the intensive care unit through the use of a special pulmonary artery catheter that has a fiberoptic lumen. This fiberoptic lumen monitors the percent of hemoglobin with oxygen mixed in venous blood.Continuous monitoring of mixed venous oxygen saturation (Svo_2) provides ongoing evidence between oxygen supply and demand. The Svo_2 returning to the right ventricle reflects the oxygen consumption of body tissues. The normal range of Svo_2 is 60 to 80 percent (Mims, 1989). When the Svo_2 drops below 60 percent, it reflects an imbalance of oxygen supply and demand. Either the oxygen supply to tissues has decreased (decreased CO, arterial saturation, or hemoglobin), or tissue demands for oxygen have increased (e.g., pain, fever). With an increase in Svo_2, more oxygenated blood is returning to the right ventricle. This can be related to an increased oxygen supply (high Fio_2) that is not needed by the tissues, the tissues are not extracting oxygen effectively (anaerobic metabolism), or tissue demand for oxygen has decreased (hypothermia, neuromuscular blocking agents). Thus, assessment of mixed venous oxygen saturation, or Svo_2 monitoring, indicates the adequacy of the supply of oxygen in relation to tissue demands.

In summary, cells require oxygen to synthesize ATP to provide energy to maintain their specific cell function. Cells of different organs have different oxygen demands to meet their needs and, therefore, extract different amounts of oxygen from hemoglobin. Oxygen consumption is a measurement of the amount of oxygen used by tissues. Several clinical conditions are known to alter oxygen consumption. When tissues need more oxygen, CO increases to increase the oxygen supply as tissues attempt to extract more oxygen from the blood. If these compensatory mechanisms fail, ATP production is altered, anaerobic metabolism ensues, and lactic acid is produced. A continuous assessment of oxygen supply and demand can be made in the intensive care unit by using a Svo_2 pulmonary artery catheter.

Section Two Review

1. Oxygen consumption is
   A. the difference between oxygen content of arterial blood and venous blood
   B. a measurement of the amount of oxygen used by the body
   C. dependent on arterial oxygen content and cardiac output (CO)
   D. the product of CO and venous oxygen content

2. Which one of the following conditions increases oxygen consumption?
   A. pancuronium 10 mg IV
   B. MSO_4 5 mg IV
   C. bedrest
   D. temperature of 102F

3. Which of the following conditions decreases oxygen consumption?
   A. temperature of 102F
   B. 75 percent full-thickness burn
   C. MSO_4 5 mg IV
   D. respiratory rate of 50/minute

4. Which of the following organs extracts the most amount of oxygen from blood?
   A. heart
   B. brain
   C. lungs
   D. kidneys

5. Severe infections can increase oxygen consumption by
   A. 100 percent
   B. 60 percent
   C. 5 percent
   D. 20 percent

Answers: 1, B. 2, D. 3, C. 4, A. 5, B.

Section Three: Functional Classifications of Shock States

At the completion of this section, the learner will be able to describe the mechanism of impaired oxygen delivery and consumption for each of the four functional classifications of shock.

Common to all shock states is impaired oxygen delivery with altered oxygen consumption. Traditionally, shock states have been classified according to their etiology, e.g., septic shock, hemorrhagic shock, neurogenic shock. More recently, shock has been categorized into four functional states, a classification that is useful for critical care nursing (Clochesy, 1988). The functional classifications of shock states are hypovolemic, transport, obstructive, and cardiogenic. These classifications are grouped not according to the cause of the shock state but according to similar mechanisms responsible for impaired oxygen delivery. Hypovolemic shock states have impaired oxygen delivery because of inadequate intravascular volume, resulting in decreased CO. Transport shock states have impaired oxygen delivery due to a diminished supply of hemoglobin in which to carry oxygen to tissues. Obstructive shock states have impaired oxygen delivery because of a mechanical barrier impeding blood flow to tissues. Cardiogenic shock states have impaired oxygen delivery because the heart fails to function as a pump to deliver oxygenated blood into the systemic circulation. The functional states, causes, and mechanisms of impaired oxygen delivery are summarized in Table 8–3.

Hypovolemic Shock States

Hypovolemia can result from two conditions: the fluid volume in the circulation has decreased or the size of the intravascular compartment has increased in proportion to the fluid volume. When either or both of these conditions occur, there is decreased venous return to the right heart. This reduces ventricular filling pressure, stroke volume, CO, and blood pressure.

Loss of intravascular volume can be caused by loss of blood volume (hemorrhage) or as a result of loss of intravascular fluid from the skin (as with dehydration or burns), loss of fluid from persistent vomiting or diarrhea, or loss of fluid from the intravascular compartment to interstitial spaces (third spacing). A diminished fluid volume leads to a decreased CO, resulting in impaired oxygen delivery.

Hypovolemic shock states also can be caused by an abnormal placement of vascular volume. The blood volume may be normal, but the intravascular volume is maldistributed because of alterations in the size of the blood vessels (Rice, 1991a). Persistent arterial vasodilation causes the intravascular compartment to increase without a corresponding increase in volume. Arterial vasodilation is seen with neurogenic shock, anaphylactic shock, and septic shock.

Neurogenic shock may occur with a spinal cord injury. When there is injury to the spinal cord above the midthoracic region, impulses from the sympathetic nervous system cannot reach the arterioles. The loss of sympathetic nerve innervation prohibits vasoconstriction of blood vessels, but blood vessels

---

TABLE 8–3. FUNCTIONAL STATES OF SHOCK, CAUSES, AND PATHOLOGIC MECHANISMS

Functional State	Etiology	Mechanism of Impaired O_2 Delivery
Hypovolemic	Fluid volume loss (dehydration, burn injuries, third spacing)	Loss of intravascular volume
	Vasodilation (neurogenic shock, anaphylactic shock, septic shock)	Increase in vessel diameter Loss of sympathetic tone Histamine release Endotoxin release
Transport	Hg unable to carry O_2 (anemia, hemorrhage, carbon monoxide poisoning)	Dysfunction or inadequate amount of RBCs and or Hg Inadequate amount of RBCs and Hg Carbon monoxide preferentially bound to Hg
Obstructive	Mechanical barriers to blood flow (pulmonary embolism, tension pneumothorax, cardiac tamponade)	Barrier to blood flow Pulmonary artery blocked Great vessels kinked Ventricles unable to fill or eject blood volume
Cardiogenic	Heart fails to function as a pump (myocardial infarction, dysrhythmias)	Ischemic muscles fail to contract Irregular rate/rhythm causes heart to fail its function as a pump

Adapted from *Essentials of critical care nursing*, p. 127, edited by J.M. Closchesy, 1988, Rockville, MD: Aspen Publishing Inc.

continue to receive parasympathetic innervation allowing vasodilation. Blood then pools in the dilated peripheral venous system. The right heart receives an inadequate venous return, and CO decreases. As CO decreases, delivery of oxygen-carrying blood decreases.

Anaphylactic shock occurs in response to a severe allergic reaction. Massive amounts of vasoactive substances (e.g., histamine, serotonin, prostaglandins) are released, causing vasodilation and increased capillary permeability. Vasodilation increases the intravascular compartment. The increased capillary permeability allows fluid to move from intravascular spaces to interstitial spaces. As fluid is lost from the vascular compartment, a relative hypovolemia develops. The net consequences of combined massive vasodilation and increased capillary permeability alter peripheral blood flow and decrease tissue perfusion (Rice, 1991a).

Septic shock is a systemic response to invading microorganisms of all types: gram-positive and gram-negative bacteria, fungi, or viruses. The most common causative organisms in septic shock are gram-negative bacteria. These organisms release endotoxins that invade the bloodstream and stimulate the release of mediators, such as histamine, kinins, leukotrienes, and prostaglandins. These substances produce vasodilation and increased capillary permeability. This reduces venous return and lowers diastolic filling pressures in the heart. A second fluid alteration seen in septic shock is a maldistribution of circulating blood volume. Some organs receive more blood than needed as a result of vasodilation, whereas others (skin, lungs, kidneys) do not receive the blood flow they need. Altered fluid volume related to vasodilation, increased capillary permeability, and maldistribution of circulating volume characterize septic shock.

Transport Shock States

The common pathologic mechanism in transport shock states is a diminished supply of hemoglobin available to carry oxygen to tissues. With anemia and hemorrhage, there are less red blood cells and thus less hemoglobin for oxygen to bind to. Carbon monoxide has a higher affinity for hemoglobin than does oxygen. When carbon monoxide is inhaled, it binds rapidly and specifically with hemoglobin. The affinity of carbon monoxide for hemoglobin is over 200 times that of oxygen (Wruk, 1990). This reduces the carrying capacity of blood for oxygen, inhibits unloading of oxygen to all tissues, and results in hypoxia, especially to the brain and heart. With carbon monoxide poisoning, an adequate amount of oxygen

may be available to bind with hemoglobin, but it is prevented from binding with hemoglobin because carbon monoxide has preferentially bound to the hemoglobin. A shock state occurs as the supply of oxygen to tissues is severely restricted.

Obstructive Shock States

Obstructive shock states occur as a result of a mechanical barrier to blood flow that blocks oxygen delivery to tissues. Causes may be attributed to pulmonary embolism, tension pneumothorax, or cardiac tamponade.

Emboli resulting from a venous thrombosis usually are large to moderate in size and can occlude a major pulmonary artery. This can result in occlusion of a substantial portion of the pulmonary circulation, which eliminates a significant portion of the gas-exchanging area. Blood cannot receive oxygen from the lungs, and, thus, oxygen delivery to meet tissue demands cannot occur.

A tension pneumothorax occurs when air enters the pleural space during inspiration but cannot leave during expiration. The progressive accumulation of air within the thoracic cavity leads to a shift of the mediastinal structures and compression of the opposite lung. The increased pleural pressure decreases venous return to the heart.

Cardiac tamponade is caused by bleeding into a nonflexible pericardial sac. The accumulating pressure around the heart increases intracardiac pressures, impairing ventricular filling and decreasing cardiac output.

Cardiogenic Shock States

Cardiogenic shock states are produced when the heart fails in its pumping function. Dysfunction of either the right or left ventricle can lead to cardiogenic shock. Failure can occur when the right ventricle fails to pump the volume of venous blood returned to it or when the left ventricle fails to pump oxygenated blood to the systemic circulation. Causes of cardiogenic shock, in order of frequency, include severe left ventricular failure (as a result of a myocardial infarction), acute mitral regurgitation, ventricular septal defect, and right ventricular infarction (Demling, 1988).

A left ventricular myocardial infarction produces a necrotic area that impairs contractility and CO. Severe left ventricular failure occurs when greater than 40 percent of the left ventricular myocardium is necrosed (Daily, 1989). As the right ventricle pumps blood into the pulmonary vasculature, the pulmonary vasculature becomes engorged because the left ventricle cannot effectively pump out the volume it has received. As the CO and stroke volume decrease, systemic blood pressure and oxygen delivery decrease.

Right ventricular infarction occurs in approximately one third to one half of all patients with an inferior myocardial infarction (Daily, 1989). In cardiogenic shock caused by dysfunction of the right ventricle, the right ventricle is unable to pump adequate amounts of blood into the lungs. Filling of the pulmonary vasculature decreases, filling of the left ventricle decreases, and, consequently, CO decreases.

In summary, shock states can be classified according to the common pathologic mechanisms that produce the impaired oxygen delivery: hypovolemic, transport, obstructive, and cardiogenic shock states. Independent of etiology or pathologic mechanisms, altered tissue perfusion with impaired oxygen delivery in relation to oxygen consumption is common to all forms of shock.

Section Three Review

1. Which of the following conditions produces a hypovolemic shock state?
   A. carbon monoxide poisoning
   B. tension pneumothorax
   C. pulmonary emboli
   D. third spacing
2. Which of the following conditions can produce a transport shock state?
   A. carbon monoxide poisoning
   B. dehydration
   C. cardiac tamponade
   D. anaphylactic shock
3. Which of the following conditions can produce an obstructive shock state?
   A. myocardial infarction
   B. anemia
   C. pulmonary emboli
   D. sepsis

4. Which of the following statements characterizes septic shock?
   A. occurs as a result of fluid shifts and vasoconstriction
   B. inadequate oxygen delivery and impaired oxygen consumption
   C. loss of sympathetic nerve innervation prohibits vasoconstriction
   D. occurs in response to an allergic reaction
5. The most common cause of cardiogenic shock is
   A. right ventricular failure
   B. left ventricular failure
   C. acute mitral valve regurgitation
   D. ventricular septal defect

Answers: 1, D. 2, A. 3, C. 4, B. 5, B.

Section Four: Physiologic Response to Shock

At the completion of this section, the learner will be able to describe the compensatory mechanisms that occur in response to shock states.

When oxygen delivery does not support tissue metabolic demands, shock occurs. In an attempt to stabilize this life-threatening situation, a pattern of responses, or compensatory mechanisms, occurs.

Compensation in Shock

Complex neuroendocrine responses are triggered to overcome ineffective circulating blood volume. Low pressure stretch receptors in the right atrium sense a decreased circulating blood volume when there is a decreased venous return to the right atrium. Baroreceptors in the aorta and carotid arteries sense a decrease in blood volume and cardiac output. Carotid body chemoreceptors sense alterations in pH and Pco_2. These receptors all alert the hypothalamus to what could be a life-threatening situation.

The hypothalamus releases adrenocorticotropic hormone (ACTH), which activates the adrenals to secrete aldosterone. Aldosterone causes sodium and water retention in efforts to increase the blood volume and blood pressure. Sodium and water retention stimulates the release of antidiuretic hormone (ADH), which prevents reabsorption of water in the

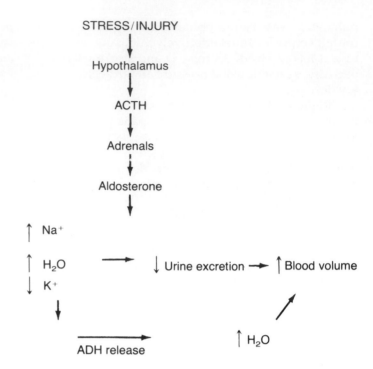

Figure 8–2. ACTH, aldosterone, and ADH release.

kidney tubules and thus increases the blood volume. The goal of the release of these hormones is to preserve blood volume by conserving the amount of fluid excreted by the kidneys. This process is summarized in Figure 8–2.

The baroreceptors and chemoreceptors alert the hypothalamus to activate the sympathetic nervous system's fight-or-flight response. This system releases a massive amount of norepinephrine, which produces several compensatory mechanisms (Table 8–4).

CO must be augmented in shock to ensure adequate tissue perfusion. CO is proportional to venous return. To increase venous return, sodium and water are retained by ACTH, aldosterone, and ADH. In addition to these hormones, another mechanism, the renin-angiotensin-aldosterone cycle, is activated to increase blood volume and venous return. As a result of decreased blood flow to the kidneys, the juxtaglomerular cells in the kidneys excrete renin. Renin catalyzes angiotensinogen in the liver, which then converts to angiotensin I in the circulation. Once in the lungs, angiotensin I converts to angiotensin II, which is a potent vasoconstrictor. The vasoconstriction produced by angiotensin II increases blood pressure by increasing afterload. Angiotensin II is converted to angiotensin III, which stimulate the release of aldosterone. The renin-angiotensin-aldosterone cycle is depicted in Figure 8–3.

TABLE 8–4. SYMPATHETIC NERVOUS SYSTEM'S FIGHT-OR-FLIGHT RESPONSE

Physiologic Response	Physiologic Rationale
Increased blood pressure	Due to vasoconstriction
Increased heart rate	For rapid delivery of needed oxygen
Increased respiratory rate	Bronchodilation occurs to receive more oxygen and correct acidosis
Increased glycolysis	To increase availability of glucose for energy
Decreased urinary output	To conserve fluid volume, return more blood volume to cardiovascular system to increase volume and blood pressure
Decreased blood flow to internal organs (i.e., kidneys, gastrointestinal tract, liver)	To allow more blood flow to more vital organs (i.e., heart and lungs)
Decreased intestinal peristalsis	Shunting of blood to vital organs, no need for digestion as body energy is redirected to life-saving measures
Cool skin	Alpha receptors produce peripheral vasoconstriction to shunt blood to more vital organs
Diaphoresis	To release heat as a by-product of energy use

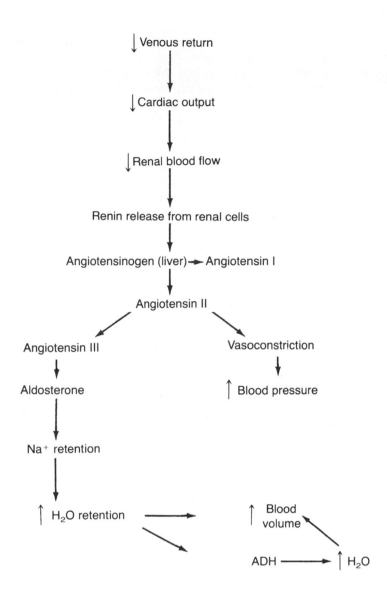

Figure 8–3. Renin-angiotensin-aldosterone cycle.

The cardiovascular response to shock is designed to restore blood volume and pressure toward normal. The mechanisms responsible for restoring cardiovascular homeostasis include augmentation of CO, redistribution of blood flow, and restoration of blood volume.

Phases of Shock

There are three stages of shock: nonprogressive, progressive, and irreversible. In the nonprogressive stage, tissue perfusion is altered, and the compensatory mechanisms occur to prevent further deterioration and restore homeostasis. During the progressive stage of shock, shock has progressed to a point of cardiovascular collapse, and if it is left untreated, death occurs. In the irreversible phase, the body has become resistant to treatment, and death is inevitable.

When shock is so severe that the compensatory mechanisms cannot restore homeostasis and if prompt and proper treatment of shock has not been instituted, nonprogressive shock becomes progressive shock. Compensatory physiologic changes that initially were helpful in shunting blood to vital organs become ineffective in the progressive phase of shock (Rice, 1991b). Progressive shock results in major dysfunction of many organs. The continued low blood flow, poor tissue perfusion, inadequate oxygen delivery, and buildup of metabolic wastes over time lead to multisystem organ failure (MSOF). Dysfunction of organ systems can occur alone or in combination. Usually, MSOF occurs as a series of events in a vicious cycle. When these organs fail in succession, mortality greatly increases.

As cerebral blood flow decreases, the patient's level of consciousness deteriorates. When renal blood flow is diminished long enough, renal failure occurs as a result of acute tubular necrosis. Toxic wastes, such as urea and creatinine, cannot be excreted and remain in the blood. The liver, because of its high metabolic rate, depends on an adequate blood supply of oxygen and an adequate circulatory system in which to excrete its metabolic wastes. With continued inadequate oxygenation, the liver cannot metabolize drugs and waste products, such as ammonia and lactic acid, which then accumulate in the blood. Since the liver normally filters debris and bacteria, these materials are allowed to accumulate in the circulation. Poor liver function also leads to fibrinolysis and the development of disseminated intravascular coagulation, which can cause an uncontrollable massive bleeding syndrome. Prolonged hypoperfusion leads to ischemia and ulceration of the stomach. Accumulation of gastric acid erodes gastric mucosa, causing a stress ulcer, and may precipitate gastrointestinal hemorrhage. Decreased perfusion and oxygenation of the pancreas activates some of the pancreatic enzymes, one of which is myocardial depressant factor (MDF). MDF depresses myocardial contractility. Decreased pulmonary capillary blood flow impairs gas exchange. Arterial oxygen levels decrease, and carbon dioxide levels increase. Surfactant keeps alveoli open, but in progressive shock, ischemic alveolar cells reduce its production. The alveoli collapse and produce massive atelectasis and decreased pulmonary compliance. The combination of massive atelectasis, interstitial edema, and reduced pulmonary compliance has a profound effect on ventilation and gas exchange. Respiratory failure in progressive shock is very common and is termed adult respiratory distress syndrome (ARDS) (Rice, 1991b).

If the reduction in oxygen supply continues in proportion to oxygen demand, metabolic wastes continue to accumulate, MSOF continues to progress, tissues become irreversibly damaged, and the shock has progressed to a stage where it is considered to be irreversible. Signs and symptoms of cardiac, pulmonary, hepatic, renal, neurologic, and gastrointestinal failure may be present. At this phase of shock, any type of treatment becomes incapable of sustaining life.

In summary, compensatory mechanisms occur in response to shock in an attempt to prevent further deterioration and restore homeostasis. Complex neuroendocrine responses are triggered to overcome ineffective circulating blood volume. The hormones ACTH, aldosterone, and ADH are released to increase blood volume. The sympathetic nervous system releases a massive amount of norepinephrine, which produces multiorgan responses in an effort to sustain a life-threatening situation. The cardiovascular system tries to restore arterial blood pressure and blood volume by augmenting CO through increased venous return. The renin-angiotensin-aldosterone cycle is initiated to enhance preload through increased venous return and increased afterload through vasoconstriction. When compensatory mechanisms cannot restore the system to normal, shock can progress to a phase of continued inadequate tissue oxygenation in relation to demand. Cells become ineffective and die, metabolic wastes accumulate, and MSOF occurs. Eventually, shock can progress to an irreversible phase where death is inevitable.

Section Four Review

1. Aldosterone increases blood volume by
   A. increasing sodium retention
   B. increasing water retention
   C. decreasing potassium retention
   D. all of the above
2. Angiotensin II
   A. is a vasoconstrictor
   B. is a vasodilator
   C. is released by ADH
   D. causes the release of ACTH
3. ACTH, aldosterone, and ADH
   A. sense alterations in pH and P_{CO_2}
   B. alert the hypothalamus to what could be a life-threatening situation
   C. conserve the amount of fluid excreted by the kidneys
   D. increase the heart rate for rapid delivery of O_2

4. Norepinephrine produces which of the following compensatory mechanisms?
   A. decreased blood pressure
   B. increased intestinal peristalsis
   C. increased glycolysis
   D. decreased heart rate

5. Continued low blood flow, poor tissue perfusion, and inadequate oxygen delivery cause
   A. multisystem organ failure
   B. the hypothalamus to release ACTH
   C. the release of renin from renal cells
   D. decreased urinary output

Answers: 1, D. 2, A. 3, C. 4, C. 5, A.

Section Five: Clinical Findings Associated with Shock States

At the completion of this section, the learner will be able to list the clinical manifestations for each of the functional shock states.

Clinical manifestations of all shock states are the result of inadequate oxygen delivery and the compensatory mechanisms of the neuroendocrine and cardiovascular systems. The clinical findings correlate with organs that have a compromised blood flow (as blood flow to the skin decreases, the skin will be cold and cyanotic; as blood flow to the kidneys decreases, urinary output will be decreased and so on).

Hypovolemic Shock States

In hypovolemic shock states due to fluid loss, the signs and symptoms are related to the degree of volume depletion. The skin will be cool, and capillary refill will be poor. Depending on the amount of fluid volume lost, the blood pressure may be low, and orthostatic changes in blood pressure may be noted. Tachycardia will be evident, and urinary output will be low. Hemodynamically, as less volume is returned to the right atrium, the right atrial pressure (RAP) will be low. As less fluid is delivered to the pulmonary vasculature and the left ventricle, pressures will be low, as evidenced by a low pulmonary artery wedge pressure (PAWP), low pulmonary artery pressure (PAP), and low CO. The systemic vascular resistance (SVR) will be elevated as vasoconstriction occurs in efforts to increase venous return and CO. The skin is cool and clammy: cold because of compensatory vasoconstriction, and clammy secondary to the release of catecholamines.

In neurogenic shock, signs and symptoms are related to the loss of sympathetic innervation. Persistent vasodilation produces a decreased SVR. Pooling of blood in dilated vessels results in diminished venous return, producing a lower RAP, PAP, PAWP, and CO. Heart rate (HR) will be decreased as a result of parasympathetic innervation. Peripheral vasodilation produces warm skin. Hypothermia and absence of sweating below the level of the spinal cord injury may be present.

With anaphylactic shock, chemical mediators cause vasodilation and increased capillary permeability. As fluid leaves the vascular compartment and seeps into interstitial spaces, signs of hypovolemia occur: decreased BP, RAP, PAP, PAWP, and CO, with an increased HR. The vasodilation produces a decreased SVR and warm skin. Angioedema (edema in membranous tissues) can be seen in the eyes, mouth, and tongue. As fluid shifts from the capillaries into interstitial spaces, edema of the uvula and larynx can occur, which may produce an acute respiratory obstruction. Laryngeal edema is accompanied by impaired phonation and a high pitched cough.

The pathophysiologic changes of septic shock evolve to produce two distinct phases. Clinical manifestations of septic shock will depend on what phase of septic shock the patient is in. The first phase is termed *warm* or *hyperdynamic*. In this phase, there is a general vasodilation as evidenced by warm skin and a temperature greater than 102F. A moderate tachycardia, less than 120 bpm, is accompanied by an increased CO and stroke volume (Langfitt, 1984). The mediators released in response to the infectious organisms produce vasodilation. This is clinically manifested by a decreased SVR and afterload. The vasodilation reduces venous return. The reduction in SVR lowers afterload, which enhances CO. RAP, PAP, and PAWP may be low, depending on the patient's volume status. Intermittent temperature spikes also may be present. As the septic shock progresses, different clinical manifestations may be seen. The second phase of septic shock is termed the *cold* or *hypodynamic* phase. As the shock progresses from warm to cold, continued fluid shifts create a hypovolemia, and CO decreases. CO is decreased because of reduced preload and decreased force of ventricular contractions (Rice, 1991a). Extreme vasoconstriction occurs due to an increase in epinephrine and norepinephrine. The skin is cold, pale, and clammy. Subnormal temperatures indicate that the body is unable to maintain metabolic heat production (Langfitt, 1984).

Transport Shock States

The diminished hemoglobin supply produces the clinical manifestations seen in transport shock states. In shock caused by anemia or hemorrhage, a low hematocrit and hemoglobin will be present. RAP and PAWP may be normal, depending on the patient's volume status. In shock produced by carbon monoxide poisoning, a low Pao_2 will be evident. The patient may complain of a severe headache. An increased heart rate and respiratory rate will be present. In severe carbon monoxide toxicity, altered level of consciousness from syncope to coma with convulsions may occur (Wruk, 1990).

Obstructive Shock States

The clinical manifestations of obstructive shock states are the result of a mechanical barrier to blood flow resulting in inadequate oxygen delivery and hypoperfusion.

Pulsus paradoxus is one of the classic signs of cardiac tamponade. Pulsus paradoxus is an exaggerated decrease (greater than 10 mm Hg) of the systolic blood pressure during inspiration. Tense fluid accumulation within the pericardial sac impairs left ventricular filling during inspiration when right ventricular filling is increased (Sulzbach, 1989). This causes an exaggerated reduction in systolic blood pressure during inspiration. Another clinical manifestation of cardiac tamponade is distant heart sounds (muffled by the increased pericardial fluid and a pericardial friction rub). In tamponade, RAP usually is elevated and is equaled by the PAWP. Beck's triad, consisting of elevated RAP, decreased BP, and muffled heart sounds, may be present (Joiner and Kolodychuk, 1991).

Increased pleural pressure as a result of a tension pneumothorax puts direct pressure on the heart, vena cava, and contralateral lung. As a result, there will be decreased breath sounds, tracheal deviation, and bradycardia. This results in poor ventilation, decreased venous return, and decreased CO.

The clinical manifestations of pulmonary embolism depend on whether a massive or submassive embolism develops. A massive embolism occurs suddenly. The patient may complain of crushing, substernal chest pain and shortness of breath. The blood pressure may be low, and the patient may be cyanotic. A submassive embolism may produce clinical symptoms as it occludes a medium-sized artery. The patient's heart rate and respiratory rate may be elevated. Generalized chest discomfort, fever, cough, and hemoptysis may develop. Elevation of PAP is secondary to increased pulmonary vascular resistance. Elevation of PAP is directly related to the size of the embolus (Daily, 1989). The PAWP can be normal but usually is low as a result of decreased filling of the left atrium secondary to the obstruction.

Cardiogenic Shock States

Clinical manifestations produced in cardiogenic shock states depend on whether there is left-sided heart failure or right-sided heart failure.

Left ventricular failure produces clinical manifestations associated with hypoperfusion and pulmonary congestion, including dyspnea, bilateral rales, diastolic gallop (S_3), S_4, and a systolic murmur (Daily, 1989). Hemodynamic alterations include an elevated PAWP (greater than 24 mm Hg) secondary to decreased ventricular compliance (Daily, 1989). The PAP is elevated secondary to pulmonary venous hypertension. The RAP may be low, depending on the patient's volume status. Arterial pressure is markedly reduced with a narrow pulse pressure. Pulsus alternans, with regular, alternating changes in the pulse pressure irrespective of the respiratory cycle often is present. The CI is very low (less than 2.4 L/minute/m²) in severe left ventricular failure (Daily, 1989).

Clinical manifestations of right ventricular failure are associated with systemic venous congestion. A right ventricular gallop, a split second heart sound, and hepatojugular reflex usually are present. The RAP can be elevated above 10 mm Hg and is directly related to the degree of right ventricle damage (Daily, 1989). The PAP may be elevated, but in severe right ventricular failure, it may be low. The PAWP may be normal or low, reflecting the decreased left ventricular filling as a result of decreased right ventricular ejection. PAWP is usually lower than RAP.

In summary, clinical manifestations associated with shock states are the result of inadequate oxygen delivery and the compensatory mechanisms of the neuroendocrine and cardiovascular systems. In hypovolemic shock states due to fluid loss, the signs and symptoms are related to the degree of volume depletion. In neurogenic shock, anaphylactic shock, and septic shock, signs and symptoms are related to vasodilation. A diminished supply of hemoglobin produces the clinical manifestations seen in transport shock states. The clinical manifestations of obstructive shock states are the result of a mechanical barrier to blood flow. Clinical manifestations of cardiogenic shock states depend on whether there is left or right ventricular failure. Right ventricular failure produces signs associated with systemic venous congestion. Left ventricular failure produces clinical manifestations associated with hypoperfusion and pulmonary congestion.

Section Five Review

1. The signs and symptoms of anaphylactic shock are
   A. related to the loss of sympathetic tone
   B. related to the release of chemical mediators
   C. decreased SVR, PAWP, and increased temperature
   D. decreased RAP, increased CO, and increased temperature
2. A low Hct and Hg will be present in shock caused by
   A. a pulmonary embolism
   B. volume depletion
   C. anemia
   D. right ventricular failure
3. Mr. G was involved in a motor vehicle accident. He sustained a spinal cord injury. Which of the following are clinical manifestations of a spinal cord injury?
   A. increased heart rate, SVR, and RAP
   B. decreased heart rate, decreased SVR, and increased RAP
   C. increased heart rate, increased SVR, and decreased RAP
   D. decreased heart rate, SVR, and RAP

4. Mr. T has candida sepsis. Which of the following clinical manifestations would he likely demonstrate in the warm phase?
   A. decreased SVR, decreased CO
   B. increased SVR, decreased CO
   C. decreased SVR, increased CO
   D. increased SVR, increased CO
5. Which of the following would characterize right-sided heart failure?
   A. RAP will be high and greatly higher than PAWP
   B. RAP will be low
   C. PAWP will be high and greatly higher than RAP
   D. RAP and PAWP will be greatly elevated

Answers: 1, B. 2, C. 3, D. 4, C. 5, A.

Section Six: Treatment of Shock

At the completion of this section, the learner will be able to list the medical and nursing interventions that optimize oxygen delivery and decrease oxygen consumption.

The primary goals of treatment are to identify and treat the underlying cause of shock, optimize oxygen delivery, and decrease oxygen consumption.

Interventions To Optimize Oxygen Delivery

Supplemental oxygen may be administered in an attempt to improve oxygen delivery to hypoxic tissues. For patients who are conscious, spontaneously breathing, and have adequate arterial blood gases, oxygen delivered by nasal cannula or mask may be all that is necessary. However, in the unconscious patient or in the patient demonstrating respiratory distress, intubation and mechanical ventilation may be required.

Administration of IV fluids assists in restoring optimal tissue perfusion by restoring preload and increasing the CO component of oxygen delivery. The fluid best suited for shock states remains controversial. Usually, a combination of crystalloids and colloids is administered. Crystalloid solution (i.e., lactated Ringers solution) replete interstitial and intravascular fluid volumes and increase preload and CO. Administration of colloids enhance the blood's oxygen-carrying capacity. Colloids have oncotic capabilities not inherent in crystalloids. Whole blood is administered in a volume of 500 mL and can increase the Hct by 2 to 3 percent. Packed red blood cells are administered in a volume of 250 mL and can elevate the Hct by 3 to 4 percent (Greenburg, 1988). Packed red blood cells usually are given to provide adequate hemoglobin concentration and are supplemented with crystalloids to maintain an adequate circulatory volume. Autologous blood can be administered in hemorrhagic shock. Inotropic support may be necessary if volume administration is not sufficient to maintain oxygen delivery.

Positive inotropic drugs increase contractility by stimulating the beta$_1$-receptors in the heart. Increased contraction results in increased stroke volume as the ventricles eject more completely and reduce preload (Halfman-Franey and Bergstrom, 1989). Reducing preload can decrease pulmonary congestion and lower myocardial oxygen demand. Inotropic drugs that increase CO and enhance tissue perfusion include dopamine, dobutamine, norepinephrine, and isoproterenol. Dopamine has both alpha- and beta-receptor effects. In low doses (1–2 μg/kg/minute), it causes renal vasodilation, improves renal blood flow, and increases urinary output. In moderate doses (2–5 μg/kg/minute), beta$_1$-receptors are activated, and CO increases. Larger doses stimulate alpha-receptors and increase blood pressure. Dobutamine selectively acts on beta$_1$-receptors to increase contractility and CO. Dobutamine also decreases SVR. Isoproterenol acts on beta$_1$- and beta$_2$-receptors to increase CO, increase heart rate, and decrease SVR. All inotropic drugs must be used with caution, since they increase myocardial oxygen consumption.

Vasoactive drugs are drugs that act on the smooth muscle layer of blood vessels, which affects preload and afterload. These drugs are either vasoconstrictors or vasodilators. Vasoconstrictors, or vasopressors, mimic the sympathetic nervous system to increase blood flow to vital organs by increasing blood pressure and CO. Vasopressors include epinephrine, norepinephrine, metaraminol bitartrate, isoproterenol, dopamine, and dobutamine. These drugs increase SVR and blood pressure. Vasopressors should not be given unless the SVR is abnormally low, as in septic shock or anaphylactic shock. These drugs should be given only when the patient's volume status is adequate (as reflected by RAP or PAWP or both).

Afterload reducing (vasodilating) drugs produce vasodilation, which improves cardiac performance and assists in perfusing tissues. Peripheral arterial vasodilators (nitroprusside, nitroglycerine) can decrease SVR and reduce myocardial oxygen demand. When afterload is decreased, stroke volume is improved. The ventricles have less resistance to overcome and eject blood with less force. These drugs decrease preload as well as afterload. Therefore, these drugs should be used with caution in shock.

Afterload reducing drugs should be given only to patients with a PAWP of at least 15 to 18 mm Hg who have adequate fluid volume (Rackow, 1984). The patient must be monitored carefully so that the blood pressure does not become so low that reflex tachycardia occurs and coronary perfusion suffers.

In most circumstances, a combination of drugs may be advantageous. Combining an inotropic drug with a vasodilating drug can maximize oxygen delivery by increasing contractility and decreasing afterload. Sympathomimetic drugs are temporary agents, since they do not treat the underlying cause of shock. They have a relatively short half-duration of action and can be easily titrated to the patient's rapidly changing condition.

Placing the patient in Trendelenburg position is an intervention frequently used for the treatment of hypotension. It is believed that this position displaces blood from the systemic venules and small veins into the right heart and thus serves to increase stroke volume and CO. However, Holcroft and Blaisdell (1986) have found the Trendelenburg position to be ineffective in treating shock because it impairs left ventricular function.

The pneumatic antishock garment (PASG) or military antishock trousers (MAST) are an intervention used for hemorrhage control and blood pressure support. The PASG is a trouserlike suit that encloses the legs, thighs, and trunk and exerts a variable degree of compression on the underlying tissues. Theoretically, it empties veins in these portions of the body and returns more blood to the systemic circulation. Use of PASG is reserved for hypovolemic shock from hemorrhage. It is used primarily in prehospital management of trauma victims.

The patient's response to treatment must be assessed frequently for signs of improved oxygen delivery. Signs of improved oxygen delivery include a CI of 4 to 4.5 L/minute/m^2 urinary output greater than 30 mL/hour or 0.5/mL/kg/hour, pulse < 120 bpm, and MAP greater than 80 mm Hg (Demling, 1988).

Interventions to Decrease Oxygen Consumption

In addition to optimizing oxygen delivery, interventions also should include measures to decrease oxygen consumption. Interventions to decrease oxygen consumption should be directed toward decreasing total body work, decreasing pain and anxiety, and decreasing temperature.

Decreasing total body work is an attempt to decrease oxygen demands of all tissues. Shock states can increase oxygen consumption to double that of normal. Hyperventilation occurs in an effort to increase oxygen delivery to meet demands, but this requires a great deal of effort, and the patient can rapidly develop respiratory acidosis and respiratory distress. Effective ventilation is ensured with intubation and mechanical ventilation. Mechanical ventilation also decreases the respiratory muscle oxygen demands. A tidal volume of 9 to 13 mL/kg (twice the norm) often is needed to respond to increased metabolic and oxygen demands. Decreasing oxygen consumption of voluntary muscles can be achieved with neuromuscular blocking agents, pancuronium (Pavulon) or vecuronium (Norcuron). These drugs eliminate unnecessary muscle activity and allow oxygen to be redirected for use in involuntary muscles, such as the heart.

Pain and anxiety initiate the sympathetic nervous system's fight-or-flight response, which causes the release of catecholamines. Catecholamines increase metabolic rates and oxygen consumption. Measures should be taken to minimize pain and anxiety. Appropriate analgesics should be administered. It is important to recognize that pain and anxiety may be present in the paralyzed patient.

Hyperthermia increases metabolic demands and oxygen requirements. This should be controlled with antipyretic drugs, such as acetaminophen, and a cooling blanket.

Interventions to optimize oxygen delivery and minimize oxygen consumption should be applied to all patients in shock. Individualized interventions should be initiated to treat the underlying cause of shock. These interventions are described briefly in the following paragraphs.

Hypovolemic Shock States

The treatment goal for hypovolemic shock states is restoration of fluid volume. In hypovolemic shock, the source of the fluid loss should be identified and controlled. Increasing the volume of a hypovolemic patient by 25 to 35 percent can increase the CO to 100 percent (Greenburg, 1988). The patient in hypovolemic shock is initially given 2L to 3L of crystalloids. The nurse should assess for a response in heart rate, blood pressure, and urinary output. If no response is noted, additional fluids may be required.

The goal of treatment in neurogenic shock is to maintain stability of the spine and provide cardiovascular (blood pressure and HR) stability. Because of unopposed parasympathetic intervention, patients with complete, high spinal cord injuries have a decreased blood pressure and pulse. These patients often require fluid administration to establish preload or a vasopressor if adequate volume has been given. A slight bradycardia requires close monitoring. If a marked bradycardia occurs, appropriate medications to increase heart rate and avoid hypoxia will be necessary (Langfitt, 1984).

The treatment goals for septic shock are to identify and treat the infecting organisms and to restore adequate tissue perfusion. Volume replacement in the septic patient attempts to replace fluid lost into the interstitium from the vascular compartment. Volume replacement may be supplemented with the administration of vasopressor drugs to increase afterload, blood pressure, and CO. Broad-spectrum antibiotics usually are initiated as soon as septic shock is suspected. It is necessary to monitor drug levels, especially aminoglycosides, to maintain adequate bacterial killing while minimizing toxicity. Treatment of hyperthermia with antipyretics (aspirin, acetaminophen) will decrease oxygen consumption.

Transport Shock States

The treatment goal in transport shock states is to optimize the hemoglobin concentration and restore oxygen-carrying capacity. For the treatment of anemia or hemorrhage or both, packed red blood cells may be administered in efforts to provide an adequate hemoglobin concentration. The goal in treatment is to achieve a serum hemoglobin level greater than 12 g/100 mL.

The treatment for carbon monoxide poisoning consists of the administration of oxygen. The administration of 100 percent oxygen will eliminate the carbon monoxide poisoning within 40 to 90 minutes. Hyperbaric oxygen will eliminate the carbon monoxide within 30 minutes (Wruk, 1990). Carboxyhemoglobin level determinations should be repeated every 2 to 4 hours until the level reached is less than 15 percent (Wruk, 1990).

Obstructive Shock States

The treatment goal in obstructive shock states is to remove the mechanical barrier to blood flow. For a tension pneumothorax, trapped air is decompressed by a physician with the insertion of a 14-gauge needle, a chest tube, or both. Needle pericardiocentesis may decompress the pericardium for cardiac tamponade. This decompression should improve the heart's pumping ability. If not, a thoracotomy may be required to surgically control and decompress the tamponade.

Treatment of a pulmonary embolus consists of definitive therapy to remove the obstruction, usually administration of tissue plasminogen activator (tPA), streptokinase, or urokinase, followed by heparin therapy (Daily, 1989).

Cardiogenic Shock States

The specific treatment for cardiogenic shock is based on the cardiac abnormality and whether the shock is caused by left-sided or right-sided heart failure.

The treatment goal in right-sided heart failure is to augment preload by volume expansion. Volume expansion will increase right ventricular output. Sufficient fluid is given to maintain the RAP between 10 and 15 mm Hg (Daily, 1989). Vasodilators can decrease the SVR, but adequate preload is essential to prevent further declines in CO. Positive inotropes (dopamine, dobutamine) may be necessary to improve contractility and help restore systemic perfusion.

The treatment goal in left-sided heart failure is to improve ventricular function and prevent the progression toward right heart failure. If excess preload is the cause, administration of venodilators and diuretics is indicated. By decreasing preload, the volume of blood entering the right atrium and stress on the left ventricle will be reduced. Afterload reducers will increase the CO and decrease pulmonary congestion. Inotropic drugs will increase cardiac contractility and increase CO. Intra-aortic balloon counterpulsation (IABP) may be useful when there is an inadequate response to pharmacologic agents. IABP will decrease afterload, augment coronary blood flow and CO, and decrease myocardial oxygen demands. IABP decreases the strain on the left ventricle by reducing afterload. With a lower pressure, the ventricle does not have to contract forcibly to expel blood into the aorta. The IABP is inserted into the femoral artery and advanced until it is in the descending thoracic aorta. The IABP is synchronized with the patient's heart rate. During ventricular diastole, the balloon inflates. With the balloon inflated, the blood distal to the balloon is forced back toward the aortic valve. This supplies the coronary arteries with additional oxygenated blood to meet myocardial oxygen needs. Before ventricular systole, the balloon deflates, which decreases pressure in the aorta. This makes it easier for the left ventricle to contract and expel its oxygenated blood.

In summary, the primary goals for treatment of shock are to optimize oxygen delivery and decrease tissue oxygen consumption. Interventions that optimize oxygen delivery include supplemental oxygen administration, restoration of intravascular fluid volume, administration of inotropic and vasoactive drugs, Trendelenburg position, and MAST trousers. Improved oxygen delivery should be assessed in terms of improved CO, increased urinary output, a decrease in heart rate, and an increase in blood pressure. Interventions that decrease oxygen consumption include decreasing total body work through adequate ventilation and neuromuscular blocking agents, minimizing pain and stress, and correcting hyperthermia. Further and more individualized interventions are directed toward treating the underlying cause of shock for the four functional shock states.

Section Six Review

You have been assigned to provide nursing care to Mr. J, a 74-year-old male with a diagnosis of septic shock of unknown etiology. During the change of shift report, you are given the following information.

- Vital signs: BP 70/42, pulse 140 sinus tachycardia, respiration 38, temperature 103F
- Recent laboratory results: ABGs: pH 7.25, Pco_2 30, Po_2 60, HCO_3^- 18, base deficit 8, Hct 27, Hg 8, Na^+ 140, K^+ 4.5
- Hemodynamic readings: MAP 51, RAP 3, PAP 18/8, PAWP 8, CO 4, SVR 356
- IV fluids: D_5 and 1/2 NS + 20 mEq KCl at 100 mL/hour
- Urinary output past 8 hours: 160 mL/hour

As you walk to Mr. J's bedside, you note that he is pale and restless. He is lying in the semi-Fowler's position.

Answer the following questions based on the information provided about Mr. J.

1. Which of the following could best increase Mr. J's CO and restore preload?
   A. D_5 and 1/2 NS + 20 mEq KCl at 75 mL/hour
   B. D_5 and 1/2 NS + 20 mEq KCl at 100 mL/hour
   C. Lactated Ringer's (LR) at 50 mL/hour
   D. LR at 200 mL/hour
2. Which of the following would indicate that Mr. J's oxygen delivery was improving?
   A. urinary output of 50 mL/hour
   B. RAP 1 mm Hg
   C. Hct 27
   D. respiratory rate of 38/minute

3. Mr. J currently is receiving a total volume (TV) of 350 mL/hour. Based on what you know about oxygen consumption during shock, which of the following orders might you expect the physician to write?
   A. decrease the TV
   B. increase the TV
   C. eliminate the TV
   D. leave the TV at 350
4. Which of the following drugs would NOT decrease Mr. J's oxygen consumption?
   A. norepinephrine
   B. pancuronium
   C. acetaminophen
   D. MSO_4

5. What effect would be produced if dopamine 1 μg/kg/minute was added to Mr. J's treatment?
   A. increased myocardial oxygen demands
   B. increased blood pressure
   C. decreased urinary output
   D. increased urinary output

Answers: 1, D. 2, A. 3, B. 4, A. 5, D.

Posttest

1. Which of the following factors does not control oxygen delivery?
   A. the heart's pumping ability
   B. core body temperature
   C. local tissue autoregulation
   D. sympathetic nervous system regulation
2. Stimulation of a dopaminergic receptor would produce
   A. renal vasodilation
   B. suppression of norepinephrine
   C. increased vascular resistance
   D. decreased airway resistance
3. Which of the following increases oxygen consumption?
   A. temperature of 97F
   B. pancuronium 10 mg IV
   C. MSO_4 2 mg IV
   D. anxiety
4. Which of the following decreases oxygen consumption?
   A. respiratory rate of 42/minute
   B. temperature of 102F
   C. MSO_4 4 mg IV
   D. septic shock
5. Transport shock states have impaired oxygen delivery because
   A. a barrier impedes blood flow to tissues
   B. there is a loss of intravascular volume
   C. hemoglobin is unavailable to carry oxygen
   D. decreased sympathetic tone produces vasoconstriction

6. Vasodilation and maldistribution of circulating volume characterize
   A. anaphylactic shock
   B. septic shock
   C. neurogenic shock
   D. obstructive shock
7. ACTH and ADH
   A. cause sodium and water depletion
   B. are chemoreceptors that sense alterations in pH and Pco_2
   C. release norepinephrine
   D. preserve blood volume by conserving fluid.
8. Clinical signs of hypovolemic shock include
   A. cool skin, increased pulse, and low RAP
   B. warm skin, decreased pulse, and decreased CO
   C. cool skin, increased pulse, and increased CO
   D. warm skin, increased pulse, and low RAP
9. Systemic venous congestion is a manifestation of
   A. left ventricular failure
   B. right ventricular failure
   C. anaphylactic shock
   D. cardiac tamponade
10. Crystalloid solutions
    A. can increase the Hct by 2 to 3 percent
    B. are given to supplement hemoglobin concentrations
    C. replete fluid volumes and increase preload
    D. possess oncotic capabilities

11. Afterload reducing drugs
    A. increase blood pressure and CO
    B. restrict blood flow to internal organs
    C. produce vasodilation and improve cardiac performance
    D. produce vasoconstriction and increase myocardial oxygen consumption

12. Common to all shock states is
    A. decreased blood pressure, heart rate, and urine output
    B. increased oxygen delivery with increased oxygen consumption
    C. impaired oxygen delivery with altered oxygen consumption
    D. decreased blood pressure, increased heart rate, and decreased urine output

Posttest Answers

Question	Answer	Section	Question	Answer	Section
1	B	One	7	D	Four
2	A	One	8	A	Five
3	D	Two	9	B	Five
4	C	Two	10	C	Six
5	C	Three	11	C	Six
6	B	Three	12	C	Three

REFERENCES

Buran, M.J. (1987). Oxygen consumption. In J.V. Short and M.R. Pinsky (eds). *Oxygen transport in the critically ill*, pp. 16–21. Chicago: Year Book Medical Publishers.

Clochesy, J.M. (1988). Understanding shock states. In J.M. Clochesy (ed). *Essentials of critical care nursing*, pp. 16–21. Rockville, Maryland: Aspen Publishers, Inc.

Daily, E.K. (1989). Use of hemodynamics to differentiate pathophysiologic causes of cardiogenic shock. *Crit. Care Clin. North Am.* 1(3):589–602.

Demling, R.H. (1988). *Decision making in surgical critical care*. Toronto: B.C. Decker, Inc.

Greenburg, A.G. (1988) Pathophysiology of shock. In T.A. Miller (ed). *Physiologic basis of modern surgical care*, pp. 154–172. St. Louis: C.V. Mosby Co.

Halfman-Franey, M., and Bergstrom, D. (1989). Clinical management using direct and derived parameters. *Crit. Care Clin. North Am.* 1(3): 547–561.

Holcroft, J.W., and Blasidell, F.W. (1986). Shock: Causes and management of circulatory collapse. In D.C. Sabiston (ed). *Textbook of surgery*, 13th ed., (pp. 38–63). Philadelphia: W.B. Saunders Co.

Joiner, G.A., and Kolodychuk, G.R. (1991). Neoplastic cardiac tamponade. *Crit. Care Nurse.* 11(2):50–58.

Langfitt, D.E. (1984). Shock states. In D.E. Langfitt (ed). *Critical care: Certification and Review*, pp. 481–488. Bowie, Maryland: Brady Communications.

Mims, B.C. (1989). Physiologic rationale of SvO$_2$ monitoring. *Crit. Care Clin. North Am.* 1(3):619–628.

Rackow, E.C. (1984). Of shock and vasoactive drugs. *Emerg. Med.* 16:115–123.

Rice, V. (1991a). Shock: A clinical syndrome. An update. Part I. *Crit. Care Nurse.* 11(4):20–27.

Rice, V. (1991b). Shock: A clinical syndrome. An update. Part 2. *Crit. Care Nurse.* 11(5):74–82.

Shoemaker, W.L. (1987). Circulatory mechanisms of shock and their mediators. *Crit. Care Med.* 15:787–794.

Sulzbach, L.M. (1989). Measurement of pulsus paradoxus. *Focus Crit. Care.* 16(2):142–145.

Von Rueden, K.T. (1989). Cardiopulmonary assessment of the critically ill trauma patient. *Crit. Care Clin. North Am.* 1(1):33–44.

Wruk, K.M. (1990). Drug overdose and poisoning. In C.M. Hudak, B.M. Gallo, and J.J. Benz (eds). *Critical care nursing: A holistic approach*, 5th ed., pp. 780–800. Philadelphia: J.B. Lippincott Co.

ADDITIONAL READING

Collins, J.A. (1986). Blood transfusions and disorders of surgical bleeding. In D.C. Sabiston (ed). *Textbook of surgery*, 13th ed., pp. 99–115. Philadelphia: W.B. Saunders Co.

Goldberg, H.S. (1978). Control of cardiac output by the circuit. In J.V. Snyder and M.R. Pinsky (eds). *Oxygen transport in the critically ill*, pp. 36–45. Chicago: Year Book Medical Publishers Co.

Goldberg, H.S., and Pinsky, M.R. (1987). Ventricular pump function. In J.V. Snyder and M.R. Pinsky (eds). *Oxygen transport in the critically ill*, pp. 25–35. Chicago: Year Book Medical Publishers Co.

Guyton, A.C. (1982). Cardiac output and circulatory shock. In A.C. Guyton (ed). *Human physiology and mechanisms of disease*, 3rd ed., pp. 187–200. Philadelphia: W.B. Saunders Co.

Kandel, G. (1983). Mixed venous oxygen saturation. *Arch. Intern. Med.* 143(July):1440–1402.

McQuillan, K.A., and Wiles, C.E. (1988). Initial management of traumatic shock in V.C. Cardonna, et al. (eds). *Trauma nursing: From resuscitation through rehabilitation*, pp. 160–182. Philadelphia: W.B. Saunders Co.

Osterfield, G. (1989). Shock. In B.C. Long and W.J. Phipps (eds). *Medical-surgical nursing: A nursing process approach*, 2nd ed., pp. 144–166. St. Louis: C.V. Mosby Co.

Parrillo, J.E. (1989). Septic shock in humans: Clinical evaluation, pathogenesis and therapeutic approach. In W.C. Shoemaker et al. (eds). *Textbook of critical care*, 2nd ed., pp. 1006–1024. Philadelphia: W.B. Saunders Co.

Rajfer, S.I., and Goldberg, L.I. (1989). Sympathomimetic amines in the treatment of shock. In W.C. Shoemaker et al. (eds). *Textbook of clinical care*, 2nd ed., pp. 438–440. Philadelphia: W.B. Saunders Co.

Savino, J.A. (1987). Hemodynamic monitoring in trauma. *Trauma Q.* 3(3):13–31.

Shoemaker, W.C. (1989). Shock states: Pathophysiology, monitoring, outcome prediction and therapy. In W.C. Shoemaker et al. (eds). *Textbook of critical care*, 2nd ed., pp. 977–993. Philadelphia: W.B. Saunders Co.

Urban, N. (1988). Integrating hemodynamic parameters with clinical decision making. *Crit. Care Nurse.* 6(2):48–61.

Vary, T.C., and Linberg, S.E. (1988). Pathophysiology of traumatic shock. In V.C. Cardonna et al. (eds). *Trauma nursing: From resuscitation to rehabilitation*, pp. 127–158. Philadelphia: W.B. Saunders Co.

White, K.M. (1985). Completing the hemodynamic picture: Svo$_2$. *Heart Lung.* 14(3):272–280.

Wilmore, D.W. (1986). Homeostasis: Bodily changes in trauma and surgery. In D.C. Sabiston (ed). *Textbook of surgery*, 13th ed., pp. 23–37. Philadelphia: W.B. Saunders Co.

Module 9

Nursing Care of the Patient with Altered Tissue Perfusion

Pamela Stinson Kidd

Nursing Care of the Patient with Altered Tissue Perfusion is designed to integrate the major points discussed in the four modules, *Perfusion, Hemodynamic Monitoring, Cardiac Monitoring and Related Interventions,* and *Shock States.* This module summarizes relationships between key concepts and assists the learner in clustering information to facilitate clinical application. The module is divided into four parts. Part I discusses assessment data frequently used in deriving appropriate nursing diagnoses for a patient with a perfusion problem. Part II applies the content in an interactive learning style. The learner is encouraged to identify nursing actions based on assessment of a patient in a case study format. Part III discusses nursing care of a patient being hemodynamically monitored. Nursing care of a patient with a fluid volume excess condition is addressed in Part IV. Consequences of selecting a particular action are discussed, and the rationale for correct actions is presented. The module ends with a summary of nursing priorities in caring for a patient with an altered tissue perfusion.

Objectives

Following completion of the module, *Nursing Care of the Patient with Altered Tissue Perfusion,* the learner will be able to

1. Identify relationships between cardiac output (CO), ECG patterns, and hemodynamic readings
2. Cluster assessment data to formulate perfusion patterns
3. Appraise a patient's perfusion status based on a nursing assessment
4. Identify priorities in nursing care for a patient experiencing an alteration in perfusion
5. Explain rationale for nursing actions that support perfusion
6. Explain nursing responsibilities associated with hemodynamic monitoring

Glossary

Edema. Accumulation of excessive fluid in the interstitial spaces

Murmur. An audible vibration produced by turbulent blood flow in the heart

Palpitation. Cardiac rhythm abnormalities that produce a skipping sensation in the heart

Phlebostatic axis. An area located at the fourth intercostal space of the lateral chest wall that anatomically corresponds with the placement of a pulmonary arterial catheter

S_1. Heart sound produced by closure of the mitral and tricuspid valves

S_2. Heart sound produced by closure of the aortic and pulmonic valves

S_3. Abnormal heart sound in persons over the age of 30 produced by ventricular filling against increased ventricular pressure; appears immediately after S_2 in the cardiac cycle

S_4. Abnormal heart sound produced by decreased ventricular compliance; appears immediately before S_1 in the cardiac cycle

Syncope. A temporary loss of consciousness usually related to decreased cardiac output

Abbreviations

AST. Aspartate aminotransferase, previously referred to as SGOT (serum glutamic oxaloacetic transaminase)

CO. Cardiac output

CPK. Creatinine phosphokinase

CVP. Central venous pressure

IABP. Intra-aortic balloon pump

LDH. Lactic dehydrogenase

MAST. Military antishock trousers also known as pneumatic antishock garment

PAP. Pulmonary arterial pressure

PCWP. Pulmonary capillary wedge pressure

SVR. Systemic vascular resistance

THE FOCUSED PERFUSION ASSESSMENT

Nursing History

Precipitating Event

It is considered a priority to assess perfusion whether or not your patient has a history of a perfusion abnormality. Airway, breathing, and circulation (A, B, C,) should be assessed before eliciting a nursing history. A brief, limited assessment can be performed systematically in less than 60 seconds. A head to toe format or systems approach can be used to cluster assessment data. Regardless of the format used, the nurse is assuring that the patient is able to provide subjective information without further compromising his or her physical integrity.

It is important to focus on the event that led to the present admission of the patient. Focusing on this area will provide information on the patient's ability to compensate to a cardiovascular stressor. Nursing interventions are targeted toward increasing myocardial oxygen supply while decreasing myocardial demands. Information about the precipitating event can be used to identify areas where the patient needs external support in order to compensate.

Past Medical History

The patient's past medical history is important. Certain conditions, such as hypertension, diabetes, congenital heart anomalies, mitral valve prolapse, and rheumatic fever, may produce vascular changes that impede the patient's ability to compensate. Medical management of previous perfusion abnormalities is important to note. A history of cardiac surgery, angioplasty, or administration of thrombolytics can alert the nurse to the patient's state of cardiovascular health and the patient's potential to compensate to an additional cardiovascular stressor.

It is essential to differentiate chronic symptoms from current symptoms. This is especially true in the elderly patient. For example, an elderly patient may have chronic pedal edema secondary to a decreased glomerular filtration rate or decreased venous compliance associated with normal aging. The edema may not be related to acute cardiovascular changes.

Diet History

A diet history should be elicited in a patient with a perfusion disorder. Cholesterol, fat, sodium, and potassium intake may be related to a hypertensive episode or a dysrhythmia. If the patient is on cardiovascular medications or thiazide diuretics, a diet history is crucial to assessing the patient's degree of compliance with the long-term management plan and perhaps understanding of the perfusion disorder and treatment modalities.

Medication History

A medication history will help the nurse evaluate the patient's response to interventions as well as identify potential sources for assessment findings. If the patient is taking beta-blockers, such as propranolol (Inderal), depolarization is depressed. Beta-blocking agents inhibit sympathetic nervous stimulation and atrium-ventricle conduction and decrease cardiac contractility and arterial pressure. Thus, the cardiac rhythm is slower than what the patient may have experienced previously. If the patient's rhythm converts to complete heart block, a ventricular pattern, or asystole, it may be more difficult to convert the pattern to a sinus rhythm. The beta-blocking agent decreases the ability of the cardiac cells to respond to cardiac stimulating drugs. If the patient has been using over-the-counter stimulants, drinking or eating excessive caffeine-containing substances, or has a history of smoking tobacco, tachydysrhythmias and hypertension may result. These symptoms may occur in direct response to previous treatments or lifestyle patterns and not as a result of the presenting perfusion disorder.

In summary, a pertinent nursing history of a patient with a perfusion disorder includes a brief history of the present event, previously diagnosed conditions and medical management, comparison of current symptoms with previous symptoms, dietary intake, use of prescribed and over-the-counter medications, and a smoking/lifestyle profile.

Frequent Symptoms Associated with Perfusion Disorders

If a perfusion disorder is suspected, the nurse should focus on eliciting the most common circulatory complaints: pain, edema, palpitations, and a change in level of consciousness (Gawlinski, 1988).

Pain

Although chest pain is discussed in Module 4, *Nursing Management of A Patient with Altered Respiratory Function*, it warrants further discussion in order to discriminate pain of cardiac origin from that of pulmonary origin. The mnemonic PQRST is helpful in organizing assessment data related to pain. Eliciting information about precipitating factors (P), quality, (Q), radiation and region (R), associated symptoms (S), and timing and treatment strategies (T) will clue the nurse to the origin of the pain. Table 9–1 compares pain assessment data.

The pain associated with perfusion disorders usually is related to an imbalance between myocardial oxygen supply and myocardial oxygen demands. This imbalance may be due to coronary artery vasoconstriction, coronary artery occlusion, or a chronic narrowing of the coronary artery. Myocardial oxygen supply also can be decreased because of decreased hemoglobin or decreased oxygen saturation of the hemoglobin. Fluid volume excess conditions can produce pain because the myocardium cannot permanently circulate the additional volume, and the oxygen demands of the myocardium increase. Although there may not be changes in the coronary arteries or hemoglobin, the normal supply may be inadequate to meet the increased demand. The pain associated with perfusion disorders must be relieved, since it is an indirect measurement of myocardial oxygen. Pain relief usually is achieved by using a combination of vasodilators and narcotics.

Edema

Edema may be manifested directly (as in shortness of breath) in a patient with a perfusion disorder. Increased ventricular and atrial pressures eventually result in heart failure (Starling's law) that leads to increased hydrostatic pressure due to fluid stasis.

TABLE 9–1. COMPARISON OF PAIN ASSESSMENT DATA

	Cardiac Origin	Pulmonary Origin
Precipitating factors	Activity Changes in environmental temperature Eating Emotional stress Hypertension Traumatic injury to heart Infection	Immobility Fractures of ribs or long bones Upper or lower respiratory infection
Quality	Pressurelike tightness Burning nature Stabbing and sharp may increase with anxiety	Changes with respiratory cycle May increase with cough May increase with activity
Region and radiation	Substernal Precordial Radiation to neck, arms, back, and abdomen	Lateral chest Radiation to shoulder and neck
Associated symptoms	Diaphoresis Nausea and vomiting Dyspnea Change in level of consciousness Abnormal heart sounds Apprehension	Dyspnea Cough Decreased or adventitious breath sounds Apprehension (but usually less than that seen with cardiac origin)
Timing and treatment strategies	May be sudden or gradual May be relieved with rest or vasodilators	May be sudden or gradual May be relieved with change in position Usually not relieved with rest or vasodilators

Venous obstruction, as in the case of thrombosis, can also increase hydrostatic pressure (Guyton, 1986). Elevated hydrostatic pressure in the capillaries produces fluid movement out of the capillary and into the interstitial spaces. Edema is usually not detectable until the interstitial fluid volume is 30 percent above normal (Gawlinski, 1988). This translates approximately to a 5 to 10 pound (2.3 to 4.5 kg) weight gain (Roberts, 1985).

Shortness of breath results from fluid movement out of the pulmonary capillaries and into the lung interstitial space, thereby decreasing oxygen diffusion from the alevoli into the pulmonary capillaries. The presence of crackles or rales on auscultation of the lungs indicates pulmonary edema. Severe pulmonary edema will be associated with frothy, pink sputum production.

Edema is measured on a 1 to 4 scale, with 4 being most severe (Bates, 1986). It is described as pitting or nonpitting in nature. Nonpitting edema is associated with protein coagulation in the tissue and is seen more frequently in conditions of decreased plasma proteins. Pitting edema, interstitial fluid with less protein content, is frequently associated with perfusion disorders. Assessment of edema includes direct observation and palpation of the skin, particularly in the sacrum and lower legs.

Edema has been discussed as a distribution problem. There are other signs of distribution abnor-

malities that should be evaluated in a patient with a perfusion problem. Jugular venous distention (JVD) may indicate a fluid distribution problem. The venous system is a low pressure system, and it is sensitive to right atrial pressure. Retention of blood in the right side of the heart (as in the case of heart failure or cor pulmonale) will increase right atrial pressure and subsequently produce jugular venous distention due to backflow through the vena cavae. In assessing for venous distention, elevate the head of the bed to approximately 45 degrees. The patient's head should be turned slightly away from the examiner. A penlight can be used to shine a light tangentially across the neck. Figure 9–1 illustrates measurement of JVD.

Invasive measurement of fluid distribution can be obtained through a pulmonary arterial catheter. An elevated pulmonary capillary wedge pressure (PCWP) indicates left ventricle failure (increased left heart preload) and may be associated with crackles or rales because of backflow of blood into the lungs and subsequent fluid shifts. An elevated right atrial pressure (increased right heart preload) is seen commonly in right heart failure (cor pulmonale) and may be associated with jugular venous distention and peripheral edema. In cases of severe heart failure, the PCWP, RAP, and PAP will remain elevated while the CO decreases secondary to decreased contractility (Starling's law).

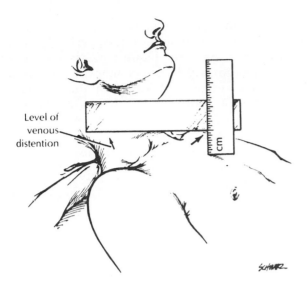

Level of
venous
distention

Figure 9–1. Measurement of jugular venous distention. (*Reproduced by permission from Malasanos, Lois, Barkauskas, Violet, and Staltenberg-Allen, Kathryn: Health assessment, ed. 4, St. Louis, 1990, The C.V. Mosby Co.*)

Palpitations

A patient with a perfusion disorder may complain of his or her heart "skipping" or "thumping." This symptom is related to the occurrence of premature cardiac beats. The best way of detecting premature beats is by obtaining an ECG and monitoring the patient's cardiac rhythm. However, at times, the patient may be removed from the cardiac monitor in anticipation of transport out of an intensive or intermediate care setting. Palpation of the pulse will reveal premature beats. There will be irregular pulse amplitude due to the decreased blood volume associated with premature beats and larger than normal volume of the beat immediately after the premature beat related to prolonged diastolic filling.

Auscultation of heart sounds can confirm the presence of extra beats. S_1 represents ventricular systole and occurs at the closure of the mitral and tricuspid valves. It is heard best at the apex of the heart because of the direction of blood flow during systole. The blood flow is out of the right ventricle into the pulmonary artery and out of the left ventricle into the aorta. S_2 is the end of systole and represents the closure of the aortic and pulmonic valves. It is heard best at the aortic area. Diastole is longer than systole, so the pause between S_1 and S_2 is shorter than the pause between S_2 and S_1.

Extra heart sounds may appear during diastole because of rapid deceleration of blood against increased ventricular pressure, as encountered in heart failure. This increased pressure is due to remaining blood volume that is not ejected, related to overstretching of the myocardium. An S_3 occurs imme-

diately after the S_2 and is associated with heart failure and cardiomyopathy in individuals over 30 years of age (Gawlinski, 1988). An S_4 occurs immediately before an S_1. An S_4 may be present in the elderly patient due to decreased distensibility of the left ventricle associated with aging. An S_4 usually is associated with hypertension or myocardial infarction. In severe failure, both an S_3 and S_4 may be heard.

It is important to auscultate for the presence of murmurs in the patient with a perfusion disorder. A cardiology consultation and additional cardiovascular diagnostic tests may be necessary to determine the exact cause and classification of a murmur. The nurse should note the appearance of a new murmur, especially in patients who have experienced a myocardial infarction. A murmur in this situation may indicate abnormal atrium-ventricle venous communication due to ventricular septum rupture or acute mitral regurgitation due to papillary muscle rupture.

It is impossible to confirm the type or pattern of premature impulse by palpation alone. Only an ECG tracing will identify the number of premature beats occurring and their origin.

Change in Level of Responsiveness

A patient with a perfusion disorder may experience a change in level of responsiveness related to a decreased CO or blockage of cerebral circulation. Dysrhythmias, heart failure, myocardial infarction, or a cerebrovascular attack may be the initial event that precipitated the circulatory changes. The brain receives blood flow from the carotid and vertebral arteries. Fifteen percent of the total CO goes to the brain each minute (Guyton, 1986). If the arterial pressure falls below 60 mm Hg, cerebral blood flow is compromised. A fluid volume deficit or a blood distribution problem ultimately can compromise cerebral blood flow. Changes in level of responsiveness can be subtle and may range from reduced wakefulness and decreased concentration to coma (Mitchell et al, 1984). The patient may experience syncopal episodes (a temporary loss of consciousness, followed by complete, spontaneous recovery).

The Perfusion Assessment

As stated earlier, the assessment begins with the primary survey that focuses on the assessment of airway, breathing, and circulation. Circulation is assessed initially by palpation of a pulse. If a pulse is absent, cardiopulmonary resuscitation and advanced life support measures are initiated. These measures include insertion of an IV catheter and use of IV cardiac medications. The learner is referred to the American Heart Association's textbook *Advanced Cardiac Life Support* (1987) for a complete discussion of cardiopulmonary resuscitation. In cases of traumatic injury and subsequent perfusion emergencies, the learner is referred to Module 10 of this book, *Trauma Assessment and Resuscitation*, the American College of Surgeons' *Advanced Trauma Life Support Manual* (1989), and Rea's *Trauma Nursing Core Course Association Manual* (1991) for additional resources.

When a pulse is verified as present, the nurse completes a rapid perfusion assessment. This assessment includes determining the degree of patient responsiveness, assessing for bleeding from invasive lines or tubes, examining the neck veins for distention, and inspecting the skin for adequate perfusion. Inspecting the skin involves assessment of capillary refill, the presence of peripheral pulses, and skin temperature.

Vital Signs

The nurse obtains a full set of vital signs. In the acutely ill patient, baseline vital signs are essential in order to determine the trend of subsequent data. The pulse can be evaluated using auscultation. The integrity of the heart sounds and the presence of extra heart sounds can be assessed at the same time. When a patient is on a mechanical ventilator and has a restrictive pulmonary disorder (presence of crackles and rhonchi), it may be impossible to hear heart sounds adequately. Palpation is used to calculate the heart rate and to assess the pulse integrity. Even in situations when the pulse can be auscultated, the pulse should also be palpated. This provides data about the pulse amplitude and can provide clues to the presence of a fluid volume deficit condition (weak, thready pulse) or a fluid volume excess disorder (bounding pulse). A rhythm strip from the cardiac monitor should be obtained and interpreted. The strip usually is placed on the nursing assessment record. Additionally, peripheral pulses in all extremities should be assessed.

The patient's blood pressure can be obtained by using a variety of methods. An arterial line may be present to provide a direct measurement of arterial pressure. A mechanical external cuff blood pressure device may be used that records the blood pressure automatically. A traditional stethoscope and sphygmomanometer can be used. A Doppler device may be used to amplify sound in low flow states or noisy environments. Finally, the blood pressure can be obtained by using a sphygmomanometer and palpation, especially in noisy environments where it is difficult to hear, for example, during ground and air transport or in a busy emergency department. In patients with hypovolemia, increased systemic vascular resistance, or both, indirect measurements of blood pressure may be lower than invasive intraarterial measurements because of diminution of sounds. Systolic pressure may be underestimated, and diastolic pressure may be overestimated (Rebenson-Piano et al, 1987).

A patient may have invasive measurement of heart pressure if a central venous line or a pulmonary arterial catheter is in place. Module 6, *Hemodynamic Monitoring*, discusses these heart pressures in detail. If either of these lines is present, the nurse should obtain measurements of RAP, PAP, PCWP, CO, and CI after the equipment is checked and calibrated. Strips of these hemodynamic patterns may be obtained and placed in the nursing assessment record for future comparison.

Temperature should be assessed. Fever increases myocardial oxygen demands and may precipitate an acute perfusion problem in a patient who has a history of cardiac disease. Fever should be treated with antipyretics, and the patient's temperature should be reevaluated to determine the degree of effectiveness of the medication.

Respirations are assessed for rate and character. Shortness of breath may accompany perfusion disorders, as in left ventricular failure. A detailed review of breath sounds is provided in Module 4, *Nursing Care of the Patient with Altered Respiratory Function*.

Skin Integrity

The skin is assessed for temperature, edema, open wounds, and color. Pale, cool, clammy skin occurs from decreased peripheral perfusion, usually related to hypovolemia. These symptoms are in direct response to the sympathetic nervous system's attempt to maintain CO with a decrease in stroke volume. Pale, hairless skin that is taut from edema accompanies decreased peripheral perfusion related to the presence of fluid in the interstitial spaces. Edema is discussed in greater detail earlier in this module. The presence of nonhealing wounds may indicate decreased tissue perfusion from either a blockage of peripheral vessels or decreased CO. Capillary refill can be examined as a method of determining adequacy of peripheral perfusion. Normal refilling time of the nailbeds can fluctuate dramatically based on sex, history of peripheral vascular disease, and temperature of the extremities. The following parameters can be used for a standard of comparasion: 2 seconds for adult male and pediatric patients, 2.9 seconds for adult female, and 4.5 seconds for the elderly patient (62 years of age or greater) (Schriger and Baraff, 1988).

Urine Output

Since 21 percent of a person's CO is distributed to the kidneys, renal perfusion is affected directly by decreased CO (Guyton, 1986). Patients who are hemodynamically unstable should have their urine measured precisely. Urimeters may be placed on the urinary collection device to monitor output. A urine output of less than 30 ML/hour in the acutely ill adult patient indicates decreased blood renal perfusion.

In summary, an acute perfusion abnormality may occur rapidly. The nurse must know the patient's baseline data in order to appreciate changes in perfusion status. The following assessment data indicate an acute alteration in circulatory function.

- Presence of uncontrolled external bleeding
- Decreasing level of responsiveness, restlessness (decreased cerebral perfusion)
- Irregular, thready pulse
- Resting pulse rate of greater than 120 bpm
- Chest pain with shortness of breath
- Flat or distended neck veins (may indicate hypovolemia or pericardiac tamponade)
- Cool, clammy, pale skin
- Changing trends in vital signs and hemodynamic readings
- Presence of complete heart block, ventricular dysrhythmia, or sustained supraventricular tachycardia as evidenced by ECG

Appropriate nursing diagnoses for a patient experiencing a perfusion disorder include

- **Fluid volume deficit**
- **Fluid volume excess**
- **Alteration in tissue perfusion**
- **Decreased cardiac output**
- **Ineffective breathing patterns**
- **Pain**

CASE STUDY 1

——— SUE S, A PATIENT WITH A FLUID VOLUME DEFICIT ———

Sue S is a 24-year-old, gravida 1 female who is 12 weeks pregnant. Her husband brought her to the emergency department when Sue passed out at home. Sue began vomiting en route and complaining of severe, continuous right lower quadrant pain that extended to her suprapubic area. She also complained of pain in the right shoulder area. Sue is admitted into your zone by the triage nurse.

The Initial Appraisal

On walking into Sue's patient care area, you note the following.
General Appearance. Sue is diaphoretic. She is of moderate stature. Weight is appropriate for height. She is fully clothed.
Signs of Distress. Sue is moaning. She is lying on her left side with her knees drawn to her chest. She is clutching a man's hands.
Other. You do not note any IV lines or oxygen in use. The man identifies himself as her husband.

Focused Circulatory Assessment

You quickly place Sue in a hospital gown, noting her profuse diaphoresis and cool and clammy skin. Because Sue appears to be in acute distress, you immediately perform a rapid assessment focusing on her perfusion status. The results are as follows.

Sue is restless but alert and oriented to person, place, time, and reason for being at the hospital. Her blood pressure is 90/70 (baseline according to her husband is 128/70), pulse is 126/minute, respiratory rate is 28/minute. Her respirations are shallow. Sue's radial pulse is regular. S_1 and S_2 are present without murmur. No extra heart sounds are auscultated. Breath sounds are clear bilaterally. Her capillary refill is 3 seconds. Her nailbeds are dusky. No bowel sounds are auscultated after 1 minute. Her abdomen is firm. Sue's pain increases dramatically on palpation of any part of her abdomen. She complains of increased pain unrelieved by change in position. Her oral temperature is 99F.

After this initial assessment, you alert the emergency physician, Dr. P, who is busy examining a patient who is experiencing an acute myocardial infarction. Until she is able to examine Sue, Dr. P orders

- 1,000 mL lactated Ringer's solution to be infused at 200 mL/hour through a large-bore IV line
- Stat. CBC
- Type and crossmatch for four units of blood
- Cardiac monitor
- Foley catheter to straight drain
- Urinalysis and urine for pregnancy test
- Serum hCG
- Electrolyte panel
- CT scan of the abdomen
- Oxygen 2 L per nasal cannula

QUESTION

Considering Sue's presenting symptoms, prioritize the following orders. Which order should be implemented first?
1. CT scan of the abdomen
2. Serum hCG
3. Cardiac monitor
4. IV access

ANSWER

The correct answer is 4. Since Sue's blood pressure is low, compared to her normal value and she has had an episode of syncope at home, the IV line should be initiated first. IV access will provide a means of administering fluid boluses or volume expanders if necessary. Blood can be obtained at the same time for the laboratory tests. Oxygen should be administered next, since tachycardia increases myocardial demands for oxygenation. Next, Sue should be connected to the cardiac monitor because of her fast heart rate. The CT scan should be ordered to help determine the source of Sue's hypotension. Finally, the urinalysis should be obtained. The status of Sue's pregnancy can be determined by the serum hCG. The urine pregnancy test and urinalysis will provide supplemental data.

Stat. Test Results
CBC (Normal values are from Alspach and Williams, 1985.)

WBC = 15,000	(Normal range 5,000–10,000/μL)
RBC = 5.0	(Normal range 4.2–5.4 × 10^6/μL)
Hb = 12	(Normal range 12–16 g/dL in females)
Hct = 37%	(Normal range 28–47% in females)

Electrolytes
Sodium (Na) = 146   (Normal range 136–146 mEq/L)

Potassium (K) = 3.5	(Normal range 3.5–5.5 mEq/L)
Chloride (Cl) = 95	(Normal range 96–106 mEq/L)
Calcium (Ca) = 8.8	(Normal range 8.5–10.5 mg/dL)
Glucose = 140	(Normal range 80–120 mg/dL)

Serum hCG
 Pending
CT abdomen
 Scan positive for diffuse abdominal bleeding

QUESTION

What is the significance of the laboratory and radiographic data?

ANSWER

The WBC is elevated, perhaps in response to abdominal infection secondary to bleeding. The CBC, Hb, and Hct are on the low side of normal because of abdominal bleeding. It generally takes 6 hours after hemorrhage begins to detect a noticeable decrease in the Hct (Gawlinski, 1988). The high normal sodium is related to an increase in aldosterone secretion to maintain blood volume. Thus, renal excretion of sodium decreases. Renal excretion of potassium increases because of this same response as evidenced by Sue's low normal level. Her glucose is elevated due to sympathetic stimulation. The CT scan suggests a ruptured ectopic pregnancy originating in the right fallopian tube. This finding is consistent with Sue's history of being 3 months pregnant. Ectopic pregnancy is a life-threatening event because of associated internal bleeding. The results of the CT scan confirm that Sue requires surgical intervention.

Focused Nursing History

While Sue is in the radiology department with the emergency medicine resident, you speak with her husband to obtain the most critical historical data that may have an impact on Sue's present situation. The comprehensive nursing database will be completed within 24 hours postadmission. Her husband gives the following history.

Sue diagnosed her pregnancy using an over-the-counter pregnancy detection kit. Both she and her husband are excited about the pregnancy, since they have tried to conceive for over 2 years. Sue has not had any problems during the pregnancy. Before trying to conceive, Sue was using birth control pills. Her last menstrual period was 86 days ago. She has not had a previous pregnancy. For the last 2 days, she has complained of abdominal pain that has gradually increased in intensity. She has had nausea but did not begin vomiting until in the car on the way to the emergency department. Sue fainted when she got up to answer the phone after lying on the couch to try to relieve her abdominal pain. She has never fainted before. Sue does not have any medical conditions. She is not allergic to any

medication. Her last meal was 6 hours ago. She has had two glasses of water since her last meal.

The Systematic Bedside Assessment

Sue returns from having a CT scan. You will complete a head-to-toe assessment, since you will be caring for Sue until the operating suite is ready and the general surgeon completes his present case. Sue signs a permit for an exploratory laparotomy.

Head and Neck. Sue remains oriented, but she is restless. She has a nasal cannula present that is delivering 2 L of oxygen. Her neck veins are slightly filled at an angle of 30 degrees. No other abnormalities of the head and neck are noted.

Chest. Cardiac Status. As previously noted. Apical heart rate is 138. The pattern that is present on the cardiac monitor is shown in Figure 9–2. Blood pressure is 88/70. Lactated Ringer's solution is being infused at 200 mL/hour via a No. 16 IV catheter in the right forearm. The IV site is negative for edema and redness.

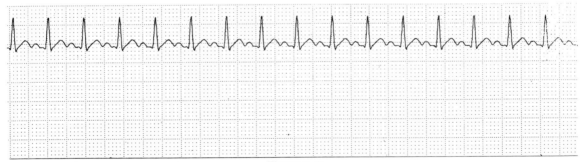

Figure 9–2.

QUESTION

The pattern in Figure 9–2 is
1. Normal sinus rhythm
2. Sinus tachycardia
3. Supraventricular tachycardia
4. Atrial fibrillation

---

2. Sinus tachycardia is indicated because the rate is greater than 100 and P waves precede the QRS complex.

Pulmonary Status. As previously noted. The respiratory rate has increased to 32/minute. Respirations remain shallow.

Abdomen. The adbomen is firm and tight. No bowel sounds are auscultated. Sue complains of increased pain in all quadrants and in her right shoulder on light palpation.

Pelvis. A No. 16 Foley catheter is in place draining light, yellow urine, 40 mL in the first hour of placement. Reagent strip is negative for hematuria, ketones, and glucose.

Extremities. The skin is diaphoretic, cool, and clammy. The nailbeds are dusky. Capillary refill is sluggish. Peripheral pulses are palpable but faint (1+) in all extremities.

Posterior. Posterior breath sounds are diminished in bilateral lower lung fields. No sacral edema is noted.

Development of Nursing Diagnoses

Clustering Data. You have just completed your head-to-toe assessment and are ready to list appropriate nursing diagnoses for Sue. To cluster the data, look for abnormal results found during the assessment. Sue's major symptoms at this time are her intense pain and hypotension. These primary symptoms can initiate your first cluster of critical cues (Carpenito, 1987).

CLUSTER 1

Subjective data. Sue complains of continuous abdominal pain unrelieved with change in position. Pain has increased over the last 2 days. The pain increased with abdominal palpation and radiates to all four quadrants and the right shoulder (Kehr's sign). Nausea and vomiting are present, and the patient fainted once at home.

Objective data. Blood pressure is 88–90/70. The heart rate is 126 to 138. Respirations are 28. Hb and Hct are borderline low. Potassium is borderline low, and sodium is borderline high. Urine output low is at 40 mL/hour. The last menstrual period was 86 days ago, and she had a positive over-the-counter pregnancy test. The CT scan was positive for adbominal bleeding.

QUESTION

Based on these data, which of the following nursing diagnoses would you select as being appropriate in planning Sue's care?
1. **Fluid volume, deficit, actual**
2. **Cardiac output, altered: decreased**
3. **Tissue perfusion, altered: renal, peripheral**
4. **All of the above**

ANSWER

The correct answer is 4. All three are present in Sue's case. However, the decreased CO and tissue perfusion are directly related to the actual fluid volume deficit. Therefore, focusing your nursing interventions on addressing the fluid volume status will improve her CO and tissue perfusion. The most appropriate of the three diagnoses is ***Fluid volume, deficit, actual*** related to adbominal bleeding.

Expected patient outcomes for Sue would include

1. Systolic blood pressure greater than 90 mm Hg
2. Heart rate between 60 and 100 bpm
3. Respirations 12 to 16/minute
4. Absence of abdominal pain
5. Urine output of at least 30 mL/hour
6. Absence of dizziness and syncope (Ulrich et al, 1986)

For the purposes of Sue's case study, only the perfusion-related nursing diagnosis will be developed further. In a true clinical situation, however, other clusters would be developed based on primary critical cues from the collected data. If data are insufficient, you should collect additional data to confirm or refute your hypotheses.

Based on Sue's available data, these additional nursing diagnoses also pertain to her case.

- **Infection** related to adbominal irritation as evidenced by elevated WBC
- **Impaired gas exchange** related to decreased cellular oxygenation
- **High risk for alteration in urinary elimination,** related to decreased renal perfusion
- **Alteration in nutrition: less than body requirements** related to increased metabolic rate
- **Acute pain** related to adbominal irritation
- **High risk for disturbance in self-concept, role performance, and body image** related to surgical incision, loss of pregnancy, and potential loss of reproductive abilities

Sue's fluid volume deficit is related to hemorrhage. Excessive diuresis and severe dehydration also may produce a fluid volume deficit. Sue's treatment goals will focus on stopping the source of her bleeding, restoring vascular volume, and optimizing perfusion. These general goals should be reflected in the nursing diagnoses and expected patient outcomes. For example, restoring vascular volume is addressed in the nursing diagnosis: ***Fluid volume deficit.*** Accomplishment of this goal will be measured in such criteria as systolic blood pressure greater than 90 mm Hg, heart rate between 60 and 100 bpm, and urinary output of at least 30 mL/hour.

Development of the Plan of Care

Nursing interventions will be based on activities that will help Sue meet her expected patient outcomes. They will consist of collaborative interventions that are both mutidisciplinary and interdisciplinary (Leuner et al, 1990). Independent interventions are activities that are within the scope of nursing practice and do not require a physician's order.

Collaborative Interventions Related to Circulatory Status. The physician's orders may include the following.

1. *Volume replacement.* Crystalloids or colloids may be used to expand the vascular volume. Usually, lactated Ringer's solution is used initially because it contains potassium and calcium as well as lactate. Lactate is converted to bicarbonate to provide additional compensation for acidosis, which is encountered commonly in shock states. Whole blood will be administered once the typing and crossmatching are performed. In circumstances where the patient has a history of heart or renal failure, packed red blood cells may be given instead of whole blood to improve the oxygen-carrying capacity of the blood without reversing the volume deficit so quickly that a fluid overload condition may develop. Albumin and plasma may be administered in situations when the fluid volume deficit is related to fluid shifting from the vascular space into the interstitial space. Synthetic volume expanders (Dextran and Hespan) may be used to rapidly expand volume until crossmatching is completed or blood is available. For additional information, refer to Module 8, *Shock States.* This module further addresses fluid replacement.

2. *Vasopressor therapy.* Vasoconstrictors may be ordered to increase venous return and, ultimately, CO. The most commonly used vasoconstrictor is norepinephrine. The major problem associated with the use of vasoconstrictors is decreased renal perfusion, since the patient is already vasoconstricted due to sympathetic stimulation. Inotropes also may be administered. High-dose dopamine (greater than 10 μg/kg/minute) may be given to produce peripheral vasoconstriction and increase venous return. Although in low

doses dopamine has a dopaminergic action resulting in increased urinary output, high doses counteract this effect of increased renal circulation.

3. *Oxygen.* Oxygen is administered to ensure that the blood that reaches the tissues is adequately oxygenated. High-flow oxygen is preferred in hypovolemic states. A nonrebreather mask connected to 10 L of oxygen will promote hemoglobin saturation and help prevent respiratory acidosis (Rea, 1991). Since Sue's condition has not improved, the physician probably will change the route and amount of oxygen she is receiving.

4. *Military antishock trousers.* A MAST garment is used to control internal bleeding. The exact mechanism by which MAST work is not known. Originally, it was thought that core circulation was promoted by redistributing peripheral blood flow. MAST are used also to tamponande bleeding in some situations. MAST may be used preoperatively to maintain a systolic blood pressure over 90 mm Hg. If Sue's blood pressure continues to drop, the trousers may be applied and inflated. The trousers are placed under Sue as a precautionary measure in anticipation of the need for inflation.

5. *Hemodynamic monitoring.* A central venous pressure line or a pulmonary arterial catheter may be inserted to provide direct measurements of CO and preload. Placement of a central line will provide another access route for IV fluid replacement and blood specimen removal as well as pressure monitoring.

6. *Laboratory and X-ray testing.* Serial Hb and Hct levels will be obtained to monitor the degree of hemorrhage. A chest x-ray will be obtained preoperatively for baseline purposes or after placement of a central IV line to ensure proper placement. Arterial blood gases will be determined if Sue's level of responsiveness changes. A lactic acid level also would be obtained at that time to monitor acidosis.

Independent Nursing Interventions

1. Elevate Sue's legs to promote venous drainage from the legs.
2. Facilitate and maintain a position of comfort to decrease Sue's pain and anxiety and thus oxygen use.

3. Maintain accurate intake and output records.
4. Keep Sue NPO in anticipation of surgery.
5. Monitor vital signs continuously.
6. Monitor the effects of drug therapy and fluid replacement.
7. Monitor test results (report abnormal results).
8. Keep the patient and husband informed about the plan of care.
9. Assess for decreased perfusion (report abnormal results)
   - Systolic blood pressure less than 90 mm Hg
   - Narrowing of pulse pressure
   - Respirations less than 8 or greater than 30/minute
   - Presence of bradycardia, tachycardia, or premature beats
   - Change in responsiveness
   - Urine output less than 30 mL/hour
   - Flat neck veins

Plan Evaluation and Revision

Sue's perfusion plan of care is now developed and ready to be executed. Her progress will be monitored at regular intervals to evaluate the effects of the various therapeutic actions. If progress is not being noted toward attainment of Sue's expected patient outcomes, her plan may need revisions, examining alternative interventions that may be more effective.

Sue's condition worsens. Her blood pressure is 66 mm Hg and obtainable only by Doppler. She is unresponsive. You call for the physician and adjust her IV fluids to a wide open rate. The runner from the blood bank has just arrived with four units of crossmatched blood. Dr. P decides to insert a pulmonary arterial catheter and a peripheral arterial catheter. You assist her with the procedures while another nurse hangs the blood through the peripheral IV line. Dr. P gives an order to inflate the leg compartments of the MAST suit until the systolic blood pressure reaches 90 mm Hg.

NURSING CARE OF A PATIENT BEING MONITORED HEMODYNAMICALLY

The goals and outcome criteria that are appropriate to the management of Sue while she is being hemodynamically monitored can be divided into two major groupings: support of her physiologic needs and support of her psychosocial needs.

Support of Physiologic Needs

Sue's physiologic needs will be met through nursing interventions that promote adequate fluid volume and distribution and prevent infection and hemodynamic monitoring complications. Sue's nursing management will be planned around interventions to attain these goals. These goals are addressed through the nursing diagnoses of **Alteration in cardiac output: decrease, Fluid volume deficit, Alteration in tissue perfusion: peripheral, Potential for infection,** and **Potential for injury.** Before addressing these diagnoses, the pulmonary and arterial catheters must be inserted. The nurse caring for a patient undergoing invasive monitoring must prepare the patient and the equipment as well as monitor the patient during insertion.

Prepare the Patient

An alert patient may be sedated before the procedure. Sue is unresponsive, and sedation will not be provided. It is important to explain to the patient and family why invasive monitoring is necessary and what it entails. Another nurse has discussed with Sue's husband, who is now in the waiting area, the rationale for inserting a pulmonary arterial catheter and initiating an arterial line. He has signed the permit allowing insertion. It is helpful to explain to the patient what to expect during insertion. During insertion, the patient may be placed in reverse Trendelenburg position with the patient's face turned away from the insertion site if the subclavian or internal jugular vein is used for entry. This facilitates passage and decreases the risk of air embolism. The phelbostatic axis (fourth intercostal space) should be marked on the patient's lateral chest wall to serve as a landmark for obtaining readings. This point is thought to approximate the catheter tip. It is extremely important that measurements are obtained using the same point of reference in order to identify changes in readings related to the patient's physiologic condition and not an artifact related to technique. Baseline vital signs should be obtained to use as a comparison with patient values during insertion.

Prepare the Equipment

The type of equipment needed depends on the monitoring system used by the facility as well as the type of catheter used. A monitor (usually with an amplifier, oscilloscope, and digital display) is necessary. A transducer is used to convert the mechanical signal transmitted by the fluid-filled tubing to an electrical signal that can be understood by the monitor. Transducers may be disposable or nondisposable. A water manometer may be used instead of a transducer for obtaining central venous pressure (CVP) readings if waveform depiction is not necessary. The effects of atmospheric and hydrostatic pressure must be eliminated before obtaining pressure readings from the patient. Zeroing the monitor will negate other pressure influences. Since the exact procedure used to zero a monitor depends on the manufacturer, this module does not discuss specific details. The reader is instead referred to the appropriate user's manual. The monitor should be zeroed (1) before critical measurements are taken, (2) when there is a sudden change in pressure readings, (3) when there is a change in transducer reference placement, and (4) every 4 hours (Daily, 1990). Calibration of the monitor should be checked by turning the calibration knob. The nurse is checking to see if the monitor can read a predetermined value. Usually the knob can be adjusted. Adjustments are made until there is congruency between the actual monitor reading and the precalibrated value. Nondisposable transducers may need to be calibrated also. The reader is again referred to the appropriate user's manual for the calibration procedure.

Catheters differ according to size and number of lumens. The number of lumens determine the capabilities of the catheter. Sue is receiving a triple-lumen pulmonary arterial catheter equipped with a side port and a thermistor for CO measurements. The side port will provide additional access for volume replacement. A multiple-lumen catheter allows for pressure monitoring and medication/fluid administration. Some catheters are equipped with pacing capabilities or fiberoptics, permitting continuous monitoring of the oxygen saturation of mixed venous blood. A flush system is necessary for each lumen used for pressure monitoring purposes. Most flush systems consist of heparinized 5 percent dextrose in water solution and pressure tubing. The solution is maintained at 300 mm Hg by inserting the bag into a pressure infusor cuff. The tubing must be primed, and all air must be removed before connecting the tubing to the catheter port. Unused ports may be capped and heparinized periodically. If the catheter is capable of obtaining CO measurements, the thermistor hub of the catheter must be connected, by cable, to the CO computer. The CO computer may be located in the same monitor used for pressure monitoring, or it may be a separate device. Injectate solution and tubing (after priming) are connected by stopcock to the proximal lumen port of the catheter. A percutaneous vascular access tray may be used for instruments.

Insertion Responsibilities

During insertion, the nurse should observe the patient's cardiac rhythm. The patient may experience premature ventricular contractions (PVC), especially as the catheter is advanced into and through the right ventricle. IV lidocaine should be kept at the bedside to treat ventricular tachycardia and multiple PVCs. Defibrillation may be necessary if the patient develops ventricular fibrillation. Initial pressures should be recorded as the catheter is advanced. This is the only time pressures will be recorded in the right ventricle. Module 6, *Hemodynamic Monitoring*, provides pictorial and verbal descriptions of the waveforms, normal pressure measurements, and basic troubleshooting. The nurse will connect the catheter lumens to the appropriate tubing as blood exits the catheter. The physician usually sutures the catheter in place and applies the dressing. Sue did not experience any dysrhythmias during insertion. Her initial readings were CVP 2, RVP 16/0, PAP 17/6, PAP mean 8, PCWP 3.

A portable chest x-ray should be obtained postinsertion to validate catheter placement and to examine lung expansion. A pneumothorax may occur during insertion using the subclavian or jugular vein, since the lung extends above the clavicle.

Obtaining Measurements

Much controversy is present in the literature about the influence of variables (i.e., medications and patient position) on the accuracy of pressure readings (Chulay and Miller, 1984; Laulive, 1982; Nemens and Woods, 1982; Woods and Mansfield, 1986). Generally, readings should be obtained with the patient supine and the transducer positioned at the phlebostatic axis. The most important factor is to document the position in which the reading is obtained. Documentation of the bed position during recording of pressures is necessary to help ensure consistency. If the bed is elevated, the same degree of elevation should be used for subsequent readings. Readings may be taken when the patient is on his or her side as long as the transducer is rezeroed and adjusted to the phlebostatic axis. Because Sue was unresponsive, her readings were obtained in the supine position.

It is beyond the scope of this book to discuss advanced waveform interpretation. For additional information in this area, the learner should refer to an outside resource. Waveforms may be dampened or have decreased amplitude if a clot is forming at the catheter tip. Figure 9–3 is an example of a dampened arterial pressure waveform. Air bubbles in the system also will produce damping. Remove all air bubbles by closing the system off to the patient and flushing the line or withdraw the bubbles with a needle and syringe. Having the patient cough or change position also may increase the amplitude and sharpness of the waveform. Catheter fling is a waveform that is noisy or accentuated from excessive movement of the catheter. This condition may result from use of excessive tubing. Decreasing the tubing length and using stiff connecting tubing usually will relieve this problem.

Physiologic factors may influence pressure readings. Intrapleural pressure may falsely elevate readings. Measurements should be obtained at end-expiration, when there is no air flow, and the intrapleural pressure remains stable. Newer monitoring systems include an algorithim to identify the pressure at end-expiration (Ellis, 1985). End-expiratory measurements are very important when the patient is being ventilated mechanically. The ventilator delivers positive pressure breaths as compared to nega-

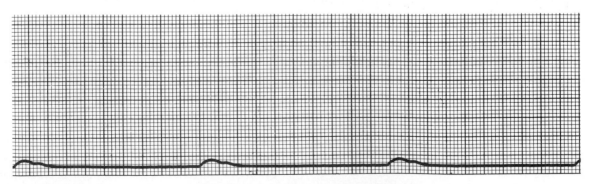

Figure 9–3. Dampened arterial waveform.

tive pressure spontaneous breathing. Hemodynamic pressures may be elevated artificially because of this positive pressure breathing. When a patient is receiving positive end-expiratory pressure (PEEP) as a ventilatory adjunct, the hemodynamic readings may be falsely elevated to a greater degree. Module 4, *Nursing Care of the Patient with Altered Respiratory Function*, discusses hemodynamic trends of a patient being ventilated mechanically. Institutions vary regarding the policy used to obtain hemodynamic measurements in a patient on the ventilator. Patients who can tolerate removal from the ventilator may be removed to obtain readings. However, readings obtained while the patient is on the ventilator tend to reflect the actual circumstances under which the cardiovascular system is operating. Consistency in obtaining readings is important so that patient's trends can be evaluated.

In summary, the following guidelines can be used when interpreting readings.

1. Always look at patient trends and not an isolated reading.
2. Question abnormal readings. Recheck the reading after zeroing and calibrating the equipment. Assess the patient for additional data to support the reading.
3. Compare the patient with his or her normal values and not the textbook.
4. Do not be fooled by normal readings. The patient may have normal readings temporarily because of compensatory mechanisms. Continue to assess the patient.
5. Assess the interrelationships between the readings. You are trying to obtain a picture of the patient's hemodynamic status and not just a PCWP or a CVP reading.

Interpreting Trends

Module 6, *Hemodynamic Monitoring*, discusses each hemodynamic pressure and etiologies of high and low readings. Nursing interventions for patients with high and low readings are discussed. Derived parameters also are addressed. Knowledge of cardiopulmonary anatomy and circulatory flow through the heart and the lungs is essential to understanding the implications of a composite of hemodynamic readings. For example, an elevated CVP reading associated with normal PCWP and PAP readings indicates that a problem is present with either the pulmonary valve, right ventricle (cor pulmonale), or tricuspid valve. An elevated CVP pressure in conjunction with elevated PCWP and PAP pressures is indicative of fluid overload, left heart failure, or pul-

monary disease. An elevated PAP reading with a normal CVP reading may exist in early pulmonary disease. Hemodynamic readings are altered in shock states. In hypovolemic and cardiogenic shock, the systemic vascular resistance (SVR) is increased as a compensatory mechanism, and the CO is decreased. The same is true in late septic shock. In early septic shock, CO is increased and SVR is decreased as a response to vasodilation and enhanced cardiac contractility. Neurogenic shock resembles early septic shock because of the unopposed parasympathetic stimulation. Thus, SVR is decreased and CO is increased. Sue's initial readings were low, indicating a fluid volume deficit. Her cardiac output was 3.2 L/minute. The mean arterial pressure reading was 65. Her SVR was 1,575 dynes/second/cm^{-5}, indicating that her sympathetic nervous system is trying to compensate for the low venous return.

Potential Complications

Several complications may occur from invasive hemodynamic monitoring. Infection may result. Air emboli or thromboembolism can occur from loose connections or improper flushing, respectively. Never flush a port if resistance is met. Fluid overload may result from fluid infusion through multiple lumens or lack of surveillance of IV pumps. Exsanguination may occur from any hemodynamic monitoring line if a stopcock remains open or tubing becomes disconnected.

Pulmonary infarction can result from leaving the pulmonary artery balloon inflated or when a deflated balloon becomes lodged in the pulmonary capillary bed. A wedging waveform will appear on the monitor (Figure 9–4). The patient should be turned or made to cough to relieve a lodged balloon. Open the stopcock on the port and remove the syringe to allow passive deflation of the balloon. The balloon may rupture from repeated overfilling of the balloon. If you are unable to obtain a wedge waveform after instilling the proper amount of air through the PA catheter balloon port, turn the lumen off to the patient, mark the line *Do not use*, and notify the physician.

Nursing Diagnoses

Since the pulmonary and arterial catheters are in place, we can address Sue's physiologic needs as previously identified in the nursing diagnoses of (1) **Alteration in cardiac output: decreased**, (2) **Fluid volume deficit**, (3) **Alteration in tissue perfusion:**

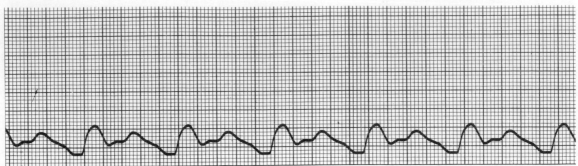

Figure 9–4. Pulmonary capillary wedge pressure waveform.

peripheral, (4) **Potential for infection,** and (5) **Potential for injury.**

Alteration in Cardiac Output: Decreased

Obtaining Sue's CO, CI, and SVR measurements will provide information about her response to fluid and medication administration. Sue's SVR reading will indicate the degree to which her sympathetic nervous system is trying to compensate for the low stroke volume. Her heart rate and pattern should be assessed to determine her hemodynamic response to changes in rate or rhythm. Dysrhythmias and tachycardia will further diminish her CO. Improvement in Sue's level of responsiveness would indicate improvement in her CO. Her urine output provides another parameter for monitoring CO, since 20% of the CO goes to the kidneys (Guyton, 1986).

Fluid Volume Deficit

Sue's preload will need to be monitored to determine her response to volume replacement. The impact of inotropes and vasopressors on Sue's preload can be examined by comparing CVP and PCWP readings after medication administration with baseline measures. Hemoglobin and hematocrit values will provide information regarding how much volume has been lost. Because Sue is being hemodynamically monitored, she is at risk for exsanguination if the tubing becomes disconnected or a stopcock is left open. To prevent this from occurring, keep all catheter connecting sites visible and reassess frequently. Keep monitor alarms on to detect changes in blood pressure. In addition, the assessment data that helped you evaluate Sue's cardiac output status will also help you evaluate her fluid volume status.

Alteration in Tissue Perfusion: Peripheral

Since Sue has a fluid volume deficit, her tissue perfusion is compromised. Because she also has a pulmo-

nary arterial and peripheral artery catheter in place, she is at risk for further compromise in her peripheral perfusion. Thrombus formation or thrombophlebitis may occur. The insertion site should be examined at least every 8 hours for tenderness, redness, and skin temperature. A loss in arterial pulsation distal to the placement of the catheter may indicate arterial insufficiency related to thrombus formation.

High Risk for Infection

The catheter dressing, tubing, stopcocks, and transducer should be changed according to institution protocol. Aseptic technique should be used when obtaining blood specimens and flushing the catheter. Ports should be cleansed of all blood after obtaining samples. Sue's WBC is already elevated and should be monitored for further increases. Her temperature should be evaluated. If an infection is suspected related to the hemodynamic monitoring, the catheter may be removed or changed and cultures may be obtained from Sue's blood and the catheter.

High Risk for Injury

If Sue becomes restless, she may pull out her pulmonary or arterial catheter. She may need to be restrained or sedated if a change occurs in her responsiveness level. If the pulmonary arterial catheter tip falls into the right ventricle, Sue may experience life-threatening dysrhythmias. If you notice a right ventricular waveform pattern, the physician should be notified. The balloon will need to be inflated through the pulmonary artery balloon port by either the physician or nurse (depending on hospital policy). This should allow the catheter to float back into the pulmonary artery. If Sue has hemoptysis and abnormal ABGs and respirations, she may be experiencing a pulmonary infarction from permanent wedging of the balloon or lodging of the deflated balloon in the pulmonary capillary bed. Open the stopcock on the pulmonary artery balloon port and remove the syringe to allow for passive deflation of the balloon.

Support of Psychosocial Needs

Support of Sue's psychosocial needs will center around interventions that reduce anxiety and promote a balance between sleep and activity.

Anxiety Related to Equipment

Most patients identify that the monitoring of rhythms and patterns on oscilloscopes is equivalent to being critically ill. Granted, hemodynamic monitoring is used most frequently in the unstable patient, but it can be used also for patients who require frequent blood specimens and multiple medications. Catheters may be left in place for fluid and medication administration after cardiac pressures are unable to be obtained due to catheter malfunction. Sue went from having one pattern monitored, her cardiac rhythm, to having four patterns monitored: cardiac rhythm, CVP, PAP, and arterial pressure. Family members may become alarmed when they notice the oscilloscope at the patient's bedside. Most individuals are accustomed to peripheral IV lines, but insertion of a catheter into the neck may be a foreign concept. Sue was unresponsive at the time that the catheter was inserted. When she becomes responsive, the nurse will need to explain the purpose of the catheters and warn Sue not to touch any of the tubing or connections.

High Risk for Sleep Pattern Disturbance

Periodic assessment of hemodynamic readings may interrupt Sue's rest and sleep. Decreasing the light in her room at night while providing adequate lighting for obtaining measurements will foster Sue's rest. While Sue is in the emergency department, it will be difficult for her to rest because of the noise and constant patient flow. However, the priority in the emergency department is to improve Sue's fluid volume so her surgical procedure will be less stressful. After surgery, the nurse can obtain hemodynamic measurements in Sue's position of comfort (or sleep) as long as the nurse rezeros the transducer and maintains the transducer at the phlebostatic axis. Sue's position while the readings were obtained should be documented.

The operating suite is ready for Sue. Here hemodynamic lines are secured. Blood and lactated Ringer's are infusing through her CVP port and side port, respectively. The leg components of the MAST suit remain inflated, since her mean arterial pressure is 60. She is still receiving 10 L of oxygen through a non-rebreather mask. Sue remains in sinus tachycardia. The report is given to the operating room nurse. Sue's husband is escorted to the surgical waiting area.

CASE STUDY 2

—— DELORES GARCIA, A PATIENT
EXPERIENCING FLUID VOLUME EXCESS ——

You are the nurse assigned to care for Mrs. Garcia. Mrs. Garcia was admitted to the telemetry floor with a diagnosis of **Angina: rule out myocardial infarction.** She was admitted through the emergency department 16 hours previously.

The Initial Appraisal

On walking in the room you note the following.
General Appearance. Mrs. Garcia is a Hispanic female of moderate stature. She is overweight and tidy in apprearance.
Signs of Distress. Mrs. Garcia is diaphoretic. Her respirations are fast and shallow. She is sitting upright in bed.
Other. You note that she is receiving oxygen by nasal cannula. An IV solution of D_5W is infusing.

Focused Respiratory and Circulatory Assessment

Because Mrs. Garcia appears to be in acute distress, you immediately perform a rapid assessment focusing on her cardiopulmonary status. The results are as follows.

Mrs. Garcia is restless but oriented to person, place, time, and reason for hospitalization. Her respiratory rate is 28/minute, shallow and regular. On auscultation of her chest, you note bilateral medium crackles in the lower lung fields, left greater than right. S_1 and S_2 are present. No murmurs are noted, but an S_3 is auscultated. Her blood pressure is 156/106, and her pulse is 104 bpm. She is complaining of chest pain, sharp in nature, that is radiating down her left arm. She is in the cardiac rhythm shown in Figure 9–5.

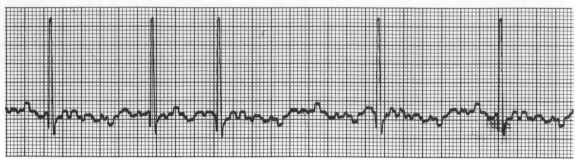

Figure 9–5.

QUESTION

The pattern in Figure 9–5 is
1. Atrial flutter
2. Complete heart block
3. Atrial fibrillation
4. Artifact

ANSWER

3. P waves are not distinquishable. The R to R interval is irregular.

Following this initial assessment, you check her admission orders. Mrs. Garcia has the following medications ordered.

- 10 mg Nifedipine SL PRN systolic blood pressure greater than 140 mm Hg or diastolic blood pressure greater than 100 mm Hg

- Nitroglycerin grain 1/150 SL PRN chest pain
- Morphine sulfate 4 mg IVP PRN every 2 to 3 hours for chest pain

---

QUESTION

What effect will these medications have on Mrs. Garcia's perfusion status?

ANSWER

All of the medications will help improve Mrs. Garcia's CO. Nitroglycerin is a fast-acting drug that will produce peripheral vasodilation, thus redistributing blood away from the congested pulmonary bed. Nitroglycerin also may increase collateral circulation to the myocardium. The vasodilation should decrease her pain. Nifedipine could be administered next. This is a calcium channel blocking agent that has both arterial and venous vasodilating effects. It will help to relieve the coronary vasospasm that is probably producing Mrs. Garcia's pain. Morphine decreases preload by producing peripheral vasodilation. It decreases anxiety, which increases myocardial oxygen consumption. Morphine also relaxes airway smooth muscle, so it may decrease Mrs. Garcia's respiratory rate by improving gas exchange.

You administer all three of the medications and place a call to her cardiologist. In the interim, Mrs. Garcia's morning laboratory results come back.

Electrolytes
(Normal ranges are from Alspach and Williams, 1985.)

Sodium (Na) = 142	(Normal range 136–146 mEq/L)
Potassium (K) = 3.5	(Normal range 3.5–5.5 mEq/L)
Chloride (Cl) = 104	(Normal range 96–106 mEq/L)
Calcium (Ca) = 9.0	(Normal range 8.5–10.5 mg/dL)

(Normal ranges are from Pagana and Pagana, 1986.)

Creatinine phosphokinase (CPK) = 20 mU/mL	(Normal range 5–75 mU/mL)
Serum aspartate aminotransferase (AST) (previouosly SGOT) = 24 IU/L	(Normal range 5–40 IU/L)
Lactic dehydrogenase (LDH) = 120 ImU/mL	(Normal range 90–200 ImU/mL)

QUESTION

What is the significance of these laboratory results?

ANSWER

Mrs. Garcia's electrolyte values are within normal limits. Thus, she should not be prediposed to cardiac dysrhythmias resulting from electrolyte disturbances. However, her potassium level is borderline low. You will need to check her chart to see if she has been taking diuretics at home for chronic medical conditions. If digitalis is prescribed because of her beginning pulmonary edema (as suspected based on the presence of crackles on pulmonary auscultation), Mrs. Garcia may be predisposed to digitalis toxicity.

The normal cardiac enzyme levels indicate that Mrs. Garcia has not experienced a myocardial infarction. When the heart muscle is damaged, enzymes are released. The CPK level rises within 6 hours, peaks in 18 hours, and declines to normal in 2 to 3 days postinfarction (Pagana and Pagana, 1986). If the CPK level was elevated, isoenzymes would be ordered to determine the cause of the elevation. CPK-MB is the isoenzyme associated with cardiac cells. The CPK-MB level will begin to rise 3 to 6 hours postinfarction. It does not rise during angina. After myocardial infarction, the AST (SGOT) level will increase within 10 hours, peak in 48 hours, and return to normal by 4 days (Pagana and Pagana, 1986). An elevated LDH level also requires isoenzyme analysis. There are five LDH isoenzymes. Isoenzyme LDH-1 is located in the heart and red blood cells. LDH-2 is the most predominant LDH isoenzyme. When the LDH-1 level is greater than the LDH-2 level, it is indicative of a myocardial infarction (Pagana and Pagana, 1986). If Mrs. Garcia's LDH level had been elevated, isoenzymes would have been obtained.

Mrs. Garcia's pain has not decreased. She is complaining of being short of breath. Her blood pressure has dropped to 114/72. Her heart rate is 92. Respirations remain at 28/minute. Her daughter arrives in the room to see you administering a second grain 1/150 nitroglycerin tablet SL to her mother.

Focused Nursing History

Since Mrs. Garcia is still experiencing pain, you decide to speak with her daughter to obtain the most important critical historical data that may have an impact on Mrs. Garcia's present situation. The comprehensive nursing database has not yet been completed but will need to be finished within 24 hours of Mrs. Garcia's admission. Her daughter gives the following history.

Mrs. Garcia started experiencing chest pain the morning of her admission after she had moved a piece of bedroom furniture. She had been complaining of "heartburn" after eating heavy meals intermittently for the last 6 months. The pain yesterday would not go away after Mrs. Garcia rested. She called her daughter, who drove over to her house and convinced her to go to the hospital. Mrs. Garcia is not allergic to any medicine. She has a history of smoking 1 pack of cigarettes a day for 20 years. She is 47 years old and has a history of hypertension. She takes Lasix 10 mg orally daily for her blood pressure. She does not take potassium supplements, but her daughter states that Mrs. Garcia eats many bananas.

Even though most of this information should already be recorded in Mrs. Garcia's chart, you have not had time to read her chart. This information was important to obtain and will help you as you perform your systematic assessment.

The Systematic Bedside Assessment

Head and Neck. Mrs. Garcia has an olive complexion. Perspiration is on her forehead. She remains oriented and alert. Oxygen is infusing through her nasal cannula at 2 L/minute. She is in a semi-Fowler's position at 30 degrees. Her jugular veins are full but not distended.

Chest. Pulmonary status. Her crackles have increased since your initial assessment. Crackles in her right and left lung fields are equal in intensity. Respirations are 26/minute.

Cardiac status. It is more difficult to hear her heart sounds because of the crackles. However, S_1, S_2, and S_3 are still audible. Her apical heart rate is irregular without a distinctive pattern. Her blood pressure is 92/70.

Abdomen. Her abdomen is soft and/obese. Hy-poactive bowel sounds are auscultated. No pain is elicited on palpation. Liver borders are nonpalpable.

Pelvis. Mrs. Garcia is voiding per bedpan and voided 100 mL in the last hour. Her urine has been yellow and clear. Reagent strips are negative for glucose, ketones, and blood.

Extremities. She has bilateral 2+ nonpitting pedal edema. Pedal pulses are faint (1+) but palpable. Capillary refill is 2 seconds in all extremities. Her skin is damp from perspiration.

Posterior. No sacral edema is noted. Posterior breath sounds reveal bilateral course crackles lower to midlung fields.

Development of Nursing Diagnoses

Clustering Data. You are now ready to develop nursing diagnoses based on the available subjective and objective data. To cluster your data, look for abnormal values discovered during the assessment. Mrs. Garcia's major symptoms at this time are chest pain, decreasing blood pressure, and increasing pulmonary crackles. Thus, these primary symptoms can initiate your first cluster of critical cues (Carpenito, 1987; Kersten, 1989).

CLUSTER 1

Subjective data. The patient is complaining of increasing chest pain not relieved with nitroglycerin SL × two or morphine sulfate 4 mg IVP. She also is complaining of shortness of breath despite oxygen administration at 2 L per nasal cannula. She has a previous history of hypertension and heartburn.

Objective data. Mrs. Garcia is diaphoretic with full neck veins, 2+ bilateral pedal edema. Crackles are auscultated in the bilateral posterior lung fields. S_3 is auscultated. Atrial fibrillation with rapid ventricular response is noted. On admission, cardiac enzymes were normal.

QUESTION

Based on the above data, which of the following nursing diagnoses is the priority diagnosis at this time for Mrs. Garcia?
1. **Alteration in cardiac output: decreased**
2. **Impaired gas exchange**
3. **Alteration in tissue perfusion: peripheral**
4. **Fluid volume excess**

ANSWER

The correct answer is 4. Although you might expect a decreased CO to be present, you lack data to confirm this diagnosis, since Mrs. Garcia is still voiding an appropriate amount and she remains alert. It is true that her blood pressure has decreased, but it may be decreased as a normal response to the vasodilating medications. Arterial blood gases have not been obtained, so impaired gas exchange cannot be supported. However, if Mrs. Garcia's tachypnea continues and her crackles continue to increase, impaired gas exchange probably will be present. Alteration in peripheral tissue perfusion cannot be supported adequately because even though her pedal pulses are faint (1+), they are present, and capillary refill is normal. Fluid volume excess is the most plausible diagnosis because of her increasing crackles and shortness of breath associated with increasing chest pain. She is also in atrial fibrillation, a pattern commonly associated with heart failure. Mrs. Garcia's admission diagnosis of angina and history of hypertension suggests that she is susceptible to congestive heart failure. Several factors can contribute to fluid overload: increased fluid intake, decreased fluid elimination, or decreased fluid distribution. Mrs. Garcia's fluid volume overload is related to distribution. The volume has remained unchanged. Her left ventricle has decreased contractility due to distention probably related to chronic hypertension.

The physician calls, and you inform him of Mrs. Garcia's present status. He orders a stat. ECG, portable chest film, cardiac enzymes, and arterial blood gases. He wants you to initiate a nitroglycerin IV drip at 5 μg/minute. He is coming to see Mrs. Garcia. She will be transferred to the coronary care unit as soon as a bed is available.

When you return to Mrs. Garcia's room, you notice that she is less responsive and responds to touch instead of verbal stimuli. Her daughter is crying and saying, "Momma don't die!" Mrs. Garcia's cardiac rhythym in lead II has changed to that shown in Figure 9–6.

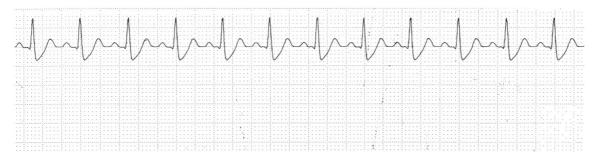

Figure 9–6.

QUESTION

The pattern in Figure 9–6 indicates which of the following?
1. ectopic pacemaker
2. infarction
3. conduction abnormality
4. ischemia

ANSWER

4. You recognize this pattern as indicating myocardial ischemia. The ST segment should be isoelectric. An alteration from isoelectric occurs from delayed repolarization.

You rush to start the IV nitroglycerin drip. You push the nurse call light to get extra help into the room. Another nurse enters and escorts Mrs. Garcia's daughter to the central waiting area. Fortunately, Mrs. Garcia's vital signs have not changed. The stat. ECG and portable chest x-ray are completed. A blood specimen for enzyme analysis is obtained. An arterial stick is performed for blood gas analysis.

The physician arrives and reads the ECG and portable chest film. Based on her history and the ECG, Mrs. Garcia is diagnosed as having an acute anterolateral infarction. Cardiomegaly is present with bilateral infiltrates on the chest film. Congestive heart failure with acute pulmonary edema also is diagnosed. She is transferred immediately to the coronary care unit.

QUICK REVIEW

Mrs. Garcia's initial symptoms demonstrated compensatory efforts to maintain CO, which is determined by stroke volume and heart rate. The changes in the ECG indicate that myocardial oxygen supply is diminished, probably due to a blockage in the coronary arteries. Mrs. Garcia's pain is secondary to a decreased myocardial oxygen supply. Injured myocardial tissue cannot contract adequately, and blood remains in the left ventricle. As the left ventricle becomes stretched, contractility further decreases once the point of maximum elasticity is reached. Starling's law addresses the limits of cardiac compensation. The heart rate initially will increase in an effort to maintain CO. The sympathetic nervous system is stimulated, and peripheral vasoconstriction produces the symptoms of nausea and diaphoresis. Mrs. Garcia's CO has now decreased, as evidenced by her decreased responsiveness.

Since more data are available, it is time to reassess nursing diagnoses appropriate for Mrs. Garcia. Mrs. Garcia's perfusion problem is complex. Because the perfusion problem involves a fluid volume excess related to decreased fluid distribution and decreased CO related to decreased myocardial contractility, it is suggested that you join them together to address them.

Expected patient outcomes for Mrs. Garcia would include

1. Absence of crackles on auscultation
2. Absence of dyspnea
3. Stable vital signs: systolic blood pressure >90 <140
4. Absence of S_3
5. Absence of jugular venous distention
6. Absence of ascites and abdominal tenderness
7. Usual mental status
8. Urine output >30 mL/hour
9. Arterial blood gases within normal limits (WNL) for Mrs. Garcia
10. Cardiac enzymes WNL
11. Absence of chest pain

For the purposes of Mrs. Garcia's case study, only the perfusion-related nursing diagnoses are further developed. However, in a true clinical situation, as the nurse creating Mrs. Garcia's plan of care, you would continue to develop other clusters based on assessment data. If data are insufficient, you should follow through on collecting the necessary data to confirm or refute your hypotheses.

Based on the preliminary data that has been collected on Mrs. Garcia, there is sufficient support to state the following nursing diagnoses.

- **Chest pain** related to myocardial ischemia
- **Alteration in tissue perfusion: cerebral** related to decreased myocardial contractility

- **High risk for impaired gas exchange** related to pulmonary interstitial fluid
- **High risk for anxiety** related to impending transfer to coronary care unit
- **High risk for fear** related to severity of illness

Treatment goals for Mrs. Garcia will focus on increasing the blood supply to the heart, decreasing the demands placed on the heart, and improving the blood flow distribution. These general goals should be reflected in the nursing diagnoses and expected patient outcomes on the nursing care plan. For example, decreasing the demands placed on the heart is addressed in the nursing diagnosis of fluid volume overload. Accomplishment of the goal will be measured in such criteria as *Patient will be pain free.*

Development of the Plan of Care

Nursing interventions will be based on activities that will help Mrs. Garcia meet her expected patient outcomes. They will consist of collaborative interventions ordered by the physician but require nursing action and independent interventions that the nurse implements without a physician's order.

Collaborative Interventions Related to Perfusion Status. The physician's orders may include the following.

1. *Cardiovascular drug therapy.* Mrs. Garcia will be receiving several drugs while hospitalized. Thrombolytics may be ordered to dissolve a thrombus and thereby improve coronary artery perfusion, limit the extent of the myocardial ischemia, and improve left ventricular function. These agents usually are initiated in the early stages of an acute myocardial infarction. Streptokinase, eminase, and tissue plasminogen activator are commonly used thrombolytic agents. These drugs are contraindicted if the patient has a bleeding disorder, potential for bleeding, a recent surgery or cerebrovascular accident, and uncontrolled hypertension. The major nursing concern associated with administering thrombolytic agents is to monitor for complications. The most frequent complications are bleeding, allergic reaction, and reperfusion dysrhythymias.

Inotropic agents, such as dopamine, dobutamine, and digitalis, may be administered. These agents will increase myocardial contractility and improve ventricular function. A negative effect of these agents is that they increase myocardial oxygen consumption.

Vasodilators may be ordered. Frequently used IV vasodilators are nitroprusside, nitroglycerin, and phentolamine. These drugs indirectly improve stroke volume and CO by decreasing afterload. The heart is able to eject against less resistance.

QUESTION

Which of the following may be an undesirable side effect of vasodilators?
1. Decreased systemic vascular resistance
2. Decreased CO
3. Increased PCWP
4. Increased CVP

ANSWER

2. Hypotension and a further decrease in CO may occur if preload is diminished due to venous pooling.

A diuretic is ordered for Mrs. Garcia to
1. Prevent renal failure
2. Increase the PCWP
3. Decrease vasoconstriction
4. Reduce preload

4. Diuretics may be given to reduce preload and pulmonary venous congestion.

Loop diuretics are the preferred drug of choice in cases of acute congestive heart failure. Furosemide has vasodilating and diuretic properties and thus has a greater potential of decreasing preload (Wallace, 1990). The nurse must monitor for fluid volume deficit that may occur with over diuresis and electrolyte abnormalities.

Oxygen therapy is ordered to reduce myocardial workload and to meet cellular energy requirements.

2. *Mechanical support.* If Mrs. Garcia's heart failure worsens, she may need an intra-aortic balloon pump (IABP). This device improves coronary artery perfusion by inflating during diastole and increasing the coronary artery perfusion pressure. It deflates during systole, rapidly decreasing the coronary artery pressure and ventricular ejection resistance. The nurse caring for a patient with an IABP requires special preparation in order to adjust balloon inflation/deflation correctly.

3. *Dietary restrictions.* Mrs. Garcia may be placed on a sodium restricted diet. Use of table salt and salt in food preparation may need to be eliminated. She may also be placed on fluid restriction until her fluid distribution problem is under control. The nurse would need to monitor Mrs. Garcia's sodium level and intake and output record and ensure that she receives the correct meal tray. Family members need to be made aware of dietary restrictions so they do not bring food that would be detrimental to Mrs. Garcia's fluid volume status.

4. *Hemodynamic monitoring.* Mrs. Garcia may have a pulmonary arterial catheter placed once she is in the coronary care unit. Nursing responsibilities associated with hemodynamic monitoring have been discussed earlier in this module. You would expect Mrs. Garcia's hemodynamic readings to be abnormal because of her fluid volume overload. Before initiation of drug therapy, Mrs. Garcia's CVP, PAP, and PCWP readings would be elevated due to increased volume. Her CO and CI would be decreased. Mrs. Garcia's SVR would be elevated initially to try to compensate for her decreased stroke volume. However, her blood pressure has been decreasing, and a nitroglycerin IV drip was initiated. Her SVR should now be decreased. Medications will be administered and titrated to decrease her CVP, PAP, and PCWP while increasing her CO. The combination of inotropes and vasodilators can be confusing to a novice nurse, since they appear to have opposite actions. However, the goal of using both of these agents is the same, improvement of CO.

5. *Laboratory and x-ray testing.* Cardiac enzymes probably will be ordered at least every 6 hours to determine the severity of Mrs. Garcia's myocardial infarction. ABGs will be ordered intermittently to monitor gas exchange. If a thrombolytic agent has been administered, ABGs may not be ordered to prevent repeated puncture or repeated arterial manipulation (via arterial line). Pulse oximetry may be used to monitor gas exchange noninvasively. Periodic chest x-rays will

assist in determining the effects of interventions. The cardiomegaly and pulmonary infiltrates should diminish in size.

Independent Nursing Interventions Related to Perfusion Status

1. Assess for decreased perfusion
   - Systolic blood pressure <90 mm Hg
   - Heart rate <60 or >100
   - Urine output <30 mL/hour
   - Decreased responsiveness
   - Diminished peripheral pulses
   - Capillary refill >2.9 seconds
   - Pedal edema
   - Dysrhythmias
2. Assess for fluid overload
   - Metabolic or respiratory acidosis
   - Dyspnea
   - Abnormal breath sounds
   - Extra heart sounds
   - Jugular venous distention
   - Ascites
   - Weight gain
   - Abnormal electrolyte levels
3. Implement measures to reduce cardiac workload
   - Place Mrs. Garcia in semi-Fowler's position
   - Allow for frequent rest periods
   - Monitor intake and output
   - Monitor for side effects of drug therapy
   - Keep oxygen device on patient
   - Administer pain medication as ordered and use imagery and other diversional activities
   - Decrease patient anxiety
     a. Refer to support services as necessary (i.e., chaplain, social services)
     b. Assist patient with identifying coping behaviors
     c. Explain procedures, environment, and equipment to degree of patient satisfaction

Plan Evaluation and Revision

Mrs. Garcia's plan of care is now ready to be executed by the coronary care unit nurse. Her progress will be monitored at regular intervals to evaluate the effects of various therapeutic actions. If progress is not being noted toward attainment of her expected patient outcomes, Mrs. Garcia's plan of care may need to be revised.

Summary

This module has addressed the nursing care of a patient who is experiencing an alteration in perfusion. Concepts from the perfusion-related modules, *Perfusion, Hemodynamic Monitoring, Cardiac Monitoring and Related Interventions,* and *Shock States,* have been applied in a case study approach. It is impossible to address specifically each perfusion problem a nurse may encounter in the clinical setting. However, these problems can be managed by applying basic principles. These principles can be classified into fluid volume excess and fluid volume deficit situations. Two case studies were used to illustrate nursing care responsibilities in these situations. Review questions were intergrated throughout the case study to encourage application of material in other modules and assimilation of content within this module. Nursing interventions for a patient being hemodynamically monitored were addressed specifically because of the frequency with which this intervention is used and its use in patients experiencing both fluid overload and fluid excess.

REFERENCES

Alspach, J., and Williams, S. (1985). *Core curriculum for critical care nursing.* Philadelphia: W.B. Saunders Co.

American College of Surgeons (1989). *Advanced trauma life support course manual.* Chicago: American College of Surgeons.

American Heart Association (1987). Advanced cardiac life support course manual. Dallas: American Heart Association.

Bates, B. (1986). *A guide to physical examination,* 3rd ed. Philadelphia: J.B. Lippincott.

Carpenito, L. (1987). *Nursing diagnosis: Application to clinical practice,* 2nd ed. Philadelphia: J.B. Lippincott.

Chulay, M., and Miller, T. (1984). The effect of backrest elevation on pulmonary artery and capillary wedge pressures in patients after cardiac surgery. *Heart Lung.* 13:138–140.

Daily, E. (1990). Hemodynamic monitoring. In J. Dolan (ed). *Critical care nursing: Clinical management through the nursing process,* Chap. 41. Philadelphia: F.A. Davis.

Ellis, D. (1985). Interpretation of beat-to-beat blood pressure valves in the presence of ventilatory changes. *J. Clin. Monitoring.* 1:65.

Gawlinski, A. (1988). Cardiovascular physical assessment. In N. Holloway ed. *Nursing the critically ill adult,* 3rd ed, Chap. 10. Menlo Park: Addison-Wesley.

Guyton, A. (1986). *Textbook of medical physiology,* 3rd ed. Philadelphia: W.B. Saunders Co.

Kersten, L. (1989). *Comprehensive respiratory nursing.* Philadelphia: W.B. Saunders Co.

Laulive, J. (1982). Pulmonary artery pressures and position changes in the critically ill adult. *Dimensions Crit. Care Nursing.* 1:28–34.

Leuner, J., Manton, A., Kelliher, D., Sullivan, S., and Doherty, M. (1990). *Mastering the nursing process: A case method approach.* Philadelphia: F.A. Davis.

Mitchell, P., Cammermeyer, M., Ozuna, J., and Woods, N. (1984). *Neurological assessment for nursing practice.* Reston, Virginia: Prentice-Hall.

Naji, P. (1990). Nursing management of the patient with coronary artery disease, angina pectoris or myocardial infarction. In J. Dolan ed. *Critical care nursing: Clinical management through the nursing process,* Chap. 43. Philadelphia: F.A. Davis.

Nemens, E., and Woods, S. (1982). Normal fluctuations in pulmonary artery and pulmonary capillary wedge pressures in acutely ill patients. *Heart Lung.* 11:393–398.

Pagana, K., and Pagana, T. (1986). *Diagnostic testing and nursing implications.* St. Louis: C.V. Mosby Co.

Rea, R. (ed). (1991). *Trauma nursing core course association manual.* Chicago: Emergency Nurses Association.

Rebenson-Piano, M., Holin, K., and Powers, M. (1987). An examination of the differences that occur between direct and indirect blood pressure measurement. *Heart Lung* 16:285–293.

Roberts (1985). *Physiological concepts and the critically ill patient.* Norwalk, Connecticut: Appleton & Lange.

Schriger, D., and Baraff, L. (1988). Defining normal capillary refill: Variation with age, sex, and temperature. *Ann. Emerg. Med.* 17:932–935.

Ulrich, S., Canale, S., and Wendell, S. (1986). *Nursing care planning guide: A nursing diagnosis approach.* Philadelphia: W.B. Saunders Co.

Wallace, P. (1990). Nursing management of the patient with heart failure. In J. Dolan, ed. *Critical care nursing: Clinical management through the nursing process.* Chap. 44. Philadelphia: F.A. Davis.

Woods, S., and Mansfield, L. (1986). Effect of patient position upon the pulmonary artery and pulmonary capillary wedge pressures in acutely ill patients. *Heart Lung.* 13:83–90.

PART III

Trauma

Module 10

Trauma Assessment and Resuscitation

Colleen H. Swartz

The module, *Trauma Assessment and Resuscitation,* is intended to facilitate the learner's understanding of trauma. Focused attention is given to mechanism of injury for both blunt and penetrating trauma as an assessment factor to raise the learner's index of suspicion for certain injuries. The module is composed of eight sections. Sections One through Four focus on mechanism of injury and kinematics of trauma. Section Five presents specific clinical and age-related variances that may mediate injury response. Sections Six and Seven focus on the trauma assessment and resuscitative principles based on primary and secondary survey, and Section Eight summarizes key points in the mediation of life-threatening injury related to trauma with a brief discussion about traumatic shock. Each section includes a set of review questions to help the reader evaluate understanding of section content before proceeding to the next section. All section reviews and the pretest and posttest in the module include answers. It is suggested that the learner review those concepts that have been missed in the review questions before proceeding to the next section.

Objectives

At the completion of this module, the learner will be able to

1. Define injury, potential mechanisms of injury, and risk factors that influence injury patterns

2. Define the forces most often applied when considering the kinematics of blunt injury

3. Define the forces most often applied when considering the kinematics of penetrating injury

4. Describe the relationship between identified force eliciting an injury and suspected resultant injury pattern

5. Apply clinical and age-related variances that may influence or mediate the host's response to injury

6. Identify the clinical assessment format used to identify life-threatening injuries: the primary survey

7. Identify the clinical assessment format used to identify all injuries sustained: the secondary survey

8. Discuss the trimodal distribution of trauma-related mortalities and the importance of early recognition and intervention with traumatic shock

---

Pretest

1. The most common cause of injury is
   A. falls
   B. motor vehicle crashes
   C. gunshot wounds
   D. near drowning
2. The typical profile of a trauma victim would be
   A. male, 15–24 years of age, intoxicated
   B. female, 15–24 years of age, intoxicated
   C. female, 24–32 years of age, intoxicated
   D. male, 24–32 years of age, not intoxicated
3. The most common force associated with blunt trauma is
   A. acceleration/deceleration
   B. compression
   C. shearing
   D. axial loading
4. The best definition of tensile forces is
   A. forces opposing one another across a plane
   B. squeezing/compartmentalization of tissue
   C. forces precipitating laceration, avulsion
   D. drawing out/extending tissue
5. The process of temporary displacement of tissue forward and laterally by a penetrating missile is
   A. tensile forces
   B. cavitation
   C. yaw
   D. tumbling
6. The extent of cavitation and tissue deformation produced by a missile is determined by
   A. yaw
   B. tumbling
   C. missile caliber and velocity
   D. all of the above
7. Secondary missiles often are created with penetrating trauma involving which two types of tissue?
   A. teeth and bone
   B. brain and soft tissue
   C. abdominal organs and vessels
   D. great vessels and brain
8. The most frequently seen pattern of injury for a pedestrian child hit by an automobile is
   A. fractures of femur, tibia, and fibula on side of impact
   B. fracture of femur, chest injury, and injury to contralateral skull
   C. pelvic fractures, compression fractures
   D. fractured spleen or liver, upper extremity fractures

9. Impairment of judgment occurs with blood alcohol content as low as
   A. 100 mg/dL
   B. 20–80 mg/dL
   C. 200 mg/dL
   D. 300 mg/dL
10. Cocaine usually manifests itself as a
    A. CNS depressant
    B. sympathomimetic
    C. hallucinogenic
    D. antidepressant
11. When assessing a pediatric trauma patient, one must consider
    A. increasing frequency of multiorgan injuries
    B. decreasing frequency of multiorgan injuries
    C. decreased risk of hypothermia
    D. increased ability of the skeleton to absorb significant forces
12. The center of gravity in a child is considered to be the
    A. head
    B. pelvis
    C. lower extremities
    D. abdominal area
13. The immediate nursing intervention for the hypotensive pregnant trauma patient should be
    A. turning the patient to the right lateral decubitus position
    B. turning the patient to the left lateral decubitus position
    C. high flow oxygen
    D. Trendelenburg position
14. Ordered priorities in the primary survey are
    A. disability, airway, breathing
    B. cervical spine immobilization, circulation, breathing
    C. hemorrhage, fractures, chest trauma
    D. airway, breathing, circulation, disability, and exposure
15. In maintaining the pediatric airway, all the following are true EXCEPT
    A. the tongue is small and unlikely to cause airway obstruction
    B. the glottic opening is more anterior and cephalad
    C. the trachea is short and narrow
    D. hypoxemia is very poorly tolerated

16. In the early shock state (blood volume loss less than 25 percent), the blood pressure usually will be
    A. normal
    B. slightly elevated
    C. slightly decreased
    D. markedly decreased

17. The distribution of trauma-related mortalities is
    A. modal
    B. bimodal
    C. trimodal
    D. quasimodal

18. The intraabdominal organ most frequently associated with exsanguination is
    A. liver
    B. spleen
    C. small bowel
    D. colon

Pretest answers: 1, B. 2, A. 3, A. 4, D. 5, B. 6, D. 7, A. 8, B. 9, B. 10, B. 11, A. 12, A. 13, B. 14, D. 15, A. 16, A. 17, C. 18, A.

Glossary

Acceleration. A change in the rate of velocity or speed of a moving body

Blast effect. Phenomenon of structure injury outside the direct missile path in penetrating injury

Blood alcohol content (BAC). Measurement of intoxication in mg/dL or g/dL; a BAC indicating legal intoxication is usually 100 mg/dL or 0.100 g/dL

Blunt injury. Injury without interruption of skin integrity

Caliber. The diameter of a bullet expressed in hundredths or thousandths of an inch

Cavitation. Creation of a temporary cavity as tissues are stretched and compressed and displaced forward and laterally, creating a tract from a penetrating missile

Chance fracture. Distraction or tension fractures of the thoracolumbar spine usually between L1 and L4

Compression. Ability of an object or structure to resist squeezing forces or inward pressure

Contrecoup injury. Injury to parts of the brain located on the side opposite that of the primary injury

Coup. Injury to parts of the brain located on the side of primary injury

Crepitus. A grating sound heard on movement, as with ends of broken bone

Cribriform. The thin, perforated, medial portion of the horizontal plate of the ethmoid bone

Cricothyroidotomy. A surgical airway created by division and cannulation of the trachea between the cricoid and thyroid cartilage

Exsanquination. The most extreme form of hemorrhage, with an initial loss of blood volume of 40 percent and a rate of hemorrhage exceeding 250 mL/minute

Force. A physical factor that changes the motion of a body either at rest or already in motion

Injury. Any body trauma caused by violence or other forces

Kinematics. The science or study of motion

Penetrating injury. Injury produced by foreign objects sent into motion violating the integrity of the skin

Shearing. Structures slipping relative to each other across a plane

Subcutaneous emphysema. Distention of subcutaneous tissues by gas or air in the interstices

Synergistic. The harmonious action of two agents, such as drugs, producing an effect that neither could produce alone or an effect that is greater than the total effects of each agent operating by itself

Tensile forces. Forces that draw out or extend tissues

Tracheostomy. A surgical airway created by cutting into the trachea below the cricothyroid membrane

Trauma. Body injury caused by violence or other forces

Tumbling. The forward rotation of a missile around the center of mass (somersaulting)

Velocity. The speed of a moving object on a ratio of distance and time

Waddell's triad. A defined triad of injury associated with an automobile hitting a pedestrian

Yawing. Deviation of a missile from its straight path

Abbreviations

BAC. Blood alcohol content

CNS. Central nervous system

COPD. Chronic obstructive pulmonary disease

CVA. Cerebrovascular accident

mph. Miles per hour

MVC. Motor vehicle crash

psi. Pounds per square inch

Section One: An Overview of the Injured Patient

At the completion of this section, the learner will be able to define injury, potential mechanisms of injury, and personal and environmental factors that influence injury patterns.

Historically, injuries or accidents were viewed as a result of random chance that was beyond human control. Now, injury is viewed as an event with an identifiable cause via the interaction of energy and force with a recipient. The recipient may be an inanimate object, such as a car, or may be a human being. *Webster* identifies injury as "that which causes harm or damage, the damage, or hurt done." Another definition of trauma is "any body injury caused by violence or other forces." Understanding injury (or trauma as we often call it) will enable you to approach a patient in crisis with a level-headed, systematic plan based on your body of nursing knowledge surrounding the concept.

Injury results from acute exposure to energy, such as kinetic (crash, fall, bullet), chemical, thermal, electrical, or ionizing radiation, or from a lack of essential agents, such as oxygen and heat (drowning and frostbite) (Waller, 1985). Motor vehicle crashes (MVCs) are the most common cause of injury, followed by falls. The injury occurs because of the body's inability to tolerate excessive exposure to the energy source. Effects of injury on the human body vary depending on the injuring agent. For our purposes, we concentrate on two major categories of injury: blunt and penetrating.

Blunt trauma is considered injury without interruption of skin integrity. Blunt trauma may be life threatening because the extent of the injury may be covert, making diagnosis difficult. Blunt forces transfer their energy by tissue deformation. The nature of the injury is related to both the transfer of injury and the anatomic structure involved.

Penetrating trauma refers to injury produced by foreign objects set into motion. Whereas blunt trauma produces tissue deformation via energy transference, penetrating trauma produces actual tissue penetration and may also cause surrounding tissue deformation based on energy transferred by the penetrating object.

Since energy transference occurs with both blunt and penetrating injury, deformation and displacement of body tissue and organs occur. Injury takes place as the structural limits of the organ are exceeded. Damage may be localized, such as hematoma formation, or systemic, as in shock states. The local response of the patient varies according to the organ involved. Additional examples are fractures of bone, bleeding of vessels, or edema of tissues (Salandar and Bingham, 1991).

Injuries, like other diseases, do not occur at random. Identifiable risk factors are present that predispose individuals to certain injury patterns. A brief discussion of a few of these risk factors is presented.

Age

The death rate from injury is highest for patients 75 years and older. However, injury is the leading cause of death in all Americans ages 1 through 44. The lowest injury death rate is for patients aged 5 through 14. The highest injury rate is for patients aged 15 through 24 because of their exposure to high-risk activities (including poor judgment with the use of alcohol, drugs, and driving practices). The highest homicide rate occurs among people between 20 and 29 years of age (Baker et al, 1984).

Sex

Injury rates are highest for 15 to 24-year-old males. The risk for males is 2.5 times that of females, possibly because of male involvement in hazardous activities (Withers and Baker, 1987).

Alcohol

The use and abuse of alcoholic beverages influence the likelihood of virtually all types of injury, even among young teenagers. Over 50 percent of all trauma is reported to occur in the presence of high blood alcohol concentrations (BACs). Approximately 30 to 40 percent of vehicular crashes can be associated with significant elevations in BAC. Thirty percent of individuals with gunshot wounds have BAC of 0.03 g/dL or higher. An increase in the severity of injury is associated with an increase in blood alcohol level.

Race, Income, Geography

Native Americans have the highest death rates from unintentional injury, blacks have the highest homicide rates, and whites and Native Americans have the highest suicide rates. An inverse relationship between income levels and death rates exists for blacks and whites. There is a higher unintentional injury rate in rural areas and a higher intentional injury rate in urban areas. Mechanisms of rural unintentional injuries commonly are MVCs, lightning, and chemical exposure. Urban intentional injuries usually are related to homicide attempts.

This section has discussed common variables associated with injury patterns. Injuries were discussed as events with identifiable causes, contrary to the public's view of injuries as accidents.

Section One Review

1. The two major categories of injury are
   A. chemical and thermal
   B. fractures and burns
   C. blunt and penetrating
   D. MVAs and gunshot wounds
2. The death rate from injury is highest for
   A. patients 24–42 years
   B. patients 15–24 years
   C. patients 5–14 years
   D. patients 75 years and older
3. The highest injury rate occurs in which age group?
   A. 15–24 years
   B. 1–5 years
   C. 24–32 years
   D. ≥ 75 years

4. The risk for males vs females for injury is
   A. 2.5 times lower
   B. 2.5 times higher
   C. 5 times higher
   D. equal
5. Over ____ percent of all trauma is reported to occur in the presence of high blood alcohol content ratios.
   A. 10
   B. 25
   C. 50
   D. 75

Answers: 1, C. 2, D. 3, A. 4, B. 5, C.

Section Two: Kinematics of Blunt Trauma

At the completion of this section, you will be able to define and apply clinically the forces most often reflected during assessment of blunt injury.

Force is a physical factor that changes the motion of a body either at rest or already in motion. Force is calculated by the following equation.

$$\text{Force} = \text{mass} \times \text{acceleration}$$

The more slowly the force is applied, the more slowly energy is released, with less subsequent tissue deformation. The forces most often applied are acceleration, deceleration, shearing, and compression (Weigelt and McCormack, 1988).

Acceleration is a change in the rate of velocity or speed of a moving body. As velocity increases, so does tissue damage. The following example illustrates the concept of acceleration. Acceleration is operationalized. On impact with a solid object (e.g., another car, brick wall, telephone pole), the driver is suddenly propelled forward. He experiences a sudden acceleration of body mass determined by the rate of speed at which he was traveling and his body mass. This relationship is reflected in the following formula.

$$\text{Body weight} \times \text{mph} = \text{psi of impact}$$

A person weighing 100 pounds, traveling at 35 mph, will hit at 3,500 pounds per square inch (psi).

This is equivalent to jumping, head-first from a three story building!

Deceleration is a decrease in the velocity of a moving object. The same driver in the example given who is moving forward after hitting a solid object will experience a sudden deceleration after he comes into contact with the mass that impedes his forward (or backward) progression, e.g., the steering wheel, a tree, the road, or another passenger.

Shearing refers to structures slipping relative to each other across a plane. Think of the shearing or slipping of internal organs, such as the liver, spleen, or spinal cord, as they experience the acceleration/deceleration of a MVC.

Compression is the ability of an object or structure to resist squeezing forces or inward pressure. Imagine compression of an extremity under a car or the compression of the liver and spleen by the steering wheel against the abdomen.

Acceleration and deceleration injuries are most common with blunt trauma. An example of this mechanism of injury is injury to the thoracic aorta. Typically, MVCs and falls from 20 feet or higher precipitate stretching, bowing, and shearing in major vessels, such as the aorta. The damage from this vessel shearing can cause damage to any or all layers of the vessel wall (intima, media, adventitia). The vessel wall can tear, dissect, rupture, or form an aneurysm immediately or at any time postinjury. The shearing damage occurs in the vessels as they decelerate at a different rate from the rest of the body's internal structures. The aorta is affixed posteriorly to the chest wall at the isthmus just below the subclavian artery origin. The rest of the aorta is free to move above and below this point of fixation during acceleration/deceleration. This movement produces shearing, causing aorta injury that has a mortality of 80 percent (Weigelt and McCormack, 1988). (Are you beginning to understand how mechanism of injury can tremendously influence your assessment for certain injuries?)

Other injuries associated with blunt trauma forces are head injuries (think about the movement of the brain inside the skull with acceleration, deceleration, and shearing—remember coup and contrecoup injuries), spinal cord injuries (the cervical spine is predisposed to shearing and acceleration/deceleration because of its instability and poor support, since it is weakest at cervical vertebrae 5, 6, and 7), fractures (from shearing and compression), and abdominal injuries (abdominal organs, especially spleen and liver are very vascular, and trauma patients may exsanguinate from shearing and disruption of major vessels supplying these areas).

Tissue responsiveness to applied forces varies, creating characteristic limits of the tissues' ability to withstand the forces of acceleration, deceleration, compression, and shearing. Tissue deformation is generally the result of tensile forces or shear forces. Tensile forces draw out or extend tissues and create injury, whereas shear forces create injury when forces oppose each other across a plane. The coup and contrecoup injury is an example of application of both tensile and shear forces. As the brain moves within the bony skull during injury, the brain moves in one direction as the skull and dura move in another. Shear forces cause the coup injury as tensile forces precipitate the contrecoup injury (Salander and Bingham, 1991).

Tissue, organ, and systemic responses to the forces applied with blunt trauma often present a complex interrelationship of potential injury manifestation. Trauma patients with similar mechanisms of injury typically have different combinations of organ and systemic injury based on individual variances in ability to withstand the forces applied. A myriad of potential injury combinations, manifestations, and outcomes exists, prompting the clinician to approach the patient in a systematic fashion.

In this section, different types of forces related to blunt injury were identified. A brief discussion of tissue and organ response to applied forces was presented, as was the relationship between force and injury.

Section Two Review

1. Acceleration is a change in the rate of velocity or speed of a moving body. As velocity increases, tissue damage
   A. decreases
   B. increases
   C. remains constant
   D. cannot be determined

2. A decrease in the velocity of a moving object is
   A. acceleration
   B. deceleration
   C. compression
   D. shearing

3. Structures slipping relative to each other across a plane is
   A. acceleration
   B. deceleration
   C. compression
   D. shearing
4. The ability of an object or structure to resist squeezing forces or inward pressure is
   A. acceleration
   B. deceleration
   C. compression
   D. shearing
5. You are traveling on the interstate at 65 mph and you weigh 120 pounds. You lose control of the car and hit a telephone pole. The acceleration of body mass you will experience on impact equals
   A. 3,000 psi
   B. 120 psi
   C. 6,500 psi
   D. 7,800 psi

6. Mass × acceleration =
   A. force
   B. psi
   C. velocity
   D. shearing

Answers: 1, B. 2, B. 3, D. 4, C. 5, D. 6, A.

Section Three: Kinematics of Penetrating Trauma

At the completion of this section, you will be able to define and apply clinically the forces most often reflected during assessment of penetrating injury.

Penetrating trauma refers to injury produced by foreign objects set into motion. Tissue or organ penetration occurs, and the severity of injury is manifested by structures damaged. The amount of kinetic injury lost by the missile has a direct relationship with tissue damage. The energy lost by the missile is transferred to the tissue. As the missile penetrates tissue, the tissue is temporarily displaced forward and laterally, creating a tract. The tissue acceleration creates a temporary cavity as tissues are stretched and compressed, a process called cavitation. Cavitation has a direct relationship to the amount of kinetic energy transmitted to tissue. The size of the cavity may be many times the diameter of the missile. The tissue surrounding the missile tract stretches, compresses, and shears, which produces damage outside the direct path of the missile. Thus, vessels, nerves, and other structures that were not directly damaged by the missile may be affected. The phenomenon of structure injury outside the direct missile path is referred to as a blast effect (Weigelt and McCormack, 1988; Swan and Swan, 1989).

The extent of cavitation and tissue deformation produced by a missile is determined by the velocity of the missile. Lower velocity missiles tend to produce a path of tissue disruption only slightly greater than the diameter of the missile. Thus, tissue disruption and blast effect are minimized. However, high velocity missiles lose more kinetic energy, creating an intense blast effect. At higher velocities, the missile creates a tremendous disruption of tissue, with the acceleration and compression of tissues away from the missile creating greater cavitation. Cavity enlargement continues even after the missile has passed through the tissue. You can see where higher velocity missiles will produce more serious injury owing to the destructive process of cavitation and blast effect to surrounding tissue and organs. With high velocity missiles, the cavity diameter might be 30 to 40 times the missile diameter (Weigelt and McCormack, 1988).

Consider a missile moving in stable flight toward the host (for our purposes, the patient). The missile passes from air into the human tissue, which is several hundreds times more dense than air. As the missile passes into the tissue, the surrounding environment changes and precipitates an instability of the missile. The unstable missile may yaw, tumble, deform, or fragment or a combination of these.

Yawing is the deviation of a missile from its straight path. Tumbling is the action of forward rotation around the center of mass (somersaulting) (Figures 10–1 and 10–2). Yawing and tumbling increase the area of the missile as tissue is hit, thus increasing

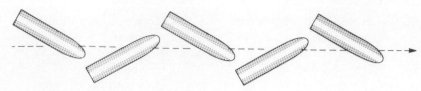

Figure 10-1. Yawing is the deviation of a bullet in its longitudinal axis from the straight line of flight. (*From* Gunshot wounds: Pathophysiology and management, *2nd ed., p. 13, edited by K.G. Swan and R.C. Swan, 1989, St. Louis: Mosby Year Book.*)

the area of destruction. Higher velocity missiles have a greater propensity for yaw and tumble.

Another principle to consider when analyzing the effects of penetrating injury is the creation of secondary missiles by the penetrating agent. A missile or its fragments may impart sufficient kinetic injury to dense tissue, such as bone or teeth, to create highly destructive secondary missiles. These secondary missiles may take erratic, unpredictable courses, resulting in additional injury. Secondary missiles also may be created by fragmentation of the primary missile. Thus, the anticipated missile path may be compounded, complicated, or enhanced by tissue damage precipitated by a secondary missile.

Assessment of entry and exit wounds is critical in assessment of the patient with penetrating injury. With high velocity injuries, the entrance wound may be larger than the bullet diameter (i.e., caliber, expressed in two hundredths or thousandths of an inch, such as 22 caliber, which means 22 hundredths of an inch caliber). Cavitation with higher velocity missiles tends to form early and close to the point of impact. If the path traversed by the high velocity missile is short, the exit wound may be large and ragged as the missile exits just as the maximum loss of kinetic energy occurs. Not all penetrating injuries result in exit wounds, since the missile may fragment and remain inside the body.

Should a high velocity missile take a longer path of destruction, entrance and exit wounds may appear small and apparently innocuous. However, typically, the tissue destruction and cavitation have occurred deep within the patient, especially if yawing, tumbling, and fragmentation have occurred. Tissue destruction and injury cannot be predicted based solely on appearance of entry and exit wounds (Swan

and Swan, 1989). A summary of velocity, cavitation, and blast effect is depicted in Figure 10-3.

Penetrating injuries, such as stab wounds and impalements, are typically considered low velocity injuries. Injuries produced usually can be anticipated based on underlying structures. It is critical that impaled objects be immobilized and left in place until definitive surgical intervention is available. The impaled objects actually may be controlling hemorrhage from damaged structures, and removal may precipitate exsanguination.

Typically, damage to structures remains localized, but special consideration must be given when injury occurs where body cavities lie in close proximity to one another. This principle is of critical importance when considering the close proximity of the thoracic and abdominal cavities, especially those occurring near the diaphragm, which offers very little resistance to the penetrating agent.

Penetrating injuries to the chest below the nipple line anteriorly, the sixth rib laterally, or the inferior point of the scapula posteriorly may involve not only intrathoracic but also intraabdominal structures (Kerr and Sood, 1989). The right diaphragm may rise as high as the fourth intercostal space and the left diaphragm to the fifth intercostal space (the right hemodiaphragm is slightly elevated by the liver) during maximum expiration, rendering the contents of the abdominal cavity exposed to injury with lower chest trauma (Figure 10-4). During maximum inspiration, the diaphragm recedes as low as the sixth intercostal space at the midclavicular line and the eighth intercostal space at the midaxillary line. Although stab wounds or impalement wounds are considered low velocity injury, the potential extent of damage should not be underestimated.

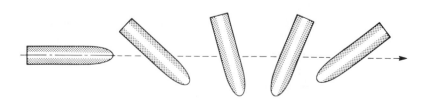

Figure 10-2. Tumbling is the action of forward rotation around the center of mass. (*From* Gunshot wounds: Pathophysiology and management, *2nd ed., p. 13, edited by K.G. Swan and R.C. Swan, 1989, St. Louis: Mosby Year Book.*)

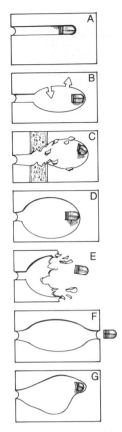

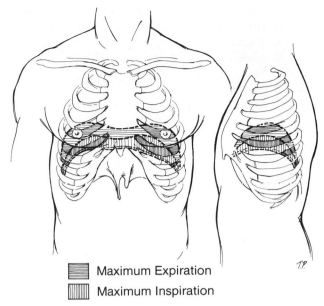

Maximum Expiration

Maximum Inspiration

Figure 10–4. Diaphragmatic excursion during the respiratory cycle. Injury to lower chest or upper abdomen can occur, with penetrating injury dependent on the phase of the respiratory cycle and the site of injury. (*From* Trauma nursing from resuscitation through rehabilitation, *p. 120, edited by V.A. Cardona et al, 1988, Philadelphia: W.B. Saunders Co.*)

Figure 10–3. Patterns of injury in animal tissue secondary to variations in missile ballistics and tissue characteristics. **A.** Low velocity, no cavitation, minimal blast effect, small entrance and exit wounds. **B.** Higher velocity, cavity formation, blast effect likely. Arrows show direction and magnitude of tissue acceleration. **C.** Higher velocity, as in **B**, but with bullet deformation and creation of secondary missiles on penetration of bone, increasing the likelihood of blast effect. **D.** Very high velocity, large cavity, likely blast effect with small entrance. Exit wound may be small. **E.** Very high velocity, thin target. Small entrance with large and ragged exit. **F.** Cavitation and blast effect occurring deep inside, with small entrance and exit wounds. **G.** Asymmetrical cavitation as bullet begins to deform and tumble. (*From* Trauma nursing from resuscitation through rehabilitation, *p. 118, edited by V.A. Cardona et al, 1988, Philadelphia: W.B. Saunders Co.*)

This section has reviewed the kinematics of penetrating injury. Velocity, cavitation, yaw, and tumbling were reviewed for their influence on ultimate injury of structures. Critical application of these concepts will maximize the clinician's ability to evaluate penetrating traumatic injury based on mechanism.

Section Three Review

1. As a missile penetrates, the tissue is temporarily displaced forward and laterally, creating a tract. This process is known as
   A. velocity
   B. yaw
   C. tumbling
   D. cavitation

2. Cavitation demonstrates a(an) _____ relationship with the amount of kinetic energy transmitted to tissue.
   A. inverse
   B. direct
   C. insignificant
   D. diagonal

3. The phenomenon of structure injury outside the direct missile path is referred to as
   A. cavitation
   B. blast effect
   C. yaw
   D. tumbling

4. Yaw and tumble will _____ the area of tissue destruction precipitated by a missile.
   A. decrease
   B. increase
   C. minimize
   D. not affect

5. A patient has an impaled knife in the upper abdomen. You should immediately
   A. remove the knife and apply pressure
   B. manipulate the knife to facilitate assessment of injured organs
   C. stabilize the knife without removal and minimal manipulation
   D. leave the knife alone

6. The diameter of a missile in hundredths or thousandths of an inch is expressed as
   A. caliber
   B. velocity
   C. blast effect
   D. force

Answers: 1, D. 2, B. 3, B. 4, B. 5, C. 6, A.

Section Four: Translating Principles of Mechanism of Injury

At the completion of this section, you will be able to translate mechanism of injury into potential injury patterns manifested by the patient for both blunt and penetrating injuries.

Certain mechanisms result in predictable injury patterns. Thus, the history of the event preceding the injury should elicit a raised index of suspicion for certain combinations of injured structures. Some commonly seen injuries resulting from blunt and penetrating trauma and their injury mechanism are listed.

Mechanism of Injury	Potential Structure Injury
Pedestrian hit by automobile	
Adult (Waddell's triad, Figure 10–5)	Fractures of femur, tibia, and fibula on side of impact; ligamental damage to impacted knee; mild contralateral head injury
Child (Waddell's triad)	Fractures of femur, chest injury, contralateral head injury
Unrestrained driver (Figure 10–6)	Head and/or facial injury, fractures of ribs, sternum with underlying myocardial or pulmonary contusion, cervical spine fractures, laryngotracheal injuries, spleen, liver, small bowel injuries, posterior fracture–dislocation of hip, femur fractures
Unrestrained front seat passenger	Head and/or facial injuries, laryngotracheal injuries, posterior fracture–dislocation of femoral head, femur/patellar fractures

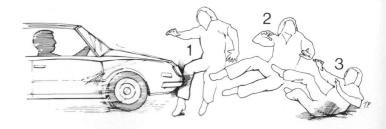

Figure 10–5. Waddell's triad in adult pedestrians. Impact (**1**) with the bumper or hood and lateral rotation (**2**) produce injury to the upper or lower leg and contralateral skull (**3**). (*From* Trauma nursing from resuscitation through rehabilitation, *p. 107, edited by V.A. Cardona et al, 1988, Philadelphia: W.B.Saunders Co.*)

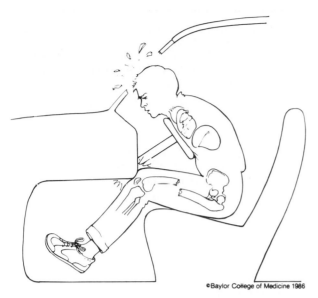

©Baylor College of Medicine 1986

Figure 10–6. Unrestrained driver in motor vehicle crash may sustain injuries to the cranium, face, sternum, ribs, myocardium, lung parenchyma, cervical vertebrae, spleen, liver, small bowel, pelvis, and lower extremities. (*From* Trauma, *2nd ed., by Moore et al, 1991, Norwalk, Connecticut: Appleton & Lange.*)

Restrained driver (lap and shoulder harness)	Contusions of structures underlying harness, i.e., pulmonary contusion, contusion of small bowel
Restrained passenger (lap belt only)	Flexion/distraction fractures (Chance fractures), especially lumbar vertebrae (L1–L4), duodenal injuries, cervical spine injuries
Fall injuries	Compression fractures of lumbosacral spine and calcaneus fractures; fractures of radius/ulna, patella if victim falls forward
Vehicular ejection	Multiple injuries, especially head and cervical spine injuries
	Injury risk increases by 300% when ejection occurs
Low velocity impalement	Local tissue/organ disruption, little or no cavitation
High velocity	Entrance wound larger
missile, short missile path	than missile caliber; large ragged exit wound with cavitation
High velocity missile, long missile path	Entrance wound larger than missile caliber; exit wound slightly larger than or equal to missile caliber; extensive cavitation (blast effect to deep structures absorbing lost kinetic energy)
High velocity missile hitting bone or teeth	Entry wound larger than missile caliber; possibly no exit wound with missile fragmentation; secondary missile injury in unpredictable, erratic pattern

An example illustrating the importance of the application of mechanism of injury follows. A 21-year-old male, unrestrained driver hits another vehicle head on. Traveling speed was in excess of 95 mph. The steering wheel was broken, as was the windshield. Potential injuries involved include

1. Intracranial injury, indicated by the high rate of speed and shattered windshield
2. Cervical vertebrae injury, indicated by suspected acceleration/deceleration at the high rate of speed
3. Intrathoracic injuries, indicated by the broken steering wheel—suspect rib fractures, myocardial, pulmonary contusions, great vessel injury
4. Intraabdominal injuries, indicated by the broken steering wheel and acceleration/deceleration; injuries could include splenic/liver lacerations, small bowel injuries, great vessel injuries
5. Long bone fractures, especially femur fractures or posterior hip fracture–dislocation, because of impact of knees with dashboard
6. Multiple skin lacerations, avulsions, punctures from impact

The importance of mechanism of injury in anticipation of the injury pattern has been stressed in this section. Both blunt and penetrating injuries were addressed.

Section Four Review

1. Waddell's triad is a characteristic injury pattern exhibited by
   A. unrestrained driver in MVC
   B. unrestrained passenger in MVC
   C. victims of gunshot wounds
   D. pedestrians injured by vehicular contact
2. A restrained passenger (lap belt only) may exhibit flexion/distraction fractures of which area of the vertebral column?
   A. cervical
   B. lumbar
   C. thoracic
   D. sacral
3. The intraabdominal organ injury usually associated with Chance fractures is the
   A. liver
   B. duodenum
   C. colon
   D. spleen
4. A 24-year-old male weighing 100 pounds is admitted after sustaining a gunshot wound to the chest with a high velocity missile. You would expect the entrance and exit wounds to appear as
   A. entrance: larger than missile caliber
      exit: larger, ragged, with cavitation
   B. entrance: smaller than missile caliber
      exit: slightly larger than missile caliber
   C. entrance and exit wounds equal in size: slightly larger than missile caliber
   D. entrance: large, ragged
      exit: small, minimal cavitation
5. Which of the following is true?
   A. vehicular ejection increases the risk for potential injury
   B. vehicular ejection decreases the risk for potential injury
   C. vehicular ejection is not related to the risk for potential injury
   D. vehicular ejection is associated with seat belt use

Answers: 1, D. 2, B. 3, B. 4, A. 5, A.

Section Five: Mediators of Injury Response

At the completion of this section, you will be able to state some of the conditions that could mediate the patient's response to injury. There are some clinical conditions you must consider that could very well mediate the patient's response to injury. These include underlying medical conditions, drug ingestion, and physiologic alterations based on age and body size.

Underlying Medical Conditions

Underlying medical conditions are extremely important to identify when considering the patient's physiologic and hemodynamic response to trauma. The most commonly encountered conditions include chronic obstructive pulmonary disease (COPD), heart disease, and underlying cerebral insufficiency, such as with cerebrovascular accident (CVA). These conditions or the medication used to control their effects may very well alter the physiologic response to trauma. The patient with COPD who sustains a minor pulmonary contusion related to blunt trauma may require prompt, life-saving intubation because of the alteration in the ventilation-perfusion ratio and effects on the resilience of affected lung tissue. Beta blockade used for coronary artery disease to minimize oxygen demands by the heart could prevent a normal response to hypovolemia (i.e., tachycardia). The patient with a head injury who has had a CVA in the past may experience an altered level of consciousness, difficulty in communication, or sensorimotor dysfunction due to the CVA and not due to the acute head injury. Eliciting a complete medical history is crucial during the initial assessment.

Drug Ingestion

The high incidence of alcohol as a contributing factor to injury has already been demonstrated. How is injury affected by alcohol ingestion? The most common effect is the inability to clearly establish a baseline level of consciousness. As a CNS depressant, the effects of alcohol on the brain are concentration dependent. The most sensitive tool for evaluation of brain injury is level of consciousness. Therefore, alcohol involvement is a critical consideration.

Blood alcohol content (BAC) is a measurement of intoxication. Measurement is conducted in milligrams per deciliter or grams per deciliter, varying from institution to institution. Legal intoxication in most states is 100 mg/dL or 0.100 g/dL. However, impairment of judgment occurs at a level of 50 mg/dL or 0.05 g/dL. A history of alcohol use should be obtained, since a degree of tolerance ensues with frequent alcohol ingestion. The effects of alcohol on motor, sensory, and memory functions are summarized here (McCabe and Hassan, 1988).

Alcohol (Ethanol) Concentration (mg/dL)	Effects
20–80	Impairment of judgment, thought processes, reaction time, suppression of inhibition
100 (legal intoxication)	Further impairment of judgment, increased reaction time, decreased motor control
200–300	Gross intoxication evident ataxia, diplopia, vomiting
300–400	Stuporous, hypothermic, amnesic
400–500	Death may result from respiratory arrest

The concomitant use of alcohol and other CNS depressants (e.g., barbiturates, opiates, sedatives–hypnotics) may result in potentiation of each drug's effects, creating a synergistic effect.

CNS stimulants, such as cocaine, also can alter the level of consciousness in the injured patient. Cocaine use mimics and intensifies a sympathetic stimulation or the fight-or-flight response in the patient. Notably, increases in heart rate and blood pressure occur along with vasoconstriction, dilated pupils, tremors, excitability, and restlessness. Ventricular dysrhythmias, tachypnea, or Cheyne-Stokes respirations may occur with large doses. Neurologically, mental status changes range from anxiety to acute paranoid psychosis. Seizure activity also may occur after cocaine ingestion (McCabe and Hassan, 1988).

You can begin to appreciate the difficulty in obtaining a baseline level of consciousness when the patient is intoxicated with alcohol or other drugs, which cloud his sensorium.

Age-Related Variances in Children

Age-related variances are especially important in the pediatric population. The injured child possesses unique characteristics that should alter your initial assessment. The primary mechanism of injury to children in the United States is blunt trauma. Automobiles cause the most significant injury to children, who suffer as passengers, pedestrians, and bicyclists. Falls and vehicular collisions account for almost 80 percent of all pediatric injuries. The most common injuries sustained by children requiring admission to a trauma center are head trauma, followed in frequency by fracture of the extremities and injury to the torso (Eichelberger, 1991). Multisystem injury is the rule rather than the exception, and, therefore, all organ systems must be assumed injured until proven otherwise. The following unique aspects must be considered during the initial assessment.

Size and Shape

Smaller physical size is the most obvious difference between children and adults. The applied energy from trauma dissipates over the smaller mass of the child, resulting in greater force over a smaller area. This more intense energy dissipation is applied to a body with less fat, less elastic connective tissue, and closer proximity of multiple organs, resulting in a high frequency of multiorgan injuries (American College of Surgeons Committee on Trauma, 1989a).

The normal blood volume of a child is 7 to 8 percent of his or her body weight (corresponding to a 20 to 25 percent larger blood volume than that of an adult, whose normal volume is 5 to 6 percent of body weight). Thus, blood loss considered negligible in an adult can produce shock in a child. Children also tend to have lower hemoglobin and hematocrit levels than adults, even into the teenage years (Eichelberger, 1991).

Skeleton

The child's skeleton is incompletely calcified, contains multiple active growth centers, and is very resilient. Thus, it is less able to absorb significant forces during a traumatic event. This results in internal organ damage without overlying bony fractures. For example, rib fractures are unusual, but pulmonary contusion is common (American College of Surgeons Committee on Trauma, 1989a). The elasticity of the child's developing bones requires significant stress for fracture.

Surface Area

The ratio between the child's body surface and body volume is highest at birth and diminishes throughout infancy and childhood. There are two implications of the relatively large body surface area to mass ratio in children: (1) increased susceptibility to dehydration due to greater insensible water loss and (2) increased risk of hypothermia from increased conductive and corrective heat losses. This factor is of crucial importance in a child ≤ 6 months of age, who lacks the insulation of subcutaneous fat and the involuntary shivering mechanism of older children (Eichelberger, 1991).

Other Considerations (Eichelberger, 1991)

Renal Function. Renal function in children less than 1 year of age is immature. The infant possesses only half the urine-concentrating capabilities of the adult kidney.

Alteration in Center of Gravity. The head of a child is relatively large compared to the rest of the body. A higher center of gravity results, which leads to increased frequency of head trauma.

Sensitivity to Hypoxia. The child's CNS is exquisitely sensitive to hypoxia. Hypoxia is very poorly tolerated in the pediatric population.

Mediastinum Mobility. The mediastinum is not well fixed in the child, resulting in wide swings of the heart and great vessels during trauma.

In children who die soon after injury, the primary mechanisms causing death are airway compromise, hypovolemic shock, and CNS damage. All of these mechanisms impair adequate tissue perfusion, precipitating a shock state. Prompt recognition and intervention for the aforementioned life-threatening conditions are addressed in later sections. The reader is referred to Module 23, *Nursing Care of the Acutely Ill Pediatric Patient,* for additional pediatric considerations.

The Pregnant Patient

The pregnant trauma patient also presents unique aspects of care that must be considered carefully.

Anatomic Changes

Anatomic rearrangement as pregnancy progresses is inevitable and may cause confusion in physical diagnosis. Depending on the gestational size of the uterus, different patterns of injury may occur to the mother as well as to the fetus. The liver and spleen of the gravid patient do not enlarge. However, they are compacted, or confined to a space that is continuously decreasing in size. As energy is dissipated

via the uterus to these organs, a predisposition for organ rupture is evident. A decrease in lower esophageal sphincter tone results in reflux and predisposes the pregnant patient to aspiration. The bladder, attached to the lower uterus, concomitantly rises out of the pelvis as the pregnancy progresses, increasing the bladder's vulnerability to injury. Diaphragmatic displacement causes a decrease in residual lung volume, ventilatory reserve, and Pao_2. Minute ventilation increases by 40 percent, with increasing tidal volume and diaphragmatic excursion. These changes result in chronic respiratory alkalosis, with Pco_2 averaging 30 mm Hg (Mauro et al, 1990).

Hemodynamic Changes

By the tenth week of pregnancy, CO is increased by 1.0 L to 1.5 L/minute. A high-output, low-resistance hemodynamic state is characteristic in pregnancy. Plasma volume increases 50 percent between 10 and 30 weeks. Physiologic anemia results from a hypervolemic and hemodiluted state. By the end of the second trimester, average hemoglobin decreases from 13.7 to 14.0 g/dL to 11.0 to 12.0 g/dL, and hematocrit decreases from 39.8 percent to 33 to 34 percent. Leukocytosis (16,000–18,000/mm³) is present. Maternal heart rate increases throughout pregnancy, with a slight increase in stroke volume. During the third trimester, it reaches 15 to 20 bpm more than in the nonpregnant state. An important fact to remember is that some women experience profound hypotension when placed in the supine position (especially during the third trimester). This is known as the vena cava syndrome and is caused by the enlarged uterus compressing the inferior vena cava, decreasing venous return and preload. The hypotension can be relieved by turning the patient to the left lateral decubitus position or by shifting the weight of the uterine contents to the left (Mauro et al, 1990).

Blood Volume and Composition

The pregnant trauma patient responds very differently to stress than the nonpregnant patient. Because of the hypervolemic state associated with pregnancy, a 30 to 35 percent blood loss may occur in a pregnant patient without hypotension. A low peripheral vascular resistance fosters warm, dry periphery vs the typical cool, moist skin associated with shock.

The pregnant trauma patient exhibits a hypercoagulation state. Clotting factors I, VII, VIII, IX, and X are increased. Because of the changes in coagulation state, the pregnant trauma patient is predisposed to disseminated intravascular coagulation (DIC), particularly postoperatively, after massive fluid resuscitation, or after penetrating or significant blunt abdominal injury (Mauro et al, 1990). The reader is referred to Module 22, *Nursing Care of the Acutely Ill Obstetric Patient*, for additional considerations.

The Elderly Patient

The elderly trauma patient should be evaluated carefully during the initial and ongoing assessment. Special considerations for the elderly trauma patient include the following.

Chronic Disease States

The elderly (ages 65 and older) may have chronic disease states that could exacerbate or compound the trauma. Common underlying medical conditions include COPD, coronary artery disease, diabetes mellitus, congestive heart failure, hypertension, and conditions leading to diminished neurologic acuity (e.g., CVA and carotid insufficiency). The patient not only may have a chronic medical condition but also could be treated with a polypharmaceutical regimen that may affect the response to a traumatic injury (Bobb, 1988).

Deterioration in Body Systems

Age-related deterioration in body systems is normal. The deterioration is noted most often in the cardiorespiratory, neurologic, and musculoskeletal systems. Cardiorespiratory effects include decreased distensibility of blood vessels, increased systolic blood pressure and systemic vascular resistance, increased vascular resistance, decreased CO, decreased respiratory muscle strength, limited chest expansion, and decreased number of functioning al-veoli. Neurologic effects of aging include short-term memory loss, reduced cerebral blood flow, and decreased visual acuity. Musculoskeletal effects include bone loss and increased risk of fracture, loss of muscle strength, and increased wear on joints.

Difficulties during the initial assessment related to normal aging may present themselves to the clinician. Because of the decline in gag and cough reflexes, airway integrity may be difficult to maintain. Detection of shock may be difficult because of the propensity toward hypertension. Thus, normal blood pressures actually may indicate low perfusion states in the elderly. Altered sensorium may be due to short-term memory loss or auditory or visual impairments (Andrews, 1990).

Altered Perceptions

Alterations in perception and delayed response time to stressors may also contribute to injury. Alterations include diminished or impaired proprioception, visual acuity, temperature sensation, and hearing.

The following example illustrates the concepts discussed. A 72-year-old male is involved in an MVC. He has a previous history that includes myocardial infarction and hypertension and currently is taking inderal. A syncopal episode precipitated the MVC. The patient arrives with a blood pressure of 105/60, heart rate 65, and initial hematocrit 25 percent. A CT scan of the abdomen reveals a complex splenic laceration. Although the patient was in hypovolemic shock, the tachycardia usually associated with the shock state was prevented by the beta blockade and the diminished cardiorespiratory responsiveness.

This section has addressed individualizing the patient's response to injury based on a variety of factors. Age-related variances across the life span were discussed briefly.

Section Five Review

1. Alcohol use in the trauma patient acts as a CNS
   A. stimulant
   B. depressant
   C. vasoconstrictive agent
   D. vasodilator
2. Cocaine use in the trauma patient acts as a CNS
   A. stimulant
   B. depressant
   C. vasodilator
   D. vasoconstrictor
3. Impairment of judgment occurs with blood alcohol content of _____, whereas legal intoxication in most states is considered a blood alcohol content of _____.
   A. 0.05 g/dL, 0.10 g/dL
   B. 0.20 g/dL, 0.10 g/dL
   C. 100 mg/dL, 0.10 g/dL
   D. 300 mg/dL, 400 mg/dL

4. _____ and _____ account for almost 80 percent of all pediatric injuries.
   A. gunshot wounds and abuse
   B. falls and vehicular crashes
   C. near drowning and falls
   D. recreational injuries and vehicular crashes
5. The most common injury to a child precipitating admission to a trauma center is
   A. pulmonary contusion
   B. head injury
   C. rib fractures
   D. femur fractures
6. The normal blood volume for a child is _____ percent of body weight compared to that of an adult, which is _____ percent of body weight.
   A. 5–6, 8–10
   B. 7–8, 7–8
   C. 7–8, 5–6
   D. 8–10, 12–15
7. In children, the injury pattern of internal organ damage without overlying bony fracture is related to
   A. an incompletely calcified, resilient skeleton
   B. diminished body surface area
   C. increased elastic connective tissue
   D. increased fat
8. The immediate nursing intervention for a pregnant woman in her third trimester who is hypotensive after an MVC is
   A. administering vasopressors
   B. colloid transfusion
   C. turning the patient to the left lateral decubitus position, maintaining immobilization
   D. placing the patient in Trendelenburg

9. Increasing progesterone levels causing smooth muscle relaxation may elicit esophageal reflux in the pregnant woman. Thus, a predisposition to _____ may occur.
   A. aspiration
   B. increased gastric motility
   C. difficulty in intubation
   D. gastritis
10. By the tenth week of pregnancy, CO is increased by _____ L/minute.
    A. 0.5–1.0
    B. 1.0–1.5
    C. 1.5–2.0
    D. 2.0–2.5
11. A 24-year-old female, 7 months pregnant, victim of an MVC, has arrived. Her initial hematocrit is 31 percent. You should
    A. check fetal heart tones
    B. check for vaginal bleeding
    C. anticipate transfusion
    D. consider this normal

Answers: 1, B. 2, A. 3, A. 4, B. 5, B. 6, C. 7, A. 8, C. 9, A. 10, B. 11, D.

Section Six: Trauma Assessment and Resuscitation—The Primary Survey

At the completion of this section, you will be able to identify the specific clinical assessment format used to determine the effects of injury.

Because of the unpredictable effects of trauma-related injury on the patient, you must develop a rapid, systematic approach to each patient to ensure that no effects of injury will be overlooked. You must remember, trauma should never be approached as a unisystem disease but a multisystem disease. If one body system is injured, you must ensure that no other body system has been adversely affected. Thus, a rapid systematic approach with establishment of management priorities is essential.

Trauma presents a myriad of potentially life-threatening injuries. The life-threatening injuries must be evaluated quickly, with immediate intervention. The trauma assessment is divided into three phases: primary survey, resuscitation, and secondary survey.

The primary survey and resuscitation are the focus of this section, and a subsequent section addresses the secondary survey. The purpose of the primary survey is to identify life-threatening conditions and intervene appropriately. Primary survey is done via the A, B, C, D, E approach as outlined.

- A, Airway (with cervical spine immobilization). Ensure that the patient has an open airway.

- B, Breathing. Is the patient breathing? Are respirations effective? Does the patient need assistance via Ambu-bag or mechanical ventilation?
- C, Circulation. The trauma patient is at very high risk for hypovolemic shock from acute blood loss and third spacing of fluid with soft tissue damage. You must identify hypovolemia quickly and search for the etiology.
- D, Disability. Do a quick neuroexamination of the patient's level of consciousness and motor function.
- E, Exposure. The patient should be completely undressed to provide for visualization of external causes of injury (Rea, 1991).

Each of the components of the primary survey is explored in detail to ensure that you have all the information necessary to approach the multiply injured patient using critical thinking and problem-solving strategies. Pediatric variances in approach are addressed under each heading.

Airway and Cervical Spine

The first step in the primary survey of a trauma patient is assessment for the patency of the patient's airway. An injury to the cervical spine should always be assumed in the patient with multisystem trauma, especially in the patient with an injury above the clavicle. Excessive manipulation of the head, face, or neck, precipitating hyperextension or hyperflexion of the cervical spine, may convert a fracture without neurologic manifestations into a fracture–dislocation with spinal cord contusion, laceration, compression, or transection.

The goal of airway management is optimization of ventilation and oxygenation, with cervical spine protection. Remember, however, that airway integrity does not ensure adequate ventilation. The airway must be opened and secured, and then ventilation can be addressed.

Potential causes of airway obstruction include the tongue falling back into the oropharynx, obstructing the airway, blood, vomitus, secretions, or foreign objects obstructing the airway, fractures of the facial bony structures, or crushing injuries of the laryngotracheal tree. You should be alerted to actual or potential airway obstruction based on the following symptoms.

1. Dyspnea
2. Diminished breath sounds despite respiratory effort
3. Dysphonia (hoarseness, stridor)
4. Dysphagia
5. Drooling

Airway management techniques range from simple positional maneuvers to complex surgical procedures. During all maneuvers, it is critical that the cervical spine be maintained by inline immobilization with the head in the neutral position. Cervical spine immobilization can best be achieved by manual inline axial traction by a caregiver or by a hard cervical collar, sandbags on either side of the victim's head, and tape across the victim's forehead, securing the head to the backboard. This prevents forward flexion, hyperextension, and lateral rotation of the cervical spine.

The first, and most simple, maneuver to attempt in opening the airway is a chin lift or modified jaw thrust, maintaining the head in a neutral position. This maneuver may very well open the airway adequately and allow ventilation to take place. The pediatric airway is easily obstructed, especially in the child with an altered level of consciousness. Loss of muscle tone in the oral pharynx results in the tongue falling posteriorly, causing airway obstruction. In comparison to an adult, the following pediatric considerations apply in regard to airway management.

1. The child's tongue is proportionally larger and is housed in a smaller oral cavity.
2. The glottic opening is more anterior and cephalad.
3. The trachea is short and narrow (Eichelberger, 1991).

Along with the modified jaw thrust/chin lift, the airway can be suctioned for debris, secretions, blood, or vomitus. An oropharyngeal or nasopharyngeal airway may be used to facilitate airway maintenance.

The oropharyngeal airway should be used only in patients who are unconscious and have an absent gag reflex. Using this airway in a conscious patient may precipitate gagging, vomiting, and potential aspiration. Improper placement of the oropharyngeal airway actually may cause airway obstruction. The nasopharyngeal airway also may be used to facilitate airway integrity in the conscious victim with an intact gag reflex.

If the aforementioned procedures are inadequate in establishment of an airway, more aggressive measures must be taken. The patient should be hyperventilated with a bag-valve-mask with 100 percent oxygen to facilitate tolerance of the procedure. A frequent complication of hyperventilation in children with this technique is gastric distention. Increased risks secondary to the distention include vomiting, aspiration, and diaphragmatic impingement. Appropriate placement of a gastric tube orally or nasally will prevent these complications.

Endotracheal intubation can be achieved either orally or nasally. Nasotracheal intubation is preferred in the injured patient, since hyperextension of the neck is minimized. However, a patient must have spontaneous respiratory effort for placement of the tube. With this method, the tube should be advanced during the inspiratory effort when the epiglottis is open. Orotracheal intubation is necessary when the patient is apneic or cribriform plate fracture is suspected in the injured patient, as with basilar skull fractures. With fractures of the cribriform plate, the nasally inserted endotracheal tube could pass into the cranial vault, injuring brain tissue. Should orotracheal intubation be necessary, absolute and vigilant care must be taken to avoid hyperextension of the cervical spine. After intubation is achieved, breath sounds anteriorly and laterally should be ausculated to confirm tracheal intubation. The clinician also should ausculate over the epigastrium to rule out esophageal intubation, which would be lethal in the acute trauma situation. Tube displacement may occur during transport, especially in children, since the endotracheal tubes used for children are uncuffed, thereby more mobile. Right mainstem bronchus intubation occurs occasionally, since the right mainstem is straighter than the left as it branches from the trachea, facilitating passage of the tube into its lumen. Continuous reassessment of breath sounds in any intubated patient, adult or pediatric, is a crucial nursing intervention.

The only indication for creating a surgical airway is inability to intubate the trachea. Inability to intubate the trachea may result from edema of the glottis, larynx fracture, severe oropharyngeal hemorrhage, or gross instability of the midface due to trauma. A surgical airway can be achieved via a cricothyroidotomy or tracheostomy. Surgical cricothyroidotomy is performed by making an incision through the cricothyroid membrane and into the trachea. Surgical cricothyroidotomy is not recommended for children less than 12 years of age because the cricoid cartilage is the only circumferential support to the upper trachea. Thus, tracheostomy must be performed should a surgical airway become necessary (American College of Surgeons Committee on Trauma, 1989a).

Tracheostomy must be considered in the child less than 12 years of age and in the patient with suspected laryngeal trauma. Symptoms of laryngeal injury include tenderness, hoarseness, subcutaneous emphysema, and intolerance of the supine position. The supine position is poorly tolerated by these patients because on assuming the position, the airway is allowed to collapse where the laryngeal injury has occurred. By the patient's sitting upright, the airway is maintained even though the larynx is injured.

Aggressive airway management is critical in the trauma population. Assurance of airway integrity is the priority in the primary survey, with techniques ranging from a simple modified jaw thrust to a complex surgical procedure. The clinician must be ready for anything to ensure optimal patient management.

Breathing

The next step in the primary survey is to address the adequacy of ventilation in the injured patients. The primary goal of ventilation is to achieve maximum cellular oxygenation by providing an oxygen-rich environment. Thus, all trauma patients should receive high flow oxygen during the initial evaluation.

Breathing should be evaluated by the look, listen, and feel parameters. Look to detect the presence of respiratory excursion, listen for breath sounds, and feel for breathing. Positive pressure ventilation may be required in some patients and can be provided in a number of ways: mouth-to-mask, bag-valve-mask, or positive pressure ventilator.

Confirmation of the adequacy of ventilation is best achieved by obtaining an arterial blood gas determination or continuous monitoring of end-tidal CO_2 and arterial oxygen saturation by noninvasive measures. If arterial blood gases are inadequate, the airway should be reevaluated, and the patient should be evaluated for the presence of pneumothorax, hemothorax, hemopneumothorax, or tension pneumothorax. Tube thoracostomy would be indicated for any of these conditions, since they are all considered life threatening. Refer to Module 14, *Nursing Care of the Patient with Multiple Injuries*, for assessment guidelines in evaluating these clinical conditions.

Circulation

The next step in the primary survey after airway and breathing have been adequately addressed is circulation. Inadequate circulation occurs as shock. Shock is a clinical state characterized by inadequate delivery of oxygen and metabolic substrates to meet the increased metabolic demands of the tissues (Eichelberger, 1991).

Assessment of circulation adequacy should include palpating for strength, rate, rhythm, and symmetry of carotid, radial, femoral, and pedal pulses. Skin temperature also should be evaluated, as should capillary refill centrally and peripherally. Mucous membranes can be inspected as well. The adequacy of tissue perfusion is reflected sensitively by the patient's level of consciousness.

Successful treatment of shock depends on early recognition and aggressive fluid resuscitation to prevent the development of hypotension. IV access is critical for volume infusion. Two large bore IVs should be established (16 gauge or larger in adults, 18 gauge or larger in children), and crystalloid administration should ensue promptly. Lactated Ringer's solution is the solution of choice for adults and children. Lactated Ringer's solution can be infused at a wide open rate in the adult and should be bolused in children at 20 mL/kg of body weight. If the child shows no improvement, a second bolus can be administered at 20 mL/kg of body weight. If signs of shock persist, a 10 mL/kg bolus of packed red blood cells can be transfused.

Remember that the early signs of shock are subtle in children. Normal blood volume in the child varies from 7 percent to 8 percent, or 70 to 80 mL/kg body weight. A small volume loss for an adult can precipitate shock in the child. Early shock from acute blood loss of up to 25 percent of blood volume (20 mL/kg body weight) generally is well tolerated in healthy children. Signs and symptoms based on shock stages are as follows (Eichelberger, 1991).

Shock Stage	Signs and Symptoms

Early shock
    Blood volume loss
    less than 25%
	Mild tachycardia (greater than 130 bpm), peripheral vasoconstriction, normal blood pressure (greater than 80 mm Hg systolic), dyspnea, tachypnea, agitation, lethargy, or hypotonia

Worsening shock
    Blood volume loss
    greater than 25%
	Persistent tachycardia, decreasing pulse pressure (less than 20 mm Hg), poor peripheral perfusion, prolonged capillary refill (longer than 2 seconds)

Profound shock
    Blood volume loss
    greater than 50%
	Profound hypotension, vasoconstriction

Recognition of the site of blood loss is critical in the mediation of shock. Blood volume loss in quantities enough to produce a shock state can occur in one or more of the following five areas.

1. Chest. In the adult, 2.5 L of blood can be lost in each hemothorax. Thus, a total of 5 L can be lost inside the chest.
2. Abdomen. As much as 6 L of blood can be lost via intraperitoneal bleeding from damaged organs or vessels.
3. Pelvis and retroperitoneum. An unstable pelvic fracture, especially those involving the posterior elements of the pelvis, can precipitate liters of blood loss. A patient actually may exsanguinate from an unstable pelvic fracture involving posterior bony elements.
4. Femur fractures. For each femur fracture, 500 to 1,000 mL of blood can be lost.
5. External hemorrhage. Wounds are especially a consideration in children. A scalp laceration particularly requires proper hemostasis, since it can lead to a shock state in young children.

Among the causes of early postinjury deaths in the hospital that are amenable to effective treatment, hemorrhage is predominant. The most common cause of shock in the injured patient is hypovolemia resulting from acute blood loss. Fluid resuscitation is the fundamental treatment for hypovolemic shock until definitive surgical intervention is available to treat the site (or sites) of injury.

Current controversies in circulation management include choice of fluid for resuscitation (hypertonic saline, crystalloid vs colloid, hetastarch, albumin, lactated Ringer's solution, normal saline), the use of the pneumatic antishock garment (PASG) or military antishock trousers (MAST), and the use of open resuscitative thoracotomy in the emergency department. These controversies are beyond the scope of this module, and additional reading on each topic is recommended.

Disability

After airway, breathing, and circulation are managed adequately, the next step is evaluation of neurologic disability. The purpose of the neurologic examination in the primary survey is to establish quickly the patient's level of consciousness and pupillary size and reaction.

The patient's level of consciousness can best be determined by the AVPU method.

- A, *A*lert
- V, Responds to *V*erbal stimulation
- P, Responds to *P*ainful stimulation
- U, *U*nresponsive

A more detailed examination should be included in the secondary survey.

Exposure

At this point in the primary survey, the patient should be completely disrobed in preparation for the secondary survey.

This section has given you a broad overview of the primary survey conducted during the initial phase of trauma evaluation. Special considerations for children were presented.

Section Six Review

1. The following are true concerning the pediatric airway EXCEPT
   A. the glottic opening is more anterior and cephalad
   B. the trachea is short and narrow
   C. the child's tongue is proportionately smaller and usually has little to do with airway integrity
   D. cervical spine immobilization requires meticulous attention

2. Contraindications to the use of an oropharyngeal airway include
   A. consciousness/presence of gag reflex
   B. unconsciousness
   C. absence of gag reflex
   D. questionable airway integrity

3. A frequent complication of hyperventilation, especially in children, is
   A. vomiting
   B. increased airway pressures
   C. gastric distention
   D. increased pulmonary compliance

4. Your patient has just been intubated for progressive respiratory failure. On ausculation of breath sounds, you note present breath sounds in right lung fields and absent breath sounds in left lung fields. You should anticipate the cause as
   A. right mainstem intubation
   B. esophageal intubation
   C. tension pneumothorax
   D. pericardial effusion

5. The surgical airway of choice in the child less than 12 years of age who has severe facial fractures and bleeding is
   A. tracheostomy
   B. cricothyroidotomy
   C. orotracheal intubation
   D. nasotracheal intubation

6. High flow oxygen should be used for all of the following groups of trauma patients EXCEPT
   A. acute respiratory failure
   B. normal respiratory rate, systolic blood pressure of 90
   C. hemopneumothorax
   D. patient with COPD and an isolated ankle injury

7. When bolusing the injured child with a crystalloid solution, the initial bolus should be
   A. 10 mL/kg
   B. 20 mL/kg
   C. 50 mL/kg
   D. 1 L

Answers: 1, C. 2, A. 3, C. 4, A. 5, A. 6, D. 7, B.

Section Seven: Trauma Assessment and Resuscitation: The Secondary Survey

This section outlines the conduction of the secondary survey during the initial trauma evaluation. At the completion of this section, you should have an understanding of the components of the secondary survey and a suggested format for conducting the secondary survey.

The secondary survey should begin only after the primary survey is completed and all immediately life-threatening injuries have been addressed. A head-to-toe approach is usually adopted, with thorough examination of each body system. A critical point to remember is should your patient become hemodynamically unstable at any point during the secondary survey, you should immediately return to the primary survey format (A, B, C, and D) to troubleshoot the problem. A summary of key points in the secondary survey has been adapted as follows from the American College of Surgeons Committee on Trauma Advanced Trauma Life Support Course Provider Manual (1989).

Surveyed System	Evaluated Criteria
Head	Complete neurologic examination using a tool, such as the Glasgow Coma Score, reevaluation of pupillary size and reactivity, inspection, palpation of cranium for lacerations, fractures, contusions, hemotympan-

	ium, cerebrospinal fluid leakage, and so on.
Maxillofacial	Assessment for facial fractures via inspection, palpation for open fractures, lacerations, mobility/instability of facial structures
Cervical spine/neck	Inspection and palpation of neck anteriorly (maintaining cervical spine immobilization) and palpation anteriorly and posteriorly for pain, crepitus, bony stepoffs indicating fracture–dislocation, and neck vein distention
Chest	Inspection for paradoxical movement, flail segments, open chest wounds, ecchymosis; palpation for rib fractures, subcutaneous emphysema, respiratory excursion, sternal fractures; ausculation for quality, equality of breath sounds, presence of adventitious sounds; ausculation of heart sounds for quality, extra heart sounds, murmurs, or pericardial friction rubs possibly indicating pericardial effusion
Abdomen	Inspection and ausculation before palpation to prevent precipitation of misleading bowel sounds by manual manipulation; abdomen inspection for abrasions, contusions, lacerations, distention; ausculation for bowel sounds in four quadrants, bruits, and breath sounds; light and deep palpation precipitating a painful response may indicate intraperitoneal bleeding and should be quickly attended
Pelvis, perineum, genitalia	Pelvis inspection for deformation and palpation for stability. Perineum and genitalia inspection for bleeding at the

	meatus, hematoma, vaginal bleeding, lacerations. Rectal examination to evaluate rectal wall integrity, presence of blood, position of prostate, presence of palpable pelvic fractures, and quality of sphincter tone
Extremities	Visual evaluation of extremities for contusions or deformities; palpation of all extremities for tenderness, crepitation, or abnormal range of motion may raise index of suspicion for fracture; all peripheral pulses should be evaluated
Back	All patients should be log rolled with careful attention to spinal immobilization to afford the clinician a full view of the patient's posterior surfaces, including neck, back, buttocks, and lower extremities; these areas should be carefully inspected and palpated to detect any area of injury
Complete neurologic examination	Motor and sensory evaluation of the extremities and re-evaluation of the patient's Glasgow Coma Scale score and pupils; any evidence of paralysis or paresis should prompt immediate immobilization of the entire patient if not already done

At the completion of the secondary survey, you must remember that the trauma patient demands continuous reevaluation so that any new signs or symptoms are not overlooked. Other life-threatening problems may appear, or exacerbation of previously treated injuries may occur (such as tension pneumothorax, pericardial tamponade, or intracranial bleeding). Continuous monitoring of vital signs and urinary output is critical. Urinary output should be maintained at 50 mL/hour for the adult and 1 mL/kg hour for children to ensure adequacy of tissue perfusion.

This section has outlined the format for the secondary survey to be conducted during initial assessment and resuscitation of the trauma patient. Key criteria for evaluation were identified in each area to facilitate assessment parameters.

Section Seven Review

1. During the secondary survey, your patient becomes hemodynamically unstable. You should immediately
   A. stop the secondary survey and reinstitute the primary survey
   B. finish the secondary survey, looking for potential etiologies of instability
   C. start at the beginning of the secondary survey
   D. reevaluate patency and flow rates of IVs
2. The purpose of the secondary survey is to
   A. identify and intervene with life-threatening injuries
   B. identify the existence of all injuries
   C. facilitate treatment of airway and breathing
   D. assess response of resuscitative interventions
3. The complete and immediate immobilization of the entire patient should take place with the following findings during secondary survey
   A. inability to establish airway
   B. tense, distended abdomen
   C. Glasgow Coma Scale score ≤ 8
   D. evidence of paralysis or paresis

4. Presence of abdominal pain on light or deep palpation in the injured patient usually indicates
   A. gastritis
   B. presence of intraperitoneal blood
   C. pelvic fracture
   D. intracerebral pathology
5. Rectal examination should be done to evaluate all of the following EXCEPT
   A. rectal wall integrity
   B. presence of blood
   C. bladder injury
   D. palpable pelvic fractures

Answers: 1, A. 2, B. 3, D. 4, B. 5, C.

Section Eight: Trauma Mortality and Traumatic Shock

At the completion of this section, you will be able to describe the trimodal distribution of trauma-related mortalities and how amount of time elapsed post-injury will affect your clinical assessment. A brief discussion of traumatic shock and exsanguination is presented.

Trauma Deaths

Twenty percent of trauma-related mortalities are considered preventable in our country today. This is an astounding statistic in an age of modern technology with the myriad of life-saving interventions we use. When plotted on a graph, trauma-related mortalities exhibit a trimodal distribution; that is, death from trauma has three peak periods of occurrence. The first peak occurs within minutes of the injury. These deaths usually result from injuries to the brain, upper spinal cord, heart, aorta, or other major blood vessel. The second peak occurs within 2 hours of injury, and death usually is related to subdural or epidural hematomas, hemopneumothorax, ruptured spleen, lacerated liver, fractured femurs, or other injuries resulting in significant blood loss. The third peak occurs days to weeks after the injury and usually results from complications of sepsis or multiple organ failure (American College of Surgeons, 1987).

How does the knowledge of this distribution affect your clinical practice? Again, this knowledge can empower you to anticipate the needs of the patient based on time from injury and physiologic manifestation of the injury. If you receive a patient within minutes of injury or perhaps you are the first responder as a flight nurse, what are the life-threatening injuries that may cause death in this time frame? Has the patient experienced brainstem compression or laceration resulting in respiratory center dysfunction? Perhaps the patient has experienced atlanto-occipital dislocation and severe spinal cord contusion or transection, or perhaps the heart or great vessels have been lacerated, transected, or disrupted. What assessment and intervention must be performed in order to mediate these injuries?

An unstable patient arrives within 30 minutes of injury. What conditions must you appreciate clinically in order to anticipate a life-threatening situation? Epidural or subdural hematomas (What is his level of consciousness?), hemopneumothorax (What is his respiratory effort? How are his lung sounds? Will a chest tube be necessary?), ruptured spleen or lacerated liver (Does he have a tense and painful abdomen? Is the patient hypotensive with no signs of obvious blood loss?), or fractured femurs (Is his leg painful, with an obvious fracture?)

Perhaps you are in the critical care environment with a patient 2 weeks after his injury. If he is experiencing multiple organ failure or sepsis, what could be the precipitating factors or contributing factors to his condition? Was he overhydrated during the first 24 to 48 hours and ARDS has ensued? Did he have a missed intraabdominal injury predisposing him to sepsis?

Shock from Trauma

Mortality from trauma may result from what is considered a preventable cause. One of the most frequently encountered clinical states in the injured patient is traumatic shock. Because of the frequency of traumatic shock, a brief discussion of hemorrhagic shock ensues. You should refer to Module 8, *Shock States*, for an in-depth examination of the cellular tissue, organ, and system response to shock.

The most common cause of shock in the injured patient is hypovolemia resulting from acute blood loss. Acute blood loss can occur externally, as with lacerations, open fractures, avulsion injuries, or amputations, or internally within a body cavity, as with bleeding into the chest cavity, abdominal cavity, retroperitoneum, or soft tissue. (Section Six of this module has a discussion of potential sites of blood loss in large enough quantities to precipitate shock.)

As with most body systems dysfunction, a general pattern of body compensatory mechanisms occurs in response to hemorrhagic shock in an effort to stabilize the unstable body system. Remember, shock is basically a cellular derangement, and all cells usually are affected when a shock state is encountered.

As blood loss continues in the injured patient, the compensatory mechanisms become more pronounced and eventually fail, precipitating severe problems with tissue perfusion, unless prompt recognition and intervention are conducted. A small volume of blood (approximately 10 percent of total blood volume) can be removed without significant effect on mean arterial pressure or CO. With blood loss exceeding 10 percent, decreased venous return precipitates a decreased CO and, thus, a decreased mean arterial pressure. Should 35 to 40 percent of

total blood volume be lost, both CO and mean arterial pressure fall to zero (Vary and Linberg, 1988).

The body maintains a regional distribution of blood flow in hemorrhage with greater than 10 percent loss of blood volume. The body selectively shunts blood away from nonvital tissue to critical, vital organs, such as the heart and brain. If left untreated for any length of time, the shock state will progress until it becomes refractory to any treatment.

Exsanguination is the most extreme form of hemorrhage. It is a hemorrhage in which there is an initial loss of 40 percent of the patient's blood volume, with a rate of blood loss, or a rate of hemorrhage, exceeding 250 mL/minute. If uncontrolled, the patient may lose 50 percent of the entire blood volume in 10 minutes (Asensio, 1990).

Most injuries precipitating exsanguination are from penetrating trauma. An identifiable cluster of organs and organ systems with a high incidence of exsanguination has been identified (Asensio, 1990).

I. Heart
II. Abdominal vascular system
    A. Arterial system
        1. Abdominal aorta
        2. Superior mesenteric artery
    B. Venous system
        1. Inferior vena cava
        2. Portal vein
        3. Liver

Resuscitation of the exsanguinating patient rests on the intensified basic principles of circulation management. IV access must be established quickly with adequate, large-bore catheters. The preferred fluid for resuscitation of the exsanguinating patient is lactated Ringer's solution. In the patient experiencing hemorrhage shock, the red cell mass is likely to be reduced by 50 percent, and the plasma space may be reduced to 35 percent. For adequate resuscitation to ensue, both plasma and interstitial fluid spaces must be replenished by the most appropriate electrolyte solution, lactated Ringer's solution (Asensio, 1990).

Transfusion of blood ideally should occur after the initial infusion of 2 to 4 L of lactated Ringer's solution. O-negative blood should be used during initial resuscitation until type-specific or cross-matched blood becomes available. Controversy continues about the use of packed red blood cells vs whole blood vs other component therapy.

Other adjuncts are available in the acute phase of resuscitation of the exsanguinating patient. Rapid infusion devices are available and can deliver large amounts of crystalloid and colloid incredibly quickly. The use of autotransfusion devices in major chest injury may facilitate resuscitative efforts, especially in those patients with large hemothoraces.

Emergency department open resuscitative thoracotomy also may be used to manage the exsanguinating patient, especially if exsanguination is suspected to be related to injury to the great vessels (i.e., aorta) or the heart.

Critical analysis during the primary survey and quick recognition of traumatic shock are essential skills in the resuscitative phase of trauma. The 20 percent of preventable trauma-related mortalities can be mediated with improved prehospital and hospital care in the provision of highly skilled clinicians who can evaluate the injured patient rapidly and effectively.

In summary, the process of trauma assessment can be refined and polished with the knowledge of clinical conditions that cause deaths in our trauma population. Nursing can play a key role in mediating the preventable deaths from trauma that continue to plague our modern society.

Section Eight Review

1. ___ percent of trauma-related mortalities are considered preventable.
   A. 10
   B. 20
   C. 30
   D. 50
2. Trauma related mortalities exhibit a _____ distribution.
   A. modal
   B. bimodal
   C. trimodal
   D. bell-shaped
3. The second mode occurs within 2 hours postinjury and may be attributed to all of the following EXCEPT
   A. sepsis
   B. ruptured spleen
   C. liver laceration
   D. hemopneumothorax
4. The third mode occurs within days to weeks postinjury and usually can be attributed to
   A. exsanguination
   B. multiple organ failure/sepsis
   C. brainstem compression
   D. atlanto-occipital dislocation

5. The most common cause of shock in the injured patient is
   A. hypovolemia
   B. cardiogenic
   C. neurogenic
   D. sepsis
6. The three organs and organ systems most commonly associated with exsanguination are
   A. heart, liver, abdominal vasculature
   B. lung, brain, heart
   C. brain, kidney, spleen
   D. kidney, abdominal vasculature, lung
7. The crystalloid of choice for infusion in the exsanguinating patient is
   A. normal saline
   B. lactated Ringer's solution
   C. D$_5$W
   D. hypertonic saline

Answers: 1, B. 2, C. 3, A. 4, B. 5, A. 6, A. 7, B.

Posttest

1. Typically, a trauma patient has which demographic profile?
   A. 15–24 years, male, using alcohol, lower income level
   B. 24–32 years, male, using alcohol, upper income level
   C. 15–24 years, female, using alcohol, lower income level
   D. 15–24 years, male, no alcohol involvement, lower income level

2. What are the four forces that must be considered in assessment of injury?
   A. acceleration, mass, axial loading, deceleration
   B. shearing, compression, impact, axial loading
   C. acceleration, deceleration, shearing, stretching
   D. acceleration, deceleration, shearing, compression

3. The coup and contrecoup injury is an example of application of _____ and _____ forces, respectively.
   A. shear, tensile
   B. tensile, shear
   C. compression, axial loading
   D. acceleration, tensile

4. As penetration of tissue occurs with penetrating trauma, tissues are temporarily displaced forward and laterally, creating a temporary cavity. This process is called
   A. tumbling
   B. yaw
   C. blast effect
   D. cavitation

5. The extent of cavitation and tissue deformation is most determined by
   A. yaw
   B. velocity
   C. blast effect
   D. tissue density

6. The higher the velocity of the missile, the greater the propensity for
   A. yaw
   B. tumble
   C. cavitation
   D. all of the above

7. A patient is admitted to your unit with a stab injury to the right sternal border, fifth intercostal space. Injury must be considered to the abdomen as well as to the thorax because
   A. the left diaphragm can rise as high as the fourth intercostal space during maximum expiration
   B. the right diaphragm can rise as high as the fourth intercostal space during maximum expiration
   C. the diaphragm recedes to the eighth intercostal space during maximum inspiration at the midclavicular line
   D. the diaphragm recedes to the sixth intercostal space during maximum inspiration at the midaxillary line

8. Which of the following best describes the injury pattern associated with a pedestrian (child) hit by an automobile?
   A. fractured femur, tibia, fibula on side of impact
   B. compression fractures of lumbosacral spine
   C. high cervical fractures and head injuries
   D. fracture of femur, chest injury, and injury to contralateral skull as child is thrown on impact

9. An injury pattern unique to the restrained passenger with lap belt only is
   A. pulmonary contusion
   B. cervical fractures
   C. flexion/distraction fractures of lumbar vertebrae
   D. femur fractures

10. Trauma victims who have ingested cocaine before arrival may exhibit a sympathomimetic presentation. Clinical signs may include
    A. tachycardia, dilated pupils, tremors, elevated blood pressure
    B. tachycardia, constricted pupils, tremors, elevated blood pressure
    C. bradycardia, hypotension
    D. dilated pupils, hypotension, bradycardia

11. With pediatric trauma victims, multisystem injury is the rule rather than the exception. This is due to
    A. size and shape of the child
    B. skeleton of the child
    C. surface area of the child
    D. all of the above

12. Hypothermia is critically important in trauma patients ≤ 6 months of age because
    A. they lack subcutaneous fat and involuntary shivering mechanism
    B. they poorly metabolize brown fat to conserve heat
    C. their body surface area facilitates heat conservation
    D. involuntary shivering is the only available mechanism for heat conservation

13. The metabolic derangement typically seen in the pregnant trauma patient is
    A. respiratory alkalosis
    B. respiratory acidosis
    C. metabolic alkalosis
    D. metabolic acidosis

14. The IMMEDIATE nursing intervention for a pregnant woman in her third trimester who is hypotensive after an MVC is
    A. vasopressors
    B. colloid transfusion
    C. turning the patient to the left lateral decubitus position, maintaining immobilization or leftward uterine displacement manually
    D. Trendelenburg position

15. The first three components of the primary survey are
    A. airway, circulation, cervical spine control
    B. airway, breathing, circulation
    C. circulation, cervical spine control, breathing
    D. breathing, disability, circulation

16. Airway considerations in the pediatric trauma victim include all of the following EXCEPT
    A. the child's tongue is proportionately larger and housed in a smaller oral cavity
    B. the glottic opening is more anterior and cephalad
    C. the trachea is short and narrow
    D. it is easier to intubate the left mainstem bronchus rather than the right

17. Nasotracheal intubation should be avoided in any patient where a cribriform plate fracture is suspected because
    A. the technique is extraordinarily difficult
    B. the cranial vault becomes vulnerable, and the tube could be passed into the brain tissue
    C. vocal cord visualization is difficult
    D. cervical spine injury is unlikely

18. All of the following may indicate injury to the larynx EXCEPT
    A. tenderness
    B. hoarseness
    C. subcutaneous emphysema
    D. preference for the supine position

19. The purpose of the secondary survey is to
    A. identify and intervene with life-threatening injuries
    B. identify the existence of all injuries
    C. facilitate treatment of airway and breathing
    D. assess response to resuscitative interventions

20. Any injured patient in a shock state should be evaluated for the most common etiology of traumatic shock, which is
    A. hypovolemic
    B. cardiogenic
    C. neurogenic
    D. sepsis

Posttest Answers

Question	Answer	Section	Question	Answer	Section
1	A	One	11	D	Five
2	D	Two	12	A	Five
3	A	Two	13	A	Five
4	D	Three	14	C	Five
5	B	Three	15	B	Six
6	D	Three	16	D	Six
7	B	Three	17	B	Six
8	D	Four	18	D	Six
9	C	Four	19	B	Seven
10	A	Five	20	A	Eight

REFERENCES

American College of Surgeons. (1987). *Hospital and prehospital resources for optimal care of the injured patient and appendices A through J.* Chicago: American College of Surgeons.

American College of Surgeons Committee on Trauma. (1989a). Pediatric trauma. In *Advanced trauma life support course manual*, pp. 215–233. Chicago: American College of Surgeons.

American College of Surgeons Committee on Trauma. (1989b). Trauma in pregnancy. In *Advanced trauma life support course manual*, pp. 235–242. Chicago: American College of Surgeons.

American College of Surgeons Committee on Trauma. (1989c). *Advanced trauma life support course provider manual.* Chicago: American College of Surgeons.

Andrews, J.F. (1990). Trauma in the elderly. In *Contemporary perspectives in trauma nursing.* Berryville, Virginia: Forum Medicum, Inc.

Asensio, J.A. (1990). Exsanguination from penetrating injuries. In R.F. Buckman and L.N. Manro (eds). *Trauma quarterly—Difficult problems in urban trauma, Part II*, pp. 1–25. Rockville, Maryland: Aspen.

Baker, S.P., O'Neill, B., and Karpf, R.S. (1984). Overview of injury mortality. In *The injury fact book*, pp. 17–37. Lexington, Kentucky: D.C. Heath & Co.

Bobb, J.K. (1988). Trauma in the elderly. In V.A. Cardona, P.D. Hurn, P.J. Mason, A.M. Scanlon-Schilpp, and S.W. Veise-Berry (eds). *Trauma nursing from resuscitation through rehabilitation*, pp. 692–706. Philadelphia: W.B. Saunders Co.

Eichelberger, M.R. (1991). Pediatric trauma. In D.D. Trunkey and F.R. Lewis (eds). *Current therapy of trauma, 3rd ed.*, pp. 21–39. St. Louis: C.V. Mosby Co.

Kerr, T., and Sood, R. (1989). Management of asymptomatic stab wounds of the chest. In R.F. Buckman and J.M. Strange (eds). *Trauma quarterly—Difficult problems in urban trauma, Part I,* pp. 27–32. Rockville, Maryland: Aspen.

Mauro, L.H., Cochrane, S.O., and Cochrane, P. (1990). Trauma and pregnancy in the urban environment. In R.F. Buckman and L.H. Mauro (eds). *Trauma quarterly—Difficult problems in urban trauma, Part II,* pp. 69–82. Rockville, Maryland: Aspen.

McCabe, P.E., and Hassan, E. (1988). The trauma patient with a history of substance abuse. In V.A. Cardona, P.D. Hurn, P.J. Mason, A.M. Scanlon-Schilpp, and S.W. Veise-Berry (eds). *Trauma nursing from resuscitation through rehabilitation,* pp. 759–784. Philadelphia: W.B. Saunders Co.

Rea, R.E. (ed). (1991). Epidemiology and mechanism of injury. In R.E. Rea (ed). *Trauma nursing core course association manual, 2nd ed.,* pp. 11-1–11-7). Chicago: American Nurses Association.

Salander, J.M., and Bingham, R. (1991). Mechanisms of force in trauma. In D.D. Trunkey and F.R. Lewis (eds).

Current therapy of trauma, 3rd ed., pp. 44–46. St. Louis: C.V. Mosby Co.

Swan, K.G., and Swan, R.C. (1989). Wound ballistics. In *Gunshot wounds: Pathophysiology and management,* pp. 7–20. St. Louis: Mosby Year Book.

Vary, T.C., and Linberg, S.E. (1988). Pathophysiology of traumatic shock. In V.A. Cardona, P.D. Hurn, P.J. Mason, A.M. Scanlon-Schilpp, and S.W. Veise-Berry (eds). *Trauma nursing from resuscitation through rehabilitation,* pp. 127–159. Philadelphia: W.B. Saunders Co.

Waller, J.A. (1985). *Injury control: A guide to the causes and prevention of trauma.* Lexington, Kentucky: D.C. Heath & Co.

Weigelt, J.A., and McCormack, A. (1988). Mechanism of injury. In V.A. Cardona, P.D. Hurn, P.J. Mason, A.M. Scanlon-Schilpp, and S.W. Veise-Berry (eds). *Trauma nursing from resuscitation through rehabilitation,* pp. 105–126. Philadelphia: W.B. Saunders Co.

Withers, B.F., and Baker, J.P. (1987). Epidemiology and prevention of injuries. *Emergency Med. Clin. North Am.* 2:701–715.

Module **11**

Wound Management

Karen L. Johnson

A wound presents an alteration in skin integrity, and altered skin integrity interferes with the physiologic functions of the skin. Wound healing is a complex process that begins on initiation of the wound. There are multiple factors that affect the wound healing process. Nursing has a major influence on the outcome of wound healing. When providing wound care, the nurse must assess and evaluate the wound management regimen in relation to the wound healing process. Clinical nursing assessments and appropriate nursing plans and interventions greatly affect the outcome of wound healing.

The purpose of this module is to describe the anatomic structures and physiologic functions of the skin, physiologic events that occur when an alteration in skin integrity occurs, factors that affect restoration of skin integrity, principles of wound management, and nursing assessment of and interventions for the patient with alteration in skin integrity.

To help determine your current level of understanding of this topic, the module begins with a pretest.

Objectives

At the completion of this module, the learner will be able to

1. Relate anatomic structures with physiologic functions of the skin
2. State the three phases of wound healing
3. Describe the events that occur in each phase of wound healing
4. Define three methods of wound closure
5. Recognize factors that affect the wound healing process
6. Identify conditions that predispose a patient to develop a wound infection
7. Identify criteria used to diagnose a wound infection
8. State interventions that can be used to prevent and treat wound infections
9. Describe the rationale for various treatment modalities used in wound management
10. Identify the common clinical assessments made to evaluate wound healing
11. State the mechanisms and pathophysiology of burn injuries
12. Estimate the extent and depth of a burn injury
13. State the principles of burn wound management

Pretest

1. The layer of the skin that contains connective tissue, elastic fibers, blood vessels, and nerves is the
   A. epidermis
   B. dermis
   C. hypodermis
   D. subcutaneous tissue

2. The functions of the skin include all of the following EXCEPT
   A. regulation of body temperature
   B. production of vitamin D
   C. protection from the external environment
   D. production of calcium

3. The major events that occur during the regeneration phase of wound healing include all of the following EXCEPT
   A. hemostasis
   B. epithelialization
   C. granulation
   D. collagen formation

4. The four cardinal signs of inflammation occur as a result of
   A. normal chemical and vascular events
   B. an infectious process
   C. bradykinins
   D. an increased number of white blood cells

5. Wounds that have significant contamination or significant tissue loss usually are not sutured. These wounds are left open to heal by the process of
   A. primary intention
   B. secondary intention
   C. delayed primary intention
   D. delayed secondary intention

6. Which of the following does not affect wound healing?
   A. age
   B. weight
   C. serum glucose of 450
   D. race

7. Which of the following would not predispose a patient to developing a wound infection?
   A. susceptible host
   B. compromised wound
   C. infectious organism
   D. low hematocrit

8. Which of the following is the most reliable datum in diagnosing a wound infection?
   A. WBC count of 20,000/mm³
   B. gram stain testing
   C. culture and sensitivity testing
   D. purulent drainage from a wound

9. The golden period of wound management is considered to be how many hours postinjury?
   A. 6–12 hours
   B. the first hour
   C. 1–6 hours
   D. 12–24 hours

10. A solution used for wound irrigation that aids in mechanical debridement but does not damage granulation tissue is
    A. betadine
    B. normal saline
    C. acetic acid
    D. hydrogen peroxide

11. Mr. W has an abdominal wound that is healing by secondary intention. On assessment of this wound, seropurulent drainage is noted from granulating tissue, with some necrotic tissue present. Which type of dressing would you select to remove the debris and necrotic tissue without causing harm to the granulation tissue?
    A. dry sterile dressing
    B. wet to dry dressing
    C. synthetic dressing
    D. hydrocolloid dressing

12. Topical antibiotics are applied to burn wounds because
    A. they immediately penetrate the wound at the site of bacterial invasion
    B. burn wounds are ischemic, thus preventing the use of parenteral antibiotics
    C. they are soothing for the patient
    D. they aid in cleansing and debriding bacterial debris

13. Which of the following burn injuries penetrate deep into tissues and produce necrosis for several hours postinjury?
    A. electrical burns
    B. thermal burns
    C. alkaline burns
    D. acidic burns

14. A burn wound that is white, painless, and leathery in texture describes
    A. third degree burn
    B. deep partial thickness burn
    C. second degree burn
    D. first degree burn

Pretest answers: 1, B. 2, D. 3, A. 4, A. 5, B. 6, D. 7, D. 8, C. 9, A. 10, B. 11, B. 12, B. 13, C. 14, A.

Glossary

Abrasion. Partial thickness denudation of skin caused by friction or scraping

Avulsion. Full thickness skin loss; wound edges cannot be approximated

Contusion. Injury to superficial tissues with disruption of blood vessels with extravasion into the skin

Debridement. Process of removing dead or foreign material from a wound

Delayed primary intention. Method of wound closure that uses a combination of primary and secondary intention

Dermis. Middle layer of skin, referred to as "true skin"

Endogenous. Arising from within the patient

Eschar. Hard, black, dehydrated tissue

Exogenous. Entering from external environment

First degree burn. Involves epidermis only

Laceration. Open wound causing incision or abrupt disruption of tissue

Primary intention. Method of wound closure using sutures or tape

Puncture. Deep, narrow, open wound resulting from penetrating or sharp objects

Second degree burn. Destroys epidermis and portions of dermis

Secondary intention. Method of wound closure where the wound is allowed to heal gradually using the biologic phases of wound healing to fill in a cavity or defect

Slough. Moist, stringy, thick, yellow tissue that is dying

Susceptible host. Patient with some degree of local or systemic impairment of resistance to bacterial invasion

Superficial partial thickness burn. Involves epidermis and one half or less of the dermis

Third degree burn. Destruction of epidermis, dermis, and portions of subcutaneous tissues

Wound. An alteration and disruption of the anatomic and physiologic functions of the skin

Abbreviations

CO. Carbon monoxide

E. coli. *Escherichia coli*

WBC. White blood cell

Section One: Anatomy and Physiology of the Skin

At the completion of this section, the learner will be able to identify the anatomic structures and physiologic functions of the skin.

The skin is a tough membrane covering the entire body surface. It is the largest organ of the body and is composed of three layers of tissue: the epidermis, the dermis, and the hypodermis or subcutaneous tissue. The epidermis is the outermost layer and contains epithelial cells. The middle layer, often referred to as the "true skin," is the dermis. This layer contains connective tissue and elastic fibers, sensory and motor nerve endings, and a complex network of capillary and lymphatic vessels and muscles. From the dermis arise the appendages of the skin—hair, nails, sebaceous and sweat glands—which then penetrate the epidermis. The dermis lacks exact boundaries and merges with subcutaneous tissues containing blood vessels, nerves, muscle, and adipose tissue. The anatomy of the skin is depicted in Figure 11–1.

The epidermis contains epithelial tissue that is responsible for regeneration of the skin. This tissue is composed of cells that rapidly reproduce and regenerate through the process of epithelialization.

The various components of the dermis provide elements to protect and combat foreign materials and regenerate itself after exposure to the external environment. Connective tissue and elastic fibers provide strength and pliability to protect the internal environment. Nutrients are delivered to and cellular wastes are removed by the blood and lymphatic vessels. Nerve endings, present within the dermis, respond to cold, heat, touch, pain, and pressure.

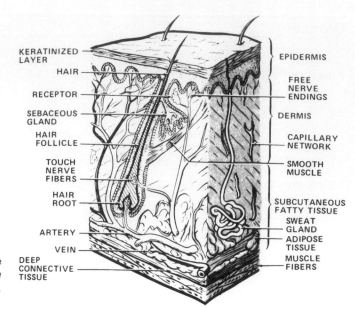

Figure 11–1. Anatomy of the skin. The skin is composed of three layers of tissue: the epidermis, dermis, and hypodermis. (*From Trauma nursing: Principles and practice, p. 155, by B.E. Knezevich, 1986, Norwalk, Connecticut: Appleton-Century-Crofts.*)

The subcutaneous tissues store caloric energy in adipose tissue and assist in regulating the body temperature by acting as insulation, acting as a cushion against external forces and providing the body with shape and substance. A summary of the physiologic functions of the skin is shown in Table 11–1.

A wound creates an alteration and disruption of the anatomic and physiologic functions of the skin. A wound can be created intentionally, as with a surgeon's knife, by accidental trauma, such as a motor vehicle crash, or by chronic forces, such as in decubitus ulcer formation.

Terms used to describe injuries to the skin are abrasions, avulsions, contusions, lacerations, and puncture wounds.

Any wound interrupts the normal skin and tissue integrity and thus the normal physiologic functions of the skin. Healing begins at the moment of injury. The healing process is discussed in Section Two of this module.

In summary, the skin is composed of three layers. The outermost layer is the epidermis, which contains epithelial tissue. This tissue rapidly reproduces when injured through the process of epithelialization. The dermis is the middle layer and contains connective tissue, nerves, blood, and lymphatic vessels. The innermost layer is the dermis, which merges with subcutaneous tissue containing adipose tissue that stores energy, regulates body heat, and acts as a cushion. The skin has more than 10 physiologic functions. An alteration of the anatomic and physiologic functions results in a wound.

TABLE 11–1. PHYSIOLOGIC FUNCTIONS OF THE SKIN

Protection
Insulation
Sensation
Excretion
Communication
Preservation of internal fluids
Production of vitamin D
Storage for calories
Provision of shape and substance to the body

Section One Review

1. Which of the following is NOT a layer of the skin?
   A. epithelial tissue
   B. epidermis
   C. dermis
   D. subcutaneous tissue

2. The components of the dermis are
   A. epithelial cells, subcutaneous tissue
   B. adipose tissue, subcutaneous tissue
   C. hair, nails, and sebaceous glands
   D. connective tissue, blood and lymph vessels

3. The physiologic functions of the skin include
   A. secretion, production of vitamin C
   B. excretion, production of vitamin D
   C. storage of information, communication
   D. regulation of body temperature, storage of vitamin A

4. Wound healing begins
   A. within an hour after injury
   B. within 6 hours after injury
   C. at the moment of injury
   D. within 24 hours of injury

Answers: 1, A. 2, D. 3, B. 4, C.

Section Two: Wound Biology

At the completion of this section, the learner will be able to state the three phases of wound healing, describe the events that occur in each phase of wound healing, and define the three methods of wound closure.

A wound disrupts the skin's integrity and its physiologic mechanisms. On injury, the body immediately begins the process of restoring its integrity and the physiologic functions of the skin. A basic understanding of the wound healing process helps to assess, diagnose, plan, and evaluate nursing interventions for the patient with alteration in skin integrity.

Wound healing is a process that includes an integrated series of physiologic, cellular, and biochemical events that begin at the moment of injury. There are three phases of wound healing: reaction, regeneration, and remodeling (Hess and Miller, 1990).

Reaction

The reaction phase occurs immediately after injury and can last up to 4 days after injury. The major events that occur in this phase are hemostasis and removal of cellular debris and infectious agents.

Immediately on injury, vascular and cellular events are initiated. Any tissue injury results in altered integrity of blood vessel walls. Vasoconstriction occurs for the first 5 to 10 minutes in an attempt to achieve hemostasis. Platelets aggregate at the injury site to form a plug to seal the break in the vessel wall. Once hemostasis is achieved, the blood vessels dilate to bring needed nutrients, chemicals and white blood cells (WBCs) to the injured area. WBCs quickly adhere to the endothelium and begin to control any bacterial contamination that has gained entry into the wound. Macrophages appear and begin to engulf and remove dead tissue. The chemical and vascular events that occur during the reaction phase of wound

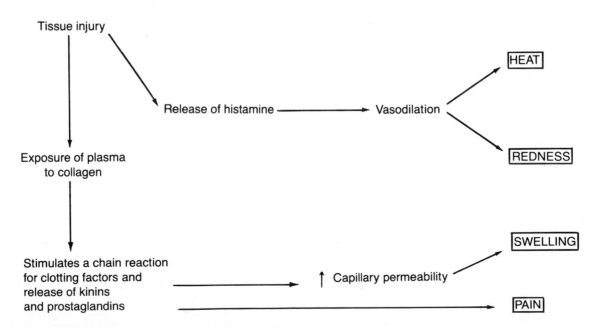

Figure 11–2. Basic inflammatory response to the four cardinal signs of inflammation. The chemical and vascular events that occur during the reaction phase of wound healing produce the four cardinal signs of inflammation.

healing produce the four cardinal signs of inflammation: heat, redness, swelling, and pain (Figure 11–2).

Regeneration

The regeneration phase occurs 4 to 24 days after injury. Major events that occur during this phase include epithelialization, collagen formation, granulation tissue formation, and contraction.

Epithelialization involves the migration of epithelial cells across a wound's surface. The cells rapidly undergo mitotic divisions and migrate along fibrin strands to reestablish layers of epithelium in an attempt to cover the defect. A moist environment enhances epithelialization. Epithelial cells cannot spread on surface laden with debris or bacteria. Therefore, the wound healing process will be inhibited by the presence of debris or bacteria. The process of epithelialization serves to provide a barrier against the external environment and further bacterial invasion.

As the epithelial surface thickens, fibroblasts appear in the wound. Fibroblasts produce collagen, the major component of new connective tissue. Fluid collections, hematomas, dead tissue, and foreign materials act as physical barriers to prevent fibroblast penetration. Therefore, removal of these materials is one of the primary goals of wound management (Section Five). The wound space fills with fiber bundles that enlarge and form a dense collagenous structure (the scar) that binds the tissues firmly together.

As the population of fibroblasts decreases, collagen fibers become dominant in the wound. Collagen requires several nutrients and minerals for its synthesis. Thus, the nutritional status of the patient becomes very important during wound healing. This is discussed in greater detail in Section Three.

At the same time that epithelialization is occurring and collagen is forming, granulation tissue also is forming. The vascular endothelium proliferates, and a great deal of capillary budding appears. These buds give the new granulation tissue its characteristic pink-red color and appearance. As new granulation tissue fills in the wound, the wound margins begin to contract or pull together, and the surface area of the wound decreases (Hess and Miller, 1990).

Contraction of a wound occurs when the wound margins begin to pull toward the center of the wound to decrease the wound surface area. Shrinkage of the wound progresses from the wound's edges to heal open defects.

Remodeling

Usually, by the third week after a disruption in skin integrity, the wound has closed, and remodeling, re-

organization, and cell differentiation begin (Hotter, 1982). The final repair process is remodeling. This phase lasts 24 days to up to 2 years. Major events of this final phase include increased collagen reorganization and increased tensile strength. The final product of all the events that occur during wound healing is the scar, which has covered the defect and restored the protective barrier against the external environment.

Methods of Wound Closure

The rate of wound healing differs depending on the method used to close the wound. The method used depends on the amount of tissue damage/loss and the potential for wound infection. Methods of wound closure include primary intention, secondary intention, and delayed primary intention (Figure 11–3).

Primary intention refers to closing the wound by mechanical means, by either sutures or tape. This method is used when there is minimal tissue loss, and skin edges are well approximated. Clean lacerations and most surgical incisions are closed using primary intention. The reaction phase resolves immediately, the regeneration phase is minimal, and

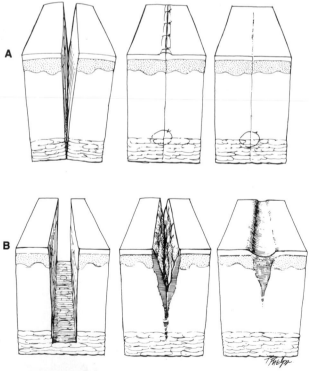

Figure 11–3. Methods of wound closure. Two methods of wound closure include primary intention (**A**) and secondary intention (**B**). (*From Trauma nursing: From resuscitation through rehabilitation, p. 275, edited by V.D. Cardona et al, 1988, Philadelphia: W.B. Saunders Co.*)

the remodeling phase is complete with a thin scar (Hess and Miller, 1990).

Wounds that heal by secondary intention usually are large wounds in which there is significant tissue loss, damage or bacterial contamination. These wound cavities heal gradually and use the biologic phases of wound healing to fill in the cavity or defect. Healing occurs by granulation, contraction, and epithelialization. Epithelialization is promoted through the use of dressing changes to provide moisture and debridement until contraction is complete.

Delayed primary intention is a method of wound closure that uses a combination of primary and secondary intention. The wound is left open for a short period of time, usually a few days, to allow edema and exudate to resolve. The wound is packed with dressings that are changed to remove any debris and is closed later by primary intention.

The expected outcome of the wound healing process is restoration of the skin and tissue integrity and its physiologic functions. The wound healing process is dependent on various factors that affect the efficiency and effectiveness of all events in the process. The next section discusses these factors.

In summary, wound healing is a complex process of events that begin at the moment of injury and continue for years after injury. These are three phases of wound healing. The first phase is the reaction phase, which lasts a few days. Hemostasis and removal of cellular debris and infectious agents are the goals of this phase. The second phase, which lasts 4 to 24 days, is the regeneration phase. Major events in this phase include epithelialization, collagen formation, formation of granulation tissue, and wound contraction. The final phase of wound healing, the remodeling phase, can last up to 2 years. During the final phase, collagen reorganization and increased tensile strength of the scar occur. The three methods of wound closure include primary, secondary, and delayed primary intention. The rate of wound healing differs depending on the method used to close the wound. An understanding of the wound healing process helps to assess, diagnose, plan, and evaluate nursing interventions to facilitate the wound healing process.

Section Two Review

1. Heat, redness, swelling, and pain occur during which of the following phases of wound healing?
   A. remodeling
   B. contraction
   C. regeneration
   D. reaction
2. Epithelialization
   A. is enhanced by a moist environment
   B. is enhanced by a dry, sterile environment
   C. occurs to remove debris
   D. spreads on surfaces laden with debris
3. Fluid collections, hematomas, and dead tissue act as
   A. scaffolds for fibroblast proliferation
   B. barriers for fibroblast proliferation
   C. protective covers for new epithelial cells
   D. a moist environment to enhance epithelialization

4. An incision for a cholecystectomy usually would be allowed to heal by
   A. delayed primary intention
   B. secondary intention
   C. primary intention
   D. delayed secondary intention
5. Delayed primary intention allows
   A. immediate resolution of the reaction phase
   B. edema and exudate to resolve
   C. for gradual healing of the wound
   D. reorganization and cell differentiation for remodeling

Answers: 1, D. 2, A. 3, B. 4, C. 5, B.

Section Three: Factors That Affect Wound Healing

At the completion of this section, the learner will be able to state physiologic and environmental factors that affect wound healing.

Generally, there are no treatments or medications that accelerate the wound healing process. However, there are factors that affect the efficiency and effectiveness of the process of wound healing. It is important for the nurse to assess the patient in relation to these factors to optimize the restoration of skin integrity.

Oxygenation/Tissue Perfusion

Many drugs and treatments have been investigated to accelerate healing. However, perfusion of injured tissue with well-oxygenated blood has been found to be most important (Hunt, 1989). A decrease in available oxygen to wounded tissues produces three major effects: (1) decrease in fibroblast reproduction rate, (2) decrease in the rate of epithelial cell reproduction, and (3) decrease in the rate of collagen synthesis and, subsequently, wound tensile strength (Epifanio, 1988). There are many conditions that can interfere with the delivery of oxygen to the wound, e.g., thrombosis, radiation, obesity, diabetes, cardiovascular disease, cigarette smoking, hypotension, hypothermia, and administration of vasoactive drugs. Smoking not only causes peripheral vasoconstriction but also alters platelet function in the wound healing process. Significant blood loss, as frequently occurs in traumatically injured patients, results in hypovolemia, hypotension, and decreased tissue perfusion. Perfusion is influenced by adequate circulating blood volume. An insufficient amount of oxygen carrying hemoglobin affects wound healing.

Nutrition

Metabolic processes involved in wound healing rely heavily on adequate nutritional substances. Physiologic and psychologic stress, traumatic injury, and fever further increase the basal metabolic rate, demanding adequate nutritional reserves. Because of these demands, malnutrition in the critically ill patient is not uncommon. A sufficient amount of protein is one of the most important nutritional substances for wound healing. Protein is required for collagen synthesis, immune responses, formation of granulation tissue, and fibroblast proliferation. Glycolysis contributes 70 percent of the energy needed for restoring tissue integrity and fighting infection (Hotter, 1982). Fats serve as building blocks

for prostaglandins, which regulate cell metabolism, inflammation, and circulation. Vitamins and trace elements are necessary for numerous events in the tissue healing and rebuilding process.

Age

It is generally believed that advancing age adversely affects wound healing. Circulation fibroblast activity, and collagen synthesis are diminished in the elderly (Smith and Cuzzell, 1988). In addition to the physiologic effects of aging, the elderly are more likely to have nutritional deficiencies, pulmonary or cardiovascular diseases, that further diminish local oxygenation to wounds, and immunologic resistance.

Diabetes

Diabetics, particularly those who are not well controlled, are particularly at risk for failure of their wounds to close (Hotter, 1982). Small vessel vascular changes occur in diabetic people that impair tissue perfusion and oxygenation. Hyperglycemia inhibits leukocyte phagocytosis.

Blood Chemistries

Normal serum electrolytes enhance wound repair. Potassium is necessary for building proteins for wound repair. Phagocytosis is inhibited by acidosis and elevated sodium and glucose levels.

Temperature

Hypothermia and its resultant vasoconstriction decrease blood supply and oxygen to wounds. WBCs become less active in lower temperatures.

Moisture

Moisture enhances epithelial growth. However, too much moisture provides an optimal medium for bacterial proliferation. In too dry an environment, granulation tissue is inhibited by fibrous tissue and heavy scabs.

Medications

Steroid therapy has a well-known inhibitory effect on wound healing. Decreased protein synthesis, delayed development of granulation tissue, inhibition of fibroblast proliferation, and reduced epithelialization are effects of steroid administration. In addition, inhibition of the inflammatory response and the immunosuppressive actions of steroids make the patient more susceptible to developing a wound infection.

Obesity

Obese patients have greater amounts of adipose tissue. Fatty tissue is poorly vascularized and is frequently the most common site of infection (Hunt, 1989). Adipose tissue is difficult to suture, which makes the obese patient at risk to develop a wound dehiscence.

Antibiotics and Infection

Traumatic wounds tend to be contaminated by the external environment. The administration of antibiotics greatly affects the outcome of healing. These two factors are so important to wound healing that they are discussed in greater detail in the next section.

In summary, there are no medications or treatments to accelerate wound healing. There are conditions and factors known to affect the wound healing process. Perfusion of well-oxygenated blood to the wound is considered to be the most important factor affecting wound healing. It is important for the nurse to assess patients for any factor that may affect wound healing. Appropriate plans and nursing interventions must be instituted to manipulate as many variables as possible to promote efficient and effective wound healing.

Section Three Review

1. Small vessel changes occur that impair tissue perfusion/oxygenation with
   A. malnutrition
   B. elevated sodium levels
   C. diabetes
   D. steroid therapy
2. The most important nutritional substance for wound healing is
   A. glucose
   B. fat
   C. vitamins
   D. protein
3. Which of the following is NOT an effect of steroid therapy on wound healing?
   A. decreased protein synthesis
   B. proliferation of fibroblasts
   C. delayed development of granulation tissue
   D. reduced epithelialization

4. The most important factor that affects wound healing is
   A. preventing infection
   B. total parenteral nutrition
   C. perfusion of injured tissues with well-oxygenated blood
   D. potassium replacements
5. Seventy percent of the energy needed for restoring skin integrity and fighting infection comes from
   A. glycolysis
   B. gluconeogenesis
   C. protein catabolism
   D. fats

Answers: 1, C. 2, D. 3, B. 4, C. 5, A.

Section Four: Etiology, Prevention, and Treatment of Wound Infections

At the completion of this section, the learner will be able to identify conditions that predispose a patient to develop a wound infection, identify criteria used to diagnose a wound as being infected, and describe interventions that may be used in preventing and treating wound infections.

Infection is a common and very effective deter-rent to effective wound healing. Any disruption of, or compromise to, the skin's integrity can result in infection. These events include physical trauma, operative and invasive procedures, and inadequate tissue perfusion (Hoyt, 1988). A wound infection develops when the body's defense mechanisms cannot eliminate the bacteria contaminating the wound or prevent further bacterial growth. Three elements predispose the patient to developing a wound infection: (1) a susceptible host, (2) a compromised wound, and (3) an infectious organism.

Susceptible Host

One of the major determinants of the subsequent infection after surgery or trauma is the patient's own ability to use defense mechanisms to resist the threat of infection. The patient who is a susceptible host has some degree of local or systemic impairment of resistance to bacterial invasion. Local impairment may be due to dead, foreign material or hematomas directly in the wound or some interference in blood supply to the area as a result of vascular disease. Systemic impairment of the patient's resistance may include diabetes, acute or chronic use of steroids, renal disease, malnutrition, cardiovascular disease, extremes of age, obesity, cancer, or the use of immunosuppressive therapies (Tobin, 1984). These patients usually have some impairment in the acute inflammatory response or phagocytic mechanisms. Any patient with altered skin integrity has lost the major mechanical barrier blocking invasion by pathologic organisms and, thus, is a susceptible host.

Compromised Wound

A compromised wound is one that contains devitalized tissue. Devitalized tissue is tissue that has been separated from the circulation and the body's antimicrobial defenses (Stevenson and Mathes, 1988). Bacteria proliferate on wounds that contain dead tissue, hematomas, or foreign material. Debridement of these materials is essential to prevent an environment conducive to bacterial growth.

Infectious Organism

Bacteria can contaminate any wound. Many different organisms are capable of initiating a wound infection. Organisms come from endogenous or exogenous sources. Endogenous sources arise from within the patient. Many organisms exist on and in the human body, on the skin, in the respiratory tract, in the gastrointestinal or genitourinary tracts. Organisms in these areas are not pathogenic until they are released from their normal inhabitant sites and allowed to proliferate in a sterile area of the body. Exogenous organisms enter the body from the external environment when the skin barrier has been broken. The external environment may be the accident scene (for trauma patients) or the health care setting.

The presence of an organism in a wound does not necessarily mean there is a wound infection. It is generally accepted that wounds can handle 100,000 bacterial organisms per gram of tissue (Robson, 1988). Infectious organisms cause clinical injury or damage to the wound when there are sufficient numbers of organisms with sufficient virulence in a susceptible host with a compromised wound.

Classification of Wounds

Classification of surgical procedures permits a more accurate assessment of the likelihood of developing wound infections. Based on this assessment, the need for further preventive measures to reduce the chance of infection can be determined. The classification system as defined by Burdon (1982) is as follows.

Class I	Clean surgical procedure: Surgical procedure in which the gastrointestinal, respiratory, and urinary tracts are not opened, and no inflammation is encountered.
Class II	Clean-contaminated surgical procedure: An operation in which the gastrointestinal tract, respiratory tract, or female genital tract is opened but no significant bacterial spillage from these tracts occurs.
Class III	Contaminated surgical procedure: An operation where significant bacterial spillage has occurred from a viscus that is colonized by bacteria. Appreciable contamination occurs whenever a viscus containing bacteria is incised even though no appreciable spillage is observed.
Class IV	Dirty surgical procedure: Surgical procedure where purulent material is encountered during surgery or when a viscus that is colonized by bacteria has been perforated.

In a prospective study of over 40,000 surgical wound infections, Cruse (1975) found that the incidence of infection was clearly related to the degree of bacterial contamination to which the wounds were exposed (Table 11–2).

TABLE 11–2. INCIDENCE OF INFECTIONS IN SURGICAL PROCEDURES

Procedure Classification	Incidence of Infection (%)
Class I	1.8
Class II	9.1
Class III	18.4
Class IV	41.8
Overall	5.1

Prevention of Wound Infections

One of the greatest priorities in wound care is prevention of infection. Prevention of wound infections begins with recognition of the three elements that predispose the patient to a wound infection (susceptible host, compromised wound, infectious organism) and knowledge of the classification of surgical procedures and wounds.

For elective surgical procedures, prevention begins preoperatively through skin preparation, mechanical and antibiotic bowel preparations, prophylactic administration of antibiotics, and sterile operative site draping. Intraoperatively, careful surgical technique minimizes injury, and aseptic technique prevents endogenous and exogenous sources of bacterial contamination.

For traumatically injured wounds, resuscitation and life-saving measures often take priority over immediate treatment of wounds. Once the resuscitative phase is completed, prompt and proper management of the wounds decreases the likelihood of subsequent infection. It is not uncommon for traumatically incurred wounds to be filled with dirt, grass, glass, twigs, leaves, knives, bullets, or stool. The presence of these and other environmental materials is important to assess as predictors of infective risk. The golden period of wound management is considered to be 6 to 12 hours postinjury (Epifanio, 1988). Wounds treated within this period have a better likelihood of healing without infection. Management of these wounds begins in the emergency department or operating room with cleansing of the wounds using high pressure irrigation and debridement to remove bacteria and foreign debris from the wounds.

The importance of handwashing to prevent the transmission of infectious organisms was determined over a century ago. Handwashing is still considered one of the most important methods to prevent wound infections (Schimpff et al, 1989). This is especially important in critical care settings where susceptible hosts, compromised wounds, and infectious organisms are in close proximity to each other.

Treatment of Wound Infections

Wound infections range from superficial cases of cellulitis to deep-seated abscesses. A wound infection is suspected if the four cardinal signs of inflammation (heat, redness, swelling, and pain) exist at the wound site, along with an elevated WBC count and fever. However, many conditions may cause these symptoms, including the inflammatory phase of wound healing. In addition, drainage from a wound does not mean it is infected. The patient's overall condition and a positive wound culture are more definitive criteria to evaluate a wound for infection. Any drainage from a wound must be sent to the laboratory for culture and sensitivity testing and gram stain. The culture and sensitivity testing will identify the specific organisms in the wound and antibiotic sensitivity of the organisms. The gram stain characterizes the nature of the drainage and provides a rapid best guess as to the identity of the organism, gram-positive or gram-negative. The culture and sensitivity testing takes 24 to 72 hours for results, which are very reliable and specific. The gram stain takes only several hours, but the results are not as specific.

Bacterial organisms contaminating wounds must be sensitive to the antibiotic administered. However, as previously stated, it may take up to 3 days to obtain this information. Thus, a knowledge of the likely wound contaminants and their established sensitivities is helpful in instituting prompt treatment. For example, organisms in the colon that have leaked into the peritoneum and are likely to cause infections in wounds in the abdomen are anaerobic organisms (bacteroides, clostridia, *Escherichia coli*), which respond to aminoglycosides. *E. coli* is most commonly found in septic wounds after colon operations or injury (Schmipff et al, 1989).

Wound infections may not be apparent until the second to seventh day postoperatively or after traumatic injury (Smith and Caswell, 1988). When a wound infection is suspected, prompt and appropriate treatment should be instituted.

In summary, it is imperative that the nurse recognize the importance of nursing's role in preventing wound infections and preventing further bacterial proliferation in already infected wounds. Nursing plans and interventions should optimize the environment to promote wound healing. Each patient must be assessed as a susceptible host for pathogenic organisms, and interventions must be instituted to promote and safeguard the patient's ability to resist infection. Astute nursing assessments can identify a compromised wound. Measures can be taken to prevent the wound from being an ideal environment for bacterial invasion and proliferation. Knowledge of the classification of surgical wounds permits the nurse to assess for the likelihood of development of a wound infection. Plans for prophylactic interventions to reduce the infective risk can be made. Ongoing nursing assessments can detect signs of infection so that prompt and appropriate treatment can be instituted.

Section Four Review

1. Which of the following would NOT predispose to the development of a wound infection?
   A. susceptible host
   B. exogenous organisms
   C. compromised wound
   D. infectious organism
2. Local impairment of resistance to bacterial invasion may be due to
   A. foreign material
   B. malnutrition
   C. cancer
   D. immunosuppressive drugs
3. Organisms from endogenous sources come from
   A. debris in the wound
   B. the accident scene
   C. the gastrointestinal tract
   D. the hospital setting

4. A surgical procedure performed for a perforated viscus would carry an incidence of infection of approximately
   A. 1.8 percent
   B. 9.1 percent
   C. 41.8 percent
   D. 75 percent
5. Which of the following diagnose a wound as being infected?
   A. purulent drainage from a wound
   B. culture and sensitivity testing
   C. the four cardinal signs of inflammation
   D. temperature of 103F

Answers: 1, B. 2, A. 3, C. 4, C. 5, B.

Section Five: Principles of Wound Management

The purpose of this section is to assist the learner in understanding treatment modalities and principles of wound management. At the completion of this section, the learner will be able to state the rationale for wound irrigation, debridement, and dressing changes and identify tube and drain placement and their indications for use in wound management.

Nursing has a major influence on the outcome of wound healing. When providing wound care, it is imperative that the wound healing process and the effectiveness of the wound management regimen be evaluated.

Irrigation

The purpose of irrigating a wound is to remove debris and bacterial contamination by the pressure in a stream of fluid (Epifanio, 1988). The wound should be irrigated with a solution under pressure. It is not the volume of the solution used but the pressure exerted that removes debris and bacteria. Solution in a 30 mL syringe can accomplish this. Irrigation can remove enough bacteria to cross the threshold to non-infective levels.

Disinfectant solutions (hydrogen peroxide, povidone-iodine) may be used as irrigating solutions. Hydrogen peroxide is used to irrigate wounds to loosen dead or dying tissue. It should be rinsed thoroughly away with normal saline (Neuberger and Reckling, 1985). Povidone-iodine (Betadine) is an antiseptic that kills bacteria and fungi. However, this solution has been shown to damage granulation tissue and irritate intact skin around the wound (Hess and Miller, 1990). Normal saline is the most commonly used and recommended solution for wound irrigation. It aids in mechanical debridement and does not damage granulation tissue.

Debridement

Wound bacteria proliferate in necrotic tissue and wound debris. The physician can debride the wound surgically, or the wound can be debrided mechanically during dressing changes. Large areas of necrotic tissue are removed more effectively by manual means. Smaller areas are debrided with dressing changes as the debris and bacteria entwine around the mesh of a gauze and are removed with the dressing change.

Dressings

Dressings are placed over wounds for multiple purposes: debridement, protection from the external environment, provision of a physiologic environment conducive to wound healing, and to provide immo-

TABLE 11–3. WOUND DRESSINGS

Type	Indication	Considerations
Wet to dry Put on wet and remove dry	Use with wounds healing by secondary intention Removes debris and necrotic materials from wounds, use as a debriding alternative	No solution should be visibly dripping from the dressing as it is placed into the wound; this retards wound closure, increases bacteria, and macerates periwound skin Gauze touching wound surfaces should be a single layer; wounds with large amounts of exudate should be dressed with gauze with large interstices; as exudate decreases, gauze with small interstices should be used If gauze is removed too dry, newly formed granulation tissue may be disrupted
Wet to damp Put on moist and remove moist	Use with wound healing by secondary intention Provides moist wound environment Absorbs debris and drainage	Packing material is soaked in a solution, wrung out until moist, and packed into the wound If packing sticks to tissue as it is removed, wet the packing with normal saline before removing it; this will preserve regenerating tissue
Dry Put on dry and remove dry	Used with wounds healing by primary intention Protects the wound during epithelialization	Carefully remove the dressing so that the incision does not reopen
Synthetic	Cutaneous wounds Minor burns Abrasions Donor sites	Requires dressing changes every 3–5 days
Hydrocolloid	Protect granulation and epithelial tissue Liquify necrotic tissue	Is water resistant and can adhere to uneven surfaces Do not use on documented or suspected infected wounds Change when it leaks, becomes dislodged, or develops an odor

bilization, support, comfort, information regarding quality and quantity of drainage, pressure, and absorption.

The type and care of the dressing play a major role in promoting effective wound healing. The purpose of the dressing must be considered carefully before a dressing is chosen for wound management. Specific types of dressings and their care and considerations are summarized in Table 11–3.

Dressings covering wounds healing by primary intention should have three layers. The layer covering the sutures and skin should be nonadhering to prevent disruption of new epithelial cells and act as a wick to remove any drainage from the incision. The layer over this should be spongy to absorb any drainage. The outer layer, which is taped, provides additional protection and strength in immobilizing the incision until the healing process is underway. These dressings usually are not removed for the first 24 hours postoperatively. If drainage seeps through to the outer layer of the dressing, a fourth layer is placed as reinforcement. Between 5 and 7 days after suturing, the accumulation of inflammatory cells and fibroblasts forms a ridge along the incision line, indicating that healing has taken place (Sieggreen, 1987).

Dressings covering wounds healing by secondary intention and delayed primary intention also should have three layers of dressing materials. The first layer is packed into the wound using a large mesh gauze dressing that has been soaked in a solution. The purpose of packing a wound is to provide a moist environment conducive to epithelialization and to remove debris and bacteria. Solutions frequently used are listed in Table 11–4. The gauze initially is soaked in a solution and wrung out until it is damp. The gauze is then unfolded and fluffed to promote maximum wound bed contact and aborption. Debris and bacteria entwine around the gauze mesh. When this dressing dries out, within 4 to 6 hours, the dressing is removed. As it is removed debridement occurs. The gauze should not be packed too tightly in a wound bed, since this inhibits the wound edges from contracting, and it also compresses wound capillaries, which then restrict the flow of oxygenated blood to the wound (Hess and Miller, 1990). Pack only to the edge of the wound, not over the wound edges, since this can cause maceration of the periwound skin.

After packing the wound with the first layer, apply a second layer. This layer should be dry sterile

TABLE 11–4. SOLUTIONS FOR WET TO DRY OR WET TO MOIST DRESSINGS

Normal saline	Most commonly used solution Aids in mechanical debridement Does not damage granulation tissue
Acetic acid	Used to treat Pseudomonas infections
Dakin's solution	Chlorine bleach compound; use in a weak solution Antiseptic that slightly dissolves necrotic tissue Can be used in dirty, malodorous wounds Can inhibit growth of granulation tissue
Betadine	Antiseptic that kills bacteria and fungi Used to pack dirty or infected wounds May damage granulation tissue and irritate periwound skin Use in diluted concentrations
Antibiotic solutions	Antibiotics in a solution that are applied topically Commonly used solutions are neomycin or bacitracin

gauze and should conform to the shape of the wound and absorb any drainage not contained in the first layer. The third layer is the outer dressing. This layer supports and protects the wound and keeps the packing in place.

Synthetic dressings, such as polyurethane film (Op-Site, Tegaderm), are semipermeable membranes that allow visualization of wounds. These dressings are occlusive but permeable to oxygen and require less frequent changes (usually every 3 to 5 days). Synthetic dressings are effective for use over cutaneous wounds, minor burns, abrasions, and donor sites (Flynn and Rovee, 1982).

Hydrocolloid dressing (DuoDERM, ConvaTec) are occlusive wafers made of a gumlike material, such as pectin or karaya. The gumlike material is covered with a flexible, water resistant outer layer. When fluid from the wound interacts with the hydrocolloid material, a gel-like substance is formed, which keeps the wound surface moist and promotes healing. Hydrocolloid dressings are changed every 24 to 72 hours. These dressings should not be used on documented or suspected wound infections, since the dressing creates an oxygen-deficient environment beneath the dressing that can potentiate anaerobic bacterial growth (Fowler et al, 1991).

Tubes and Drains

Various surgical tubes and drains are used whenever there is an actual or potential accumulation of fluid in naturally occurring or surgically created spaces. Drainage tubes can be classified into one of three categories: simple drains, closed suction drains, or sump drains (Amato, 1982). The categories and uses of drainage tubes are summarized in Table 11–5.

It is the nurse's responsibility to maintain the security, integrity, and patency of all tubes and drains.

In summary, nursing has a major influence on the outcome of wound healing through assessing the effectiveness of the wound management regimen. A wound management regimen may include debridement, irrigation, dressing changes, and placement of tubes and drains. Dressings are used in wound management for a multitude of purposes. The method of wound closure plays a large role in determining the type of dressing to be used in the regimen. Consideration must be made as to the solution to be used to irrigate, debride, or dress the wound. Various tubes and drains are used in wound management whenever there is an actual or potential accumulation of fluid.

TABLE 11–5. CATEGORIES AND USES OF DRAINAGE TUBES

Category	Purpose	Examples
Simple drains	Provide pathway to allow fluid to drain by gravity	Penrose, T-tube, gastrostomy tube, jejunostomy tube
Closed suction drains	Collapsible device attached to tube creates a negative pressure, allowing for continual removal of fluids	Jackson Pratt, Hemovac, Davol
Sump drains	Double-lumen drains; air enters drainage area and breaks the vacuum, displacing air and fluid into the outflow lumen; used in conjunction with wall suction	Salem Sump, Shirley Sump, Axion

Section Five Review

1. What size syringe would you select to irrigate a wound?
   A. 30 mL syringe
   B. 50 mL syringe
   C. 60 mL syringe
   D. 100 mL syringe
2. What type of dressing would be indicated to cover a wound healing by primary intention?
   A. dry
   B. wet to wet
   C. wet to dry
   D. polyurethane
3. The layer next to the wound in wet to dry dressings
   A. should adhere to the wound to prevent disruption of epithelial layers
   B. provides protection and strength in immobilizing the wound
   C. debrides the wound
   D. should be put on wet so the wound remains soupy

4. A solution used to treat *Pseudomonas* wound infections is
   A. Dakin's solution
   B. acetic acid
   C. Betadine
   D. half-strength hydrogen peroxide
5. An example of a closed suction drain would be
   A. gastrostomy tube
   B. Salem Sump
   C. Penrose
   D. Hemovac

Answers: 1, A. 2, A. 3, C. 4, B. 5, D.

Section Six: Clinical Assessment of Wound Healing

At the completion of this section, the learner will be able to identify the common clinical assessments to evaluate wound healing.

In assessing wound healing, it is important to assess the patient's preexisting health problems, perform a physical assessment of the wound using inspection and palpation, and collect and assess objective data to assess the patient's tissue perfusion/oxygenation and immunologic and nutritional status.

Preexisting Health Problems

In collecting the initial nursing database, it is important to assess the patient for diseases, conditions, and medications or treatments that may impair the healing process. This will assist in detecting patients at risk for delayed wound healing. It is important to assess for conditions that alter tissue perfusion/oxygenation and impair the body's resistance to infection.

Physical Examination

Physical examination of all wounds includes inspection, palpation, evaluation, and documentation (Epifanio, 1988). Evaluation of the progress, or lack of progress, the wound is making should be made with every dressing change.

Inspection

Wounds, suture lines, casts, pins, and surrounding skin integrity should be inspected for signs of infection, breakdown, and irritation. Inspect wounds to assess and evaluate the healing process and the effectiveness of wound care. Inspection should include at least the following components.

Measurement of the Wound

Measure and record the length, width, and depth of the wound. A diagram should be made in the nursing care plan for ongoing comparison of the healing process. The amount and depth of tissue loss should be assessed, since this greatly influences the choice of treatment for wound management. Depth can be determined by inserting a sterile cotton tip applicator into the deepest part of the wound and grasping the applicator where it meets the wound's edge (Hess and Miller, 1990).

Presence of Exudate or Drainage

Estimating the amount of blood and fluid loss allows for appropriate fluid and electrolyte replacement. Draining wounds produce exudate that can consist of blood, serum, pus, serosanguineous fluid, or other body fluids, including ascitic fluid, bile, feces, urine, and gastrointestinal secretions. Drainage of these body secretions from wounds usually is indicative of an anastomotic leak or development of a fistula. Documentation of all wound drainage should include color, amount, consistency, and odor. Inspect the wound dressing as it is removed from the wound. If the dressing is too dry, reevaluate how moist the packing was at the time of insertion or increase the frequency of dressing changes. If the outer layer of the dressing becomes saturated, consider increasing the frequency of dressing changes (Hess and Miller, 1990).

Appearance of Wound Tissue

Inspect the wound for the presence of foreign materials and necrotic tissue. Slough is moist, stringy, thick, yellow or tan tissue that is dying. Eschar is black, hard, dehydrated tissue (Hess and Miller, 1990). The presence of such tissue will require surgical or mechanical debridement. Assess the tissue for red-pink granulation tissue with its characteristic budding appearance.

Inspection of Wound Edges

Inspect the wound for contraction (gradual healing from the edges of the wound to the center of the wound), and assess for gradual healing from the interior to the surfaces of deep wounds. Wound margins should not be erythematous or tender.

Skin Color

Using a bright light, observe the wound and surrounding tissues for color. Compare the color with similar, uninjured areas. Distinguish erythema from ecchymosis by blanching the area. Areas of erythema will blanch, but areas of ecchymosis will not.

Palpation

Palpation of the wound and surrounding areas will assist in recognizing changes in size, consistency, moisture, and texture. To assess circulation into and from the wound, assess the proximal and distal pulses by palpation or by Doppler (auditory pulse). Proximal pulses demonstrate adequate circulation to the area. Distal pulses indicate that the wound is not interfering with distal circulation. Capillary refill time should be assessed and compared to the norm of less than 2 seconds. Compare the skin temperature bilaterally. Sensorimotor assessment distal to the wound can be done by testing for discrimination between sharp and dull.

Assessment of Tissue Perfusion/Oxygenation

Adequate tissue perfusion/oxygenation is one of the most important factors to assess for in wound healing. Local and systemic factors that alter tissue perfusion and oxygenation should be assessed. Necrotic areas, debris, and foreign materials in the wound do not allow adequate local tissue perfusion/oxygenation. Adequate systemic tissue perfusion/oxygenation is dependent on a full blood volume, adequate arterial oxygen content, and an adequate CO. Tissue perfusion/oxygenation can be assessed using invasive and noninvasive techniques. Noninvasive techniques include transcutaneous oximetry, assessment of capillary refill, skin temperature, and the presence of proximal and distal pulses around the wound. Invasive techniques may include hemodynamic readings, such as central venous pressure, CO/CI, arterial blood pressure, mean arterial pressure, pulmonary artery wedge pressure, and systemic vascular resistance. In addition, serum blood tests, including hematocrit and hemoglobin levels, should be monitored and assessed.

Assessment of Immunologic Status

An intact immunologic response to injury, irregardless of the cause of injury, is a key factor in proper wound healing. The patient should be assessed for the three elements that predispose the patient to a wound infection: susceptible host, compromised wound, and infectious organism. Factors that cause local and systemic resistance of infection (Section Four) should be assessed. Compromised wounds containing devitalized tissue, hematomas, and debris should be debrided to prevent an environment conducive to bacterial proliferation. The patient should be assessed for sources of pathogenic organisms.

Assessment of immunologic status should include at least the following.

White Blood Cell Count

The inflammatory phase of wound healing releases WBCs. It is not uncommon for patients with wounds to have WBC counts of 20,000 to 40,000 mm^3 during the initial phases of wound healing (Hoyt, 1988) as compared to a normal WBC count of less than 10,000 mm^3. Elevated WBC counts in later phases of wound healing are more indicative of an infectious process.

White Blood Cell Count Differential

Neutrophils are the primary cells involved in phagocytosis. Elevated neutrophil counts are indicative of an acute infection as mature and immature neutrophils are released in response to an increased need for phagocytosis. Neutrophils are essential in the presence of infection if wound healing is to occur.

Fibrinogen

Adequate amounts of fibrinogen are needed to convert to fibrin. This aids in localizing the infectious process by providing a matrix for phagocytosis.

Core Temperature

Body temperature, regulated by the hypothalamic thermoregulatory system, is triggered by microorganisms, bacterial toxins and antigens, and the inflammatory process. Since fever is a manifestation of the inflammatory process and the infectious process, it is important to assess the patient's overall clinical picture for etiologic factors of the fever. Patients in a hypothermic state experience decreased tissue perfusion/oxygenation and decreased leukocyte activity.

Wound Cultures

Wounds suspected as being infected should be sampled, and the samples of wound tissue should be sent to the laboratory for gram stain and culture and sensitivity testing. The nurse should be aware of all culture results.

Serum Antimicrobial Levels

Monitoring concentrations of antimicrobial agents in the blood can confirm therapeutic drug levels and determine toxicity. The best assessment of this can be made by drawing serum peak and trough samples. There are different protocols for when these samples are drawn, depending on the antimicrobial administered. The nurse must be aware of these protocols so that accurate therapeutic concentrations and toxicity can be assessed.

Assessment of Nutritional Status

The metabolic processes involved in wound healing rely on an adequate nutritional supply. Malnutrition affects the patient's ability to defend against pathogenic microorganisms. A complete and thorough nutritional assessment for all patients with altered skin and tissue integrity should be made. Nutritional assessment is discussed in detail in Module 16, *Nutrition*.

In summary, when assessing wound healing, it is important to assess the patient's preexisting health problems, oxygenation/perfusion, nutrition status, and immunologic status and to perform a physical assessment of the wound.

Section Six Review

1. In assessing wound healing, it is important to assess the patient's
   A. past medical history
   B. renal status
   C. mental status
   D. fluid and electrolyte balance

2. Physical examination of all wounds includes all of the following EXCEPT
   A. inspection
   B. palpation
   C. auscultation
   D. documentation

3. A noninvasive technique to assess tissue perfusion would be
   A. mean arterial pressure
   B. presence of proximal/distal pulses
   C. systemic vascular resistance
   D. hemoglobin levels
4. In early phases of wound healing, it is not uncommon for white blood cell counts to be
   A. 10,000–20,000 mm³
   B. 20,000–40,000 mm³
   C. 5,000–10,000 mm³
   D. 40,000–50,000 mm³

5. If a wound is suspected as being infected
   A. the WBC and core temperature will be high
   B. there will be exudate in the wound
   C. antimicrobial levels should be drawn
   D. wound cultures should be taken

Answers: 1, A. 2, C. 3, B. 4, B. 5, D.

Section Seven: Burn Wound Physiology

At the completion of this section, the learner will be able to state the mechanisms and pathophysiology of burn injuries and estimate the extent and degree of burn injury.

Mechanism of Injury

Burn injuries may occur by the following mechanisms: inhalation, thermal, electrical, or chemical contact. Inhalation burns cause injury to the respiratory system. Inhalation injury can result from inhalation of carbon monoxide, chemical toxins, or heat. Thermal burns, the most common mechanism of burn injury, are caused by heat or flames coming in contact with skin. Electrical burns result from contact with an electrical power source. Chemicals produce injury by exposure to strong acids or alkali.

Pathophysiology of Burn Injuries

Immediately after thermal burning, arterial and venous blood flow around the injury ceases. These vessels become permeable, and fluid, electrolytes, and proteins leak into the area of the wound. The inflammatory process is initiated. Local and systemic loss of fluid is tremendous, especially for burns greater than 30 percent of the body surface area (Baxter and Waeckerle, 1988). This loss of fluid leads to a systemic hypovolemic shock state.

The extent of damage caused by electrical burns is often much greater than it initially appears to be. The extent of injury is dependent on the duration of contact, intensity of current, resistance of the system, and the course that the electrical current travels through the body until it reaches a ground. Injury from high voltage usually results in an entry and exit wound. Both wounds usually are small and well circumscribed. Once through the entry site, the current travels through the body, damaging muscle, nerves, blood vessels, and bone, until it reaches a ground, at which time the current leaves the body and leaves an exit wound.

Chemical burns are the result of exposure to acid or alkaline solutions. Acidic solutions cause necrosis and loss of protein. Alkaline burns, generally more serious than aciditic burns, penetrate deeper into tissues and continue to produce tissue necrosis for several hours after contact (Baxter and Waeckerle, 1988).

Carbon monoxide (CO) gas may be inhaled during a fire. CO has a high affinity for hemoglobin and, as such, displaces oxygen from hemoglobin. Cellular tissues are deprived of oxygen, and hypoxia occurs. Thermal inhalation burns involve heat dissipating in the upper airways. Cellular and capillary damage lead to edema and potential airway obstruction. Inhalation of toxic agents destroys epithelial cells in the respiratory system and alveolar surfactant. The alveoli lose their distensibility, and normal gas exchange cannot occur. Atelectasis and edema result in adult respiratory distress syndrome (ARDS).

Classification of Burns

Burns are classified according to the extent of body surface area involved and the depth of injury. The extent of injury is expressed by the percentage of body surface burn in relation to the total body surface. A commonly used guide in determining the extent of injury is the rule of nines, as shown in Figure 11–4.

Traditionally, burns have been called as first, second, or third degree burns when describing the depth of burn injury (Baxter and Waeckerle, 1988) (Table 11–6). The depth of the burn often is difficult to

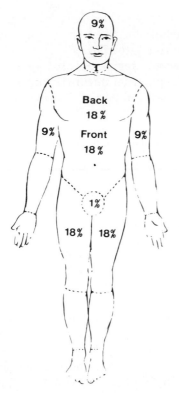

9%

Back
18%

9%   Front   9%
18%

1%

18%   18%

Figure 11–4. *The rule of nines.* The rule of nines helps determine the extent of injury expressed by the percentage of body surface area. (*From Trauma nursing: Principles and practice, p. 225, by B. Knezvich, 1986, E. Norwalk, Connecticut: Appleton-Century-Crofts.*)

TABLE 11–6. DESCRIPTION OF FIRST, SECOND, AND THIRD DEGREE BURNS

Degree of Burn	Description
First degree burn	Involves epidermis only Skin is hot, red, painful, no blisters
Second degree burn Partial thickness	Destruction of epidermis and portions of dermis
Superficial partial thickness	Involves epidermis and one half or less of dermis; blisters, blanching, extreme pain are present; skin is red and mottled
Deep partial thickness	Destruction of epidermis and deep dermal layers; skin is mottled, red/white, nonblanching, may or may not be painful
Third degree burn	Destruction of epidermis, dermis and portions of subcutaneous tissues; wound is white or charred, painless, no sensation, and skin is leathery in texture

toxic gases or heat causes injury to the respiratory system, causing atelectasis, edema, and airway obstruction. With thermal injury, blood flow around the burn ceases, the inflammatory process is initiated, and as a result, fluid loss can be tremendous. The extent of electrical burn damage can be misleading. Characteristic of electrical burns are entry and exit wounds. Chemical burns occur as a result of exposure to acidic or alkaline solutions. Burns are classified according to the extent of body surface area involved by using the rule of nines. Burns are described by the depth of a burn as first, second, or third degree burns.

assess initially. Repeated assessments over the course of several days are required.

In summary, burn injuries are the result of thermal, electrical, or chemical contacts. Inhalation of

Section Seven Review

1. Massive inflammatory response with local and systemic loss of fluid occurs with
   A. inhalation burns
   B. chemical burns
   C. thermal burns
   D. electrical burns
2. The extent of which burns is often much greater than initially assessed?
   A. thermal burns
   B. inhalation burns
   C. acidic burns
   D. electrical burns

3. Mr. R received flash burns to his anterior chest, right arm, and perineum. The estimated extent of his injury would be
   A. 50 percent
   B. 37 percent
   C. 28 percent
   D. 56 percent

4. A burn that penetrates deeply and continues to produce tissue necrosis for several hours after injury is most likely
   A. an acidic burn
   B. an alkaline burn
   C. an electrical burn
   D. a flash burn

5. White, charred, leathery textured wounds are the result of
   A. third degree burns
   B. second degree burns
   C. deep partial thickness burns
   D. superficial partial thickness burns

Answers: 1, C. 2, D. 3, C. 4, B. 5, A.

Section Eight: Burn Wound Management

At the completion of this section, the learner will be able to compare burn wound healing with other types of wound healing and state the principles of burn wound management.

Healing Process

The cellular and biochemical events that occur during the wound healing of burn injuries are similar to those that occur in the healing of other wounds. The major difference, however, is that the phases of wound healing in the burn wound occur more slowly or last longer. The inflammatory phase lasts longer, and thus overall wound repair is delayed. Neovascularization and collagen synthesis occur but, again, at a much slower rate than in wounds from other injuries. In addition, collagen layers are not as organized as they are in other wounds. Random layering of collagen occurs, which results in excessive scar tissue that produces the hypertrophic scars characteristic of second and third degree burns. Epithelialization is slowed due to the presence of necrotic tissue.

Principles of Burn Wound Management

Minor Burns

Burns involving a limited percentage of body surface area usually can be treated in the emergency department on an outpatient basis. Initial wound management of these burns focuses on the prevention of infection and additional trauma and minimizing scarring and contracture (Baxter and Waeckerle, 1988). Wound cultures should be taken.

The wound caused by thermal injury initially is cleansed using an irrigating solution. Surgical or mechanical debridement of devitalized tissue and debris is required. Blisters can be left intact, drained, or debrided. Once cleaned and debrided, the burn wounds are irrigated with normal saline. The wound is then covered with a dressing. The traditional three layer dressing usually is used. The layer next to the burn wound should be nonadherent and act as a wick to allow passage of fluid and exudate to the absorbent second layer. The outer layer should be semielastic to hold the previous layers intact. Topical antibiotics usually are used in the treatment of these burns. The topical antibiotic can be applied directly to the skin or to pads impregnated with the cream, which are then applied to the burn wound. Dressings are layered as described. Synthetic dressings can be used to cover burn wounds. Electrical burns are treated in the same manner as thermal burns.

Treatment of chemical burns requires early copious washing with saline or water to remove the chemicals. Hopefully, this was done at the injury site. Tap water should be flowed over the acid burn for 15 to 30 minutes to neutralize the acid. Initial wound care is the same as described for thermal injuries.

Major Burns

The first several hours after a major burn are consumed with life-saving resuscitative measures. Once these measures have been instituted, initial wound management begins. Initial wound management of major burns is similar to that of minor burns in that they require cleaning, debriding, irrigation, and application of topical antimicrobial dressings.

Edema presents a significant problem in the management of burn wounds. In burns that involve the entire circumference of a body part, the edema can produce a tourniquet effect. When this occurs, an escharotomy is performed. Incisions are made on the lateral and medial aspects of the affected body part to allow for expansion of the edematous body tissues.

Topical antibiotics are applied, since burn wounds are ischemic and thus do not receive any benefit from parenteral antibiotics. Mafenide acetate cream (Sulfamylon), 0.5% silver nitrate solution, and

1% silver sulfadiazine (Silvadene) are commonly used antimicrobial agents for burn wounds. A light nonocclusive dressing is applied.

Infections of burn wounds are the greatest cause of mortality in burned patients. The injury extensively alters tissue integrity and its protective barrier against environmental pathogenic invasion. The skin and exudate in the burn wound provide an excellent milieu for bacterial proliferation. Burn wounds are ischemic and do not benefit from parenteral antimicrobial agents. The burn injury itself causes severe immunosuppression. One of the primary goals of burn wound management, therefore, involves preventing or treating wound infections. Prevention of infection includes prompt removal of devitalized tissue and prompt coverage of the wound (Achauer and Martinez, 1985).

Ongoing management of burn wounds includes aggressive debridement and application of antimicrobial dressings. Hydrotherapy assists in aggressively irrigating and debriding devitalized tissue and debris. Burned patients are placed in a large tub one or two times daily. Antimicrobial topical agents are reapplied after each hydrotherapy treatment.

Aggressive removal of devitalized tissue and wound exudate is essential to maximize wound closure. Wounds can be closed surgically or with skin substitutes. There are two types of grafts used for burn wounds: biologic dressings and synthetic skin substitutes. Biologic dressings include homografts or autografts using the patient's own skin. Allografts use skin composed of donor or cadaver skin. Xenografts use skin grafts retrieved from other species, usually pig skin. Biobrane is the most commonly used synthetic skin substitute. These skin substitutes improve healing and decrease heat and evaporative losses.

Burn wound management can continue for months and even years. From the resuscitative phase to the rehabilitative phase, a multidisciplinary approach is required for the successful outcome of burn wound healing.

In summary, the phases of wound healing in the burn wound occur more slowly and last longer than in other wounds. Minor burns are cleansed, debrided, irrigated, then covered with a topical antibiotic dressing. After life-saving measures have been completed, major burns are cleansed, debrided, irrigated, and dressed with topical antibiotic dressings. Escharotomies are performed, since edema produces a tourniquet effect. Topical antibiotics are used with burns because burn wounds are ischemic. Infection of burn wounds is the greatest cause of mortality in burn patients. Ongoing management includes aggressive hydrotherapy and debridement. Wounds can be grafted using biologic dressings or synthetic skin substitutes. Burn wound management continues for months and even years.

Section Eight Review

1. Which of the following statements describes the major difference between wound healing and burn wound healing?
   A. phases of burn wound healing occur more slowly or last longer
   B. the inflammatory phase is shorter in duration
   C. neovascularization does not occur in burn wounds
   D. an organized system of layering of collagen occurs in burn wounds
2. Topical antibiotics are applied to burn wounds because
   A. they immediately penetrate at the site of bacterial invasion
   B. burn wounds are ischemic
   C. they are more soothing for the patient
   D. they aid in debriding bacterial debris
3. Hypertrophic scars characteristic of second and third degree burns are caused by
   A. lack of neovascularization
   B. lack of collagen synthesis
   C. slowed epithelialization
   D. random layering of collagen
4. Edema presents a significant problem in burn wounds because
   A. edema impedes tissue perfusion/oxygenation
   B. edema can produce a tourniquet effect
   C. edema provides a milieu for bacterial proliferation
   D. loss of protein prevents tissue repair

5. Which of the following antibiotics would NOT be chosen for burn wound management?
   A. Sulfamylon
   B. Silvadene
   C. 0.5 percent silver nitrate solution
   D. cephalosporin

Answers: 1, A. 2, B. 3, D. 4, B. 5, D.

Posttest

1. Which of the following stores energy, assists in regulating the body temperature, acts as a cushion, and provides the body with shape and substance?
   A. dermis
   B. epidermis
   C. subcutaneous tissue
   D. hypodermis

2. Epithelialization
   A. occurs even in the presence of debris
   B. spreads on surfaces laden with bacteria
   C. occurs only in healthy tissue
   D. occurs within moments after injury

3. Mr. G has undergone a cholecystectomy. Most likely his incision would be allowed to heal by
   A. primary intention
   B. secondary intention
   C. delayed primary intention
   D. delayed secondary intention

4. Of the factors that affect wound healing, which of the following has been found to be the most important?
   A. age
   B. normal serum potassium levels
   C. moisture
   D. adequate tissue perfusion

5. The golden period of wound management is
   A. the first hour after injury
   B. day 3 after injury
   C. the first 48 hours after injury
   D. the first 6 to 12 hours after injury

6. Which of the following dressing materials should NOT be used for documented or suspected wound infections?
   A. wet to dry dressings
   B. hydrocolloid dressings
   C. wet to damp dressings
   D. wet to wet dressings

7. Acetic acid is a solution used with wet to dry dressings that may be used
   A. to promote vasodilation in the wound
   B. to treat *Pseudomonas* infection in the wound
   C. to slightly dissolve necrotic debris in the wound
   D. as a fast-acting broad-spectrum antimicrobial

8. Red-pink tissue with a budding appearance is characteristic of
   A. granulation tissue
   B. imminent wound infections
   C. poor tissue perfusion
   D. the inflammatory process

9. The extent of damage caused by which burns is usually much greater than it initially appears?
   A. chemical burns
   B. thermal burns
   C. inhalation burns
   D. electrical burns

10. Which of the following criteria is most indicative of the presence of a wound infection?
    A. purulent drainage from the wound 3 days after injury
    B. core body temperature of 101.5F
    C. WBC count of 40,000/mm^3
    D. culture and sensitivity testing of wound drainage

11. To assess the extent of burn injury, one would use
    A. the rule of nines
    B. definitions of first, second, or third degree burns
    C. mechanisms of injury
    D. definitions of partial thickness burns

12. Burn wounds differ in healing from other wounds because
    A. the inflammatory phase is shorter
    B. they are ischemic
    C. collagen layering is more organized
    D. neovascularization does not occur

13. Moist, yellow, stringy tissue in a wound is
    A. a sign of epithelialization
    B. eschar
    C. slough
    D. granulation tissue

Posttest Answers

Question	Answer	Section	Question	Answer	Section
1	C	One	8	A	Six
2	C	Two	9	D	Seven
3	A	Two	10	D	Four
4	D	Three	11	A	Seven
5	D	Four	12	B	Eight
6	B	Five	13	C	Six
7	B	Five			

REFERENCES

Achauer, B.M., and Martinez, S.E. (1985). Burn wound physiology and care. *Crit. Care Clin.* (1):47–58.

Amato, E.J. (1982). Gastrointestinal tubes and drains. *Crit. Care Nurse.* Nov/Dec 2(6):50 57.

Baxter, C.R., and Waeckerle, J.F. (1988). Emergency treatment of burn injury. *Ann. Emerg. Med.* 17(2):1305–1315.

Burdon, D. (1982). Principles of antimicrobial prophylaxis. *World J. Surg.* 6(3):262–267.

Cruse, P.J. (1975). Incidence of wound infection on surgical services. *Surg. Clin. North Am.* 55(6):1269–1275.

Epifanio, P.C. (1988). Wound management. In V.D. Cardona, P.D. Hurn, A.J. Mason, A.M. Scanlon-Schilpp, and S.W. Veise-Berry (eds). *Trauma nursing: From resuscitation through rehabilitation*, pp. 224–262. Philadelphia: W.B. Saunders Co.

Flynn, M.E., and Rovee, D.T. (1982). Wound healing mechanisms. *Am. J. Nursing.* Oct 82:1544–1558.

Fowler, E., Cuzzell, J.Z., and Papen, J.C. (1991). Healing with hydrocolloid. *Am. J. Nursing.* Feb 91(3):63–64.

Hess, C.T., and Miller, P. (1990). The management of open wounds: Acute and chronic. *Ostomy Wound Management.* Nov/Dec:58–69.

Hotter, A.N. (1982). Physiologic aspect and clinical implications of wound healing. *Heart Lung.* 11(6):522–531.

Hoyt, N.J. (1988). Infection and infection control. In V.D. Cardona, P.D. Hurn, A.J. Mason, A.M. Scanlon-Schilpp, and S.W. Veise-Berry (eds). *Trauma nursing:* *From resuscitation through rehabilitation*, pp. 224–262. Philadelphia: W.B. Saunders Co.

Hunt, T.K. (1989). Critical care of wounds and wounded patients. In W.C. Shoemaker, S. Ayers, A. Grenvick, P.R. Holbrook, and W.L. Thompson (eds). *Textbook of critical care*, 2nd ed., pp. 1285–1294. Philadelphia: W.B. Saunders Co.

Neuberger, G., and Reckling, J. (1985). A new look at wound care. *Nursing 1985.* 15(2):34–42.

Robson, M.C. (1988). Disturbances of wound healing. *Ann. Emerg. Med.* 17(12):1274–1278.

Schimpff, S.C., Dejongh, C.A., and Caplan, E.S. (1989). Infections in the critical care patient. In W.C. Shoemaker, S. Ayers, A. Grenvick, P.R. Holbrook, and W.L. Thompson (eds). *Textbook of critical care*, pp. 767–779. Philadelphia: W.B. Saunders Co.

Sieggreen, M.Y. (1987). Healing of physical wounds. *Nursing Clin. North Am.* 22(2):439–447.

Smith, S.L., and Caswell, D. (1988). Infection control. In R.G. Hathaway (ed) *Nursing care of the critically ill surgical patient*, pp. 152–162. Rockville, Maryland: Aspen Publishers, Inc.

Smith, S.L. and Cuzzell, J.Z. (1988). Wound healing. In R.G. Hathaway (ed) *Nursing care of the critically ill surgical patient*, pp. 140–151. Rockville, Maryland: Aspen Publishers, Inc.

Stevenson, T.R., and Mathes, S.J. (1988). Wound healing. In T.A. Miller (ed) *Physiologic basis of modern surgical care*, pp. 1010–1018. St. Louis: C.V. Mosby Co.

Tobin, G.R. (1984). Closure of contaminated wounds. *Surg. Clin. North Am.* 64(4):639–652.

ADDITIONAL READING

Bauman, B. (1982). Update your technique for changing dressings: Wet to dry. *Nursing 82.* Feb 12(2):68–71.

Cooper, D.M., and Schumann, D. (1979). Postsurgical nursing intervention as an adjunct to wound healing. *Nursing Clin. North Am.* 14:713–725.

Dimick, A.R. (1988). Delayed wound closure: Indications and techniques. *Ann. Emerg. Med.* 17(12):1303–1304.

Edlich, R.F., Rodeheaver, G.T., Morgan R.F., Berman, D.E., and Thacker, J.G. (1988). Principles of emergency wound management. *Ann. Emerg. Med.* 17(12):1284–1301.

Hunt, T.K. (1988). The physiology of wound healing. *Ann. Emerg. Med.* 17(12):1265–1272.

Kapusnik, J.E., Sande, M.A., and Miller, R.T. (1989). Antibacterial therapy in critical care. In W.C. Shoemaker, S. Ayers, A. Grenvick, P.R. Holbrook, and W.L. Thompson (eds). *Textbook of critical care*, 2nd ed., pp. 780–801. Philadelphia: W.B. Saunders Co.

Madden, J.W., and Arem, A.J. (1986). Wound healing: Biologic and clinical features. In D.C. Sabiston (ed). *Textbook of surgery*, 13th ed., pp. 193–213. Philadelphia: W.B. Saunders Co.

Munster, A.M., and Winchurch, R.A. (1985). Infection and immunology. *Crit. Care Clin.* 1(1):119–127.

Ruberg, R.L. (1984). Role of nutrition in wound healing. *Surg. Clin. North Am.* 64(4):705–714.

Module 12

Responsiveness

Robyn Cheung

This self-study module, *Responsiveness,* was developed as a teaching guide for nurses caring for patients with alterations with a neurologic basis. Successful completion of this module will prepare you to care for these types of patients in a general care area. It will not prepare you to care for a patient in a neurologic intensive care unit.

This module contains eleven sections, beginning with a pretest and ending with a posttest. Additionally, each section ends with a test. A glossary and list of abbreviations are included.

This module begins with simple definitions of responsiveness and moves into the concept of increased intracranial pressure as a contributing factor of impaired responsiveness. A more comprehensive discussion of etiologies affecting responsiveness is provided. The module reviews common elements for assessment, in-depth assessment of impaired arousal, and how to document your assessment. The module then moves on to nursing interventions and pharmacologic therapies for patients with alterations in responsiveness. The module ends with sections on seizure disorders and select diagnostic procedures for patients with neurologic impairment.

Objectives

At the completion of this module, the learner will be able to

1. Define responsiveness and the components that make up responsiveness
2. Identify the anatomic bases that control arousal and content
3. Define the Monro-Kellie hypothesis
4. Discuss the relationship between intracranial volume and intracranial pressure
5. Discuss compensatory mechanisms for increased intracranial volume
6. Describe the outcome of uncompensated increased intracranial volume and state six contributing factors

7. State six pathologic processes that may impair arousal and content
8. Describe common elements to be evaluated in the assessment of arousal and content
9. Describe components included in an in-depth assessment of arousal
10. Document assessment of arousal and content
11. Identify nursing interventions and pharmacologic therapies for patients with an impaired level of responsiveness
12. Briefly discuss seizure disorders, and identify nursing and pharmacologic management
13. Identify selected diagnostic procedures and their clinical applications

---

Pretest

1. Responsiveness includes the functions of the cerebral hemispheres and
   A. the cerebrum
   B. the cerebellum
   C. the sensorimotor fiber tracts
   D. the reticular activating system

2. Arousal is one component of responsiveness. The other component is
   A. content
   B. intelligence
   C. wakefulness
   D. motor ability

3. The Monro-Kellie hypothesis states that volume increases in the adult intracranial vault
   A. are initially well tolerated through compensatory mechanisms
   B. are tolerated well because of the flexibility of the cranial vault
   C. can only be compensated for by cerebrospinal fluid buffering techniques
   D. usually result in death because the vault is unable to accommodate increases in volume

4. Cerebral blood vessels dilate in response to
   A. increased serum oxygen
   B. increased serum carbon dioxide
   C. decreased serum oxygen
   D. decreased serum carbon dioxide

5. Pressure regulation is an autoregulatory mechanism whereby cerebral blood vessels constrict in response to
   A. systemic hypertension
   B. hypercarbia
   C. systemic hypotension
   D. hypoxia

6. What is the cerebral perfusion pressure if MAP = 95 mm Hg and ICP = 15 mm Hg?
   A. 65 mm HG
   B. 80 mm HG
   C. 110 mm HG
   D. 125 mm HG

7. Your patient responds appropriately to stimuli, and the Glasgow Coma Scale score is 15. What would be your initial assessment and your next action?
   A. level of responsiveness is intact, vital signs would be the next logical step
   B. level of responsiveness most probably is not intact, an in-depth neurologic assessment is required
   C. you are unable to completely evaluate the level of responsiveness and need more clinical data
   D. the patient demonstrates no cognitive deficits, pupillary assessment would be the next logical step

8. The most important component of the neurologic assessment is
   A. the vital signs
   B. the level of responsiveness
   C. pupillary reactions
   D. the protective reflexes

9. A unilaterally dilated pupil is indicative of
   A. atropine or atropinelike drugs
   B. a brainstem lesion
   C. opiate overdose
   D. a cranial nerve lesion

10. The Glasgow Coma Scale assesses
    A. cognition
    B. speech patterns
    C. arousal
    D. problem-solving abilities

11. Your patient's intracranial pressure per monitor is 30 mm Hg. To assist your patient's compensatory mechanisms, your first action would be to
    A. hyperventilate the patient
    B. lower the head of the bed
    C. turn the patient to the left side
    D. drain the patient's ventricular catheter

12. Flexion of the neck or hips may cause elevations in intracranial volume by
    A. causing a decrease in venous return
    B. causing an increase in venous return
    C. causing cerebral vasodilation
    D. increasing venous outflow

13. A seizure disorder that is considered a neurologic emergency is
    A. generalized seizures
    B. partial seizures
    C. complex seizures
    D. status epilepticus

14. A disadvantage of magnetic resonance imaging (MRI) over computed tomographic (CT) scanning is
    A. MRI is an invasive procedure
    B. MRI produces results that are less refined
    C. the time required for an MRI is longer
    D. MRI is not useful for imaging anatomic location of a lesion

Pretest answers: 1, D. 2, A. 3, A. 4, B. 5, A. 6, B. 7, C. 8, B. 9, D. 10, C. 11, A. 12, A. 13, D. 14, C.

Glossary

Arousal. The component of consciousness concerned with the ability of an individual simply to respond to environmental stimuli, such as opening the eyes to speech or turning the head toward a noise

Autoregulation. Inherent property of the brain whereby cerebral blood flow is maintained at a constant rate and within normal limits by adjusting the diameter of the cerebral vessels. Pressure regulation responds to changes in systemic blood pressure; vessels constrict in response to elevated pressure and dilate in response to decreased pressures. Chemical regulation responds to blood levels of oxygen and, more strikingly, to levels of carbon dioxide; vessels dilate in response to elevated levels of carbon dioxide, less forcefully to decreased oxygen levels; vessels constrict to lowered levels of carbon dioxide

Blood–brain barrier. A network of capillary cells and membranes that provides selectivity to the substances that cross it; it serves as a control for brain volume

Cerebral blood flow. Normally is maintained at a constant rate by vasodilation of the vessels to increase the flow or vasoconstriction to decrease the flow

Cerebral blood volume. The amount of blood in the cranial vault at any given point in time; occupies about 10 percent of the total intracranial volume

Cerebral perfusion pressure. The blood pressure gradient across the brain, an estimate of the adequacy of cerebral circulation; calculated as MAP − ICP; normal is 80 mm Hg to 100 mm Hg

Consciousness. State of general awareness of oneself and the environment; made up of the components of arousal and content

Content. The component of consciousness concerned with interpreting environmental stimuli; includes thinking, memory, problem-solving, orientation, and speech

Elastance. A measure of stiffness, referring to the brain's ability to tolerate and compensate for volume increases; high elastance refers to small volume reserves in the cranial vault

Herniation. A protrusion of brain matter through a natural opening secondary to elevated intracranial pressure; carries a grave prognosis and is an ominous sign

Hydrocephalus. A clinical syndrome caused by an increased production of cerebrospinal fluid that exceeds the absorption rate

Hypercapnia. Abnormally elevated blood levels of carbon dioxide; results in vasodilation of the cerebral vessels

Intracranial pressure. Pressure exerted by the cerebrospinal fluid within the ventricles of the brain; normal pressure is 0 to 15 mm Hg

Monro-Kellie hypothesis. A principle that states that the skull is a rigid vault filled with noncompressible contents: brain, blood, and cerebrospinal fluid; if any one component increases in volume, one or both remaining components must decrease in volume for overall volume to remain constant

Responsiveness. A term synonymous with consciousness, which is a general state of awareness of oneself and the environment

Reticular activating system (RAS). A pathway of neurons and neuronal connections for transmission of sensory stimuli from the lower brainstem to the cerebral cortex; the anatomic basis of the arousal component of consciousness

Status epilepticus. A continuing series of seizures without a period of recovery or regaining of consciousness between attacks

Abbreviations

CBF. Cerebral blood flow

CPP. Cerebral perfusion pressure

CSF. Cerebrospinal fluid

CT. Computed tomography

GCS. Glasgow Coma Scale

ICP. Intracranial pressure

MAP. Mean arterial pressure

MRI. Magnetic resonance imaging

PET. Positron emission tomography

RAS. Reticular activating system

Section One: Responsiveness

At the completion of this section, you will be able to define responsiveness and the components that make up responsiveness.

Responsiveness, or consciousness, is defined as a state of general awareness of oneself and the environment and reflects the functional integrity of the brain as a whole. Responsiveness is a dynamic state that is subject to change. Level of responsiveness is the most important factor in the neurologic assessment.

Responsiveness is divided into two components: content and arousal. Arousal is concerned with the appearance of wakefulness and stimuli necessary to wake an individual. Content includes the sum of cerebral mental functions and is concerned with interpretation of the internal and external environment or the thinking processes, known as cognition.

Content and arousal are independent but interrelated components. The arousal component must be functioning for content to be experienced. An individual who is not in a state of wakefulness, or arousal, would be unable to interpret internal and external stimuli.

The arousal component of responsiveness is controlled by the reticular activating system (RAS). The RAS is a pathway of neurons and neuronal connections. It is located in the midbrain and medulla and projects into the cerebral hemispheres. The RAS receives impulses from the sense organs and transmits these impulses to the cerebral hemispheres. Thus, not only does the RAS control wakefulness or arousal, but it also has some control over content. Stimuli cannot be interpreted in the cerebral hemispheres unless they are received and transmitted to the cerebral cortex via the RAS.

The content component of responsiveness includes all functions of the brain that add quality to the arousal component and is controlled by the cerebral hemispheres. Thus, content is dependent on intact, functioning cerebral hemispheres. Functions controlled by the cerebral hemispheres include thinking, imagining, and speech.

To summarize, responsiveness is a state of general awareness of oneself and the environment and is made up of two components: arousal and content. Arousal is controlled by the RAS, and content is controlled by the cerebral hemispheres. Content and arousal are two processes that are independent, but interrelated, and together comprise the state of responsiveness.

Section One Review

1. The ascending reticular activating system chiefly is responsible for
   A. high level cognitive skills
   B. recent and remote memory
   C. level of arousal
   D. affect and mood

2. A patient making inappropriate statements and appearing disoriented would be suspected of having an impairment of
   A. the cerebellum
   B. the cerebral cortex
   C. the occipital lobe
   D. the brainstem

Answers: 1, C. 2, B.

Section Two: Monro-Kellie Hypothesis

At the completion of this section, you will be able to define the Monro-Kellie hypothesis and state the three components of the intracranial vault.

The intracranial vault is a rigid container with limited space. The contents of the intracranial vault include the brain, cerebral blood volume, and cerebrospinal fluid (CSF). The volume of each component remains relatively stable. The Monro-Kellie hypothesis states that a change in volume of any one of these components must be accompanied by a reciprocal change in one or both of the other components. If this reciprocal change is not accomplished the result is an increase in intracranial pressure (ICP).

Brain Volume

The brain is composed of neurons and glial cells. The brain volume is mainly water (80 percent), and the majority of the water is intracellular. The brain volume remains constant with the help of the blood–brain barrier.

The blood–brain barrier is a network of cells and membranes in the brain capillaries. This barrier is selective in terms of membrane permeability and molecular size of the substance attempting to enter the cerebral circulation. The blood–brain barrier is able to select which substances enter the cerebral circulation and which substances are prohibited from entering the cerebral vasculature. The blood–brain barrier is permeable to water, oxygen, and carbon dioxide and slightly permeable to the electrolytes. Most drugs are prevented from crossing the blood–brain barrier, but it depends on their molecular composi-

tion. The blood–brain barrier can be physically disrupted by trauma or functionally impaired by metabolic abnormalities, such as drug overdoses. The result is an exit of fluid from the intravascular space into the extravascular space of the brain tissue.

Cerebral Blood Volume

Cerebral blood volume is the amount of blood in the cranial vault at any point in time. Cerebral blood volume is approximately 10 percent of the total intracranial volume and is maintained at a constant level through cerebral blood flow (CBF).

Cerebrospinal Fluid

Cerebrospinal fluid (CSF) is the third component of intracranial volume and is produced in the ventricles. CSF circulates in the subarachnoid spaces of the brain and spinal cord and is reabsorbed into the venous system by the arachnoid villi. Approximately 10 percent of the total intracranial volume is CSF, which accounts for about 150 mL of CSF at any given time. Of the three components, CSF can be displaced most easily and rapidly.

In summary, the Monro-Kellie hypothesis states that the cranial vault is rigid and fixed and is made up of three compartments: the brain, the cerebral blood volume, and CSF. Brain volume is controlled by the blood–brain barrier, and cerebral blood volume is controlled by CBF. Of the three compartments, CSF is displaced most easily and rapidly and is the first reciprocal response to increase in intracranial volume.

Section Two Review

---

1. According to the Monro-Kellie hypothesis, an increase in one intracranial compartment must be accompanied by
   A. a reciprocal decrease in another compartment
   B. a reciprocal increase in the blood–brain barrier
   C. a reciprocal decrease in the blood–brain barrier
   D. a reciprocal increase in another compartment

2. Which mechanism controls brain volume?
   A. cerebral blood flow
   B. displacement of CSF
   C. blood–brain barrier
   D. vasoconstriction

Answers: 1, A. 2, C.

Section Three: Relationship Between Increased Intracranial Volume and Pressure

At the completion of this section, you will be able to describe the relationship between intracranial volume and intracranial pressure (ICP) and how this relationship is balanced through use of compensatory mechanisms.

As was discussed in Section Two, volumes in the three intracranial compartments combine to form the total intracranial volume and, ideally, to produce a normal ICP. Although units of volume can be elevated in any compartment, ICP is measured in the CSF and is defined as the pressure exerted by the CSF within the ventricles of the brain. Normal ICP ranges from 0 to 15 mm Hg. ICP greater than 15 mm Hg is abnormally elevated.

ICP is a dynamic process. It fluctuates constantly in response to changes in respiratory rate and body position and such activities as coughing and sneezing. Whereas ICP is a fluctuating phenomenon, intracranial volume is kept relatively stable and constant by reciprocal compensation, the principle outlined in the Monro-Kellie hypothesis. As this principle states, reciprocal compensation can occur in any one of the three compartments.

Cerebrospinal Fluid Volume

The first compensatory mechanism that occurs is displacement of CSF. As intracranial volume and pressure rise, CSF is shunted out of the cerebral subarachnoid space into the spinal subarachnoid space through natural openings called foramina, namely, the foramen of Magendie and foramen of Luschka. Second, as more CSF is shunted out of the subarachnoid space, the remaining CSF is absorbed at an increased rate by the arachnoid villi.

Cerebral Blood Volume

Cerebral blood volume is dependent on CBF. If CBF is increased, so too is cerebral blood volume. Cerebral blood flow is dependent upon cerebral perfusion pressure (CPP), which is defined as the pressure gradient necessary to supply adequate amounts of blood to the brain. It is the difference between mean arterial pressure (MAP) and ICP.

$$CPP = MAP - ICP$$

The normal CPP is 80 to 100 mm Hg and must be at least 50 mm Hg to provide minimal blood flow to the brain. A CPP of 30 mm Hg or less is incompatible with life and results in neuronal hypoxia and cell death.

Autoregulation is a compensatory mechanism that keeps CBF constant by maintaining an adequate CPP. Autoregulation works by automatic constriction or dilation of cerebral blood vessels in response to either changes in systemic arterial pressure or blood levels of carbon dioxide and oxygen. When systemic pressure rises, the vessels constrict to protect the brain from blood engorgement and to protect cerebral tissues from the full impact of the systemic pressure. When systemic pressure falls, the reverse occurs. Cerebral vessels dilate in an attempt to increase CBF. This compensatory mechanism is termed *pressure regulation.*

Constriction or dilation of cerebral vessels in response to blood levels of carbon dioxide and oxygen is termed *metabolic* or *chemical regulation.* Vessels dilate in response to hypercapnia, or elevated carbon dioxide levels greater than 45 mm Hg, and constrict in response to lowered levels of carbon dioxide (less than 21 mm Hg will decrease CBF to one half of normal value). Blood oxygen levels affect the diameter of cerebral vessels but are not as potent a stimulus as is carbon dioxide. Vessels dilate in response to decreased oxygen levels (less than 50 mm Hg). Oxygen levels greater than 80 mm Hg will decrease CBF slightly.

Brain Volume

As was discussed in Section Two, the blood–brain barrier acts to control brain volume by controlling the solutes and water that attempt to cross it and enter the cerebral circulation. If this controlling mechanism is disrupted, either physically or functionally, an increase in brain volume will result secondary to an escape of fluid from the intravascular space to the extravascular space. Unless there is a reciprocal decrease in either cerebral blood volume or CSF volume, an overall increase in intracranial volume and ICP will result.

Obviously, the brain is limited in its compensatory abilities. It cannot decrease its size or displace itself. The brain possesses a property called *elastance* or compliance, which is the degree of compressibility. Elastance is a measure of stiffness. If the value is high, the brain is considered tight, and the intracranial space has little volume reserve. On the other hand, compliance is a measure of slackness and is the inverse of elastance. For example, if elastance were low, the brain would be able to tolerate increases in volume for a longer period than if elastance were high.

As with all compensatory mechanisms, these mechanisms operate only within specific parameters. Autoregulation is lost when a critical point is reached, either the ICP is greater than 30 to 35 mm

Hg or systemic blood pressure is less than 60 mm Hg or greater than 160 mm Hg. If a critical point is reached, CBF will vary passively with systemic blood pressure.

In summary, this section discussed how intracranial volume influences ICP. When intracranial volume is elevated, compensatory mechanisms are activated: displacement and increased absorption of CSF and autoregulation. The brain's ability to tolerate increases in volume depends on the degree of elastance and compliance. In Section Four, the outcomes of uncompensated volume increases are discussed.

Section Three Review

1. Hypercapnea causes
   A. cerebral vasodilation
   B. cerebral vasoconstriction
   C. decreased cerebral blood flow
   D. decreased cerebral blood volume
2. Cerebral blood flow is dependent on
   A. an intact blood–brain barrier
   B. cerebral perfusion pressure
   C. serum glucose levels
   D. cerebral blood volume
3. Your patient's MAP is 80 mm Hg and the ICP is 15 mm Hg. What is the cerebral perfusion pressure?
   A. 50 mm Hg
   B. 65 mm Hg
   C. 95 mm Hg
   D. 110 mm Hg

4. Autoregulation works by
   A. increasing or decreasing blood levels of oxygen and carbon dioxide
   B. displacing CSF into the spinal subarachnoid space
   C. altering elastance and compliance properties
   D. automatically constricting or dilating cerebral blood vessels
5. In terms of increased intracranial pressure, a high measure of elastance would indicate
   A. the autoregulatory mechanism will be lost
   B. the intracranial vault has little volume reserve
   C. the brain is able to tolerate additional increases in volume
   D. the compliance measure also is high

Answers: 1, A. 2, B. 3, B. 4, D. 5, B.

Section Four: Uncompensated Increases

At the completion of this section, you will be able to describe the outcome of uncompensated compartmental volume increases and what conditions may contribute to these increases.

According to the Monro-Kellie hypothesis, any compartmental volume increase must be reciprocated by a volume decrease in one or both of the remaining compartments. If this reciprocity is not realized, total intracranial volume will increase, along with ICP. Primarily, intracranial volume is increased by any process that increases actual brain or blood volume or any process that interferes with CSF production or absorption.

Brain Volume

Space-occupying lesions and cerebral edema are the primary processes that increase brain volume. This type of lesion includes tumors, abscesses, intracerebral hemorrhage, and hematoma. Cerebral edema may occur after any type of head trauma, including surgery, brain anoxia, or ischemia. The effect of increased brain volume depends on the rate of development. Slower growing lesions, such as a chronic hematoma or slow-growing tumor, may remain asymptomatic and may be tolerated for a longer time period than an acute subdural hematoma, which develops at a faster rate.

A mass or edema that progresses and is uncompensated eventually will result in a shifting of brain tissue, or herniation, which carries a grave prognosis. This process causes displacement of brain tissue and pressure or traction on cerebral structures, which causes clinical symptoms. Herniation syndromes are described based on the end-stage of the herniation. Four herniation syndromes are as follows.

- Cingulate herniation. Lateral shift of brain tissue, usually as the result of a lesion in one of the cerebral hemispheres

- Central or transentorial herniation. Downward shift of one or both cerebral hemispheres, usually due to lesions in the frontal or parietal lobes
- Uncal or lateral transtentorial herniation. Lateral and downward shift of brain tissue, usually the temporal lobe, usually due to lesions located most laterally, such as the middle fossa in the temporal lobe. This type of herniation causes compression of the oculomotor nerve, or cranial nerve III, evidenced by the classic sign of a unilaterally dilated pupil
- Tonsillar herniation. Downward shift of brain tissue through the foramen magnum, which results in compression of the medulla and upper cervical spinal cord

Cerebral Blood Volume

Any systemic process that affects blood levels of carbon dioxide will affect CBF, cerebral perfusion pressure (CPP), and cerebral blood volume. Therefore, conditions that produce hypercapnia and hypoxemia will result in cerebral vasodilation and increased blood volume. These conditions may include chronic respiratory insufficiencies, inadequate ventilation, hypoventilation, sedation by drugs, and insufficient supplemental oxygen.

Cerebral blood volume also may be increased by any process that impedes venous outflow. This includes anything that may impede jugular circulation, such as head/neck rotation or flexion, Valsalva maneuver, and use of positive end-expiratory pressure (PEEP).

A third cause of increased blood volume is loss of autoregulatory mechanisms. Cerebral vessels become passively dependent on systemic pressure and CPP.

Cerebrospinal Fluid

Volume increases in CSF result from increased production, obstructed circulation, or decreased absorption. This is a condition termed *hydrocephalus*. Obstruction to CSF can be caused by mass lesions or infection. Decreased absorption can result from a subarachnoid hemorrhage or meningitis.

Hydrocephalus is treated surgically or mechanically. If considered to be a permanent condition, a surgical shunt is placed; if considered temporary, a ventricular drain is inserted for intermittent or continuous drainage.

The chart summarizes the causes and effects of increased intracranial volume. It must be kept in mind that any increase in brain volume, blood volume or CSF that is unchecked will result in herniation.

Component	Cause	Effect
Brain volume	Space-occupying lesion	Herniation
	Cerebral edema	
Blood volume	Hypercapnia }	Cerebral
	Hypoxemia }	dilation
	Loss of autoregulation	Passive vessels
	Venous outflow obstruction	Increased CBV
CSF	Obstruction	Hydrocephalus
	Decreased absorption	
	Increased production	

Section Four Review

1. Which of the following pathologies is NOT associated with increased intracranial volume?
   A. subdural hematoma
   B. hypotension
   C. subarachnoid hemorrhage
   D. meningioma
2. Which of the following is NOT a cause of increased CSF?
   A. meningitis
   B. venous outflow obstruction
   C. subarachnoid hemorrhage
   D. brain tumor

3. Intracranial pressure can be increased by anything that
   A. increases intracranial volume
   B. results in high compliance
   C. results in low elastance
   D. decreases carbon dioxide levels
4. Chronic respiratory insufficiency may affect
   A. brain volume
   B. brain volume, cerebral blood volume, and CSF volume
   C. CSF volume
   D. cerebral blood volume

Answers: 1, B. 2, B. 3, A. 4, D.

Section Five: Impaired Arousal and Content

At the completion of this section, you will be able to state pathologic conditions that impair the two components of responsiveness, arousal and content, and discuss how these impairments occur.

Decreased responsiveness, or consciousness, results from either diffuse impairment of cortical structures or involvement of the reticular activating system. Increased ICP is a major process that produces these impairments. These impairments result from altered CBF compression, and shifting of brain tissue. Examples of conditions that may cause these alterations include severe head trauma with cerebral edema, intracerebral or subarachnoid hemorrhage, cerebral hematomas, and obstructive hydrocephalus.

The content component of responsiveness is controlled by the cerebral hemispheres, as well as the RAS. Therefore, any process that interrupts the RAS or arousal also will affect content. On the other hand, processes that directly affect content or awareness do not necessarily impair arousal. Since content is the ability to interpret and interact and arousal merely is the ability to respond, it is possible to be awake but not aware.

Responsiveness may be altered not only by structural lesions but by metabolic and psychogenic disorders as well. The most common metabolic causes are cerebral ischemia, hypoglycemia, and sedative drug overdose. Metabolic disorders alter brain metabolism and key metabolic requirements. Examples of metabolic disorders include uremia, hepatic encephalopathy, myxedema, Cushing's disease, pheochromocytoma, and electrolyte and acid-base imbalances. Pharmacologic agents include sedatives, such as barbiturates, hypnotics, opiates, and tranquilizers, such psychotropic drugs as lithium and amphetamines, and other drugs, such as steroids, cimetidine, and salicylates. Psychogenic disorders include hysteria, catatonia, depression, and organic brain syndromes, such as dementia.

Alterations in content primarily are manifested by cognitive deficits, such as memory impairment, disorientation, impaired problem-solving abilities, and attentional deficits. It is more difficult to pinpoint the underlying cause of cognitive deficits because, generally, there is no identifiable structural or focal lesion.

In summary, any process that results in increased ICP will produce impairment of content and arousal. Thus, altered level of responsiveness may result from metabolic or psychiatric disorders primarily by impairing awareness, or content.

Section Five Review

1. Findings from your initial assessment of your patient are as follows: patient is awake, eyes are open and focusing, patient responds appropriately to verbal commands. Based on these findings, you could determine that
   A. the state of arousal is intact, but not content
   B. the state of content is intact, but not arousal
   C. not enough data have been gathered to assess content completely, but arousal is intact
   D. not enough data have been gathered to assess arousal, but content is intact
2. Your patient exhibits short-term memory deficits. This is an impairment of
   A. the cerebellum
   B. the reticular activating system
   C. the cerebral cortex
   D. cerebral blood flow

3. Content, one of the components of responsiveness, includes
   A. ability to open the eyes
   B. ability to focus the eyes
   C. ability to listen to and follow commands
   D. ability to verbalize

Answers: 1, C. 2, C. 3, C.

Section Six: Clinical Assessment

At the completion of this section, you will be able to identify common components to be assessed for arousal and content.

Arousal

The level of responsiveness is the most important factor in the neurologic assessment. The arousal component is assessed first. The first step is to determine what stimulus will arouse the patient, usually by calling his or her name. If the patient does not respond, shake the arm or shoulder gently. If no response is elicited, you must proceed from light pain to deeper pain to try to elicit a response. You should always start with the least noxious stimulus and then proceed to a more intense stimulus if necessary. An example of light pain to deeper pain is shaking the arm, to pinching the arm, to nailbed pressure, to applying pressure to the supraorbital notch. You are assessing two things: (1) Is the patient responsive to verbal stimuli? and if not (2) Does the patient exhibit purposeful movement? Purposeful movement, such as removing the stimulus or withdrawing from the stimulus, indicates functioning of sensory pathways. Abnormal posturing in response to a noxious stimulus indicates a dysfunction of either the cerebral hemispheres or brainstem. Decorticate posturing (abnormal flexion) indicates cerebral hemispheric dysfunction. Decerebrate posturing (abnormal extension) indicates brainstem dysfunction and is a more ominous sign. Patients whose extremities are restrained must be unrestrained when assessing their motor response.

Content

The content component of responsiveness is assessed by noting behavior. The patient should be assessed for orientation and should know his name, the date, and where he is. The patient is considered disoriented if unable to answer the questions cor-rectly. Testing for orientation also assesses short-term memory. Orientation can be assessed only if the patient is able to respond verbally.

After assessing orientation, ability to follow commands is assessed. Ask the patient to perform such acts as sticking out his tongue or holding up two fingers. This not only tells you if the patient is awake enough to respond but also if he is aware enough to interpret and carry out the commands.

Behavioral changes are assessed next by noting any restlessness, irritability, or combativeness. Such behavioral indicators can be caused by many things, including hypoxia, hypoglycemia, drug use, pain, or increased ICP. As the nurse, your role is to pick up clues that may point to causes for changes in behavior. A more in-depth assessment of responsiveness is discussed in Section Seven.

The last component of content that is assessed is verbal response. Assessment of speech provides information about the function of the relationship between the speech centers in the cerebrum and the cranial nerves and can help localize the area of dysfunction. The patient's speech pattern should be assessed for clarity. Is it clear or slurred and garbled? This may indicate drug use, metabolic disturbance, or cranial nerve injuries. Content of speech should be assessed for use of appropriate or inappropriate words. Confused patients may use inappropriate words. Patients with cranial nerve dysfunction usually will not give inappropriate responses, although the speech pattern may be slurred. Patients may experience receptive or expressive aphasia. Inability to understand written or spoken words is receptive aphasia. Inability to write or use language appropriately is expressive aphasia.

To summarize, the level of responsiveness is the most important part of the neurologic assessment, of which arousal is assessed first. For patients who are not in a state of wakefulness, it would be pointless to start off by assessing content. Arousal is assessed by evaluating how much stimulus, if any, is needed for the patient to respond and what type of motor responses the patient exhibits. Content is assessed by evaluating behavior and behavioral changes, ability to follow commands, and verbal response.

Section Six Review

1. What is the first component to be assessed in the neurologic assessment?
   A. content
   B. arousal
   C. behavior
   D. speech
2. During evaluation of arousal, the two things being assessed are
   A. stimuli required for the patient to respond and type of motor response
   B. behavior and behavioral changes
   C. presence of receptive and expressive aphasia
   D. presence of confusion and state of orientation

3. A decorticate motor response indicates
   A. brainstem dysfunction
   B. the patient is close to death
   C. cerebral hemispheric dysfunction
   D. arousal is intact

Answers: 1, B. 2, A. 3, C.

Section Seven: In-Depth Clinical Assessment

At the completion of this section, you will be able to identify and describe in-depth clinical assessment of patients with an alteration in arousal.

Beyond the clinical assessment of arousal and content, a more in-depth neurologic assessment includes pupillary reactions and eye movements, vital signs, and assessment of protective reflexes.

Pupillary Reactions and Eye Movements

Pupillary reactions and eye movements provide information about the location of some lesions. Pupils should be assessed for size, symmetry, shape, and reaction to light. Eye movements also should be assessed for conjugate movement. If the patient is responsive, he can be asked to look upward, downward, outward, medially inward, upward and outward, outward and downward. Deficits in eye movements usually indicate a cranial nerve dysfunction. If the patient is unresponsive, eye movements can be assessed with the oculocephalic response (doll's eyes). Full doll's eyes indicate that the lower pons is intact. The oculocephalic response can be tested only if the cervical spine is intact. This is because the rotation of the head required of this test can cause further damage to the cervical spine if any fractures have been noted.

Pupil size, symmetry, and reactiveness provide valuable information. A unilateral brain lesion can be ruled out if the pupils are equal in size. Nonreactive pupils in the midposition indicate damage to the midbrain (Figure 12–1A). Pupils that are nonreactive to light and pinpoint indicate a pons lesion or opiate drug overdose (Figure 12–1B). Pupils that are small

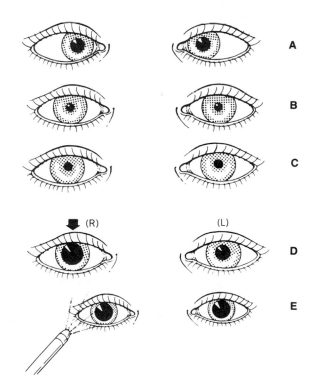

Figure 12–1. A. Unreactive pupils in midposition. **B.** Constricted unreactive pupils. **C.** Constricted reactive pupils. **D.** Unilateral dilated unreactive pupils. **E.** Dilated unreactive pupils. (*From* The clinical practice of neurologic and neurosurgical nursing, *by J. Hickey, 1986, Philadelphia, J.B. Lippincott Co.*)

but reactive to light may indicate a bilateral injury to the thalamus or hypothalamus or metabolic coma (Figure 12–1C). A unilaterally dilated and fixed pupil may indicate compression of the oculomotor nerve (cranial nerve III) (Figure 12–1D).

When both pupils are dilated and nonreactive (fixed), this requires emergency action. It may be caused by severe anoxia or ischemia. Remember that atropinelike drugs cause the pupils to dilate and this must be ruled out (Figure 12–1E) (Hickey, 1986).

Vital Signs

Vital signs are important indicators, especially in the unresponsive patient. Vital signs should be assessed not only individually but also in relationship to each other. Unfortunately, changes in the vital signs occur in the late stages of increased ICP and neurologic deterioration. Cushing's triad is a specific change in the vital signs and is evidenced by (1) an increase in the systolic blood pressure, (2) a widening pulse pressure, and (3) bradycardia. Waiting until this triad of symptoms occurs before intervening may be too late to prevent irreversible damage.

Respiration

The respiratory pattern provides the most valuable information because it can be correlated with the anatomic level of dysfunction. Respiratory rhythm and pattern are controlled by the medulla. Respirations should be assessed for rate and rhythm and should be counted for 1 full minute before stimulating the patient. Some of the more commonly described abnormal respiratory patterns found in the neurologically impaired patient are discussed in the following paragraphs. As a nurse, remember that it is more important to describe the pattern than to try to fit your patient's respiratory pattern into a category. If your patient is mechanically ventilated, it is difficult to observe these patterns, and it would be extremely detrimental to the patient to remove ventilatory support for the purpose of assessing abnormal patterns.

Cheyne-Stokes pattern indicates a bilateral lesion in the cerebral hemispheres, cerebellum, midbrain, or upper pons and may be due to cerebral infarction or metabolic diseases. This respiratory pattern is evidenced by a rhythmic waxing and waning in the depth of the respiration, followed by a period of apnea (Figure 12–2).

Central neurogenic hyperventilation indicates a lesion in the low midbrain or upper pons and may be due to infarction or ischemia of the midbrain or pons, anoxia, or tumors of the midbrain. This pattern is evidenced by respirations that have an increase in depth, are rapid (>24), and are regular (Figure 12–2).

Apneustic breathing indicates a lesion in the mid or low pons that may be due to infarction of the pons or severe meningitis. This pattern is evidenced by prolonged inspiration, with a pause at the point where the respiration is at its peak, lasting for 2 to 3 seconds. This may alternate with an expiratory pause (Figure 12–2).

Cluster breathing indicates a lesion in the low pons or upper medulla that may be due to a tumor or

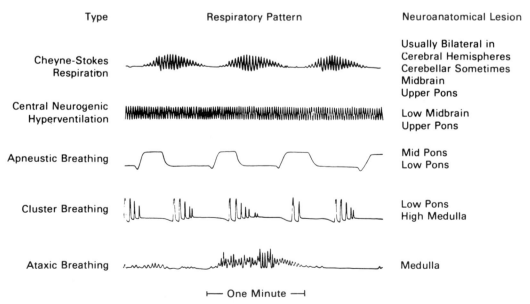

Type	Respiratory Pattern	Neuroanatomical Lesion
Cheyne-Stokes Respiration		Usually Bilateral in Cerebral Hemispheres Cerebellar Sometimes Midbrain Upper Pons
Central Neurogenic Hyperventilation		Low Midbrain Upper Pons
Apneustic Breathing		Mid Pons Low Pons
Cluster Breathing		Low Pons High Medulla
Ataxic Breathing		Medulla

├── One Minute ──┤

Figure 12–2. Abnormal respiratory patterns associated with coma. (*From Abnormal respiratory patterns in the comatose patient caused by intracranial dysfunction, by R.R.M. Gifford and M.R. Plant,* J Neurosurg Nurs 7(1):58, July 1975.)

infarction of the medulla. This pattern is described as clusters of irregular breathing with periods of apnea that occur at irregular intervals (Figure 12–2).

Ataxic breathing indicates a lesion in the medulla that may be due to a cerebellar or pons bleed, tumors of the cerebrum, or severe meningitis. These respirations are completely irregular, with deep and shallow random breaths and pauses (Hickey, 1986) (Figure 12–2).

Remember that abnormal respiratory patterns also may be initiated by such factors as acidosis, respiratory alkalosis, electrolyte imbalances, anxiety, pulmonary processes, or drugs, especially narcotics and anesthetic agents that depress the respiratory center.

Heart Rate

The pulse should be assessed for rate, rhythm, and quality. Increased heart rate may indicate poor cerebral oxygenation. Decreased heart rate is present in the late stages of increased ICP, in which case the quality will be bounding.

Blood Pressure

The medulla regulates blood pressure based on input from chemoreceptors and pressor receptors. An important response to ischemia is known as the Cushing reflex. This response is activated when pressure in the CSF system rises to a point where it equals or exceeds arterial blood pressure. In response to this increase in pressure, the systolic blood pressure rises to a level slightly higher than that of the CSF, which permits CBF to continue.

Temperature

The center for temperature regulation is in the hypothalamus, which regulates body heat via afferent impulses. Hypothermia can occur as a result of spinal shock, metabolic coma, drug overdose, especially depressants, and destructive lesions of the brainstem or hypothalamus. Hyperthermia can occur as a result of CNS infection, subarachnoid hemorrhage, hypothalamic lesions, or hemorrhage of the hypothalamus or brainstem. Temperature may fluctuate widely and may exceed 106F. Hyperthermia is treated vigorously because of the increased metabolic demands placed on the body and brain, resulting in an increase in carbon dioxide.

Protective Reflexes

Protective reflexes are cranial nerve reflexes and indicate brainstem functioning. The unresponsive patient should be assessed for the presence of intact reflexes, and if reflexes are absent or decreased, measures should be taken to protect the patient from injury. The protective reflexes include (1) corneal reflex, (2) gag reflex, (3) swallow reflex, and (4) cough reflex. Check the corneal reflex by touching the cornea with a wisp of cotton. The eye will blink rapidly if the reflex is intact. The gag reflex is checked by touching the posterior tongue with a tongue blade. If intact, the patient will gag. The cough and gag reflexes can be checked also while suctioning the intubated patient.

In summary, clinical neurologic assessment is complex, and in-depth areas commonly assessed include pupils, eye movements, vital signs, and protective reflexes. Frequently, the location of some lesions or pathologies can be determined based on the clinical assessment.

Section Seven Review

1. Which component of vital signs provides the most useful information?
   A. respiration
   B. blood pressure
   C. heart rate
   D. temperature

2. Pupils that are bilaterally pinpoint and nonreactive to light indicate
   A. unilateral brain lesion
   B. metabolic coma
   C. herniation
   D. lesion in the pons

3. The most important component of the neurologic assessment is
   A. level of responsiveness
   B. pupil reactivity
   C. cranial nerve assessment
   D. vital sign assessment

4. Protective reflexes indicate
   A. level of lesion
   B. presence of increased ICP
   C. brainstem functioning
   D. intactness of the motor tracts

Answers: 1, A. 2, D. 3, A. 4, C.

Section Eight: Documentation

At the completion of this section, you will be able to document your assessment of the arousal and content components of responsiveness.

It is important to document your assessment in a reliable and consistent manner to provide accurate transfer of information from clinician to clinician. Labels, such as comatose, lethargic, and stuporous, should be avoided because they lend themselves to subjective interpretation.

The Glasgow Coma Scale (GCS) is the most frequently used method to document neurologic assessment. The scale assesses eye opening responses and verbal and motor responses. Therefore, it assesses the arousal component of responsiveness (Table 12–1).

The GCS was developed to provide a means for objective assessment of depth of coma. It provides a way to convey quantitatively a patient's neurologic status. It is an extremely useful scale for evaluating patients at lower levels of responsiveness because it evaluates reactivity-type patterns. Higher levels of responses require cortical functioning because of the interpretation of stimuli that is required. The GCS is not a complete and valid measure of content and often misses subtle changes in cognition, such as attentional deficits. For this reason, to identify and evaluate higher order responses, additional techniques are needed.

There are certain types of patients for which the GCS is not usable. Patients with periorbital edema are unable to open their eyes and would receive an eye opening response score of 1, which may or may not be valid. Motor deficits, such as hemiparesis or paraplegia, may be overlooked, since the motor response scored is the best response elicited. Finally, it is impossible to evaluate a verbal response for patients who are intubated or have a tracheostomy.

In order to assess content, you must assess language, memory, and mood. This is possible only with the conscious patient. With an unconscious patient, you will be able to assess arousal only. Verbal response should be assessed not only for orientation but also for flow, clarity, spontaneity, and appropriateness. The patient's mood should be noted, and memory should be tested by asking the patient to name the last four or five United States presidents (remote memory). Content can be assessed using a mental status examination.

Vital signs should be documented along with

TABLE 12–1. GLASGOW COMA SCALE

Category	Score	Response
Eye opening	4	Spontaneous—eyes open spontaneously without stimulation
	3	To speech—eyes open with verbal stimulation but not necessarily to command
	2	To pain—eyes open with noxious stimuli
	1	None—no eye opening regardless of stimulation
Verbal response	5	Oriented—accurate information about person, place, time, reason for hospitalization, and personal data
	4	Confused—answers not appropriate to question but correct use of language
	3	Inappropriate words—disorganized, random speech, no sustained conversation
	2	Incomprehensible sounds—moans, groans, and mumbles incomprehensibly
	1	None—no verbalization despite stimulation
Best motor response	6	Obeys commands—performs simple tasks on command; able to repeat performance
	5	Localizes to pain—organized attempt to localize and remove painful stimuli
	4	Withdraws from pain—withdraws extremity from source of painful stimuli
	3	Abnormal flexion—decorticate posturing spontaneously or in response to noxious stimuli
	2	Extension—decerebrate posturing spontaneously or in response to noxious stimuli
	1	None—no response to noxious stimuli; flaccid

pupillary assessment. Pupil size should be assessed using a standard pupil gauge (Figure 12–3).

In summary, the GCS is a standardized and well-accepted method of assessing the arousal component but is not a valid measure of cognitive abilities or content. To evaluate content, additional methods must be employed.

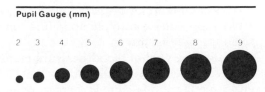

Figure 12–3. Pupil gauge in millimeters. (*From* The clinical practice of neurologic and neurosurgical nursing, *by J. Hickey, 1986, Philadelphia, J.B. Lippincott Co.*)

Section Eight Review

1. The Glasgow Coma Scale assesses
   A. cranial nerves
   B. abstract thinking
   C. arousal
   D. awareness
2. The Glasgow Coma Scale is useful because
   A. it is standardized
   B. it evaluates the ability to interpret stimuli
   C. it is subjective
   D. it evaluates vital signs and pupil reactivity

3. The Glasgow Coma Scale should not be used for
   A. quantitative evaluation
   B. evaluation of lower levels of responsiveness
   C. evaluation of attentional deficits
   D. comatose patients

Answers: 1, C. 2, A. 3, C.

Section Nine: Nursing Interventions and Pharmacologic Therapies

At the completion of this section, you will be able to identify nursing interventions and pharmacologic therapies for patients with alterations in level of responsiveness.

Alterations in level of responsiveness occur as impaired arousal or content. In general, impaired arousal is secondary to coma or a comalike state, such as occurs with increased ICP or metabolic coma secondary to drug overdose. Impaired content generally is secondary to metabolic disorders, psychiatric illnesses, and drug or alcohol abuse. Therefore, the Number One nursing intervention is to treat the primary problem.

Nursing interventions for patients with impaired arousal center around maintaining ventilation, controlling cerebral perfusion pressure (CPP), and instituting protective mechanisms and pharmacologic therapies. For impaired content, nursing interventions center around protecting the patient from injury.

Maintaining Ventilation

Patients with a decreased level of arousal frequently need to have the airway maintained because they are unable to use protective reflexes, such as coughing, or are unable to maintain an adequate respiratory pattern. Because hypoxia and hypercapnea can be better controlled with mechanical ventilation, patients may be intubated. Ventilatory rates may be set as high as 20 to blow off excess carbon dioxide and prevent cerebral vessels from vasodilating. The airway is kept patent by suctioning. Intubated patients are hyperventilated before and after suctioning with 100 percent oxygen for 60 seconds, and each suctioning pass is limited to 15 seconds (Parsons and Shogan, 1984). Keeping the patient pulled up in bed facilitates respirations, aids in keeping the patient oxygenated, and avoids carbon dioxide buildup.

Controlling Cerebral Perfusion Pressure

Because cerebral perfusion pressure (CPP) controls cerebral blood flow and cerebral blood volume, efforts to control CPP are of primary importance and include blood pressure control, temperature control, and promoting venous return.

Optimally, the goal of blood pressure management is to keep it within normal limits so that CPP is between 45 mm Hg and 160 mm Hg. Pressures above or below this range will result in loss of autoregulation and inadequate CPP. Besides pharmacologic therapy to increase or decrease blood pressure, interventions include reducing noxious stimuli and volume replacement.

Temperature control is important because hyperthermia raises cerebral metabolism. The use of antipyretics and cooling blankets helps keep body temperature controlled.

Promoting venous return is an area where nursing has a large impact through body positioning and moving. Unless the patient has a cervical spine injury, the head of the bed should be elevated to at least 30° (Mitchell, 1986). This position avoids jugular compression, promotes venous drainage, and decreases, or at least, controls ICP. Avoid neck flexion, lateral head rotation, and hip flexion of greater than 90°. This positioning avoids increasing intraabdominal or intrathoracic pressure, which can interfere with venous outflow and drainage. The body should be turned as a unit, with head, neck, trunk, and lower extremities turned in unison. This avoids head and neck rotation. Patients who are alert should be assisted in moving up in bed. Asking patients to help by pushing with their legs initiates the Valsalva maneuver, which increases intrathoracic pressure and impedes venous return.

Pharmacologic Therapy

Drug therapy will be initiated for most patients with increased ICP. The goal is to decrease intracranial volume, either by decreasing brain volume, decreasing CSF production, or decreasing the metabolic rate. Drug therapy is classified into hyperosmolar agents, steroids, diuretics, and barbiturates.

Hyperosmolar Agents

These agents act by causing movement of water from edematous brain tissue into the vascular bed, thus reducing brain volume and ICP. Rapid reduction of volume occurs within the first 15 minutes of infusion, and the effects last for 3 to 8 hours (Hickey, 1986). Mannitol and glycerol are hyperosmolic agents.

Diuretics

Diuretics, such as furosemide (Lasix) decrease brain volume and CSF production. Unlike mannitol, furosemide is selective for injured brain tissue and effectively reduces cerebral edema and ICP (Alcorn, 1983).

Steroids

The use of steroids to decrease brain volume is widely disputed. The mechanism of action is unclear, but it has been demonstrated that steroids reduce white matter edema associated with brain tumors. The drug of choice usually is dexamethasone (Decadron) (Hickey, 1986).

Barbiturates

Barbiturate therapy is not a first-line action. Barbiturates work by decreasing the metabolic rate, thereby reducing CBF and possibly reducing cerebral edema formation. This type of drug therapy produces a drug-induced coma, which makes the neurologic evaluation difficult and unreliable.

Providing a Safe and Protective Environment

The following nursing interventions are for patients with impaired content and are directed toward protecting the patient from injury, reorienting, and creating a calm, safe environment. Patients with cognitive deficits become confused easily from external stimuli. Noise should be kept to a minimum, information should be presented simply and calmly, and the amount of visitors at one time should be limited. Keeping a dim light on at night and frequent checking by the nurse will help to control confusion secondary to misperception of stimuli.

Patients with cognitive deficits often attempt to get out of bed and may pull out IV lines and catheters. Interventions, such as keeping the bed in a low position, using siderails, and frequent checks, will help keep the patient safe from harm. Frequent reorienting by the nurse will help decrease confusion and disorientation.

Trying to pick up clues that may point to the etiologies of deficits in level of responsiveness is not an easy task, especially if the cause is unrelated to increased ICP. Identifying focal injuries, such as brain tumors or hematomas, as contributing factors of altered responsiveness is a more straightforward process than identifying extracranial causes.

In summary, this section has discussed nursing interventions for patients with impaired arousal and content and has listed some of the pharmacologic therapies for patients with increased ICP.

Section Nine Review

1. Mannitol acts to decrease ICP primarily by
   A. decreasing CSF production
   B. preventing fluid absorption by cerebral cells
   C. reducing the amount of brain volume
   D. decreasing the blood–brain barrier
2. Which nursing intervention would be appropriate for a patient with intracranial hypertension?
   A. manual hyperventilation
   B. increasing the frequency of suctioning
   C. encouraging coughing and deep breathing exercises
   D. keeping the head of the bed flat
3. Which of the following pathologies may cause an impairment of content but not of arousal?
   A. drug overdose
   B. dementia
   C. expanding intracranial mass
   D. metabolic coma

4. Nursing interventions for patients with impaired content center around
   A. protection from injury
   B. maintaining the airway
   C. control of cerebral perfusion pressure
   D. drug therapy
5. Pharmacologic therapy for patients with increased ICP includes
   A. volume expanders
   B. paralyzing agents
   C. tranquilizers
   D. barbiturates

Answers: 1, C. 2, A. 3, B. 4, A. 5, D.

Section Ten: Seizure Disorders

At the completion of this section, the reader will be able to relate seizure disorders as a sequela of head trauma and discuss the nursing and pharmacologic management of seizure disorders.

A seizure disorder, or epilepsy, has a variety of etiologies. Some individuals have a genetic predisposition to seizures. In others, seizures occur as the result of a pathologic process, such as infection, brain tumors, birth injuries, cerebral circulatory alterations, or head trauma. In this section, seizure disorders are discussed as a sequela of head trauma, known as posttraumatic epilepsy.

Epilepsy is considered a syndrome and is a result of CNS irritation, characterized by recurrent paroxysmal episodes in which there is a disturbance in skeletal motor function, sensation, autonomic visceral function, behavior, or consciousness (Hickey, 1986). The dysfunction is produced by excessive and abnormal neuronal discharge.

Seizure activity may occur any time following a head injury. However, the onset of seizures appears to follow a definitive pattern. Seizure activity rarely appears before 2 months or later than 5 years after head trauma. The onset usually occurs between 6 months and 2 years posttrauma. As an acute care nurse, you probably will not witness seizure activity in the initial management stages of a head-injured

patient. Therefore, teaching patients about the potential for seizures, symptoms, and management becomes a critical part of the nursing care and management of these patients.

Some seizure activity can be triggered by identifiable stimuli; others cannot. Precipitating factors include specific odors and noises, being startled, fatigue, hypoglycemia, emotional stress, lack of sleep, fever, alcohol consumption, constipation, menstruation, and hyperventilation. Teaching patients to avoid specific circumstances or to be aware of specific precipitating factors, if there are any, is one method of teaching patients to manage a seizure disorder.

In general, seizures are classified based on the clinical nature of the onset. There are four major categories: simple partial (focal), complex partial, generalized, and unclassified. An in-depth discussion of these categories is beyond the scope of this module. The reader is encouraged to consult the references by Hickey (1986) or Marshall et al (1990).

Status Epilepticus

Status epilepticus is a neurologic emergency with potentially lethal consequences if untreated or if treatment is delayed. It is defined as a continuing series of seizures without a period of recovery or regaining of responsiveness between attacks. Status epilepticus may occur as a result of untreated or inadequately treated seizures and most commonly occurs from abrupt discontinuation of pharmacologic treatment. The continuous series of seizures can cause ischemic brain damage because of impaired respirations, producing systemic and cerebral anoxia. Therefore, immediate control of the seizures and maintaining a patent airway are critical interventions. For the patient with ICP problems, the implications are crucial. As discussed earlier, cerebral ischemia produces vasodilation, resulting in further increases in ICP. Controlling the seizure is urgent for these types of patients.

The drug of choice for status epilepticus is diazepam (Valium), given IV. Phenytoin (Dilantin) given IV also has been cited as a drug for control of status epilepticus (Marshall et al, 1990). After the seizure activity has been controlled, the patient may need to be intubated to ensure adequate oxygenation. At the least, a nasopharyngeal or oropharyngeal airway should be inserted to establish an airway. Frequent suctioning will maintain patency of the airway.

Pharmacologic Management

Anticonvulsant therapy reduces or controls seizure activity but does not cure a seizure disorder. Drug therapy is chosen based on the type of seizure and is introduced in gradually increasing doses until a therapeutic blood level is reached. Cessation of the drug is titrated in decreasing doses to prevent status epilepticus. Although many anticonvulsants currently are in use, either alone or in combination, some common drugs are phenytoin, phenobarbital (Luminal), and carbamazepine (Tegretol).

Nursing Management

The goals of nursing management of the patient with seizures are to protect the patient from injury and control the seizure and patient/family teaching.

Any patient with the potential for seizure activity should be placed on seizure precautions. This includes padding the bedrails, keeping the bedrails up, placing suction equipment at the bedside, and keeping the bed in the lowest position.

Observation and documentation of the events surrounding the seizure are important in order to identify the type of seizure and the patient's response to the interventions and to select appropriate drug therapy. Level of responsiveness immediately before, during, and after the seizure should be recorded. The time elapsed between the onset and cessation of seizure activity, the type of motor activity, and any complications, such as aspiration or apnea, should be noted also. The nurse has an important role in educating the patient and family in the management of seizure disorders. Teaching should include medication protocols, including side effects and adverse reactions, recognizing seizure activity, activity restrictions, and acute management.

In summary, seizure disorders are a common sequela of traumatic head injury. Acute management includes protection from injury, controlling the seizure, and patient/family teaching. Anticonvulsants are used for acute and long-term management.

Section Ten Review

1. In teaching a patient recovering from a head injury, the nurse would include that the onset most likely would occur
   A. within the first few weeks posttrauma
   B. within the first 6 months after head injury
   C. between 6 months and 2 years after head injury
   D. 3 to 5 years after head injury

2. An important implication for patients with increased ICP experiencing a seizure is
   A. the potential for cerebral ischemia
   B. the potential for cerebral vasoconstriction
   C. the potential for aspiration
   D. the potential for falling out of bed

Answers: 1, C. 2, A.

Section Eleven: Diagnostic Procedures

At the completion of this section, the reader will be able to discuss selected diagnostic procedures, their clinical application, advantages, and limitations.

Until the latter half of the twentieth century, the neurodiagnostic tools were crude and yielded non-specific results. Since the introduction of computed tomography (CT) scanning in the 1970s, the diagnostic methods used in neuroscience have become more refined and accurate. This section discusses some of the most recent diagnostic developments, along with their clinical applications, advantages, and limitations.

Computed Tomography Scanning

Computed tomography (CT) scanning occurs in a steplike process. The area is scanned in layers by x-ray beams that pass through the area and focus onto photographic film. This process is known as tomography. An x-ray tube is located around the area being scanned and rotates in a 180-degree arc. As the x-ray beams pass through the area, the radiation is either absorbed or transmitted onto an electronic detector. The density of the area determines whether the radiation is absorbed or transmitted, with bone absorbing the most, which will appear white on the scan, and air the least, which will appear black. Through a complex process, the radiation transmitted is converted to electric signals, which are digitalized and stored in a computer. This information is reproduced as an image on a display monitor. The area can be scanned in various thicknesses, called slices, depending on the amount of detail desired.

CT scanning of the head is useful for detecting primary injuries, such as skull fractures, hematomas, and contusions, such secondary injuries as herniation, edema, and shifting of brain tissue secondary to swelling, and abscesses and tumors.

The CT scan remains the initial procedure of choice in acute head injury because it is noninvasive, produces rapid results, is safe and painless, and has reduced the need for more invasive procedures, such as angiograms.

Magnetic Resonance Imaging

The magnetic resonance imaging (MRI) scanner is actually a large tube-shaped magnet that can create an extremely strong magnetic field. This magnetic field causes nuclei in the area scanned to line up in a uniform manner rather than spin in random directions, as is usual. Radiofrequency pulses are applied to various types of body tissue, causing body tissue nuclei to resonate. The nuclei emit energy signals, and by varying the radiofrequency pulses, different energy signals are produced. These signals are collected by a computer, which reproduces an image of the tissue scanned.

MRI is superior to CT scanning. As with CT scanning, MRI allows one to determine the anatomic location of a lesion. Additionally, MRI allows examination of the tissue itself, providing more anatomic detail than CT scanning. Therefore, detecting white matter shearing, infarction, and ischemic tissue is possible with the MRI. The MRI scan has the ability to detect pathologic processes at an earlier stage than is possible with the CT scan. Therefore, it is the procedure of choice for early diagnosis of cerebral infarction and brain tumors.

MRI carries limitations that the CT scan does not. The powerful magnetic field interferes with electrical devices. Thus, it is not an option for patients with pacemakers. Metal equipment cannot be introduced into the scanner because the magnetic field may dislodge the equipment. Patients with metal hip replacements, orthopedic pins, protheses, bullet fragments, and most ventilator equipment cannot be exposed to the MRI scanner. Obtaining an MRI takes longer than CT scanning, and MRI provides a poorer image of bone tissue. Therefore, CT scanning is the procedure of choice when time is a factor, as with the unstable trauma patient or in the detection of spinal fractures. Finally, the cost of MRI is 20 to 200 percent higher than a CT scan. The benefits of MRI must be weighed against the cost.

Positron Emission Tomography

Positron emission tomography (PET) is a new technology used to study complex physiologic processes in different body systems and is useful in detecting biochemical and physiologic abnormalities. PET has the capacity of providing measurements of regional CBF, metabolism, and biochemistry. It may prove to be useful in the evaluation of cerebrovascular disorders because of the ability to measure changes in these variables.

The patient inhales or is injected with a compound (usually carbon-11), that contains a positron-emitting nuclide. This nuclide acts as a tag on the compound, and once inside the body, the tag leaves the compound and produces two gamma-ray photons. A scanner detects the photons and codes the data into a computer, which reconstructs images of the distributed tags.

The PET scan is a much newer technology than the CT or MRI scan, and therefore, its full potential and limitations have not been studied fully. PET is being used in clinical research for the evaluation of tissue blood flow and the measurement of oxygen and glucose use. However, because of the cost (between $3,000 and $5,000) and the lengthy time involved, PET remains impractical for clinical use.

In summary, neuroscience technology is becoming more sophisticated. Not only do we now have the ability to determine the anatomic location of lesions, but with the advent of the CT scan, the MRI, and PET, we also are able to examine the tissues themselves and their metabolic and biochemical processes.

Section Eleven Review

1. CT, rather than MRI, scanning would be the procedure of choice for
   A. detecting white matter shearing
   B. detecting the early stages of brain tumors
   C. detecting cerebral infarction
   D. detecting spinal fractures

2. PET scanning is useful for detecting
   A. dementia
   B. spinal fractures
   C. skull fractures
   D. anatomic location of a brain tumor

Answers: 1, D. 2, A.

Posttest

1. The principle that explains reciprocal mechanisms involved in increased ICP is
   A. Monro-Kellie hypothesis
   B. cerebral perfusion formula
   C. autoregulation
   D. chemical regulation
2. The earliest indicator of deteriorating neurologic status is
   A. level of responsiveness
   B. motor response
   C. pupillary response
   D. vital signs
3. Hypoxemia and hypercapnea cause
   A. cerebral vasodilation
   B. decreased ICP
   C. cerebral vasoconstriction
   D. decreased CBF
4. As a compensatory mechanism, pressure regulation acts by constricting cerebral blood vessels in response to
   A. elevated blood levels of oxygen
   B. decreased blood levels of oxygen
   C. elevated systemic blood pressure
   D. decreased systemic blood pressure

5. Hyperventilating a patient results in
   A. increased CBF
   B. decreased cerebral blood volume
   C. increased elastance
   D. increased compliance
6. Which of the following may increase ICP?
   A. Valsalva maneuver
   B. raising the head of the bed
   C. manual hyperventilation
   D. use of osmotic diuretics
7. Your patient's MAP is 100 mm Hg and ICP is 10 mm Hg. What is the CPP?
   A. 80 mm Hg
   B. 90 mm Hg
   C. 110 mm Hg
   D. 120 mm Hg
8. Elastance refers to
   A. the blood vessels ability to accommodate increased volume
   B. the measure of slackness in the brain
   C. the ability of blood vessels to dilate and constrict
   D. amount of volume reserve in the intracranial vault

9. Keeping the head and neck in alignment results in
   A. decreased venous outflow
   B. increased venous outflow
   C. increased intrathoracic pressure
   D. increased intraabdominal pressure
10. Barbiturate therapy for treatment of intracranial hypertension works by
   A. paralyzing the skeletal muscles
   B. acting as a diuretic
   C. decreasing the metabolic rate
   D. sedation, thereby promoting a calm response to environmental stimuli
11. A critical nursing intervention for a patient with status epilepticus is
   A. protecting the airway
   B. padding the bedrails
   C. restraining the patient
   D. providing for privacy
12. MRI scanning, rather than CT scanning, is the procedure of choice for detecting
   A. white matter shearing
   B. hematomas
   C. bullet fragments
   D. spinal fractures

Posttest Answers

Question	Answer	Section	Question	Answer	Section
1	A	Two	7	B	Three
2	A	Seven	8	D	Three
3	A	Four	9	B	Four
4	C	Three	10	C	Nine
5	B	Nine	11	A	Ten
6	A	Nine	12	A	Eleven

REFERENCES

Alcorn, M.H. (1983). Altered levels of responsiveness: Decreased response. In M. Snyder (ed). *A guide to neurological and neurosurgical nursing.* New York: Wiley.

Hickey, J. (1986). *The clinical practice of neurologic and neurosurgical nursing.* Philadelphia: J.B. Lippincott Co.

Marshall S.B., Marshall, L.F., Vos, H.R., and Chesnut, R.M. (1990). *Neuroscience critical care: Pathophysiology and patient management.* Philadelphia: W.B. Saunders Co.

Mitchell, P.H. (1986). Intracranial hypertension: Influence of nursing activities. *Nursing Clin. North Am.* 12:563–576.

Parsons, L.C., and Shogan, J.S.O. (1984). The effects of the endotracheal tube suctioning/manual hyperventilation procedure on patients with severe closed head injuries. *Heart Lung.* 13:372–380.

Teasdale, G., and Jennett B. (1974). Assessment of coma and impaired consciousness. *Lancet.* 1:81–84.

Module 13

Impaired Physical Mobility

Kathleen Dorman Wagner

The self-study module, *Impaired Physical Mobility*, focuses on the physiologic effects of bedrest on human body systems. This module is a review of previously learned immobility concepts rather than an in-depth presentation of the topic. It presents the material in a concise, systems-oriented manner. It is included in the textbook because a major focus of care management of the acutely and critically ill centers around prevention and management of complications of immobility. Many acutely ill and the majority of critically ill patients are placed on bedrest for a prolonged period of time. Long-term immobilization places this patient population at high risk for development of serious, sometimes fatal complications of bedrest. The module consists of nine sections. Sections One and Two discuss risk factors and underlying factors associated with complications of immobility. Sections Three through Eight describe the effects of immobility on specific body systems, including cardiovascular, pulmonary, renal, gastrointestinal, integumentary, and musculoskeletal. Section Nine presents clinical implications of immobility in high acuity and critically ill patients. This section is divided into two parts: Immobility as a cumulative factor in acute illness and nursing care implications. Each section includes a set of review questions to assist the learner in evaluating understanding of section content before moving on to the next section. All reviews and the Pretest and Posttest in the module include answers. It is suggested that the learner review those concepts that were answered incorrectly before proceeding to the next section.

Objectives

At the completion of the module, the learner will be able to

1. Describe the patient who is at risk for developing complications of immobility

2. Discuss two underlying factors that cause complications of immobility

3. Describe two complications of immobility related to the cardiovascular system

4. Explain two major complications of immobility associated with the pulmonary system

5. Discuss two complications of immobility related to the renal system

6. Explain problems of the gastrointestinal tract associated with prolonged immobilization

7. Discuss the major complication of immobility associated with the integumentary system

8. Explain the complications of immobility associated with the musculoskeletal system

9. Discuss immobility as a complicating factor in the high acuity patient

10. Describe the clinical implications of immobility in the high acuity patient

Pretest

1. Factors that increase the risk of development of complications of immobility include
   A. sex
   B. ethnic background
   C. increased cardiac output
   D. preexisting conditions

2. The general term *stasis* refers to which of the following?
   A. patient condition
   B. lack of normal movement
   C. fight-or-flight mechanism
   D. movement or action

3. A thrombus is primarily composed of
   A. aggregated platelets
   B. red blood cells
   C. plasma
   D. fatty plaques

4. Effects of sympathetic nervous system stimulation include
   A. vasodilation of the mesenteric vessels
   B. vasoconstriction of the skeletal muscles
   C. vasoconstriction of the renal vessels
   D. vasoconstriction of the brain

5. Which of the following circumstances will cause thrombi to form inappropriately?
   A. when blood flow is above normal
   B. when vessels are smooth and slick
   C. when blood pressure is high
   D. when hypercoagulation exists

6. Bedrest affects ventilation by causing
   A. hypoventilation
   B. hyperventilation
   C. increased tidal volume
   D. increased minute volume

7. Absorption atelectasis is caused by
   A. reabsorption of capillary gases into the alveoli
   B. collapse of alveoli due to external pressure
   C. collapse of alveoli due to low atmospheric pressure
   D. reabsorption of alveolar gases into the capillaries

8. The major source of the mineral component of renal calculi comes from
   A. muscle
   B. fat
   C. blood
   D. bone

9. If renal calculi become lodged, they cause problems associated with
   A. obstruction
   B. circulation
   C. infection
   D. nerve damage

10. A major complication of intestinal obstruction includes which of the following?
    A. constipation
    B. diarrhea
    C. strangulation
    D. ulceration

11. Perforation of the bowel frequently leads to
    A. dehydration
    B. peritonitis
    C. ulceration
    D. ischemic bowel

12. The major etiologic factor responsible for development of a pressure ulcer is
    A. localized infection
    B. skin breakdown
    C. muscle damage
    D. compromised blood flow

13. The specific term used to describe an ulcer associated with vagal stimulation secondary to head injury is
    A. Curling's ulcer
    B. Cushing's ulcer
    C. stress ulcer
    D. gastric ulcer

14. For calcium to remain within bone, the bone is most dependent on
    A. range of motion
    B. compression load
    C. intake of sufficient calcium
    D. a high level of parathyroid hormone

15. Disuse osteoporosis is associated with an increased risk of
    A. hypocalcemia
    B. muscle atrophy
    C. hyperkalemia
    D. spontaneous fractures

16. Which of the following statements is correct regarding immobility as a complicating factor?
    A. it is composed of unique complications
    B. its effects overlap with other stressors
    C. it is not a high priority consideration as a stressor
    D. it is the most important stressor for the high acuity patient

Answers: 1, C. 2, B. 3, A. 4, C. 5, D. 6, A. 7, D. 8, D. 9, A. 10, C. 11, B. 12, D. 13, B. 14, B. 15, D. 16, B.

Glossary

Absorption atelectasis. A type of atelectasis that occurs when alveoli become obstructed by secretions

Atelectasis. A condition in which alveoli are in a collapsed state

Baroreceptors. Specialized nervous tissue located in the aorta and carotid sinus and pulmonary arteries that is sensitive to alterations in pressure and volume

Calcitonin. A hormone secreted by the thyroid gland that works in opposition to parathyroid hormone to lower serum calcium

Contracture. A condition in which there is muscle fiber shortening, causing increased resistance to passive muscle movement

Curling's ulcer. A type of stress ulcer particularly associated with severe burns

Cushing's ulcer. A type of stress ulcer particularly associated with cerebral trauma

Disuse osteoporosis. The loss of bone mass caused by immobility

Dynamic. Refers to movement or action

Mucociliary escalator. A major pulmonary defense mechanism in which foreign substances are cleared from the lower lungs by a transport system involving mucus and organized ciliary movement

Orthostatic (postural) hypotension. The significant drop in arterial blood pressure when the patient rapidly changes from a recumbent to a sitting or standing position

Paralytic ileus. An intestinal paralysis associated with acute intestinal obstruction and distention

Perforation. A complication of intestinal obstruction in which overexpansion of the intestines causes the bowel wall to tear open, dumping bowel contents into the peritoneum

Pneumonia. The presence of an inflammatory state in the lungs

Pressure ulcer (pressure sore, decubitus ulcer). Ulcer caused by pressure to a part of the body as a result of lying in bed or sitting in a chair

Stasis. Sluggish or lack of normal movement of body fluids; stagnation of secretions or airflow in the pulmonary system; decreased intestinal peristaltic activity; lack of musculoskeletal movement

Strangulation. A complication of intestinal obstruction in which capillary refill in the intestinal wall is compromised due to excessive pressure

Stress ulcers. An erosion of the intestinal mucosa associated with stress

Thrombosis. The process by which a thrombus (blood clot) is formed

Thrombus. A blood clot

Section One: Risk Factors for Developing Complications of Immobility

At the completion of this section, the learner will be able to describe the patient who is at risk for developing complications of immobility.

Virtually all patients who have been partially or completely immobilized are at risk for complications of immobility. Mobility is a relative term that occurs as a continuum ranging from complete mobility to its extreme opposite, complete immobility. Today, the completely mobile patient is rarely seen in most hospitals because of the use of outpatient facilities for this relatively well patient population. Most patients who are hospitalized are those who are experiencing a moderate to severe degree of physiologic compromise (i.e., they are classified as moderate to high acuity patients). By virtue of their degree of acuity, they generally also have some degree of impaired mobility.

There are many factors that increase the risk of development of complications of immobility (Table 13–1). These factors are integrated throughout the module. The risk of developing immobility complications increases in a fairly linear fashion with the degree of immobility and the length of time the patient has been immobilized.

TABLE 13–1. COMPLICATIONS OF IMMOBILITY RISK FACTORS

Dehydration
Decreased cardiac output states
Obesity
Malnutrition
Postoperative state
Decreased level of consciousness
Prolonged period of immobility
Stressful environment
Traumatic injury to bone or soft tissues
Preexisting conditions

Assessing for complications of immobility risk factors is an essential ongoing process. As the patient's status changes during hospitalization, risk factors may change. Early and vigorous implementation of preventive actions, both independent and collaborative, can minimize or prevent complications of immobility. Preventive measures can have a significant impact on the patient's outcome during hospitalization and beyond.

In summary, acutely ill patients are at risk for developing complications of immobility. There are multiple factors that can increase the risk of complications even further. It is crucial to assess the patient constantly for the presence of these risk factors to prevent or at least minimize the deleterious effects of prolonged immobility.

Section One Review

1. Factors that increase the risk of development of complications of immobility include
   A. sex
   B. ethnic background
   C. increased cardiac output
   D. preexisting conditions
2. The hospitalized patient population is at an increasingly high risk for development of complications of bedrest because of
   A. higher patient acuity levels
   B. overhydration problems
   C. inadequate nursing care
   D. increased admissions of males

3. The ultimate reason that risk factors are assessed continuously in the immobilized patient is
   A. to protect the patient
   B. to protect the nurse
   C. to provide adequate care
   D. to prevent multiple complications

Answers: 1, D. 2, A. 3, A.

Section Two: Underlying Factors Associated with Complications of Immobility

At the completion of this section, the learner will be able to discuss two underlying factors that cause complications of immobility.

Stasis

Stasis is a Greek word that means *standing still*. For the purposes of this module, stasis refers to sluggish or lack of normal movement of body fluids (i.e., blood or urine), stagnation of secretions or airflow in the pulmonary system, decreased intestinal peristaltic activity, and lack of musculoskeletal movement. Humans are bipedal, vertical beings. Normal body homeostatic functions are based on dynamic (pertaining to movement and action) rather than static principles, requiring regular weightbearing activities in a vertical position.

Many of the body's systems cannot adapt sufficiently to immobility and prolonged horizontal positioning. Thus, the entire body is affected when a patient is immobilized, significantly increasing the risk of developing a myriad of complications. The risk is even greater in high acuity patients, many of whom are already experiencing multisystem dysfunction.

Sympathetic Nervous System Stimulation

The sympathetic nervous system is stimulated during psychologic or physiologic stress as a natural preparation for fight or flight. Illness is a stress that triggers stimulation of the sympathetic nervous system.

When stimulated, the sympathetic nervous system causes an increase in blood pressure, pulse, and respirations. Peripheral vasoconstriction occurs to shunt blood into more vital emergency body areas, such as the heart, lungs, brain, and skeletal muscles. The sympathetic response vasoconstricts the mesenteric and renal vessels, which are not considered vital for emergency functioning, decreasing blood flow to these areas. Unfortunately, although sympathetic nervous system stimulation helps the body meet a sudden crisis, over time the effects can be deleterious to the body as a whole, causing stress-related complications, such as ulcers and hypertension.

In summary, problems involving stasis and sympathetic nervous system stimulation place all immobilized patients at risk for development of complications. Table 13–2 summarizes the major complications of immobility. Many problems can be prevented or at least minimized. However, to be able to plan and implement effective preventive actions, one must first understand the bases of the problems. This module is designed to refresh the learner about the major complications of immobility.

TABLE 13–2. SUMMARY OF THE COMPLICATIONS OF IMMOBILITY

Stasis	Sympathetic Response
Cardiovascular effects	Gastrointestinal effects
Decreased cardiac output	Paralytic ileus
Thrombus formation	Stress ulcers
Pulmonary effects	Constipation
Ventilation-perfusion ($\dot{V}/\dot{Q}$)	
abnormalities	
Absorption atelectasis	
Hypostatic pneumonia	
Genitourinary effects	
Urinary tract infection (UTI)	
Renal calculi formation	
Integumentary effects	
Pressure ulcers	
Musculoskeletal effects	
Disuse osteoporosis	
Muscle atrophy	
Contractures	

Section Two Review

1. Of the following, the sympathetic nervous system is primarily stimulated in response to
   A. stress
   B. stasis
   C. relaxation
   D. immobility
2. Effects of sympathetic nervous system stimulation include
   A. vasodilation of the mesenteric vessels
   B. vasoconstriction of the skeletal muscles
   C. vasoconstriction of the renal vessels
   D. vasoconstriction of the brain

3. The general term *stasis* refers to which of the following?
   A. patient conditions
   B. lack of normal movement
   C. fight-or-flight mechanism
   D. movement or action

Answers: 1, A. 2, C. 3, B.

Section Three: Cardiovascular Complications

At the completion of this section, the learner will be able to describe two complications of immobility related to the cardiovascular system.

Prolonged stasis of blood is associated with the development of several complications of immobility: thrombus formation and orthostatic hypotension.

Thrombus Formation

A thrombus is a blood clot. It develops through the process of thrombosis. Thrombi are composed primarily of aggregated platelets, white blood cells, and fibrin in varying quantities. In vessels where blood is flowing, platelets that have clumped together are the first to attach to the vessel wall endothelium. Once attached, the platelets begin to release certain substances, which, in turn, cause fibrin to form at the site. As the platelet and fibrin clump grows, circulating leukocytes and red blood cells also become trapped, thus increasing the thrombus size. Thrombi develop in layers, forming a tail that can be very long. Deep vein thromboses originating in the lower extremities or pelvis are seen most commonly in the immobilized patient. Should the tail of the thrombus detach, the clot (an embolus) moves through the circulation until it becomes lodged. Emboli have potentially deleterious consequences by causing obstruction of blood flow distal to the lodged embolus, causing tissue ischemia.

Ordinarily, thrombosis occurs in response to extravasation of blood due to traumatic injury or surgery. Development of blood clots normally controls bleeding and, therefore, plays an important protective role in maintaining homeostasis. There are three circumstances in which thrombus formation occurs inappropriately: first, when the vessel is no longer smooth and slick, such as is seen with atherosclerosis, second, when blood flow has been significantly reduced, and third, when the blood is in a state of increased coagulability (Price and Wilson, 1986).

Acutely ill immobilized patients are at high risk for development of a thrombosis because they generally meet at least one of the three abnormal circumstances stated. Older patients frequently have moderate to advanced atherosclerosis. Hypercoagulability is one of the many effects of the physiologic response to stress, and this group of patients generally is experiencing high stress levels. Immobilized patients have problems of venous stasis due to lack of musculoskeletal movement.

Venous stasis resulting from immobility has several etiologies. First, immobility decreases venous return to the heart. Normally, blood from the legs is pumped actively up from the lower extremities through a one-way venous valve system. This occurs primarily through a squeezing action of the leg muscles, which push against the veins during normal walking activities. Normal movement and muscle actions all over the body help keep blood in motion. When a patient is not active, this pumping action is virtually lost, which encourages blood to remain gravity dependent, thus pooling in dependent areas of the body.

Orthostatic Hypotension

Orthostatic (postural) hypotension refers to the significant drop in arterial blood pressure when the patient rapidly changes from a recumbent to a sitting or standing position. Blood pressure is controlled by three factors: arterial vasomotor tone, CO, and circulating blood volume (Hudak et al, 1990). Prolonged immobility associated with horizontal positioning may significantly decrease blood pressure because it alters cardiovascular status through several possible mechanisms: fluid shifts and diminished baroreceptor stimulation.

The Fluid Shift Theory

The fluid shift theory helps explain how cardiovascular status may be altered due to bedrest. The theory is based on the results of numerous clinical investigations showing evidence of a fluid shift from the lower extremities toward the upper extremities during bedrest. According to Winslow (1985), approximately 50 percent of blood volume is normally present in the systemic veins, 30 percent is in the intrathoracic system (heart, lungs, and great vessels), and 20 percent is located in the systemic arteries.

Standing Fluid Shift. When a person is standing up, approximately 500 mL (about 10 percent) of the blood shifts to the lower extremities due to the force of gravity. Most of this shift comes from the intrathoracic compartment. The shift is sometimes described as a "functional hemorrhage." Standing results in a reduction in venous return to the heart and decreased stroke volume, CO, and arterial blood pressure.

Horizontal Fluid Shift. When a person lies down, body fluids shift back toward the upper body, increasing intrathoracic pressure. This shift of fluids back to the body core has two physiologic effects: decreased CO and increased cardiac workload (Winslow, 1985; Ulrich et al, 1986). Increased cardiac workload generally is accompanied by an increased pulse rate of 5 to 15 bpm. During a period of prolonged immobility, the muscles in the legs lose muscle tone from lack of use. Decreased muscle tone causes pooling (stasis) of blood in the extremities, resulting in decreased CO. Diminished muscle tone also increases the response time required to adequately meet changing hemodynamic requirements when position changes are attempted, thus contributing to the development of orthostatic hypotension.

The Role of Baroreceptors

Baroreceptors are an important part of the special compensatory mechanisms activated to maintain adequate CO. When stimulated, baroreceptors trigger a reflex action of rapid peripheral vasoconstriction, which rapidly elevates the arterial blood pressure. Normally, when a person stands up, the gravity force being exerted on the blood causes it to flow away from the baroreceptors located in the aorta and carotid sinuses, decreasing baroreceptor stimulation. Hudak et al (1990) explain that orthostatic hypotension is associated with a sluggish baroreceptor reflex. When the reflex is not working properly, compensatory mechanisms are unable to respond to rapid position changes adequately. Thus, when the person attempts to stand or sit up rapidly, the blood pressure drops, causing decreased cerebral perfusion. It is the inadequate brain perfusion that accounts for the major orthostatic hypotension symptoms of dizziness, blurred vision, and syncope.

In addition to positional fluid shifts and sluggish baroreceptor response, the high acuity patient may also experience orthostatic hypotension for other reasons. Many drugs significantly manipulate the cardiovascular system, altering CO and blood pres-sure. The presence of fluid volume deficit places the patient at risk for moderate to severe CO problems accompanied by a significantly lower arterial blood pressure.

In summary, the cardiovascular system is profoundly affected by prolonged bedrest. Venous thrombosis and orthostatic hypotension are two major complications. The fluid shift theory, a sluggish baroreceptor response, fluid volume deficit, and drug therapy all are possible underlying factors in the development of orthostatic hypotension.

Section Three Review

1. Thrombus can be defined as
   A. a mass of fibrin
   B. a fatty mass
   C. a blood clot
   D. a detached plaque
2. A thrombus is formed by a process called
   A. thrombosis
   B. fibrinolysis
   C. leukocytosis
   D. thrombocytopenia
3. Which of the following circumstances will cause thrombi to form inappropriately?
   A. when blood flow is above normal
   B. when vessels are smooth and slick
   C. when blood pressure is high
   D. when blood is in a state of increased coagulability
4. A thrombus is primarily composed of
   A. aggregated platelets
   B. red blood cells
   C. plasma
   D. fatty plaques

5. Orthostatic hypotension is caused by
   A. decreased cardiac workload
   B. rapid stimulation of baroreceptors
   C. hypertonicity of lower extremity vessels
   D. diminished baroreceptor response
6. The fluid shift theory states that when a person is placed in a horizontal position, fluid
   A. is unable to shift from one compartment to another
   B. shifts from the venous supply to the arterial supply
   C. shifts from lower limb vessels back to intrathoracic vessels
   D. shifts from intrathoracic compartment to systemic vessels

Answers: 1, C. 2, A. 3, D. 4, A. 5, D. 6, C.

Section Four: Pulmonary Complications

At the completion of this section, the learner will be able to explain two major complications of immobility associated with the pulmonary system.

The pulmonary system, like the cardiovascular system, develops problems when immobility is imposed. Two of the most common problems are atelectasis and hypostatic pneumonia. Both conditions are problems of stasis. Holloway (1988) explains that pulmonary stasis is associated with the development of a state of hypoventilation (inadequate airflow). Hypoventilation results from reduced ventilatory mechanics (minute and tidal volumes) secondary to respiratory muscle wasting, a consequence of prolonged bedrest. As the muscles become weaker, the patient must work harder to maintain adequate airflow.

Altered Ventilation–Perfusion Relationship

Inspired air naturally flows toward the diaphragm, moving more air into the lung bases for optimum gas exchange. Normal aeration is physiologically designed for upright (vertical) breathing. Pulmonary perfusion is gravity dependent. This means that in an upright position, most of the pulmonary capillary perfusion is found in the lung bases. Normally, a certain relationship exists between ventilation and pulmonary perfusion (a 4:5 ratio). Ideally, airflow into the alveoli is greatest in those portions of the lungs where pulmonary perfusion is also the greatest, thus maximizing gas exchange. Significant alterations in this relationship lead to hypoxia.

Horizontal positioning interferes with the normal relationship of pulmonary ventilation-perfusion ($\dot{V}/\dot{Q}$ ratio). While horizontal, airflow continues to flow toward the diaphragm. However, since perfusion is gravity dependent, more blood moves to the dependent area of the lungs. For this reason, gas exchange is best in the dependent lung areas. For example, if the patient is positioned on the right side, the right lung is better perfused than the left lung. If both lungs are aerating equally, the right lung has better gas exchange, since it has more blood to diffuse gases across the alveolar–capillary membrane. The patient on prolonged bedrest primarily experiences an interference with ventilation due to hypoventilation problems. However, perfusion also may be altered if CO becomes diminished or if acute problems, such as pulmonary embolus or severe inflammation, interfere with pulmonary perfusion. (The concept of $\dot{V}/\dot{Q}$ ratio is discussed in detail in Module 1, *Respiratory Process.*)

Stasis of Pulmonary Secretions

Normally, pulmonary secretions are cleared from the lungs through several defense mechanisms, the mucociliary escalator and the cough reflex.

The Mucociliary Escalator

A significant portion of the lower airways is lined with pseudostratified ciliated columnar epithelium. Interspersed between the epithelial cells are mucus-producing cells that create a thin mucous layer that lines the airways. This mucous layer lies directly on top of the cilia. In the lower airways, the cilia rapidly beat in an upward motion. Secretions and foreign matter lie on the mucous layer, which is constantly being moved by cilia toward the upper airway, where it is either coughed out or swallowed.

Certain factors can reduce the effectiveness of these defense mechanisms. The mucociliary escalator is affected by such things as

1. Dehydration, which severely hampers mucous production, causing mucus to become very thick and scant in quantity

2. The presence of excessive secretions (e.g., pneumonia or chronic bronchitis), which can overburden the mucociliary escalator, thus causing pooling secretions
3. Cigarette smoking, which causes destruction of airway cilia
4. Anesthesia and certain types of drugs that decrease mucous production and ciliary action
5. High flow oxygen therapy, which decreases mucous production and decreases ciliary activity

The Cough Reflex

The cough reflex is an important pulmonary defense mechanism to clear the lower airway of foreign substances. The acutely ill immobilized patient may have a depressed cough mechanism. The ability to have an effective cough is reduced significantly by certain medications, particularly sedatives and analgesics. It also can be reduced if the patient cannot or will not use sufficient force to clear the airway (i.e., decreased level of consciousness, presence of pain, weak respiratory muscles, or diseases that restrict airflow in or out of the lungs).

Interference with either the mucociliary escalator or the cough reflex encourages pooling of pulmonary secretions. Thus, the patient becomes at risk for development of atelectasis or hypostatic pneumonia.

Atelectasis

Atelectasis is a condition in which alveoli are in a collapsed state. There are two types of atelectasis, absorption atelectasis and compression atelectasis. Compression atelectasis occurs due to pressure being placed on the alveoli, preventing them from expanding. Absorption atelectasis is the most common cause of alveolar collapse in the immobilized patient and thus is described in more detail.

Absorption atelectasis occurs when airways (bronchial or bronchiolar) become obstructed by secretions. When airway obstruction occurs, airflow distal to the obstruction ceases. Air that remains in the blocked alveoli is absorbed into the pulmonary circulation. Subsequently, with no gas present to occupy space, the alveoli collapse. Atelectic areas of the lung can no longer take part in gas exchange. Normal compensatory mechanisms shunt blood flow away from the nonfunctioning lung tissue toward better ventilated lung areas to improve the balance of ventilation to perfusion ($\dot{V}/\dot{Q}$ ratio).

Hypostatic Pneumonia

Pneumonia refers to the presence of an inflammatory state in the lung tissues. Immobilized patients are particularly at risk for developing hypostatic pneumonia. This type of pneumonia is caused by lying in one position for prolonged periods of time, accompanied by shallow breathing, causing pulmonary congestion. This, in addition to pooling of secretions, can set up an inflammatory process and encourages the invasion of infectious agents. Hypostatic pneu-

monia is noted most commonly in the lung bases (Price and Wilson, 1986).

In summary, normal pulmonary function is best when in an upright position. Prolonged immobility in a horizontal position is detrimental to normal function, placing the patient at risk for problems of stasis of gases or secretions and problems of alveolar hypoventilation. It also alters the relationship of ventilation to perfusion, which ultimately alters arterial blood gases and tissue oxygenation.

Section Four Review

1. Normally, secretions are moved up the lower airway primarily by
   A. coughing
   B. swallowing
   C. mucociliary escalator
   D. macrophage activity
2. High percentages of oxygen have what effect on mucous production?
   A. remains the same
   B. decreases production
   C. increases production
   D. initially increases, then decreases
3. Bedrest affects ventilation by causing
   A. hypoventilation
   B. hyperventilation
   C. increased tidal volume
   D. increased minute volume

4. Absorption atelectasis is caused by
   A. reabsorption of capillary gases into the alveoli
   B. collapse of alveoli due to external pressure
   C. collapse of alveoli due to low atmospheric pressure
   D. reabsorption of alveolar gases into the capillaries
5. The etiology of hypostatic pneumonia is
   A. prolonged immobility
   B. infectious agents
   C. an inflammatory process
   D. viral agents

Answers: 1, C. 2, B. 3, A. 4, D. 5, A.

Section Five: Renal Complications

At the completion of this section, the learner will be able to discuss two complications of immobility related to the renal system.

The renal system is associated with several major complications of prolonged immobility. The two problems are urinary tract infection (UTI) and renal calculi formation. Both involve problems of stasis, though the type of stasis differs.

Urinary Tract Infection

There are two major reasons why immobilized patients are at increased risk for developing urinary tract infections (UTI). First, patients who experience

prolonged immobilization also frequently require indwelling urinary catheters. Second, immobilized patients frequently are kept in a relatively horizontal position for extended periods of time. Akerly et al (1984) explain that of all nosocomial infections, approximately 40 percent are UTIs, primarily resulting from catheterization. UTIs are a contributing factor in the death of debilitated and elderly patients.

The presence of an indwelling catheter increases the risk of development of a UTI for several reasons. First, contamination may occur at the time of catheter placement by a break in aseptic technique. Second, catheter care may be inadequate. Bacteria growing on the external wall of the catheter can climb up the genitourinary tract in an ascending pattern. *Escherichia coli* commonly is the infecting agent due to fecal contamination. Catheter-related UTI is particularly a problem in women because of the close proximity of the urethra to the vagina and anus. Third, the presence of the indwelling catheter may be irritating to delicate tissues, causing development of the inflammatory response. The length of time the catheter is kept in place is an important factor in infection development. Prolonged catheter use increases both the chance of contamination and development of the inflammatory response.

Stasis of Urine Flow

The anatomic placement of the genitourinary tract causes drainage of urine by gravity-dependent flow with the body in a vertical position. Normally, urine drains from the kidneys down through the ureters and into the urinary bladder. Urine is then intermittently voided from the bladder through the urethra. When the patient is placed in a horizontal position, the gravity flow advantage is lost. Urine has a tendency to sit in kidney pelvises and in the bladder. The bladder becomes a potential reservoir for growth of infectious agents, such as *E. coli*. If an infectious process is established in the bladder, the patient's horizontal position actually may facilitate spread of the infection into the ureters and on into the kidneys. Renal calculi also may cause urinary stasis. Once formed, calculi may move down the genitourinary tract until they become lodged. Once lodged, obstruction to flow may occur, causing stasis of urine problems and possible organ damage.

Renal Calculi Formation

Several factors predispose the patient to renal calculi formation. These include urinary stasis, the quantity of calculi-producing element present (primarily calcium), and urine pH. An alkaline urine pH promotes calculi, and an acid pH inhibits formation. Most calculi are formed in the kidney itself and may be composed of calcium or other substances, such as uric acid. Price and Wilson (1986) suggest that hypercalciuria secondary to prolonged bedrest is an important predisposing cause of renal calculi formation. This is supported by the fact that approximately 90 percent of renal calculi are composed, in part, of calcium from bone calcium salts mobilization.

In summary, the renal system is susceptible to complications of immobility because of problems of stasis. First, UTIs commonly occur due to the inability to empty the bladder completely in a horizontal position. The presence of indwelling catheters is a major contributor to UTIs. Second, prolonged immobilization is associated with decalcification of bone, causing hypercalciuria. Hypercalciuria, in turn, facilitates formation of renal calculi, which can potentially damage the kidneys or other parts of the urinary tract.

Section Five Review

1. The most common infectious agent associated with indwelling urinary catheters is
   A. *Escherichia coli*
   B. *Staphylococcus aureus*
   C. *Mycobacterium*
   D. *Streptococcus*
2. Females are at higher risk for developing urinary tract infections than males because of
   A. hormonal differences
   B. increased immobility noted in females
   C. decreased immunocompetence in females
   D. anatomic differences
3. The most common causes of urinary tract infection secondary to the presence of an indwelling catheter includes all of the following EXCEPT
   A. contamination during insertion
   B. anchoring catheter to thigh
   C. inadequate perineal care
   D. tissue trauma

4. The major source of the mineral component of renal calculi comes from
   A. muscle
   B. fat
   C. blood
   D. bone
5. If renal calculi become lodged, they cause problems associated with
   A. obstruction
   B. circulation
   C. infection
   D. nerve damage

Answers: 1, A. 2, D. 3, B. 4, D. 5, A.

Section Six: Gastrointestinal Complications

At the completion of this section, the learner will be able to explain problems of the gastrointestinal tract associated with prolonged immobilization.

There are two major gastrointestinal problems that the immobilized, acutely ill patient is at risk for developing. The first is a stasis problem of decreased intestinal motility, which can cause paralytic ileus and constipation. The second problem is stress ulcers. Although stress ulcers are not caused directly by immobility, they are a common occurrence in acutely ill immobilized patients and thus are included in this module.

Paralytic (Adynamic) Ileus

Paralytic ileus is defined as an intestinal paralysis associated with acute obstruction and distention. It most commonly occurs in patients who have had abdominal surgery. Paralytic ileus is seen also in response to anesthesia and abdominal trauma. It is believed that the primary cause is overstimulation of the sympathetic nervous system through direct handling or indirect manipulation of the intestines.

Paralytic ileus generally lasts for 48 to 72 hours, resolving spontaneously. The seriousness of a paralytic ileus depends on multiple factors: whether it causes a partial or complete obstruction, to what degree it interferes with normal digestion and absorption (Brozenec and Rice, 1985), how long it lasts, and the location of the obstruction.

The major complications of intestinal obstruction include

1. Strangulation. Distention above the obstructed section of bowel can exert sufficient pressure against the intestinal wall to compromise capillary blood flow, possibly leading to eventual necrosis of tissue.
2. Perforation. If distention with gas, food, or fluids becomes severe, the bowel may become overexpanded and actually tear open, dumping bowel contents into the peritoneum.

Constipation

Intestinal peristalsis may be decreased by lack of physical activity, dehydration, lack of nutritional intake via the gastrointestinal route, anesthesia, and many drugs. As with urinary elimination, lying in a horizontal position makes bowel elimination very difficult because the gravity advantage is lost. The patient often must strain more and may not be able to fully empty the bowel. When feces are allowed to remain in the large intestine, the water content is reabsorbed back into the intestines. This dehydrates the feces, making it even more difficult to eliminate.

Stress is another component in constipation. The intestines are controlled by the autonomic nervous system. When stress is present, the sympathetic nervous system is stimulated. The intestines respond by decreased peristalsis and contraction of sphincters. Constipation also may be a symptom of paralytic ileus.

Stress Ulcer

Stress ulcer is a term commonly applied to the condition in which there is an erosion of the intestinal mucosa. Stress ulcers frequently are found in acutely ill patients who are experiencing prolonged stress, either physiologic or psychologic. Table 13–3 lists some of the common stresses associated with the development of stress ulcers, as summarized from Price and Wilson (1986).

There are two mechanisms by which stress ulcers occur, hyperacidity and tissue ischemia. Cushing's ulcers are stress ulcers that occur in the presence of hyperacidity, possibly associated with vagal stimulation secondary to head injury. Other types of stress ulcers are those in which there is no hyperacidity present. They may be associated with deterioration of the mucosal lining secondary to tissue ischemia.

Stress ulcers frequently occur in multiple areas of the stomach, though they can occur in the intestines. They generally are shallow erosions in the mucosal lining. The erosion size varies greatly. The patient often is asymptomatic for several reasons: (1) stress ulcers tend to cause a slow bleed, and (2) the serious nature of the patient's underlying condition may mask symptoms. Stress ulcers are most frequently assessed first by the discovery of positive stool or nasogastric tube aspirant guiac. Stress ulcers account for about 5 percent of all bleeding peptic ulcers (Price and Wilson, 1986).

In summary, the gastrointestinal system is susceptible to complications of bedrest in several ways. First, decreased intestinal motility, a stasis problem, can cause paralytic ileus and constipation. Second, the stress associated with acute illness can lead to development of stress ulcers.

TABLE 13–3. COMMON STRESSES ASSOCIATED WITH DEVELOPMENT OF STRESS ULCERS

Hypotensive shock
Sepsis
Severe burns (Curling's ulcers)
Hypoxia
Cerebral trauma (Cushing's ulcers)

Section Six Review

1. Paralytic ileus may be defined as
   A. an obstruction of the large bowel
   B. a paralysis of the intestines
   C. an obstruction of the small bowel
   D. a paralysis of the ileum
2. Of the following, the most common cause of paralytic ileus is
   A. hypothermia
   B. thoracic surgery
   C. inability to eat
   D. abdominal surgery
3. A paralytic ileus is believed to be caused by
   A. constipation
   B. overdistention of the bowel
   C. depression of the sympathetic nervous system
   D. overstimulation of the sympathetic nervous system

4. A major complication of intestinal obstruction includes which of the following?
   A. constipation
   B. diarrhea
   C. strangulation
   D. ulceration
5. Perforation of the bowel frequently leads to
   A. dehydration
   B. peritonitis
   C. ulceration
   D. ischemic bowel

Answers: 1, B. 2, D. 3, D. 4, C. 5, B.

Section Seven: Integumentary Complications

At the completion of this section, the learner will be able to discuss the major complications of immobility associated with the integumentary system.

Rubin (1988) explains that the skin does not normally bear any weight, with the exception of the soles of the feet. When a patient is placed in a horizontal position, a high proportion of the skin suddenly is required to bear weight. In addition, during bedrest, a large proportion of skin surface area comes into constant contact with a relatively hard surface, the bed. Horizontal positioning on a hard surface places the immobilized patient at risk for development of skin breakdown problems, such as pressure ulcers.

Pressure Ulcers

Pressure ulcers (also called decubitus ulcers or pressure sores) are ulcers caused by pressure to a part of the body as a result of lying in bed or sitting in a chair. Lying or sitting for prolonged periods of time in one position can compromise the capillary perfusion to soft tissue that is being compressed between a bony prominence (e.g., coccyx, spinal vertebra, heel) and the relatively hard surface of a bed or chair.

Capillary blood flow through peripheral soft tissues is a low pressure flow system. This is an important fact because it means that the capillaries are easily compressed together by a person's body weight. When capillaries are compressed, blood flow to the affected area is decreased or halted. Tissue that does not receive blood flow no longer receives oxygen and nutrients to the area. Compromised blood flow may cause tissue ischemia, which can then lead to breakdown of the soft tissues. Once set into motion, the damaged tissue may die and slough off, creating a pressure ulcer formation. If allowed to con-

TABLE 13–4. RISK FACTORS FOR DEVELOPMENT OF PRESSURE ULCERS

Immobility
Urinary or fecal incontinence or both
General debilitation
Advanced age
Prolonged sitting or lying
Infection, sepsis
Shearing forces of moving in bed or chair
Diminished sensation
Sensorimotor deficit

Presence of chronic conditions associated with
    Anemia, malnutrition
    Renal failure
    Diabetes mellitus
    Edema

tinue, the ulcer may destroy muscle and underlying tissues.

Stasis of blood flow is not the only contributing factor for development of pressure ulcers. Table 13–4 lists a series of risk factors showing the complexity of the problem, as summarized from Huether and Kravitz (1990). The acutely ill patient generally has multiple risk factors present.

In summary, the integumentary system is very susceptible to complications of bedrest because of its fragile nature. Being placed in a horizontal position exposes large portions of skin tissue to pressures and shearing forces that are beyond the abilities of compensatory mechanisms to deal with successfully. The major problem associated with bedrest is the development of pressure ulcers, particularly at pressure points, where the skin is pinched between two hard surfaces, such as the coccyx and the bed or chair.

Section Seven Review

1. Common locations for development of decubitus ulcers include all of the following EXCEPT
   A. head
   B. heels
   C. vertebrae
   D. coccyx
2. The major etiologic factor responsible for development of a decubitus ulcer is
   A. localized infection
   B. skin breakdown
   C. muscle damage
   D. compromised blood flow

3. Risk factors that, of themselves, increase the chances of decubitus ulcer development include all of the following EXCEPT
   A. malnutrition
   B. infection
   C. debilitation
   D. level of consciousness

Answers: 1, A. 2, D. 3, D.

Section Eight: Musculoskeletal Complications

At the completion of this section, the learner will be able to explain three complications of immobility associated with the musculoskeletal system.

In the high acuity patient, stasis of the musculoskeletal system (lack of physical activity) may result in the immobility complications of disuse osteoporosis, muscle atrophy, and contractures.

Disuse Osteoporosis

Calcium salts are a major component of bone, with calcium deposits adding strength to the bony matrix. Bone tissue is continuously being broken down and built up. The amount of bone tissue being developed is in direct relation to the amount of pressure being placed on it. For example, an athlete has bones that are heavier than the bones of a nonathlete. Normally, the calcium coming out of bone tissue is in equi-librium with calcium going into the tissue. When less of a compression load is placed on bones, the bony mass decreases in response, and bone deposition is slowed accordingly.

Prolonged immobilization causes bone loss and increased excretion of calcium through the urine. The loss of bone mass related to immobility is called disuse osteoporosis. This represents a loss of calcium from the bone faster than it is being deposited. Secretion of parathyroid hormone increases the rate of bone calcium loss as a compensatory mechanism to increase serum calcium levels, which are low due to increased urinary excretion of calcium.

Other Factors Associated with Osteoporosis

There are a variety of other factors that contribute to the development of osteoporosis. Many high acuity patients have multiple risk factors present either as preexisting states or associated with the acute illness. Older patients are at particular risk for development of complications associated with bone loss. It has

TABLE 13–5. PREDISPOSING FACTORS FOR DEVELOPMENT OF OSTEOPOROSIS

Female
Caucasian
Inadequate calcium intake
Postmenopausal
No estrogen replacement therapy at menopause
Removal of ovaries
Hyperparathyroidism
Diabetes mellitus
Sedentary lifestyle
Smoking
Others

been theorized that as one ages, there may be a natural alteration in secretion of parathyroid hormone, contributing to loss of bone calcium and bone mass (Gray, 1990). At particular risk for development of osteoporosis are postmenopausal Caucasian women who have not received estrogen replacement therapy. The hormone estrogen protects premenopausal women from bone loss. The exact nature of this protection is not well understood. Estrogen may protect either directly, through the presence of estrogen receptors in bone-producing cells, or indirectly, by stimulating the release of calcitonin, which protects against bone resorption (Holm and Hedricks, 1989). Table 13–5 lists some of the more common predisposing factors for development of osteoporosis, as summarized from Holm and Hendricks (1989) and Gray (1990).

Muscle Dysfunction

Muscle Atrophy

Muscle mass develops in response to the amount of stress placed on it. After several days of being immobilized, muscles begin to atrophy (decrease in size) through disuse. Muscle atrophy is accompanied by muscle protein loss and impaired circulation to the muscle, which further diminish strength and endurance particularly to the antigravity muscles (Muir, 1988). Muscle wasting can be severe over time, causing decreased activity tolerance and decreased joint range of motion. Muscle wasting in severe illness also occurs due to malnutrition. When the body does not receive sufficient nutrients to meet its metabolic demands, it turns to muscle protein for its source of energy, creating a catabolic state. Muscle atrophy is an important contributing factor to the inability of many patients to be weaned from mechanical ventilators. In this group of patients, respiratory muscle atrophy prevents them from being able to resume the full work of breathing.

Muscle Contractures

Prolonged immobility may result in the development of contractures (a condition in which there is muscle fiber shortening, causing increased resistance to passive movement of the muscle). Muir (1988) explains that contractures develop as a result of unopposed connective tissue shortening. Normally, the body is continuously developing and breaking down collagen fibers, which, in part, act as supportive structures to muscles and joints. This process is very active around joints, where a wide range of motion is necessary. Special meshlike collagen fibers are produced around joints. The meshlike connective tissue is less dense than connective tissue found in most other parts of the body.

Collagen fibers naturally shorten once they are produced. Active movement of the joints opposes the shortening process by causing constant stretching of the collagen meshwork, actively preventing shortening from occurring. When a patient is immobilized, the collagen meshwork develops unopposed. Dense connective tissue is laid down in place of normal collagen fibers, causing fibrosis. The rate of fibrosis development is enhanced by such problems as edema, impaired circulation, and traumatic injury (problems that commonly are associated with the acutely or critically ill patient). Disuse muscle atrophy complicated by the contracture process causes joints to contract down. The resulting reduced joint range of motion ultimately complicates the patient's complete recovery to the preadmission mobility state. Contractures are preventable through maintenance of range of motion using active or passive exercises on a daily basis (Muir, 1988).

Disuse osteoporosis and muscle atrophy are reversible problems. However, full recovery of bony mass, muscle strength, and joint range of motion takes months, assuming that the patient is able to resume a normal level of activities. Contractures can severely compromise the ability of a recovering patient to resume normal levels of mobility, requiring intense physical therapy and possible surgical interventions to relieve contracted joints.

In summary, prolonged immobility is associated with a variety of musculoskeletal problems, including disuse osteoporosis, muscle atrophy, and muscle contractures. Bones, muscles, and joints require active weightbearing activities to maintain themselves in a normal state. All three problems are reversible to some extent, with contractures requiring the most aggressive management.

Section Eight Review

1. For calcium to remain within bone, the bone is most dependent on
   A. range of motion
   B. compression load
   C. intake of sufficient calcium
   D. a high level of parathyroid hormone

2. Disuse osteoporosis is associated with an increased risk of
   A. hypocalcemia
   B. muscle atrophy
   C. hyperkalemia
   D. spontaneous fractures

3. When calcium is lost from the bony matrix, the overall effect is that the bone
   A. becomes more dense
   B. increases its collagen content
   C. becomes less dense
   D. increases its phosphorus content

4. Muscle atrophy is associated with which of the following?
   A. loss of muscle protein
   B. increased muscle lengthening
   C. loss of muscle calcium
   D. increased muscle metabolism

5. Contractures result from
   A. muscle atrophy
   B. joint calcium deposits
   C. connective tissue shortening
   D. stretching of collagen fibers

Answers: 1, B. 2, D. 3, C. 4, A. 5, C.

Section Nine: Clinical Implications of Immobility

At the completion of this section, the learner will be able to discuss the clinical implications of immobility in the high acuity patient.

Immobility: The Cumulative Factor in Acute Care

The high acuity patient often requires immobilization due to such factors as severity of condition, activity intolerance, and specific interventions. No matter what the reason is for immobilizing a patient, the potential complications remain essentially the same. As discussed earlier in the module, immobility is associated with multisystem dysfunction, and although it is not a disease entity, its complications may be fatal. Immobility is of particular concern in the high acuity patient population because their body systems are already being heavily stressed. In addition to overcoming the initial physiologic insult, they also must attempt to compensate for the adverse effects associated with many of the more aggressive medical interventions (e.g., mechanical ventilation and fluid resuscitation).

Why is immobility such an important factor in the high acuity population? It is due to the cumula-

tive nature of stress on the body systems that may lead to severe dysfunction or destruction of tissues. The following brief patient case study illustrates the overlapping nature of multiple physiologic stressors placed on the body systems.

—— CASE STUDY 1: WILLIAM PHIPPS ——

Mr. William Phipps, a 56-year-old truck driver, was brought into the emergency department after being involved in a motor vehicle accident. It is believed that he remained on the ground at the accident site for at least 1 hour before being found. He sustained multiple internal injuries and lost a significant amount of blood. When transferred to the intensive care unit, his blood pressure was still low, at 88/62. His other vital signs were pulse 132/minute, respirations 34/minute and shallow. He had a chest tube in place due to a left hemothorax. His arterial blood gas was pH 7.30, $Paco_2$ 55 mm Hg, Pao_2 54 mm Hg, HCO_3 24 mEq/L, Sao_2 76 percent. Based on the available data, it was decided that Mr. Phipps was in acute respiratory failure. Mechanical ventilation was initiated at tidal volume of 900 mL, assist/control mode at 14 breaths/minute, and oxygen concentration of 100 percent. Due to the critical nature of his condition, he was placed on strict bedrest and has remained essentially immobile for the past 5 days. Today, it was noted that he is developing a pressure ulcer on his coccyx.

Mr. Phipps has been assaulted by at least four major body stressors in addition to his initial trauma: (1) his initial prolonged hypotension, (2) acute respiratory failure, (3) mechanical ventilation, and (4) prolonged immobility. Each of these stressors by itself can cause multisystem dysfunction. When they occur together, as in the case of Mr. Phipps, they may have a cumulative effect, severely compromising organ function. Table 13–6 summarizes the multisystem effects of the four stressors.

A specific example of the cumulative nature of body stressors can be found in the problem of pressure ulcers. According to the scenario, Mr. Phipps is developing a pressure ulcer, a major complication of prolonged immobility. Pressure ulcers are caused by lack of perfusion to specific peripheral tissues. The lack of perfusion may be mechanical (due to pressure) or functional (due to low CO or poor tissue perfusion). Mr. Phipps is experiencing both problems. He has been immobilized for 5 days. His decreased CO limits the volume of blood that can move into the peripheral tissues surrounding the pressure

ulcer. In addition, the blood that is able to move into the area is poorly oxygenated due to his acute respiratory failure, causing tissue hypoxia. Tissue hypoxia, if prolonged, results in tissue ischemia and necrosis, thus contributing to the development or extension of a pressure ulcer.

Managing Immobility Complications

Prevention of the complications of immobility is a major goal in the management of the acutely ill immobilized patient and it is largely under the jurisdiction of nursing. Two activities are of particular importance based on the principle of stasis, weightbearing activities and vertical positioning. Weightbearing activities, such as early ambulation, are optimal. However, many high acuity patients are not able to ambulate. Vertical positioning, e.g., sitting in a chair or standing on a tilt board, also is beneficial.

Patients who are completely immobilized are at high risk of developing complications of immobility, requiring the nurse to use alternative interventions. Table 13–7 presents a summary of collaborative and independent nursing interventions for management of the immobilized patient.

In summary, high acuity patients, such as Mr. Phipps, are bombarded with multiple physiologic stressors, such as trauma, hypotension, acute respiratory failure, mechanical ventilation, and prolonged

TABLE 13–6. SUMMARY OF MULTIPLE STRESSORS ON BODY SYSTEMS

System	Acute Respiratory Failure	Immobility	Mechanical Ventilation	Hypotension
Cardiovascular	Myocardial tissue hypoxia; myocardial infarction	Decreased cardiac output; thrombus formation	Decreased cardiac output	Decreased cardiac output; myocardial tissue ischemia
Pulmonary	Pulmonary tissue hypoxia; adult respiratory distress syndrome (ARDS)	Atelectasis; increased $\dot{V}/\dot{Q}$ abnormalities; hypostatic pneumonia	Increased $\dot{V}/\dot{Q}$ abnormalities	Pulmonary tissue ischemia; acute respiratory failure
Renal	Renal tissue hypoxia; acute tubular necrosis (acute renal failure)	Renal calculi; urinary tract infection	Decreased urine output, sodium excretion; increased ADH and aldosterone secretion	Renal tissue ischemia
Integumentary	Skin tissue hypoxia; skin breakdown	Pressure ulcers	May decrease tissue perfusion due to lower cardiac output	Peripheral vasoconstriction
Neurovascular	Cerebral hypoxia; brain cell damage	Orthostatic hypotension	Increased intracranial pressure; decreased cerebral perfusion pressure	Cerebral tissue ischemia
Gastrointestinal	Mesenteric tissue hypoxia; ulcers; paralytic ileus	Stress ulcers; constipation; paralytic ileus	Gastric ulcers; increased liver function tests	Mesenteric vasoconstriction
Musculoskeletal	Muscle tissue hypoxia; increased muscle weakness	Disuse osteoporosis; muscle atrophy; contractures	Decreases mobility by virtue of equipment immobility	Muscle tissue hypoxia

TABLE 13–7. NURSING MANAGEMENT OF THE IMMOBILIZED PATIENT

Complication	Nursing Management	Complication	Nursing Management

Cardiovascular
Thrombus
formation
	Collaborative
	  Antiemboli hose; low-dose heparin therapy; IV therapy
	Independent
	  Monitor for signs and symptoms of deep vein thrombosis and pulmonary embolism
	  Hydration; active or passive range of motion exercises
	  Correct body alignment and neutral limb positioning (avoid bending of knees, crossing of legs)
	  If DVT is present: bedrest, leg elevation, warm moist heat
	  If pulmonary embolus is present: close monitoring of hemodynamic and respiratory status, bedrest, elevate head of bed
	Major nursing diagnosis: Alteration in tissue perfusion
			Indwelling urinary catheter vs intermittent catheterization
			  IV fluids if inadequate fluid intake
			Independent
			  Monitor for signs and symptoms of urinary tract infection
			  Hydration
			  If no indwelling catheter, sit up to urinate, if feasible
			  Meticulous, perineal or catheter care, particularly following bowel movement
			  Proper securing of indwelling catheter
			  Intake and output
			Major nursing diagnoses: Infection; Altered urinary elimination

Orthostatic
hypotension
	Collaborative
	  Antiemboli hose; if severe, tilt table may be ordered
	Independent
	  Monitor for signs and symptoms of orthostatic hypotension
	  Measure blood pressure lying and sitting (or standing)
	  Avoid rapid changes in patient position; change positions in small increments; reclining wheel chair, if necessary
	Major nursing diagnosis: Altered tissue perfusion: cerebral
		Renal calculi
		formation
			Collaborative
			  IV fluids; loop diuretics
			  Laboratory: serum calcium and phosphorus
			  Low calcium nutrition; possible acid-ash diet
			Independent
			  Monitor for signs and symptoms of renal calculi
			  Monitor urine for presence of calculi
			  Hydration; intake and output
			Major nursing diagnosis: Altered urinary elimination

Pulmonary
Atelectasis or
hypostatic
pneumonia
	Collaborative
	  Chest x-ray
	  Avoid high concentrations of oxygen
	  Bronchodilator therapy
	  Chest physiotherapy; percussion and postural drainage
	  IV fluids if intake is inadequate
	  Laboratory: sputum for culture and gram stain
	Independent
	  Monitor for signs and symptoms of atelectasis and hypostatic pneumonia
	  Deep breathing exercises or incentive spirometry
	  Frequent position changes
	  Suction if cough is ineffective
	  Hydration
	Major nursing diagnoses: Ineffective airway clearance; ineffective breathing pattern
		Gastrointestinal
		Paralytic
		(adynamic)
		ileus
			Collaborative
			  Nasogastric tube
			  Abdominal x-ray
			  Laboratory: complete blood cell count (CBC)
			  Possible IV hyperalimentation therapy
			Independent
			  Monitor for presence and quality of bowel sounds
			  Monitor for signs and symptoms of paralytic ileus
			  Avoid oral intake in the absence of bowel sounds
			Major nursing diagnoses: High risk for injury: physiologic

Renal
Urinary tract
infection
	Collaborative
	  Laboratory: urinalysis, urine culture and smears
	  Antibiotic therapy
		Constipation	Collaborative
			  IV fluid therapy
			  Laxatives
			  Diet orders: high fiber, if appropriate
			Independent
			  Monitor for signs and symptoms of constipation
			  Hydration
			  Sitting position during bowel movement, if possible
			  Encourage dietary intake
			Major nursing diagnosis: Constipation

		Stress ulcer	Collaborative
			  Endoscopy
			  Laboratory: hemoglobin and hematocrit
			  Drug therapy; antacids, histamine antagonists

(continued)

TABLE 13–7. NURSING MANAGEMENT OF THE IMMOBILIZED PATIENT (Continued)

Complication	Nursing Management	Complication	Nursing Management
	Hemorrhagic shock interventions	*Musculoskeletal*	
	Independent	Disuse osteoporosis	Collaborative
	Monitor for signs and symptoms of stress ulcer		Laboratory: serum calcium, phosphate, CBC; x-ray
	Monitor gastric secretions for pH; maintain pH >5.0		Possible vitamin D supplementation
	Administer drug therapy as ordered, monitor for effectiveness		Independent
	Major nursing diagnosis: Decreased cardiac output		Monitor for signs and symptoms of disuse osteoporosis and spontaneous fractures
			Pain relief measures
Integumentary			Careful positioning
Pressure ulcers	Collaborative		**Major nursing diagnoses: Impaired physical mobility; High risk for injury: physiologic**
	Nutritional support as appropriate to maintain healthy skin		
	Specialty bed (e.g., air flotation bed)	Muscle atrophy and contractures	Collaborative
	Independent		High nutrition diet
	Monitor for signs and symptoms of pressure ulcers		Laboratory: serum albumin, transferrin, total lymphocyte count
	Frequent position changes; careful positioning to protect pressure points		Custom-made splints (for contractures) if desired
	Avoid activities that increase friction and shearing forces:		Independent
	Lift rather than drag patient		Monitor for signs and symptoms of muscle atrophy and contractures
	Eggcrate mattress pad		Careful positioning: proper body alignment; frequent position changes
	Avoid semireclining positions		Range of motion exercises
	Meticulous skin care, focusing on pressure points		Splinting of joints into extended positions (sandbags, towels, IV armboards)
	Hydrocolloid dressings on pressure points (e.g., DuoDERM)		
	Encourage good nutrition		
	Major nursing diagnosis: Impaired skin integrity		

immobility. All of these stress factors have a cumulative effect on the body systems, perhaps severely compromising organ function. When multiple stressors are present, each affected organ system is assaulted from several sources, magnifying the insult to the organ. The cumulative nature of these complications requires close assessment and aggressive management to prevent permanent organ damage. Prevention of stasis is a major goal in planning the care of the acutely ill patient. Ideally, early ambulation and vertical positioning can be employed on a regular basis. There are a variety of alternative nursing interventions available to reduce the risk of developing many of the complications of immobility.

Section Nine Review

1. Which of the following statements is correct regarding immobility as a complicating factor?
   A. it is composed of unique complications
   B. its effects overlap with other stressors
   C. it is not a high priority consideration as a stressor
   D. it is the most important stressor for the high acuity patient

2. Respiratory failure is associated with precipitating which of the following pulmonary problems?
   A. pulmonary embolus
   B. pulmonary vasodilation
   C. pulmonary edema
   D. adult respiratory distress syndrome

3. Nursing interventions to prevent thrombus formation include all of the following EXCEPT
A. hydration
B. deep breathing
C. frequent position changes
D. range of motion exercises

4. The risk of pressure ulcers is reduced by
A. lifting
B. minimizing position changes
C. placing in semireclining positions
D. padding nonpressure point tissues

Answers: 1, B. 2, D. 3, B. 4, A.

Posttest

The following posttest is constructed in a case study format. A patient is presented. Questions are posed based on available data. New data are presented as the case study progresses.

James Erline, a 30-year-old painter, is admitted to the hospital after falling approximately 15 feet from a ladder while painting a house. James is 5 feet 8 inches tall and weighs 200 pounds. He denies any preexisting chronic conditions. He appears well nourished. His admission laboratory tests are within normal ranges. X-rays performed in the emergency department show a severe comminuted right leg fracture near the head of the femur and a right arm fracture. He requires an open reduction of the leg fracture and a closed reduction of the arm fracture. He has been placed on bedrest.

1. On admission, James has which of the following risk factors for developing a complication of immobility?
A. malnutrition
B. prolonged immobility
C. obesity
D. preexisting condition

2. During James' period of bed confinement, he needs to be assessed frequently for problems associated with immobility. The priority goal in his care management is
A. supportive care
B. preventive teaching
C. treatment of complications
D. prevention of complications

James is assessed regularly for symptoms of deep vein thrombosis (DVT) development.

3. He is most likely at risk for development of DVT because of
A. reduced blood flow
B. atherosclerosis
C. hydration state
D. nutrition state

4. Being placed in a horizontal position may alter his blood pressure because of
A. increased cardiac output
B. decreased heart rate
C. increased venous pooling
D. decreased circulating blood volume

5. Bedrest affects James' ventilation in which of the following ways?
A. minute volume is increased
B. tidal volume is decreased
C. airflow is greatest in the apices
D. maximum ventilatory capacity is increased

6. If dehydration is present, what effect would it have on James' secretions?
A. thin and increased
B. thick and increased
C. thin and decreased
D. thick and decreased

James has a urine specimen sent for analysis. A urinary tract infection (UTI) is diagnosed.

___

7. Which of the following would most likely have caused the urinary tract infection?
   A. presence of an external catheter
   B. certain dietary restrictions
   C. presence of indwelling catheter
   D. fluid intake restrictions
8. James is also at risk for developing renal calculi secondary to
   A. disuse osteoporosis
   B. muscle atrophy
   C. urinary tract infection
   D. muscle trauma

While routinely checking James' feces for occult blood, the test is noted to be guiac positive.

___

9. Stress ulcers often go unnoticed except by guiac testing because
   A. they often do not bleed
   B. they are deep, small erosions
   C. they often are slow bleeds
   D. they are caused by hyperacidity
10. If James should develop a strangulated paralytic ileus, it would mean that
    A. a bowel section has ruptured
    B. the bowel has looped around itself
    C. blood flow to a bowel section has been compromised
    D. external forces are compressing bowel, decreasing circulation

James has developed a pressure ulcer on his coccyx.

___

11. A pressure ulcer develops due to
    A. ischemic cutaneous tissue
    B. damage to fatty tissue
    C. friction skin burn
    D. damage to muscle tissue

James is developing disuse osteoporosis and a contractured right hip joint.

___

12. The optimal treatment for correcting osteoporosis is
    A. administer calcium supplements
    B. increase range of motion exercises
    C. administer parathyroid hormone
    D. increase weightbearing activities
13. Contractures are initiated by which of the following problems?
    A. muscle atrophy
    B. joint inflammation
    C. disuse osteoporosis
    D. connective tissue fibrosis
14. To protect James against the development of a severely contractured hip, the nurse should
    A. maintain the joint in an extended position
    B. administer meticulous skin care
    C. raise the head of the bed
    D. place an eggcrate mattress pad on the bed

Posttest Answers

Number	Answer	Section	Number	Answer	Section
1	C	One	8	A	Five
2	D	Two	9	C	Six
3	A	Three	10	C	Six
4	C	Three	11	A	Seven
5	B	Four	12	D	Eight
6	D	Four	13	D	Eight
7	C	Five	14	A	Nine

REFERENCES

Akerly, C.J., Blalock, T.H., Carlson, J.E., Chambers, J.K., Deminski, L.B., and Fagerness, A. (1984). Urologic disorders: Treating infection. In H.K. Hamilton (ed). *Nurse's clinical library: Renal and urologic disorders*, pp. 138–155. Springhouse, Pennsylvania: Springhouse Corp.

Brozenec, S.A., and Rice, H.V. (1985). Recognizing lower GI obstructions. In H.K. Hamilton (ed). *Nurse's clinical library: Gastrointestinal disorders*, pp. 136–161. Springhouse, Pennsylvania: Springhouse Corp.

Brunner, L.S., and Suddarth, D.S. (1988). *Textbook of medical-surgical nursing*, 6th ed. Philadelphia: J.B. Lippincott Co.

Dolan, J.T. (1991). *Critical care nursing: Clinical management through the nursing process.* Philadelphia: F.A. Davis Co.

Doyle, J., Johantzen, M., and Vitello-Cicciu, J. (1988). Vascular disease. In M.R. Kinney, D.R. Packa, and S.B. Dunbar (eds). *AACN's clinical reference for critical-care nursing.* 2nd ed., pp. 727–755. New York: McGraw-Hill Book Co.

Gray, D.P. (1990). Mechanisms of hormonal regulation. In K.L. McCance and S.E. Huether (eds). *Pathophysiology: The biologic basis for diseases in adults and children*, pp. 564–593. St. Louis: C.V. Mosby Co.

Holloway, N.M. (1988). *Nursing the critically ill adult*, 3rd ed. Reading, Massachusetts: Addison-Wesley Publishing.

Holm, K., and Hedricks, C. (1989). Immobility and bone loss in the aging adult. *Crit. Care Q.* 12(1):46–51.

Hudak, C.M., Gallo, B.M., and Benz, J.J. (1990). *Critical care nursing: A holistic approach*, 5th ed. Philadelphia: J.B. Lippincott.

Huether, S.E., and Kravitz, M. (1989). Structure, function and disorders of the integument. In K.L. McCance and S.E. Huether (eds). *Pathophysiology: The biologic basis for diseases in adults and children*, pp. 1390–1430. St. Louis: C.V. Mosby Co.

Kaldor, P.K. (1988). Pathophysiology and diagnosis of gastrointestinal problems. In M.R. Kinney, D.R. Packa, and S.B. Dunbar (eds). *AACN's clinical reference for critical-care nursing*, 2nd ed., pp. 1340–1362. New York: McGraw-Hill Book Co.

Muir, B.L. (1988). *Pathophysiology: An introduction to the mechanisms of disease*, 2nd ed. New York: John Wiley & Sons.

Price, S.A., and Wilson, L. Mc. (1986). *Pathophysiology: Clinical concepts of disease processes*, 3rd ed. New York: McGraw-Hill Book Co.

Rubin, M. (1988). The physiology of bedrest. *Am. J. Nursing.* 88(1):50–57.

Ulrich, S.P., Canale, S.W., and Wendell, S.A. (1986). *Nursing care planning guides: A nursing diagnosis approach.* Philadelphia: W.B. Saunders Co.

Winslow, E.H. (1985). Cardiovascular consequences of bedrest. *Heart Lung.* 14(3):236–246.

ADDITIONAL READING

Guyton, A.C. (1987). *Human physiology and mechanism of disease*, 4th ed. Philadelphia: W.B. Saunders Co.

Module 14

Nursing Care of the Patient with Multiple Injuries

Pamela Stinson Kidd

Nursing Care of the Patient with Multiple Injuries is designed to integrate the major points discussed in the modules, *Traumatic Assessment and Resuscitation, Wound Management, Responsiveness,* and *Impaired Physical Mobility.* This module summarizes relationships between key concepts and assists the learner in clustering information in order to facilitate clinical application. The module is divided into six parts. The first part discusses assessment data frequently used in deriving appropriate nursing diagnoses for a patient with traumatic injuries. The second part focuses on nursing care of a patient who has an intracranial pressure monitoring device. The third part and the last part apply the content in an interactive learning style. The learner is encouraged to identify nursing actions based on an assessment of a patient in a case study format. Consequences of selecting a particular action are discussed, and the rationale for correct actions is presented. Immobility concepts as they relate to the unresponsive patient are addressed next. A discussion of assessment data used in identifying complications associated with traumatic injury and the derivation of nursing diagnoses follows. The last part focuses on nursing management of a patient experiencing sequelae associated with traumatic injury. The module ends with a summary of nursing priorities in caring for a patient with traumatic injuries.

Objectives

Following completion of *Nursing Care of the Patient with Multiple Injuries,* the learner will be able to

1. Identify relationships among traumatic injury patterns, trauma assessment and resuscitation issues, and complications associated with immobility and traumatic wounds

2. Cluster assessment data to formulate nursing diagnoses associated with traumatic injury

3. Appraise a traumatically injured patient's status based on a nursing assessment

4. Identify priorities in nursing care for a patient with traumatic injuries

5. Explain the rationale for nursing actions for the patient with increased intracranial pressure

6. Explain the relationship between trauma resuscitation and complications following traumatic injury

7. Explain rationale for nursing actions that prevent complications associated with traumatic injuries

---

Glossary

A wave. Waveform pattern obtained from intracranial pressure monitoring, often referred to as plateau waves; indicative of increased intracranial pressure (greater than 15 mm Hg); predictive of cerebral hypertension; may last 5 to 20 minutes

Autocannibalism. The breakdown of skeletal muscle mass to provide nutrients during a hypermetabolic phase

Adult respiratory distress syndrome. Noncardiogenic pulmonary edema precipitated by increased pulmonary alveolar–capillary membrane permeability; fluid shifts from intravascular space into pulmonary interstitium; lung compliance is decreased related to destruction of alveolar epithelial cells (types I and II) that produce surfactant

B wave. Waveform pattern obtained from intracranial pressure monitoring associated with decreased arousal; may last up to 2 minutes; indicative of increased intracranial pressure but not as omnious as A waves

C wave. Waveform pattern obtained from intracranial pressure monitoring; low amplitude waves that occur every 4 to 8 minutes and are associated with normal intracranial pressure

Disseminated intravascular coagulation. Syndrome initiated by the release of thrombin and characterized by initial coagulation that precipitates massive lysis of clots and hemorrhage

Ectopy. Extra heart beat initiated by a focus other than the sinoatrial node

Multiple organ failure. Syndrome precipitated by hypoperfusion, usually occurs in a sequential format; lungs, liver, renal and cardiovascular system fail, respectively; may be associated with sepsis

Paradoxical pulse. A fall in the systolic blood pressure associated with inspiration due to decreased left ventricular filling because of increased intrathoracic pressure

Pericardial tamponade. Bleeding into the pericardial sac produced by a laceration of the pericardium; associated with decreased cardiac output

Sepsis. Presence of toxins in the circulation

Septic shock. Hemodynamic instability and inadequate tissue perfusion produced by toxins in the circulation

Septic syndrome. Hemodynamic instability and inadequate tissue perfusion presumed to be produced by toxins in the circulation but not confirmed by culture

Subdural hematoma. Bleeding between the dural and arachnoid layers of the brain, usually venous in nature; classification based on time from injury to onset of symptoms: acute 24 to 72 hours, subacute 72 hours to 14 days, and chronic greater than 14 days (Thelan et al, 1990)

Tension pneumothorax. Collapse of a lung that leads to collection of inspired air into the pleural space that compresses the mediastinum and decreases ventilation of the unaffected lung and cardiac output

Abbreviations

ARDS. Adult respiratory distress syndrome

ATP. Adenosine triphosphate

CPP. Cerebral perfusion pressure

CSF. Cerebrospinal fluid

CT. Computed tomography

CVP. Central venous pressure

DIC. Disseminated intravascular coagulation

F_{IO_2}. Fraction of inspired oxygen

ETOH level. Ethanol level

GCS. Glasgow Coma Scale

ICP. Intracranial pressure

MAP. Mean arterial pressure

MOF. Multiple organ failure

NG. Nasogastric

Pa_{CO_2}. Partial pressure of carbon dioxide

Pa_{O_2}. Partial pressure of oxygen

PEEP. Positive end-expiratory pressure

Sa_{O_2}. Oxygen saturation

THE FOCUSED TRAUMA ASSESSMENT

Nursing History

It is a priority to assess the trauma patient in an efficient manner that focuses on life- and limb-threatening events. Airway, breathing, and circulation (ABC) should be assessed before eliciting a nursing history. A brief, limited assessment can be performed systematically in less than 60 seconds. A head to toe format or systems approach can be used to cluster secondary assessment data later. A focused assessment concentrates on airway, breathing, circulation, disability (limited neurologic assessment), exposing the patient to locate less observable injuries, and obtaining vital signs (including temperature) (ENA, 1991). Regardless of the format used, the nurse must ensure that the patient is able to provide subjective information without further compromising his or her physical integrity. The module, *Trauma Assessment and Resuscitation,* discusses the primary survey in greater detail.

Mechanism of Injury

It is important to focus on the event that resulted in the patient's injuries. As discussed in the module, *Trauma Assessment and Resuscitation,* certain injuries can be predicted based on the combination of agent or object that produced the injury (e.g., motor vehicle, handgun), the type of energy released, (chemical, thermal, or kinetic), the force of energy (as influenced by speed, gun caliber, and so on), and use of protection devices (e.g., seatbelts, airbags, helmets). However, there are several other variables that influence the severity of the patient's injuries. The older patient may have difficulty compensating for blood loss due to decreased vascular tone and myocardial contractility. The pediatric patient may be predisposed to hypothermia because of greater body surface area and decreased thermoregulation. The length of time from the occurrence of the event to definitive treatment may increase the lethality of the event. The presence of preexisting health problems may decrease the patient's ability to meet the increased metabolic demands the traumatic injury creates. For example, a patient with congestive heart failure may not be able to compensate for hypovolemia by becoming tachycardic. Nursing interventions are targeted toward maintainence of homeostasis by ensuring that oxygen supply equals or exceeds oxygen demands. If oxygen demands are not met, the patient will enter anaerobic metabolism. Anaerobic metabolism decreases available adenosine triphosphate (ATP) to 2 moles from the 38 moles that is obtained from the breakdown of 1 mole of glucose in aerobic metabolism (Guyton, 1986).

Past Medical History and Drug Use

Certain conditions, such as hypertension, diabetes, chronic renal failure, chronic pulmonary problems, cerebrovascular attacks, and immune disorders, may produce physiologic changes that impedes the patient's ability to meet the increased oxygen demands and fight infection. Additionally, abnormalities noted on assessment may not be related to the traumatic injury but rather to previous health insults. A history of insulin use, dialysis, bronchodilators, and corticosteriod use can alert the nurse to the patient's state of health and the potential for developing complications.

It is essential to determine chronic symptoms from current symptoms. For example, an elderly patient may have an altered mental status secondary to chronic decreased cerebral perfusion and not because of an acute head injury. However, certain physiologic changes associated with aging may increase the patient's susceptibility to injury. Elderly patients have a higher incidence of subdural hematomas from falls related to increased vessel fragility, thickness of the calvaria, cerebral atrophy, visual, balance, and coordination changes, and decreased reaction time (Lehman, 1988).

A medication history will help the nurse evaluate the patient's response to interventions. If the patient is taking beta-blockers, such as propranolol (Inderal), depolarization is depressed. Beta-blocking agents inhibit sympathetic nervous stimulation and atrioevenous conduction and decrease cardiac contractility and arterial pressure. Thus, the cardiac rhythm is slower. The patient may not be able to respond to hypovolemia with a typical tachycardic response. Traumatic injury stimulates cortisol production. An insulin-dependent diabetic trauma patient may need more insulin to respond to the transient hyperglycemia. If the patient has been using illegal drugs, cardiovascular, ventilatory, and pupillary changes may occur in addition to abnormalities resulting from the injury event. Tetanus immunization history is important, since the patient may have open, dirty wounds. Elderly patients (80 years or older) who cannot recall their immunization history and do not have prior history of military service have a higher incidence of inadequate antitoxin titer when treated with 0.5 mL of tetanus vaccine (Gareau et al, 1990). Tetanus immunoglobulin is preferred for this population.

Alcohol use should be elicited in a trauma patient, since alcohol intake is associated with 20 percent of motor vehicle crashes (MVCs) involving serious injury (National Committee for Injury Prevention and Control, 1989). Positive alcohol use may produce neurologic changes that may be attributed incorrectly to the injury. For example, slurred speech may be related to alcohol intake and not to intracerebral hemorrhage. Most recent oral intake should be documented in anticipation of surgical management of the injuries. A nasogastric tube usually is placed in all trauma patients if aspiration or airway compromise is suspected or anticipated.

It is important to assess the prehospital treatment of the patient to determine the patient's response to the intervention and to obtain the baseline from which other interventions may be initiated. Any interventions provided for the patient before arrival at the hospital should be documented.

In summary, a pertinent nursing history of a trauma patient includes a brief history of the injury-producing event, previously diagnosed conditions and medical management, most recent oral intake, alcohol and illegal drug use, immunization history, use of prescribed medications, and prehospital treatment of the patient.

Frequent Symptoms Associated with Traumatic Injury

If a traumatic injury is suspected, the nurse should focus on assessing the symptoms most commonly associated with life-threatening conditions. These symptoms include ineffective breathing patterns, impaired gas exchange, altered airway clearance, hypotension, distended neck veins, decreased urine output, and a change in level of responsiveness.

Altered Airway Clearance, Ineffective Breathing Pattern, and Impaired Gas Exchange

In the trauma patient, airway is always assessed first. The airway may be compromised if the patient has a depressed mental status. The gag reflex may be absent, and foreign bodies may be present in the oropharynx. A partially obstructed airway will be noisy. Snoring, gargling, or wheezing may be present. The patient requires opening of the airway using a manual manuever (chin lift manuever if cervical spine injury has not been ruled out), immediate suctioning, and placement of an oral or nasopharyngeal artificial airway. Oral or nasotracheal intubation is another method of securing a patent airway. Facial trauma may produce copious amounts of bleeding,

and skeletal integrity of the face may be disrupted. The performance of a cricothyroidotomy is preferred to obtain a patent airway in a patient with massive facial injuries. Direct trauma to the airway may occur from blunt larnygeotracheal injuries. These patients are unable to tolerate a supine position, are hoarse, have subcutaneous emphysema, and are tender over the tracheal area. A tracheostomy is the best method of securing an airway in these patients (DeLaurier et al, 1990).

Ineffective breathing patterns are associated with tracheobronchial and thoracic injuries. The chest is observed for bruising, open wounds, and symmetry of chest wall movement. Open wounds are evaluated further by logrolling the patient and inspecting the posterior surface. No chest wall movement and the presence of abdominal breathing may indicate a cervical cord lesion (Markovchick and Anderson, 1988). The patient's respiratory rate should be noted, as should the degree of breathing effort. Paradoxical movement of the chest (inward motion with inspiration and outward motion with expiration) indicates multiple rib fractures and a flail segment. The patient with a large flail segment may require intubation and mechanical ventilation or pain control therapy in order to prevent respiratory acidosis and to promote tissue oxygenation. The chest area is palpated to detect the presence of subcutaneous emphysema, rib/sternum tenderness, or defects. Auscultation detects the presence of breath sounds bilaterally in the primary survey. Gross differences in breath sounds are important findings, since they usually indicate a pneumothorax or hemothorax. A more detailed pulmonary assessment is performed during the secondary survey (refer to Module 10, *Trauma Assessment and Resuscitation*). High-flow oxygen is administered to trauma patients before obtaining arterial blood gas results. A nonrebreathing mask or a bag-valve-mask device with an oxygen reservoir may be used depending on the patient's responsiveness level. Pulse oximetry and end-tidal CO_2 measurement may provide additional data regarding oxygenation before arterial blood gas analysis.

Aerobic metabolism is dependent on saturation of hemoglobin with oxygen. The patient's Pao_2 must be greater than 60 mm Hg on room air, respiratory rate must be between 12 and 24, and tidal volume must be 10 mL/kg to ensure aerobic metabolism (Thelan et al, 1990). The trauma patient may experience respiratory acidosis as a result of a partially obstructed airway, ineffective breathing patterns, or impaired circulation. Intubation with mechanical ventilation may be necessary to correct the acid-base imbalance. Fluid resuscitation with lactated Ringer's solution may facilitate compensation due to the solution's buffering abilities.

Hypotension and Distended Neck Veins

Peripheral vasoconstriction may artificially elevate blood pressure readings even though central arterial pressures are low. This is a short-acting compensatory mechanism. The value of clustering assessment data is to prevent misdiagnosis by focusing on one symptom while ignoring others. It is very important to monitor the trauma patient's blood pressure and at the same time assess neck veins, responsiveness level, and urine output.

Hypotension in the trauma patient usually is related to hypovolemia. Hypovolemia may result from internal bleeding or uncontrolled external bleeding. Fractures and lacerations of adbominal organs are frequent sources of bleeding in the trauma patient. For example, a fractured femur may result in 1 to 2 L of blood loss (Kosmos, 1989). However, hypotension may be related to factors that inhibit cardiac output (CO) or the loss of peripheral vascular resistance. The two most frequently encountered conditions associated with restriction of CO are cardiac tamponade and tension pneumothorax. In cardiac tamponade, hypotension occurs in response to decreased CO. A tear in the pericardium produces bleeding into the pericardial sac. The increased pressure prohibits filling of the ventricles and decreases stroke volume. The increased pericardium pressure also impedes coronary blood flow. Myocardial ischemia results and further decreases CO. Penetrating chest trauma may produce a tension pneumothorax. As atmospheric air enters the pleural cavity through the injury site, the lung on the affected side collapses while mediastinal contents and the trachea are pushed away from the injury site. The pressure placed on the great vessels inhibits venous return. Thus, the neck veins become distended.

Both cardiac tamponade and tension pneumothorax are life-threatening conditions that require immediate treatment. Blood in the pericardial sac is removed by pericardiocentesis. Insertion of a chest tube and covering the open chest wound (if present) with an impermeable dressing are appropriate interventions for the patient with a tension pneumothorax.

Hypotension also may occur in patients with spinal cord injuries who develop spinal shock. In spinal shock, the patient's blood pressure may be less than 70 mm Hg due to a loss of sympathetic tone that occurs in transection of the spinal cord (Green et al, 1987). The parasympathetic nervous system is unopposed, so peripheral vasodilation and bradycardia occur. Bradycardia is the key assessment finding that helps to differentiate spinal shock from hypovolemia. However, the patient may also be hemorrhaging but is unable to compensate by increasing the heart rate. Atropine is administered to increase the pulse rate high enough to perfuse core organs (Green et al, 1987). Fluid resuscitation is appropriate for hypovolemia but is not necessary for spinal shock, since the problem is loss of vascular tone not volume.

The presence of a radial pulse indicates an arterial pressure of 80 mm Hg. A pressure of at least 70 mm Hg is required for palpation of a femoral or brachial pulse. If a cartoid pulse can be palpated, the pressure is at least 60 mm Hg (Cavallero et al, 1988). The nurse can discriminate hypotension resulting from hypovolemia from that associated with increased pericardial pressure by assessing for the presence of a paradoxical pulse. The systolic blood pressure will fall more during inspiration if tension pneumothorax or cardiac tamponade exists. In these conditions, the increased thoracic pressure from inspiration further decreases left ventricle filling and results in blood backing up into the right heart so CO is compromised. If a central venous pressure (CVP) catheter or pulmonary arterial catheter is in place, the central venous pressure reading will be elevated due to increased right atrial filling with decreased emptying. A CVP reading of greater than 15 cm H_2O is significant (Markovchick and Anderson, 1988). Jugular venous distention will be present. Hypotension resulting from hypovolemia will be associated with flat neck veins. The value of capillary refill as an assessment parameter of hypovolemia has been questioned. However, recent research suggests that normal capillary refill is 2 seconds in the adult male and children, 3 seconds in the adult female, and 4 seconds in the elderly (Schriger and Baraff, 1988). Allowances should be made if the extremity is hypothermic, since capillary refill will be delayed. Decreased pedal pulses and pale or mottled skin also may be present.

Decreased Urine Output

The kidneys receive 20 percent of the CO, and the kidneys may reflect decreased CO earlier than other organs. In most circumstances, decreased or absent urine output in the trauma patient will indicate decreased core perfusion from an extrarenal cause. Through the process of autoregulation, the kidneys can maintain a normal urine output as long as the systolic blood pressure remains in the range of 75 to 160 mm Hg (Guyton, 1986). As the blood pressure nears 60 mm Hg, urine output ceases. The adult trauma patient should maintain an hourly urine output of at least 25 to 30 mL to ensure adequate core circulation. In rare situations, the renal artery may be lacerated from a fall or an abrupt deceleration injury.

The patient will show signs of hypovolemia, with flat neck veins and hypotension. The patient usually will be anuric.

Change in Level of Responsiveness

A change in responsiveness in the trauma patient may be related to numerous factors. In the presence of hypovolemia, cerebral blood flow decreases, resulting in stupor, unconsciousness, and eventually failure of subconscious mental processes, including vasomotor control and respiration (Guyton, 1986). The more highly specialized the tissue, the more vulnerable it is to hypoxemia. Cortical functions are lost first with cerebral hypoxia. Cerebral hypoperfusion is present when the systolic blood pressure is below 60 mm Hg (Moore, 1986). Hypoxia, hypoglycemia, and drug use also may impair responsiveness. Since a change in responsiveness may be present from cerebral injury or from systemic causes, clustering of assessment data is helpful. Responsiveness generally is evaluated at the same time that pupillary size and reaction and motor response are assessed. Module 10, *Trauma Assessment and Resuscitation,* discusses this further. If a spinal cord injury is present, the patient may not be able to respond to commands even if the patient comprehends. It is important to document the stimulus used to elicit a motor response, the exact response, and bilateral differences. The use of a standardized scale, such as the Glasgow Coma Scale (GCS) (refer to Module 12, *Responsiveness*), can facilitate monitoring of neurologic status and improve communication among multiple health care providers.

Airway protection is of major concern in a patient with decreased responsiveness. An oral or nasopharyngeal airway is inserted to maintain airway patency. Unconscious patients should be intubated endotracheally. Oxygen administration is necessary in a patient with decreased responsiveness to promote cerebral oxygenation. Traditionally, the unresponsive trauma patient has been treated with IV thiamine, naloxone, and 50 percent dextrose solution to address the possible etiologies of vitamin deficiency, opiate overdose, and hypoglycemia, respectively. Recent research suggests that naloxone may not need to be administered to all unresponsive patients, since pinpoint pupils and a respiratory rate of less than 12 are highly suggestive of opiate overdose (Hoffman et al, 1991).

Focused Assessment Findings and Nursing Diagnoses

Life-threatening conditions produce characteristic symptoms that the nurse can identify. The following cluster of data strongly suggests the presence of a life-threatening injury:

- Noisy airway
- Absent breath sounds
- Deviated trachea
- Flat or distended neck veins
- Paradoxical chest movement
- Open chest wound
- Subcutaneous emphysema
- Hypotension
- Decreased responsiveness
- Decreased urine output

Nursing diagnoses that pertain to the trauma patient can be clustered in the same manner as the assessment data. Clustering around the ABCs of airway, breathing, and circulation will assist the nurse in prioritizing nursing care.

- **Ineffective airway clearance** related to obstruction or cognitive impairment
- **Ineffective breathing pattern** related to tracheobronchial or chest wall injury, decreased area for gas exchange or pain
- **Impaired gas exchange** related to ventilation-perfusion imbalance or decreased hemoglobin
- **Decreased cardiac output** related to impairment of venous return or myocardial injury
- **Alteration in tissue perfusion** related to an imbalance between cellular oxygen demands and supply

Expected patient outcomes for the trauma patient and associated medical and nursing interventions are addressed in Module 10, *Trauma Assessment and Resuscitation.*

NURSING CARE OF A PATIENT REQUIRING INTRACRANIAL PRESSURE MONITORING

Head injury is the leading cause of all trauma-related deaths (Walleck, 1989). Thirty percent of individuals who survive the injury event require admission into a critical care unit. The recognition and treatment of increased intracranial pressure (ICP) improves the outcomes of these patients. Because of the high incidence of head injuries in trauma patients, nursing interventions for a patient with an ICP monitoring device are discussed. The next part of the module addresses nursing care of a patient being monitored invasively for changes in ICP.

The nursing care for a patient with ICP monitoring includes preparation of the patient and the equipment as well as monitoring the patient during insertion and postinsertion.

Prepare the Patient

Although patients with an elevated ICP have a decreased level of consciousness, it is better to explain the procedure to the patient assuming that the patient is able to understand. Medications to sedate and relieve pain usually are administered in conjunction with neuromuscular blocking agents before insertion of the ICP monitoring device.

Prepare the Equipment

There are three types of ICP monitoring devices currently available: epidural, subarachnoid, and intraventricular. Several new techniques, such as intraparenchymal monitoring, are in experimental phases. Monitoring of ICP from the spinal subarachnoid space through a C1–C2 lateral spinal puncture is under investigation (Wilkinson, 1987). The reader is referred to neuroscience-related literature for a comprehensive discussion of ICP monitoring techniques. This section addresses techniques encountered most frequently with the acutely ill patient.

The subarachnoid screw or bolt (Figure 14–1) is easier to place than the intraventricular catheter and does not require penetration of the brain. It is placed through burr holes in the skull. Cerebrospinal fluid (CSF) cannot be withdrawn. Brain tissue swelling may plug the device, resulting in an underestimation of ICP readings. Epidural catheters also are placed through burr holes. They do not penetrate the brain, and CSF can not be withdrawn from these devices either (Figure 14–1). An intraventricular catheter penetrates brain tissue and allows for removal of CSF

(Figure 14–1). The ability of the brain to compensate for cerebral volume changes (compliance) can be tested using an intraventricular catheter. Fluid is administered through the catheter, and the rise in ICP and changes in waveform patterns are documented. The intraventricular catheter has a higher infection rate (Smith, 1987). It may be inserted through a burr hole, but placement is more difficult. It frequently is placed in the anterior or occipital horn of the ventricle during surgery while the patient is anesthesized. Intraventricular catheters are placed in two different ways. In one, the intraventricular catheter is placed in the ventricle and is connected directly to pressure tubing by a stopcock. The tubing is connected to a transducer. IV tubing and a ventriculostomy (drainage) bag are attached to the system by a stopcock (Figure 14–2). The second device is fully implantable and consists of a catheter from the ventricular space to a subcutaneous reservoir (similar to vascular access devices) usually placed in a burr hole. Percutaneous needle entry is necessary for pressure monitoring (Figure 14–3).

The movement of the CSF is converted into electrical impulses by way of the transducer. The venting port of the transducer is placed at the level of the foramen of Monro to accurately detect pressure changes within the ventricle. The edge of the eyebrow or the tragus of the ear is a suitable external landmark. All readings are obtained with the transducer at this level. There is a 2 mm Hg discrepancy in ICP reading for every inch of discrepancy between the level of the transducer and the correct anatomic landmark (Dolan, 1991). Measurements should not be obtained while the patient is coughing, defecating, moving, or positioned with neck or hip flexion, since these activities increase ICP. Drainage of CSF is

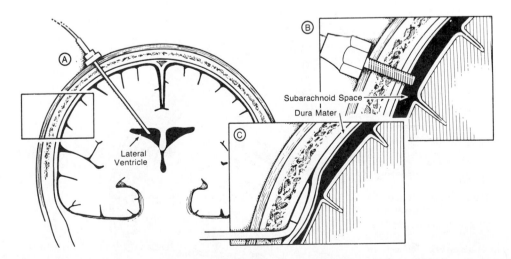

Figure 14–1. Methods employed in intracranial pressure monitoring. **A.** Intraventricular method. **B.** Subarachnoid method. **C.** Epidural method. The intraventricular method is the most invasive and has the highest infection rate of all three approaches. (*From Critical care nursing: Clinical management through the nursing process, by J. Dolan, 1991, Philadelphia: F.A. Davis Co.*)

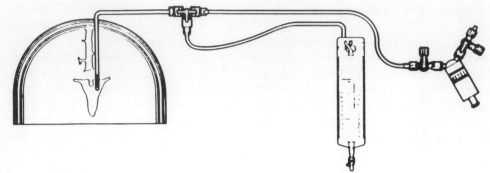

Figure 14–2. Intraventricular monitoring and drainage system. (*Courtesy of Camino Laboratories, San Diego, California.*)

determined by patient need. The level of the bag used for CSF drainage is adjusted to facilitate drainage. Generally, 0.5 to 2 mL of CSF may be drained, depending on the patient response. An order may be written to drain a certain number of drops based on ICP measurement. The amount of CSF drainage is recorded. Sterile normal saline solution is used to maintain the fluid column between the CSF and the transducer dome. A continuous flush system is not used, since even a small amount of fluid could produce lethal elevations in ICP. Some neurosurgeons may flush the system with a very small amount of antibiotic solution to prevent infection. Newer systems may use a sensor instead of a transducer that connects directly into the monitor and recorder.

Equipment for a subarachnoid or epidural device is similar to that used for an intraventricular device.

Monitor the Patient

ICP monitoring usually is used to measure ICP, promote drainage of CSF to decrease ICP, or to detect early deterioration. The normal ICP waveform is referred to as a C wave. This is a rapid, rhythmic wave with an amplitude of approximately 20 mm Hg (Figure 14–4). Early deterioration is defined as ICP greater than 20 mm Hg. Plateau waves (also referred to as A waves) (Figure 14–4) occur in response to

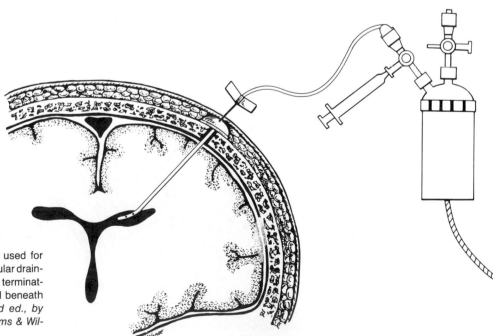

Figure 14–3. Implanted reservoir used for ICP monitoring and periodic ventricular drainage. Ventricular catheter is shown terminating in a reservoir device implanted beneath the scalp. (*From* Head injury, *2nd ed., by P. Cooper, 1987, Baltimore, Williams & Wilkins Co.*)

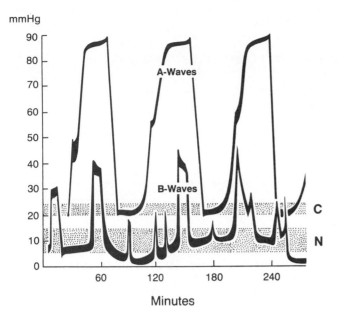

Figure 14–4. Intracranial pressure waveforms. Waveforms reflect pressure in mm HG and time in minutes. Two abnormal waveforms are depicted, including A waves and B waves. A waves reflect intracranial pressure in the range of 50 to 100 mm Hg. They have a duration of 5 to 20 minutes or longer. Their waveforms have a distinctive plateau, and they are referred to as plateau waves. B waves occur as sharp, peaked (sawtooth pattern), rhythmic oscillations, which may reach a peak pressure of 50 mm Hg. They have a duration of 1/2 to 2 minutes. N, normal intracranial pressure waveforms, reflecting a pressure within the range of 0 to 15 mm Hg. C, pressure waveform for C waves. C waves usually are rapid, rhythmic waves with an amplitude of about 20 mm Hg. They occur every 4 to 8 minutes. (*From* Critical care nursing: Clinical management through the nursing process, *by J. Dolan, 1991, Philadelphia: F.A. Davis Co.*)

rapid increases in ICP. They represent cerebrovascular dilatation. Sawtoothed waves (Figure 14–4) indicate cerebral dysfunction and may precede plateau waves. One way of remembering the differences in these waves is to recall that in the cardiac system, flutter waves (sawtoothed formation) occur before fibrillation (a more ominous pattern). They usually last for up to 2 minutes as compared to up to 20 minutes for A waves.

The ICP monitoring system remains sterile. The nurse uses sterile technique when switching ventriculostomy bags and draining CSF. The physician should be notified of the development of or any increase in fever.

In summary, nursing goals for the patient undergoing ICP monitoring focus on detecting increased ICP, treating increased ICP expeditiously, and preventing infection from the use of the monitoring devices.

CASE STUDY

——— PAM K, A PATIENT WITH DECREASED RESPONSIVENESS ———

You are the nurse assigned to admit Pam K from the postanesthesia recovery unit. Pam was transported to the emergency department by the aeromedical service. You have been informed by the postanesthesia nurse that Pam K was involved in an MVC. She was an unrestrained driver and was ejected from the vehicle. She was diagnosed with a subdural hematoma by CT scan of the head. She was taken to the operating suite, where the hematoma was drained and an intraventricular catheter was placed. Pam's intraventricular sensor was placed at the end of the craniotomy procedure. She is being mechanically ventilated. Pam is unable to ask questions about procedures, but she can feel and hear. She was awake and obeyed commands. The nurse must explain what to expect during procedures to patients receiving neuromuscular blocking agents. Because of the injury and the potential use of a neuromuscular blocking agent, it may be impossible to determine exactly what the patient can process cognitively. Pam is 25 years old. Her medical history is nonsignificant. She is being admitted with a diagnosis of closed head injury.

The Initial Appraisal

On entering Pam's intensive care unit room, you notice that she is overweight. A bulky gauze dressing is wrapped around her head. There is blood on the dressing over her forehead region.

You note that Pam is intubated and on a mechanical ventilator. In report, you were told that Pam was initially an 8T on the Glasgow Coma Scale before going to the operating suite. She tried to push the emergency department nurse's hand away when she was starting an IV line. She opened her eyes to her name. Her neurologic status later deteriorated. She has a peripheral IV line of 0.45 percent normal saline running in her right hand. She has an intraventricular ICP monitoring device. A nasogastric (NG) tube is in place. All extremities are in soft restraints. She has numerous abrasions over her body, and there is no active external bleeding. There are no signs of acute distress at present.

QUESTION

The best reason for Pam receiving a nasogastric tube in the emergency department is
1. Stress ulcers are common in head-injured patients
2. Pam may be neuromuscularly paralyzed and, if so, cannot eat
3. Spontaneous emesis is common in the head-injured patient
4. It facilitated endotracheal intubation

ANSWER

3. Spontaneous emesis is common in the head-injured patient, particularly in the first 30 to 60 minutes postinjury (Guss, 1985). If Pam vomits and aspirates, she may develop aspiration pneumonia and ultimately adult respiratory distress syndrome (ARDS). Both of these conditions decrease oxygen diffusion and ultimately decrease cerebral oxygenation.

Focused Trauma Assessment

You complete a head to toe assessment, keeping in mind your initial appraisal and the report you obtained from the postanesthesia nurse.

Head and Neck. Her neck veins are full but not distended. She has a bulky head dressing in place. The chart states that she had a 3 cm laceration of her right forehead that was sutured in the operating suite. Pam does not open her eyes, but she is tugging at her restraints. She has a 7T GCS score at present. She has an intraventricular catheter in place. No drainage is noted in the drainage bag. ICP is 15 mm Hg. C waves are present. Her number 7.5 endotracheal (E-T) tube is anchored firmly and connected to the ventilator. Her nasogastric tube is anchored and connected to low wall suction.

Chest. Because Pam was ejected from the vehicle, you know that her mechanism of injury was severe enough to produce chest and abdominal injuries. Since Pam is on the ventilator, her airway and breathing are being controlled. Breath sounds are auscultated bilaterally, indicating that the E-T tube is positioned correctly. No open chest wound or subcutaneous emphysema is noted. Ventilator settings are: mode: assist/control, rate: 20, tidal volume 750 mL FIO_2 40 percent. Her chest expansion is equal bilaterally. She is in normal sinus rhythm. At present, Pam's blood pressure is being monitored by an external cuff device. It is 100/70 mm Hg. Her pulse is 96, temperature 99.0F rectally.

Abdomen. Her abdomen is soft, without bowel sounds. There is no response when her abdomen is palpated.

Pelvis. Pam has a urinary catheter in place with a urine meter collection device. Her hourly urine output is 65 mL.

Extremities. There are no signs of external bleeding. She has a 7 cm long, 2 cm wide, deep thickness laceration of her right thigh that was irrigated, sutured, and covered with a dry sterile dressing. No blood is noted on the dressing. In report, you were told that the wound was grossly contaminated with pavement debris and dirt. Her circulation is being supported by one peripheral IV line. A solution of 0.45 percent normal saline is infusing at 50 mL/hour through a 14-gauge IV catheter in her right antecubital space. The site is patent.

Posterior. Posterior breath sounds are auscultated per ventilator cycle. No abrasions or expanding flank mass is noted.

You review her emergency department chart to identify historical data and diagnostic tests that were performed and their findings. These data will help you in planning her nursing care in the intensive care unit. You note that Pam vomited at the scene per ground emergency medical services report before the arrival of the aeromedical team.

The following laboratory studies were performed in the emergency department.

■ Arterial blood gas
■ Complete blood count with differential
■ Serum electrolyte profile with glucose
■ Type and screen
■ Serum ethanol level
■ Serum osmolality
■ Lactic acid level

- Prothrombin and partial thromboplastin times

The following radiographic studies were performed.

- Cervical spine films
- AP and lateral chest films
- CT scan of the head and abdomen

QUICK REVIEW

What is the rationale for ordering these tests in a trauma patient?

Arterial blood gas (normal values: pH 7.35–7.45, Pco_2 35–45, Po_2 75–100, HCO_3 24–28, base excess 2 to −2). In hypovolemic shock, metabolic acidosis results (for assistance in interpreting arterial blood gases, refer to Module 2). In Pam's case, baseline ABGs provide ventilatory data to use in determining ventilator settings. Her last set of gases were: pH 7.45, Pco_2 35, Po_2 96, HCO_3 25, O_2 saturation 100 percent.

CBC (normal values: female Hgb 12–16 g/dL, Hct 36–46 percent, WBC 5,000–10,000 μL, platelets 150,000–400,000 μL). The CBC provides baseline measurement of fluid loss. The hemoglobin will decrease after hemorrhage. The hematocrit will increase, indicating hemoconcentration. The WBC count may be slightly elevated due to tissue damage. A decreased platelet count will prolong clotting. Pam's hemoglobin is 11 g/dL. Her hematocrit is 47 percent. Her WBC count is 9,000, and her platelets were 300,000. These values may be indicative of hypovolemia, or they may be related to a chronic anemia.

Serum electrolyte panel (normal values: K 3.5–5.0 mEq/L, Na 135–145 mEq/L, Ca 8.5–10.5 mEq/L, Cl 95–105 mEq/L, glucose 80–120 mg/dL). Potassium levels may increase in the trauma patient due to tissue injury and hypoxia. Hyponatremia may be present if a large amount of cellular damage has occurred because sodium moves into the cell as potassium moves out. Calcium may accumulate at the injury site, producing hypocalcemia. Chloride will usually decrease, since it combines with sodium. Hyperglycemia (usually blood sugar is greater than 120 and less than 200 mg/dL) is associated with traumatic injury due to the release of corticosteroids and catecholamines. All of Pam's electrolyte values are within normal limits.

Type and screen. This is used to determine blood compatibility in case blood volume replacement is needed. Pam is typed as O+.

Serum ethanol level. Alcohol can produce vasodilation and hypotension. A change in responsiveness may be associated with ethanol use. Pam's ethanol level is 100 mg/dL, indicating positive use. This level is considered a legally intoxicated level in most states. It is not high enough to produce massive vasodilation.

Serum osmolality (normal value: 280–300 mOsm/kg H_2O). This is an indication of body fluid concentration. If fluid loss has occurred, serum osmolality is increased. Pam's serum osmolality level is 300 mOsm/kg H_2O. She may have lost some volume.

Lactic acid (normal value: 5–20 mg/dL). Lactic acid accumulation is directly related to cellular hypoxia and may increase before hypotension and decreased urine output occurs (Kee, 1991). An elevated lactic acid level (greater than 25 mg/dL) indicates acidosis. Pam's lactic acid level is normal.

Prothrombin and partial thromboplastin times (normal values: PT 11–15 seconds, PTT 60–70 seconds). These are ordered to provide baseline data on the patient's ability to clot in case hemorrhaging occurs. Pam's clotting times are normal.

Cervical spine films. Spinal cord injuries are accompanied by head injuries in 19 percent of cases (Swain et al, 1985). To rule out a cervical spine fracture, all seven cervical and T1 vertebrae must be visualized on the film. Head and spinal cord injuries are more likely to be present when the patient has been ejected from a vehicle, as in Pam's case. Pam's spinal films were negative.

AP and lateral chest films, abdominal CT scan. Head trauma rarely occurs alone. Thoracic and abdominal injuries frequently are associated with head injuries (Epstein and Hamilton, 1983). Pam's films are negative. This is important, since there was a report of emesis at the scene. However, an aspiration pneumonia will not be readily apparent on chest x-ray initially.

Head CT scan. This is the procedure of choice in the initial assessment of the head-injured patient.

Noncontrast scanning is used most frequently for the head unless a tumor is suspected. MRI is not feasible for the initial assessment of the trauma patient because of the metal associated with stabilization equipment and the length of time required for the procedure. Pam's head CT scan revealed a small, acute subdural hematoma without mass effect. Her injury was classified as moderate, since she does not respond spontaneously and she does not obey motor commands. The neurosurgeon decided to operate and relieve the hematoma.

Development of Nursing Diagnoses

Clustering Data. You have just completed your head to toe assessment and are ready to list the appropriate nursing diagnoses for Pam. To cluster the data, look for abnormals found during the assessment. Pam's major symptom at this time is her decreased responsiveness. This symptom can initiate the cluster of critical cues.

CLUSTER 1.

Subjective data. Involved in MVC as unrestrained driver ejected from the car.

Objective data. GCS score on arrival 8T, 7T at present. ICP monitoring device in place. Craniotomy for draining of subdural hematoma. Present ICP measurement is 15 mm Hg. C waves present.

Pam's decreased responsiveness is related to numerous factors. The primary injury to her head as well as the secondary cerebral edema contribute to her decreased responsiveness. The anesthesia used during the craniotomy procedure and the alcohol she drank before the MVC are also contributing factors. Hypovolemia, hypoglycemia, or hypoxia does not appear to be a factor at this time based on laboratory analysis.

CLUSTER 2.

Subjective data. Report that Pam vomited at the scene.

Objective data. Chest film clear. ABGs suggest borderline respiratory alkalosis. No adventitious breath sounds noted. Several invasive tubes present: IV line, intraventricular catheter, E-T tube, NG tube, and urinary catheter. Repair of two contaminated lacerations. Surgical incision from craniotomy. WBC = 9,000.

CLUSTER 3.

Subjective data. Unrestrained, ejected driver in MVC.

Objective data. Hgb 11 g/dL. Hct 47 percent. Serum osmolality 300 mOsm/kg H_2O. Blood pressure 100/70 mm Hg. Pulse 96 normal sinus rhythm (NSR). No active bleeding noted. Abdomen soft and appears nontender.

It is important to look at the pattern of laboratory data instead of isolated findings. At first glance, it may appear that Pam is losing volume because of her low hemoglobin and high hematocrit. An adult head trauma patient cannot be hypotensive due to blood loss from a closed head injury (Bires, 1987). Thus, other sources of bleeding should be suspected. Since her abdominal CT scan and chest films were normal, internal bleeding has initially been ruled out. External sources of bleeding, such as lacerations, may be the culprit. In Pam's case, she has a 3 cm laceration of the forehead. The bleeding was controlled by application of a pressure dressing in the field. She also has a 7 cm long, 2 cm wide, and 2 cm deep laceration to the right thigh that was bleeding. This laceration may have produced the decreased hemoglobin, although it is not likely. Changes in hemoglobin and hematocrit related to active bleeding usually require hours to manifest postinjury. Her serum osmolality is borderline high and could be related to hydration status before injury. Since Pam's other laboratory values are within normal limits, she is probably not hypovolemic. Her decreased hemoglobin may be related to a chronic condition, such as menstruation. However, if Pam had been hypovolemic, which method of fluid resuscitation would have been preferred?

QUESTION

Hypovolemia associated with a closed head injury is treated by
1. Massive volume replacement with lactated Ringer's solution
2. Combination therapy with lactated Ringer's solution and mannitol
3. Use of whole blood
4. Application of military antishock trousers

ANSWER

2. Mannitol is administered to hypovolemic patients in combination with fluid resuscitation (Bires, 1987). Since cerebral perfusion pressure (CPP) is dependent on the mean arterial pressure (MAP) as well as ICP, hypovolemia must be corrected. Fluid should be administered if the systolic blood pressure is less than 100 mm Hg. Two large-bore IV lines should be initiated, and 2 L of lactated Ringer's solution should be given. If Pam's hemoglobin or hematocrit demonstrated a deficit of 20 percent, O+ (Pam's blood type) packed cells would be given. In these cases, a pulmonary arterial catheter should be placed. The placement of a pulmonary arterial catheter provides data that can be used to determine the minimal amount of fluid that needs to be administered to maintain the MAP and, thus, CPP. (Calculation of CPP is discussed in Module 12, *Responsiveness*.)

Recent research has focused on the use of hypertonic saline solution for fluid resuscitation of head-injured patients. Use of hypertonic saline is limited to experimental situations at present. A 7.5 percent hypertonic saline solution produces a smaller increase in ICP than lactated Ringer's solution and achieves hemodynamic stability with less total fluid administration (Battistella and Wisner, 1991).

Based on the obtained data, the following nursing diagnoses are appropriate for Pam.

- **Alteration in tissue perfusion:** Cerebrovascular related to cerebral edema
- **Potential fluid volume deficit** related to undetected concomitant injuries
- **Potential for infection** related to intraventricular catheter, lacerations, aspiration, and placement of invasive tubes

Expected patient outcomes for Pam would include

1. ICP returns to 10 mm Hg
2. Pao_2 remains greater than 80 torr
3. Pco_2 remains between 25 and 30 mm Hg
4. Systolic pressure remains in the range of 100 to 160 mm Hg to maintain CPP at a level greater than 50 mm Hg
5. GCS improves to 11T
6. No drainage is noted in CSF drainage bag while catheter is patent
7. Absence of A and B ICP waves
8. Urine output remains greater than 30 mL/hour
9. Negative cultures (wound, blood, sputum, urine)
10. Temperature less than 100F rectally
11. WBC less than 10,000 μL

Based on Pam's available data, additional nursing diagnoses pertain to her case even if they are not a priority at this time.

- **Body image disturbance** related to shaving of head, forehead, and thigh laceration
- **High risk for disturbance in role performance** related to hospitalization and neurologic deficit
- **Pain** related to surgical incision and ejection from vehicle

Development of the Plan of Care

Nursing interventions will be based on activities that will help Pam meet her expected outcomes. They will consist of collaborative interventions that are both multidisciplinary and interdisciplinary. Independent interventions are activities that are within the scope of nursing practice and do not require a physician's order.

Collaborative Interventions Related to Decreased Responsiveness. The neurosurgeon orders include the following.

1. *Hyperventilation.* Because Pam's Pco_2 level was 35, the physician adjusts the ventilator settings to: tidal volume 750 mL, rate 24, mode assist/control, and Fio_2 40 percent. ABGs are ordered for 30 minutes after ventilator changes.

QUESTION

Pam's ventilator settings were changed because
1. She was in respiratory alkalosis
2. It is desirable to stimulate her respiratory drive
3. Her P_{O_2} level was too low for adequate cerebral perfusion
4. Her P_{CO_2} level was too high

ANSWER

4. A P_{CO_2} of 25 to 30 is considered optimal for maximum reduction of ICP (Jagger and Bobovsky, 1983). Pam's P_{CO_2} level is 35. Hyperventilation promotes cerebral vasoconstriction for 3 to 4 hours after a head injury. This treatment strategy has been used to prevent vasodilation and increased cerebral edema, thus decreasing cerebral perfusion to the injured tissue. However, vasoconstriction decreases cerebral oxygen delivery as well to the injured tissue. Future research may demonstrate that the benefits of vasoconstriction may be limited. If Pam was hypovolemic in addition to hypercapneic, increasing the ventilator rate could cause additional problems. Hyperventilation increases intrathoracic pressure and decreases venous return and CO. Thus, the body may be sacrificed for the head. In these cases, the rate (or tidal volume) is increased slowly, and the patient response is evaluated.

2. *Diuretic therapy.* A mannitol IV bolus of 0.15 g/kg is ordered prn for ICP greater than 15 Hg. A one-time dose of furosemide (Lasix) 60 mg intravenous push (IVP) is ordered.

QUESTION

Mannitol is a hyperosmolar agent. It is used in a head-injured patient to
1. Promote renal perfusion
2. Enhance renal excretion of drugs
3. Correct acid-base imbalances
4. Promote cerebral tissue fluid movement

ANSWER

4. Mannitol can lower ICP and increase cerebral blood flow. The effectiveness of mannitol has long been debated in the literature. The latest research supports the idea that mannitol removes water from normal brain tissue rather than the injured tissue (Walleck, 1989). The net effect is decreased ICP, but the long-term effects of dehydration of normal brain tissue are unknown. The drug is most effective when administered by bolus than by continuous IV drip. This drug further decreases ICP by reducing total body volume and inhibiting cerebrospinal fluid production. Furosemide (Lasix) may be administered in conjunction with mannitol (as in Pam's case).

3. *Neuromuscular blocking agent.* An order for vecuronium 0.1 mg/kg IVP initially, followed by 0.015 mg/kg 40 minutes later and prn was written.

QUESTION

Vecuronium is ordered for a head-injured patient because it
1. Stimulates smooth muscle contractions
2. Prevents muscular depolarization
3. Promotes spinal cord impulse transmission
4. Prevents apnea

ANSWER

2. Vecuronium (Norcuron) is a neuromuscular blocking agent. This agent prevents acetylcholine from binding with nicotinic receptors, and muscular contraction is blocked. It produces paralysis of skeletal muscles, including those necessary for ventilation. The patient is able to see, feel, and hear but is unable to move or speak. Pam will still require sedation and pain relief. Ideally, the patient is sedated and receives pain medication before administration of the neuromuscular blocking agent. Since she is endotracheally intubated, her airway is secured. Once the neuromuscular blocking agent is administered, the patient is unable to ventilate without external support. The major adverse reaction of these agents is prolonged paralysis after the medication has ceased to be administered. Electrolyte abnormalities and fever increase the likelihood of prolonged paralysis (Shlafer and Marieb, 1989). Thus, the nurse must monitor vital signs and laboratory values closely. Vecuronium will keep Pam from fighting the ventilator and treatment and helps to insure that she will receive adequate cerebral oxygenation. If Pam requires another CT scan to monitor the size of the subdural hematoma, motion artifact will be eliminated, and the obtained films may be clearer and easier to interpret.

4. *Anticonvulsant therapy.* A loading dose of 10 mg/kg of IV phenytoin also is ordered, followed by 100 mg IV every 8 hours.

QUESTION

A nursing implication associated with phenytoin administration is
1. Administer phenytoin in D_5W
2. Phenytoin is poorly soluble
3. Phenytoin metabolizes quickly and should be administered over 2 minutes
4. Phenytoin produces hypertension

ANSWER

2. Phenytoin should not be mixed with other drugs or solutions (including dextrose solutions) because it is poorly soluble and may produce a precipitate. It should be administered in a large-bore IV line, and the line should be flushed with saline postadministration. The dose should be given slowly, at a rate of 50 mg or less per minute. Rapid administration may produce hypotension and cardiovascular collapse. Pam is receiving phenytoin because it inhibits the spread of seizure activity and depresses brainstem centers responsible for seizures (Shlafer and Marieb, 1989). Seizure activity would further decrease Pam's cerebral perfusion and increase cerebral oxygen demands.

The following additional collaborative interventions have not been ordered for Pam at this time but may be necessary if Pam's neurologic status deteriorates.

5. *Fluid restriction.* Fluid may be restricted to 2 L/day to decrease the potential of cerebral edema. As used in Pam's case, 0.45 percent normal saline is the preferred IV solution, since this concentration decreases the likelihood of cerebral edema (Walleck, 1989). The patient's serum osmolality is used to titrate fluid volume. The head-injured patient's se-

rum osmolality should be maintained between 305 and 315 mOsm/L (Walleck, 1989).

6. *Glucocorticosteroids.* There is great controversy concerning the effect of steroids in the management of a patient with a head injury. They are hypothesized to stabilize the cell membranes, thus improving cerebral blood flow and ultimately restoring autoregulation (refer to Module 12, *Responsiveness,* for further discussion of autoregulation). Steroids also may produce negative effects because of their immunosuppresion function. Since Pam had a grossly contaminated wound and a surgical procedure, she may be predisposed to infection. Steroids may not be the best choice of therapy for her.

7. *Barbiturate therapy.* High-dose barbiturates may be administered to reduce cerebral metabolism and cerebral blood flow by inducing coma. Although this therapy is effective in reducing ICP, it does not decrease mortality (Walleck, 1989). Narcotic sedation and neuromuscular blocking agents may be better choices in controlling agitation and decreasing ICP.

Independent Nursing Interventions. There are independent interventions the nurse can make that focus on the identified nursing diagnoses.

1. *Positioning.* Pam should be positioned with her head elevated 30 degrees and in straight alignment. This promotes venous drainage and cerebral blood flow. Hip flexion should be avoided, since this can increase ICP. Research has demonstrated that position changes can increase ICP significantly if the patient's baseline ICP is greater than 15 mm (Parsons and Wilson, 1984). At least 15 minutes should be allowed between position changes to prevent accumulative increases from ICP (Mitchell et al, 1981).

2. *Suctioning.* Pam will require suctioning because she is being ventilated mechanically. Lidocaine (1.5 mg/kg IV) (per physician order) has been administered to head-injured patients before suctioning to suppress the cough reflex and thus produce arterial hypertension and decrease CPP (Yano et al, 1986). The patient should be hyperoxygenated first, and the suctioning should be confined to 10 seconds. Manual hyperventilation should be extended after the third suctioning. Patients with ICP measurements less than 20 mm Hg can be suctioned safely (Parsons et al, 1985). Research is being conducted to determine if manual hyperventilation is as effective as using the ventilator to hyperventilate and maintain CPP. Suctioning increases ICP on the average of 12 mm Hg above the baseline level (Reimer, 1989).

3. *Interaction.* In 1981, Bruya noticed that the patient's ICP dropped when the family approached the patient or touched the patient's arm. Family visits have been associated with decreases in ICP (Hendrickson, 1987). Other studies did not show a decrease in ICP, but family visits have not been associated with increases in ICP (Prins, 1989). Conversation about the patient or directed to the patient without touching the patient has been related to increases in ICP (Mitchell and Mauss, 1978). Therefore, the nurse caring for Pam should touch her while speaking and encourage visits by her family.

4. *Nutrition.* The head-injured patient is hypermetabolic and hypercatabolic. Nutritional interventions should be initiated in the acute phase of treatment and may take the form of total parenteral nutrition (TPN) or early nasointestinal feedings. Although the physician will order the nutritional route and solution, the nurse must ensure that the feeding is administered correctly. Often, these patients require IV medications by way of a central line. A total parenteral feeding may be stopped inappropriately to allow medication administration if there are multiple medications to give at one time and there are too few IV ports. The nurse must treat the feeding as an essential component of the patient's therapy and be meticulous about its administration. This includes restarting the TPN in a timely fashion after medication administration or serving as a patient advocate to get another access port for medication administration so that the feeding is not interrupted.

In summary, independent nursing interventions for Pam include the following.

1. Keep the head of the bed 30 degrees elevated
2. Keep Pam's head in straight alignment and prevent hip flexion
3. Administer nutritional therapy as ordered
4. Suction prn, monitoring ICP waveform and reading during the procedure. Complete the procedure within 10 seconds. Hyperoxygenate and hyperventilate before each suctioning pass and after the final pass for a longer time period
5. Allow family visitation and interaction
6. Use touch when talking to the patient
7. Monitor ICP readings and waveforms and ventricular drainage
8. Monitor effects of drug therapy
9. Maintain accurate intake and output records
10. Prevent increase in ICP
    - Decrease stimulation
    - Allow at least 15 minutes between nursing interventions
    - Prevent constipation and increase in intraabdominal pressure
    - Drain CSF as indicated per physician order

Pam's plan of care is developed and ready to be executed. Her progress will be monitored at regular intervals to evaluate the effects of the various therapeutic actions. If progress is not noted toward attainment of Pam's expected patient outcomes, her plan may need revision, examining alternative interventions that may be more effective.

IMMOBILITY AND THE UNRESPONSIVE PATIENT

A nursing conflict in caring for head-injured patients is to minimize the ICP level and at the same time prevent the complications of immobility. Keep in mind that many of the activities performed to prevent these complications increase ICP, such as range of motion exercises, bathing, oral care, catheter care, and pulmonary hygiene measures. Immobility complications are discussed in this section according to the affected body system. Module 13, *Impaired Physical Mobility,* discusses further complications.

Complications of Immobility

Pulmonary System

Proper suctioning technique was discussed earlier in the module. Research has shown that the Trendelenburg position increases ICP but not to a level where CPP is altered negatively (McQuillan, 1987). Therefore, it may be possible to perform chest physiotherapy without compromising CPP. Further research is necessary in this area.

Elimination

Constipation will increase the intraabdominal pressure and eventually increase ICP. The nurse must monitor bowel movements to detect consistency and urge associated with defecation. The physician may need to be consulted regarding the use of stool softeners, fiber agents, or stimulants. If the patient is on fluid restriction, he or she may be predisposed to the formation of urinary calculi. Urine output, BUN, and creatinine levels are monitored to detect urinary tract changes.

Musculoskeletal System

Positioning was discussed earlier in the module. Patients with ICP readings of 15 mm Hg or less can have passive position changes with 1 minute rest periods between position change to allow recovery of ICP (Parsons and Wilson, 1984). It is still believed that vigorous range of motion exercises increase ICP to an unsafe level, but this has not been tested in research. The use of a kinetic bed may prevent pooling of pulmonary secretions, tissue breakdown, and osteoporosis.

QUESTION

Which of the following would indicate that Pam was experiencing increased ICP during range of motion exercises?
1. Decreased Sao_2 according to pulse oximetry
2. Stimulation of low pressure alarm on the ventilator
3. Presence of B waves on the pressure monitor
4. A 10 mm Hg drop in blood pressure

Complications of immobility may delay the recovery and subsequent hospital discharge of a head-injured patient. Research exploring the effects of nursing measures designed to decrease immobility complications have been limited in this population.

TRAUMA SEQUELAE

As discussed in Module 10, *Trauma Assessment and Resuscitation*, trauma deaths occur in three peaks. The first peak is within the first hour postinjury, and the major causes of death are massive bleeding secondary to great vessel tears and head injuries. The second peak occurs during the initial hours post-event in the resuscitation phase. Deaths in this phase generally are attributed to internal bleeding. The final peak of trauma-related deaths occurs days to weeks after the injury event. Infection is the major cause of death in the final phase.

The primary responsibility of the nurse caring for a trauma patient in this final phase is in the area of prevention and surveillance. Treatment of trauma sequelae is controversial and primitive, since research in this area is still in its infancy as compared with trauma resuscitation research. Therefore, the goal of nursing care is to prevent that which you may not be able to treat adequately once it is present. Major medical complications in the trauma patient are septic shock/septic shock syndrome, multiple organ failure (MOF), disseminated intravascular coagulation (DIC), and ARDS. Since ARDS is discussed in Module 4, *Nursing Care of the Patient with Altered Respiratory Function*, it is not discussed in depth in this section.

Injury Event

Several types of injuries predispose the trauma patient to complications. Table 14–1 summarizes injuries and their associated sequelae. Thoracic trauma may produce massive hemorrhage in addition to disruption in the lung parenchyma. Thus, the thoracic trauma patient is at high risk for DIC and ARDS. Abdominal trauma increases the likelihood of hemorrhage and infection. Orthopedic trauma predisposes the patient to pulmonary emboli and prolonged

TABLE 14–1. TRAUMATIC INJURIES AND ASSOCIATED SEQUELAE

Condition	Pathophysiology	Complication
Thoracic trauma		
Great vessel tears Hemothorax	Hemorrhage	DIC
Tension pneumothorax	Decreased gas exchange	ARDS
Open pneumothorax	Decreased gas exchange	ARDS
	Disruption in skin integrity	Sepsis
Abdominal trauma		
Perforation of intestine	Extravasation of gastrointestinal contents into peritoneum	Sepsis
Liver/splenic laceration	Hemorrhage	DIC
Orthopedic trauma		
Femur/pelvis fracture	Hemorrhage	DIC
Longbone fractures	Disruption of fat containing tissue, increased flow of fat globules in microcirculation	ARDS
Open fractures	Disruption in skin integrity	Sepsis

immobility, which may compound the effect on gas exchange. Head injuries also may result in prolonged immobility plus local tissue destruction. The physiologic complications of trauma are intimately related. It is common for a patient to have a combination of these disorders. Although the etiologies of these conditions may differ slightly, the result is the same: inadequate oxygen delivery to the tissue. For this reason it is important to keep in mind when reading Table 14–1 that the patient may be at higher risk for one of these disorders because of the initial injury, but, in reality, any one of and more than one of these conditions may occur.

Hypoperfusion

Hypoperfusion is a precursor to all of the complications discussed in this section. In sepsis and MOF, the hypoperfusion may be distributional and secondary to vasodilation and not actual loss of volume. In DIC, hypoperfusion occurs because of diffuse hemorrhage and destruction of RBCs as they become trapped in fibrin strands. Increased alveolar capillary permeability as well as overzealous fluid resuscitation predispose the patient to ARDS. The treatment of hypovolemic shock previously has focused on improving systems (i.e., preload and contractility). The nurse should view hypovolemia from a cellular perspective in order to appreciate the cellular changes that predispose the trauma patient to complications.

Poor cellular perfusion results in a shift to anaerobic metabolism. As mentioned earlier, anaerobic metabolism is an inefficient system, since 2 adenosine triphosphate (ATP) as compared to 38 ATP with aerobic metabolism are created for energy use. Anaerobic metabolism increases the production of acids as waste products. This increased acid (such as lactic acid) produces a chemical insult that triggers the inflammatory/immune response, which activates other systems. The humoral immunity system is activated to produce vasodilation and to increase capillary permeability. Initially, this is a local response to enhance tissue repair. Cellular immunity is activated to eliminate wastes from the dying hypoxic cells. The cellular immunity system includes polymorphonuclear granulocytes, monocytes, and lymphocytes. Other biochemical substances are activated. These substances include but are not limited to oxygen radicals, tumor necrosis factor, and interleukins. The purpose of these substances is to facilitate the humoral and cellular immunity systems and to serve as transporters and mediators in cellular reactions. Overall, their net response is vasodilation.

Inflammatory/Immune Response

The functions of a local inflammatory/immune response are

1. Improvement of oxygen supply and decrease of oxygen demand at the cellular level
2. Redistribution of circulatory blood volume to injured area
3. Correction of metabolic alterations
4. Killing of microorganisms

The inflammatory/immune response is intended to be protective for the patient. If the local response becomes systemic (through what is yet an unknown process), the process is no longer compensatory but becomes pathologic. Tissue destruction continues because of massive vasodilation. Hypoperfusion produces cellular death. If enough cells die, organs die (MOF), and the patient dies.

The trauma patient must be assessed for risk factors associated with a malfunction of the compensa-

TABLE 14–2. RISK FACTORS ASSOCIATED WITH COMPLICATIONS POSTTRAUMA

Risk Factor	Rationale
Elderly	Decreased production of lymphocytes may increase susceptibility to infection Decreased microcirculation may impair cellular oxygen delivery
Malnutrition (obesity, chronic illness, alcoholism)	Decreased available protein to produce immunoglobulins and cells
Systolic blood pressure < 80 mm Hg (massive transfusion greater than 6 L within 6 hours of injury)	Hypovolemia decreases cellular oxygen supply and results in compensatory vasoconstriction that further destroys cells
Large wounds, burns	Destruction of skin as first defense against infection Increased capillary permeability in an attempt to provide nutrients and remove wastes from injured areas
Previous history of organ transplants (immunosuppression therapy) or chronic use of antibiotics	Inability to initiate local inflammatory response allows for microorganism invasion and ultimately systemic infection Decreased sensitivity to medications used for microorganism resistance
Prolonged time between injury and treatment (exact time is unknown but longer than 1 hour has been associated with increased morbidity and mortality)	Delayed volume resuscitation results in additional cellular death Delayed wound debridement results in higher microorganism invasion

tory inflammation/immune response. Table 14–2 summarizes the risk factors and the rationale for their association with complications posttrauma. The nurse should suspect the presence of complications in the older, malnourished patient with a history of chronic illness as well as the younger, healthy patient who has sustained massive injuries and has had a delay in initial treatment.

QUESTION

Which of the following events could place Pam at the highest risk for development of posttrauma complications?
1. Craniotomy
2. History of aspiration
3. Intraventricular catheter
4. Immobility

ANSWER

2. Although all of these factors increase Pam's risk for complications, aspiration places her at the highest risk for several reasons. The introduction of foreign substances in the lung fields precipitates an inflammatory response. Initiation of the inflammatory response with increased capillary permeability can produce ARDS and pulmonary edema. She has required anesthesia and mechanical ventilation. Anesthesia and mechanical ventilation prevent Pam from coughing and clearing her own airway. Coughing would be a compensatory mechanism for managing the inflammation from the aspiration. She is dependent on suctioning. In addition, suctioning can introduce pathogens. Even though Pam's chest film is clear at present, patchy infiltrates may develop later.

The rest of this section discusses each complication independently. The section ends with an overview of assessment data and nursing care for all of the complications, since the patient responses to the pathologic changes form a similar pattern.

Sepsis/Septic Shock/Septic Syndrome

Sepsis is the presence of microorganisms in the blood. Septic shock is the physiologic response to microorganisms in the blood that results in hemodynamic instability. For the diagnosis of sepsis to be made, a pathogen is identified in the body from cultures. The pathogens may be part of the patient's normal flora or may be present in the external environment. Gram-negative and gram-positive bacteria, viruses, and fungi can produce sepsis. There are several portals of entry for these microorganisms. Table 14–3 summarizes these entry points. Gram-negative bacteria produces endotoxins that cause direct cellular damage in addition to the release of vasoactive proteins (humoral response) that result in

TABLE 14–3. COMMON PORTALS OF ENTRY OF MICROORGANISMS

Entrance Point	Predisposing Agent
Urinary tract	Urinary catheters
	Suprapubic tubes
	Cystoscopic examination
Respiratory tract	Endotracheal tubes
	Tracheostomy tubes
	Mechanical ventilation
	Suctioning
	Inhalation therapy
	Aspiration
Gastrointestinal tract	Peritonitis
	Abdominal abscess
	Cirrhosis
	Ascites
	Peptic ulcers
Skin	Surgical wounds
	Burns
	Traumatic injury
	Intravenous catheters
	Intraarterial catheters
	Invasive monitoring
	Decubitus ulcers

Adapted from Dolan, Joan: *Critical care nursing: Clinical management through the nursing process,* by J. Dolan, 1991, Philadelphia: F.A. Davis Co.

vasodilation, increased capillary permeability, and activation of the clotting cascade. Although other microorganisms may not produce endotoxins, other vasoactive substances are released through a yet to be confirmed mechanism. *Septic syndrome* is a term for the condition in which the patient exhibits the symptoms of sepsis but the cultures are negative. Most clinicians believe that a microorganism is present but not in a sufficient cluster to produce a positive finding. The patient's WBC may be elevated because of the total number of microorganisms.

Septic shock (or sepsis) is characterized by two different phases: high output and low output. Both phases are related to a systemic response to microorganisms that produces cellular damage. The high output phase is the body's initial response to massive vasodilation. The CO reading (when available) may increase to 15 L/minute (Littleton, 1989). The patient's skin is warm and flushed (similar to that seen in neurogenic shock, another condition due to vasodilation from unopposed parasympathetic stimulation). Most patients will be tachypneic, which leads to respiratory alkalosis. Fever is usually present. The systemic vascular resistance is low and the CO is high, since afterload is diminished. Hypotension may result from inadequate preload due to decreased venous return. As preload decreases, CO ultimately will decrease, and the patient enters the second phase of septic shock. During this phase, the sympathetic nervous system attempts to enhance compensation. Tachycardia, peripheral vasoconstriction,

and decreased urine output occur in an attempt to restore core circulation. The patient will have a low CO reading, a high systemic vascular resistance level, and decreased preload (central venous pressure) if the patient has a pulmonary arterial catheter in place. The signs can be detected in the patient even if pulmonary arterial readings are unavailable. The patient is cold, diaphoretic, oliguric, and nonresponsive to verbal stimuli. Failure to mount a fever or to increase the WBC are poor prognostic signs (Luce, 1987).

Adult Respiratory Distress Syndrome

ARDS is characterized by the presence of pulmonary infiltrates and hypoxemia despite high concentrations of inspired oxygen. Concentrations of inspired oxygen in excess of 50 percent in conjunction with PEEP do not correct the hypoxemia (Littleton, 1989). Increased pulmonary capillary permeability results in pulmonary edema and impaired gas exchange. Pulmonary hypertension stimulates the synthesis of thromboxane. Thromboxane produces regional vasoconstriction in the lungs. Pulmonary shunting occurs in response to ventilation-perfusion mismatchs. The trauma patient is vulnerable to ARDS because of volume resuscitation and untreated hypoxia related to direct thoracic injury or indirect thoracic injury, such as that from aspiration.

QUESTION

Which of the following interventions during the trauma resuscitation phase would increase the risk of the patient developing ARDS as a complication of trauma?
1. Administration of 6 L/min of oxygen via nonrebreather mask
2. Prolonged supine positioning of the patient on a backboard
3. Administration of IV lactated Ringer's solution at 500 mL/hour
4. Performance of endotracheal suctioning

ANSWER

3. In most circumstances, administering IV fluids at 500 mL/hour could precipitate interstitial fluid shifting. This is especially true if the patient is elderly or has a history of chronic pulmonary disease or congestive heart failure, when 500 mL/hour may not be tolerated. Prolonged supine positioning by itself should not increase the likelihood of ARDS occurring unless the patient vomits in this position and aspirates. Administration of oxygen should not be detrimental unless the patient has chronic airflow limitations and depends on low oxygen levels to stimulate respirations. Endotracheal suctioning, if performed aseptically, should not significantly increase the patient's risk.

Multiple Organ Failure

MOF accounts for up to 10 percent of deaths in patients with multiple injuries (LeKander and Cerra, 1990). If MOF follows ARDS, mortality increases to 80 percent. The occurrence of MOF after the presence of septic shock is associated with a 90 percent mortality rate. MOF may occur early after the traumatic insult, but it does not become progressive until later in the hospitalization (LeKander and Cerra, 1990). This pattern involves coagulation abnormalities, the presence of a low grade fever, tachycardia and dyspnea (pulmonary insufficiency), and alteration in responsiveness. CO increases, and systemic vascular resistance decreases as in the early phase of septic shock. The patient is hypermetabolic, with elevated blood glucose and lactic acid levels. Later, renal and hepatic failure occur. A delayed and different pattern of MOF may occur in association with a primary pulmonary event and may not be apparent until late in the hospitalization. This pattern of MOF is associated with sepsis. ARDS may follow the sepsis. Liver failure occurs next and is followed by renal and cardiovascular failure. Delayed wound healing is present.

Criteria exist for defining organ failure. Acute renal failure may occur because of intracellular electrolyte imbalances that result from ischemia or from deposition of cellular debris, i.e., myoglobins, resulting in tubular obstruction. A serum creatinine level greater than or equal to 2 mg/dL is diagnostic. Liver failure is defined as a serum bilirubin level greater than 3 mg/dL of 2 days duration. Liver enzymes also will be elevated. There will be reduced levels of hepatic proteins (albumin, transferrin, and prealbumin). Cardiovascular failure is the inability to maintain a cardiac index greater than 2.5 L/minute despite vasopressor support. Hematopoietic failure occurs when the platelets decrease below 60,000/mL. Fibrin split products greater than 10 μg/mL also indicate failure.

The pattern of failure is not significant in terms of treatment and nursing care. These remain the same for both types of MOF. It is difficult to predict susceptibility to MOF using severity of injury, since cellular injury may not be detected if compensation is adequate. However, the ratio of arterial oxygen tension (Pao_2) to the fraction of inspired oxygen (Fio_2) on day 1 of injury (detection of persistent hypoxemia), plasma lactic acid levels on day 2, serum bilirubin levels on day 6, and serum creatinine levels on day 12 are indicative of the progression of MOF (LeKander and Cerra, 1990). It is not clear why a patient may progress from a hypermetabolic state to MOF. A persistent perfusion deficit, inflammation, and infection are related to the occurrence of MOF. The hypermetabolism eventually results in a phenomenon referred to as *autocannibalism*. Skeletal muscle mass is used as a nutritional source. Both muscle wasting and an associated peripheral neuropathy with skeletal muscle denervation have been associated with mechanical ventilator dependency (LeKander and Cerra, 1990).

QUESTION

Which of the following statements best describes the relationship between ARDS and MOF?
1. Decreased ventilation leads to decreased tissue oxygenation and cellular death
2. Pulmonary edema produces a fluid volume deficit and hypoperfusion of tissues
3. Organ death releases endotoxins that kill pulmonary epithelial cells
4. Increased carbon dioxide retention stimulates peripheral vasodilation and hypoperfusion of tissue

---

ANSWER

1. ARDS usually precedes MOF. The lungs may be the first organ of many to fail. A ventilation-perfusion mismatch is present in ARDS due to its restrictive disease nature. There is less surface area for oxygen exchange to occur. Thus, oxygenation of tissue is decreased, promoting tissue death. 3 is partially correct in that as MOF progresses, further deterioration occurs in pulmonary status due to the vasodilatory effect of toxins and destruction of types I and II epithelial cells that produce surfactant.

Disseminated Intravascular Coagulation

Disseminated intravascular coagulation (DIC) is another complication of trauma. This disorder is characterized by simultaneous bleeding and clotting. Initially, the patient will demonstrate signs of coagulation. Excess thrombin activates fibrinogen. Fibrin is deposited, and platelets group to form clots. Red blood cells are destroyed as they get trapped in the clots. Circulation is slowed due to the clots, and cells die from lack of oxygen and nutrients. The excessive clotting stimulates fibrinolysis. Lysis is stimulated by the intensity of the coagulation. In addition to activation of the clot-destroying process, as clotting factors get used up or consumed, a deficiency develops. Later, hemorrhage will become apparent. The skin, lungs, and kidneys are most commonly involved. The nurse should assess the skin carefully. Symptoms can be detected here when they are not apparent internally. Another reason for assessing the skin is that peripheral changes will occur first. Table 14–4 compares symptoms and the underlying process responsible for the symptoms. Diagnosis is made through laboratory testing. Fibrin split products are formed during lysis. Thrombocytopenia is present because platelets are depleted as they aggregate, and production is unable to keep pace with demand. Prothrombin time is prolonged. Often these values will be elevated before the patient shows symptoms. The nurse must review the patient's history because liver disease or multiple blood transfusions may lower these values as well as DIC.

TABLE 14–4. SYMPTOMS ASSOCIATED WITH DISSEMINATED INTRAVASCULAR COAGULATION

System	Ischemic Changes Related to Clotting	Hemorrhagic Changes Related to Lysis
Gastrointestinal	Gastric distention (infarcted bowel)	Hematemesis, melena
Pulmonary	Dyspnea, hypoxemia, pulmonary embolus	Hemoptysis
Renal	Oliguria, azotemia	Hematuria
Central nervous system	Coma, seizures	Headache (intracerebral bleeding)
Skin	Acral cyanosis Gangrene (generalized diaphoresis with mottled, cool extremities)	Petechial ecchymoses

As with MOF, DIC is an exaggeration of a normal response. Normal clotting is a localized reaction to injury, whereas DIC is a systemic response. The healthy individual maintains a balance between clot formation and lysis. In trauma, both the extrinsic and intrinsic pathways of coagulation may be stimulated. Head injury can precipitate the release of tissue thromboplastin (extrinsic pathway). Hypoxia and acidosis also stimulate the extrinsic pathway. Crush injuries, burns, and sepsis result in blood cell injury as well as platelet aggregation (intrinsic pathway).

QUESTION

The bleeding in DIC is attributed to
1. Administration of heparin
2. An abnormal hemorrhagic response
3. Decreased amount of clotting factors
4. Blocking of the clotting cascade

ANSWER

3. The major problem in DIC is an insufficient number of clotting factors, as evidenced by the decreased platelet count and prolonged prothrombin time. Clotting factors are overworking by forming clots in the microcirculation and cannot keep pace with demand stimulated by lysis of the developed clots. It is an exaggeration of a normal response.

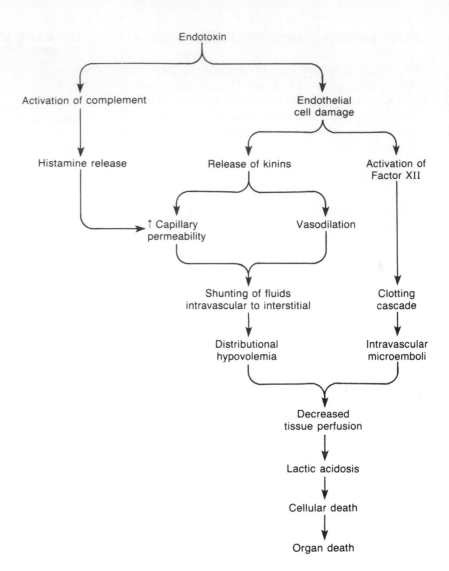

Figure 14–5. Interrelationship between multiple organ failure, adult respiratory distress syndrome, disseminated intravascular coagulation and sepsis. (*From* Critical care nursing: Clinical management through the nursing process, *by J. Dolan, 1991, Philadelphia: F.A. Davis Co.*)

Assessment and Nursing Diagnoses

Each of the posttrauma complications discussed in this section is related to hypoperfusion and decreased oxygen delivery to the cells. These conditions may coexist, and one may be the precursor to another. There are numerous physiologic relationships among the conditions. Figure 14–5 illustrates these relationships. The complement cascade is initiated as a normal response to microorganism invasion. Granulocyte aggregation is stimulated, resulting in slowing of microcirculation. Tissue hypoxia and cellular death occur. Thus, activation of the complement cascade also initiates MOF. Gram-negative sepsis can initiate both fibrinolysis and coagulation, linking sepsis with DIC. In MOF and sepsis, alveolar type 1 pneumocytes are destroyed by endotoxins. Thus, surfactant is diminished and a ventilation-perfusion mismatch occurs, resulting in the development of ARDS. An astute nurse assesses for symp-

toms that are common to all of these conditions and relies on laboratory testing to confirm which disorder is present.

Complications may occur at any time in the postinjury phase. It should be clear from this discussion why baseline laboratory and diagnostic data are so important in the trauma patient. Remember Pam with her closed head injury and multiple lacerations. Since Pam's baseline data are available, the nurse will be able to monitor for subtle changes that indicate that a complication is occurring. The following assessment data would indicate the presence of a posttrauma complication.

■ Elevation of WBC
■ Fever
■ Change in characteristics of wound drainage (foul odor, thick, and colored)
■ Inability to tolerate movement, nursing procedures (i.e., decreasing Sao_2, Pao_2)

- Decreasing level of responsiveness (related to decreased oxygenation or increased serum ammonia levels)
- Decreased urine output
- Diaphoresis
- Cool, mottled skin
- Presence of bleeding (melena, hemoptysis, hematemesis, petechiae, hematuria)
- Changing trends in vital signs/hemodynamic readings (e.g., elevated CO, decreased SVR)

Nursing diagnoses that pertain to the patient can be clustered mainly into the two broad areas of ventilation and perfusion.

Ventilation

- **Impaired gas exchange** related to increased capillary permeability and decreased surface area for gas exchange or obstruction in pulmonary capillary perfusion
- **Ineffective breathing patterns** related to decreased skeletal muscle mass and denervation
- **Ineffective airway clearance** related to fatigue, and artificial airway placement with mechanical ventilation

Perfusion

- **Fluid volume deficit** related to vasodilation, bleeding, or interstitial fluid shift
- **Decreased tissue perfusion** related to capillary obstruction and vasodilation
- **Increased cardiac output** related to catecholamine excretion and decreased systemic vascular resistance
- **Decreased cardiac output** related to decreased vascular volume

Additional nursing diagnoses would include

- **Alteration in urinary elimination patterns** related to obstruction (microemboli and myoglobin) of renal blood flow and tissue necrosis
- **Alteration in nutrition: less than body requirements** related to catecholamine release, activation of inflammatory response resulting in a hypermetabolic state, and decreased or absent oral intake
- **High risk of infection** related to open wounds, invasive procedures, and surgical incisions, debilitated state, and altered nutrition

Interventions for Posttrauma Complications

This section focuses on nursing and collaborative interventions for the trauma patient experiencing complications discussed previously and addresses interventions that are used most often. The reader is referred to the critical care literature for information on experimental interventions, such as tumor necrosis factor antibody, prostaglandins, and oxygen free radical scavengers.

Collaborative Interventions Related to Hypoperfusion from Traumatic Injury Complications

Antibiotics

Third generation cephalosporins (cefotaxime sodium and claforan) are being used more frequently to treat gram-negative infections. They have less nephrotoxicity than the aminoglycosides (gentamicin and garamycin). Combination antibiotic therapy may be used in cases of mixed infections. Usually, two antibiotics are ordered, and one of them is an aminoglycoside.

Antibodies

Research is being conducted to determine the effect of antibodies on endotoxins. This may be effective in the treatment of gram-negative sepsis. Tumor necrosis factor antibodies are being tested for their efficacy against multiple microorganisms associated with sepsis.

Computed Tomography Scanning

Radiographic studies may be completed to locate abscesses, a source of infection, which can be drained percutaneously.

Volume Resuscitation

There is a great deal of controversy concerning the best method of improving venous return. Vasopressors as well as volume replacement may be used. Volume replacement must be monitored carefully because of the increased capillary permeability, which may produce fluid shifting and pulmonary edema. Both crystalloids and colloids may be used. In the case of DIC, platelets may be administered if the level falls below 30,000 μL. Figure 14–6 illustrates the relationship between DIC pathology and the target areas of interventions. Fresh frozen plasma contains all clotting factors and may be used for volume expansion.

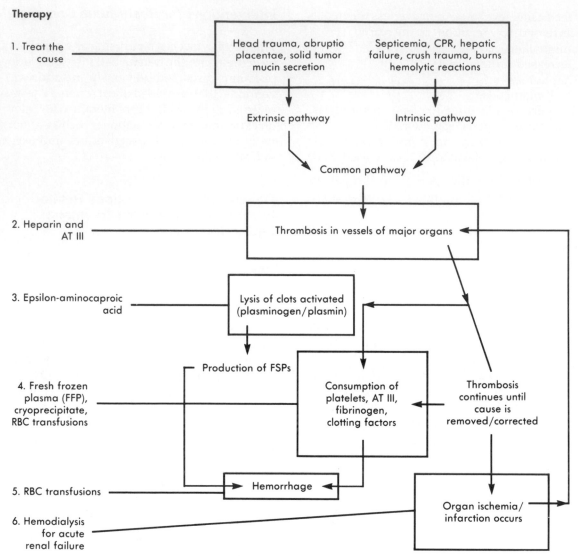

Figure 14–6. Intended sites of action for therapies in DIC. (*From* Textbook of critical care nursing, *by L. Thelan et al, 1990, St. Louis: C.V. Mosby Co.*)

Vasopressor Therapy

Dopamine may be administered to maintain renal blood flow and prevent acute tubular necrosis. Dobutamine is used to improve CO. Norepinephrine and isoproterenol are not preferred because of associated decreased renal blood flow and a further reduction in systemic vascular resistance, respectively (Luce, 1987).

Hemofiltration

Hemofiltration has been used to eliminate toxins and vasoactive mediators. There is no biochemical evidence that these substances are indeed removed. Hemofiltration may be used when other renal therapies have failed.

Endorphin Antagonists

Beta-endorphins are among the vasoactive substances in sepsis that produce vasodilation. Administration of naloxone (Narcan), an endorphin antagonist, has been associated with improvement in CO and blood pressure in animal models. The effect of naloxone for treatment of septic shock in humans has not yet been confirmed (Luce, 1987).

Heparin Therapy

Heparin inhibits thrombin action. It does not have any action on already formed clots, but it does help prevent additional clotting and the use of clotting factors. This drug is most effective when administered early in the course of DIC. The efficacy of heparin has not been proven, but it is used when signs of thrombosis are present.

Antithrombin III

This naturally occurring substance binds with thrombin to make it inactive, thus preventing clotting. It may be administered to patients with DIC.

Early Stabilization of Fractures and Debridement

The physician may stabilize fractures early to prevent further damage and stimulation of the inflammatory response. Early stabilization also promotes early ambulation and may decrease complications associated with immobility. Surgical debridement of wounds, necrotic tissue, and abscesses promotes wound healing and decreases the activity of the immune response.

Independent Nursing Interventions

Promote Ventilation and Oxygenation

Careful monitoring of arterial blood gases, end-tidal CO_2, oxygen saturation, and lactic acid levels is necessary. Most patients will require a higher than atmospheric concentration of inspired oxygen to maintain tissue oxygenation. Thus, patients will receive high flow supplemental oxygen. Most patients will require mechanical ventilation. Chest physiotherapy may be used to mobilize secretions. Endotracheal suctioning is necessary to remove excessive secretions and to promote oxygenation.

Provide Nutritional Support

Although the physician will order the nutritional supplement, it is a nursing responsibility to ensure that the patient receives the supplement in spite of multiple incompatible medications being administered simultaneously. Medication administration schedules must be planned to maintain therapeutic serum levels and adequate nutritional support. Additional side ports, stopcocks, and peripheral IV lines are used to provide IV access. An excess of total calories and carbohydrate sources is avoided because of the adverse effects on the liver, serum osmolality, carbon dioxide production, and oxygen consumption. Insulin may have to be administered to facilitate glucose uptake. The administration of amino acids will increase protein synthesis to equalize catabolism. Thus, treatment is aimed at increasing anabolism and not at decreasing catabolism. Adminis-

tration of amino acid solutions and additional nutritional support measures is a nursing priority. Serum albumin, prealbumin, and transferrin levels are monitored to determine the patient's nutritional response. Early initiation of enteral feedings has been speculated to decrease bacterial translocation across the gut wall and decrease the incidence of sepsis while at the same time improving the patient's nutritional status. Research has not confirmed the usefulness of this treatment (LeKander and Cerra, 1990).

Prevent Increased Oxygen Demand

Since the common thread of most posttrauma complications is inadequate delivery of oxygen to the tissues, activities, procedures, and conditions that increase oxygen demands should be minimized. The nurse must treat fever, seizures, and pain expeditiously. Nursing activities should be paced to allow resting periods. The nurse must weigh carefully the benefits and costs associated with physical mobilization by monitoring oxygen saturation during patient movement. Research is needed to provide empirical information about how to pace nursing interventions.

Assess for and Prevent Bleeding

Since DIC may occur separately or in conjunction with MOF and sepsis, the nurse must assess all drainage for the presence of blood. Mucous membranes, including the eyes, mouth, and nose, should be assessed. The presence of decreasing blood pressure, narrowing pulse pressure, rapid and thready pulse, and decreased level of responsiveness may be indicative of occult bleeding. Gentle technique should be used when moving the patient, performing activities of daily living, and completing procedures, since minor effort can produce major bleeding. The nurse should avoid sharp and rough objects when performing such interventions as shaving and mouth care. Prevention of constipation is another priority, since straining may produce bleeding. Intramuscular injections should be avoided.

Prevent Infection

Since several posttrauma complications are related to an exaggeration of the inflammatory/immune response, the nurse should try to decrease further stimulation of this system by preventing contamination of wounds, lines, and tubes. Invasive nursing procedures, such as suctioning, must be performed aseptically. An overreliance on the effectiveness of antibiotics should be avoided. Antibiotic therapy has associated complications, for example, diarrhea and skin breakdown. In addition, microorganisms develop resistance to antibiotics relatively quickly, diminishing their effectiveness.

Surveillance: Beware of Compensation

Compensatory responses of the patient may fool the novice nurse. The body will attempt to save the heart and brain at the expense of the liver and kidneys. The effects of hypoperfusion may not be apparent until weeks after the initial hypovolemic episode. For example, the patient's ABGs may be normal because the patient is working extra hard and depleting oxygen reserves and subsequent oxygen delivery to the tissues. The nurse should try to differentiate between an improvement in the patient's status vs a compensatory effort when the status is deteriorating. A change in the PCWP reading from 20 to 12 may not indicate correction of overzealous volume resuscitation through renal excretion but may indicate shifting of volume into the interstitial spaces, predisposing the patient to necrosis and skin breakdown as well as hypotension if the shift continues. The nurse must cluster symptoms and seek the origin of the change. Since gross clinical changes may not appear until a loss of 30 percent of blood volume occurs, the nurse must monitor the patient who looks good for subtle changes and trends in readings instead of absolute values.

QUESTION

The best reason that vasopressors may be ordered to treat hypotension for the patient with posttrauma complications is because they
1. Increase renal blood flow
2. Promote vasoconstriction
3. Increase contractility
4. Increase myocardial oxygen demands

ANSWER

2. The major problem with posttrauma complications is hypoperfusion of organs. Vasodilation occurs in response to substances associated with the inflammatory response. Vasopressors produce vasoconstriction, increasing venous return. The administration of fluid may increase venous return, but a large amount of fluid would be required because of the massive vasodilation. This large amount of fluid could precipitate pulmonary problems.

Although this section has emphasized physical manifestations of posttrauma complications, psychosocial aspects should not be ignored. The reader is referred to Module 21 for additional information. Patients who have complications posttrauma remain in the critical care unit for prolonged periods and are susceptible to sensory disturbances. Quality of life issues need to be considered by the patient and the family. Extensive rehabilitation may be necessary to regain skeletal muscle mass and neurologic function. The family's standard of living may decrease because of financial factors related to change in the role of the patient as well as health care costs.

NURSING CARE OF A PATIENT EXPERIENCING A POSTTRAUMA COMPLICATION

As discussed earlier in the module, Pam was admitted into ICU postcraniotomy for drainage of a subdural hematoma. The last time that Pam's case was discussed she was a 3T on the GCS and was receiving a neuromuscular blocking agent. Her ICP was being monitored by an intraventricular catheter. Since that time, Pam has made considerable progress. The intraventricular catheter was removed 48 hours postsurgery. She is extubated and on nasal cannula at 2 L/minute. Pam is alert and oriented, with a GCS score of 15. Her NG tube was discontinued. A peripheral IV line is in her left hand, and D_5W 0.45 percent normal saline is infusing at 100 mL/hour. Her Foley catheter is still in place because she gets fatigued and dyspneic at times when placed on the bedpan. Gentamicin 100 mg every 6 hours was ordered today because her WBC has increased to 14,000, and she has a fever of 100.6F orally. Pam is to be moved out of the unit to the general trauma floor today as soon as the bed is ready. It has been 6 days since her injury.

As the nurse caring for Pam, you are notified that the floor bed will be ready in 45 minutes. You go to Pam's bedside to relay the message. Pam is lethargic and diaphoretic. She responds appropriately when stimulated by shaking. Her GCS score is 14. Her blood pressure is 90/66 by the automatic external blood pressure cuff device. Her extremities are warm, and her skin is flushed. You suspect that her blood sugar may be a little low, since Pam's oral intake has been poor. Before performing a fingerstick and checking her blood glucose, you obtain a full set of vital signs. These measurements will provide a basis from which to evaluate the effect of subsequent nursing interventions.

Pam's heart rate is 106, her blood pressure is 90/66, oral temperature is 101.6F and her respirations are 28. Before proceeding further with the assessment, you put down the head of Pam's bed. You scan her nursing record and note that her blood pressure was 126/86. Her blood pressure has changed and may indicate a perfusion abnormality. You perform a fingerstick to obtain a blood glucose measurement. While waiting for the results, you keep speaking with Pam, who remains alert. Her blood glucose is 150 mg/dL by visual determination. You have ruled out the hypothesis of hypoglycemia. The remaining potential causes of hypotension in Pam's case are hypovolemia or an alteration in blood volume distribution.

You notify the physician about the change in Pam's status. The physician requests the following interventions.

- D_5W 0.45 percent normal saline IV at 150 mL/hour
- ECG
- ABGs
- Cefotaxime (Claforan) 2 g intravenous piggyback (IVPB) every 8 hours
- Stat. CBC, electrolyte panel
- 200 mL fluid bolus stat.
- Blood cultures before antibiotic administration
- Acetaminophen 325 mg orally every 4 hours for fever greater than 100F orally

---

QUESTION

Which of these orders is of the highest priority to implement based on Pam's condition?
1. Administer the fluid bolus
2. Administer the cefotaxime
3. Obtain ECG
4. Obtain CBC and electrolytes

ANSWER

1. You administer the fluid bolus. Blood for the CBC and electrolyte panel can be obtained later, since another antibiotic has been ordered regardless of the results. The hemoglobin and hematocrit levels will be helpful in assessing blood loss as a potential source of the hypotension. However, Pam needs to have her hypotension treated immediately in order to prevent decreased cerebral perfusion. If she

responds to the fluid bolus, hypovolemia is the origin of her hypotension. It is possible that a dysrhythmia may be producing decreased CO. However, she is in sinus tachycardia, without ectopy, on the cardiac monitor Although Pam has healing wounds that may be infected, an alteration in perfusion has taken precedence. The antibiotic can be initiated later.

After these interventions are performed, you reassess Pam's vital signs.

- Heart rate = 100
- Blood pressure = 72/60
- Respirations = 18

Pam is easily aroused, but she is less alert. Her blood pressure has not improved with position change or IV fluid bolus. The ECG confirms that Pam is in sinus tachycardia. The CBC results are

WBC = 22,000   (Normal range 5,000–
                10,000/L)
RBC = 4.0   (Normal range 4.2–5.4
                × 10⁶/L)
Hb = 15   (Normal range 12–
                16 g/dL in females)

Hct = 46%   (Normal range 38–47%
                in females)

The electrolyte panel results are

Sodium (Na) = 144   (Normal range 136–
                       146 mEq/L)
Potassium (K) = 4.0   (Normal range 3.5–
                       5.5 mEq/L)
Chloride (Cl) = 104   (Normal range 96–
                       106 mEq/L)
Calcium (Ca) = 8.8   (Normal range 8.5–
                       10.5 mg/dL)
Glucose = 142   (Normal range 80–
                       120 mg/dL)

QUESTION:

Which of the following reasons best explains Pam's lack of response to the fluid bolus?
1. Her blood volume is adequate
2. The source of her problem is decreased cardiac contractility
3. Her hypotension may be related to vasodilation
4. She is actively bleeding

ANSWER

3. This is a tough question, since all of the answers in certain situations are correct. Pam's CO is not adequate, as evidenced by her decreased responsiveness. Decreased CO may be related to an actual decreased blood volume, decreased contractility, or redistribution (vasodilation) of an adequate blood volume. In each situation, her stroke volume would be low, and her heart rate is increasing to maintain CO. It is possible that Pam may be so volume depleted that 200 mL does not restore preload to a level to maintain CO. However, at this point in her hospitalization, internal bleeding is unlikely unless a stress ulcer has developed. Since her skin is warm and flushed, you should suspect vasodilation. During hypovolemic shock, vasoconstriction occurs, making the skin cool and clammy. The elevated WBC is consistent with the presence of infection. The high normal hemoglobin is reflective of dehydration. The high normal sodium and chloride levels are consistent with dehydration/fluid shifts. The elevated glucose level may be related to infection. The ECG validates the increased heart rate, but it also indicates that myocardium is not ischemic from lack of oxygen or decreased contractility, since there are no T or ST changes, blocks, or changes in amplitude of the complexes.

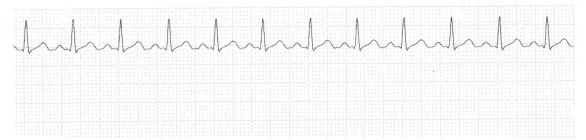

Figure 14–7.

You call the physician and notify her of the laboratory results, Pam's blood pressure postfluid bolus, and her decreased responsiveness. The decision is made to keep Pam in the intensive care unit. The physician arrives and orders a dopamine drip at 4 μg/kg/minute to be titrated until the systolic blood pressure remains at 90 mm Hg. The decision is made to intubate Pam and place her on the ventilator because her oxygen saturation continues to drop, and her ABG results were pH 7.29, $Paco_2$ 49, PaO_2 68, HCO_3 20. Pam has had 40 mL of urine output in the last hour. She is less responsive, and she reacts to pain by withdrawing. Her GCS score is 8T. She has the ECG pattern shown in Figure 14–7.

QUESTION

This pattern is
1. Atrial tachycardia
2. Normal sinus rhythm
3. Sinus tachycardia
4. Atrial flutter

ANSWER

3. Sinus tachycardia is defined as greater than 100 bpm. The sinoatrial node is serving as pacemaker, as indicated by the uniformity in the P wave configuration. In Pam's case, this is a compensatory effort to maintain an adequate CO.

QUESTION

Pam's blood gas results indicate that she is in
1. Respiratory acidosis
2. Respiratory alkalosis
3. Metabolic acidosis
4. Mixed acidosis

ANSWER

1. Pam is in respiratory acidosis because her pH is low, her $Paco_2$ is high, and her bicarbonate is normal.

Focused Nursing History

You review Pam's chart to identify her course of illness. You recall that Pam was not hypotensive in the field, but she did aspirate before her arrival at the hospital. Pam's first day in the intensive care unit was uneventful. She had one episode of increased ICP, 12 mm Hg, that lasted 2 minutes after she was suctioned. No A or B waves were noted. The intraventricular catheter was pulled 48 hours after insertion. She was weaned from the ventilator without difficulty the third day of her admission. Pam did not complain of dyspnea and had one episode of her oxygen saturation dropping to 80 percent when she tried to use the bedpan and missed. Her bed had to be changed, and the procedure fatigued her. She complained of difficulty using the incentive spirometer. Last night, the nurse noted medium rales in her right lower lung fields. Today's morning chest film detected small patchy infiltrates in her right lung fields with questionable areas in her left lung fields. The radiologist questioned the beginning of ARDS but stated that it was unlikely based on her ease of weaning. Antibiotic therapy was initiated by the physician in response to the chest film and the increased WBC. Pam's fever also began today.

The Systematic Bedside Assessment

Because of the change in Pam's status, you initiate a head to toe assessment.

Head and Neck. Pam responds to pain by withdrawing. She is intubated. Her ventilator settings are FIO_2 80 percent, tidal volume 750 mL, rate 20, and mode assist/control. No venous distention is noted. Her neck veins are one-third filled at an angle of 30 degrees.

Chest. Coarse crackles are auscultated bilaterally, with the right being greater than the left. Breath sounds are diminished in the lower lung fields. Pam's pulse oximeter finger reading is SaO_2 of 90 percent. S_1 and S_2 are auscultated. No extra heart sounds or murmurs are noted. Heart rate is 110. Her blood pressure is 84/60 after initiation of the dopamine drip.

Abdomen. Pam's abdomen is soft and supple. Bowel sounds are present in all four quadrants. Her liver area is nontender, and the liver border is nonpalpable.

Pelvis. Pam has voided 40 mL in the last hour. It is dark amber, and the specific gravity is 1.019.

Extremities. Pam is flushed, and her skin is warm. She is diaphoretic. Pam's right thigh wound is draining nonodorous yellow liquid. Her scalp incision and facial laceration are not draining. Her capillary refill is 2 seconds. Peripheral pulses are palpable in all extremities.

Posterior. No sacral edema is present. Posterior breath sounds are diminished in bilateral bases, and coarse rales is noted, with the right greater than the left.

Development of Nursing Diagnoses

Clustering Data. You have just completed your head to toe assessment and are ready to develop nursing diagnoses. To cluster your data, focus on abnormal findings found during the assessment. Pam's major symptoms at this time are decreased blood pressure, impaired gas exchange, and decreased responsiveness.

CLUSTER 1.

Subjective data. History of aspiration in the field before arrival at the hospital. Charted episodes of dyspnea on exertion and decreased oxygen saturation.

Objective data. Decreased oxygen saturation. Elevated temperature. Blood sugar elevated. Elevated WBC. Patchy infiltrates noted on chest film. Course crackles noted bilaterally on auscultation. Presence of respiratory acidosis. Right thigh wound draining yellow material.

QUESTION

Based on these data, which of the following nursing diagnoses would you select as being the priority for Pam?
1. **Decreased cardiac output**
2. **Fluid volume deficit**
3. **High risk of infection**
4. **Impaired gas exchange**

ANSWER

4. All of these diagnoses are appropriate. However, airway and breathing always take priority. Vasoactive substances and catecholamines are released in response to cellular damage from bacteria. Vasoactive substances increase capillary permeability, producing extravasation of volume into the pulmonary interstitium. The hyperglycemia is characteristic of a hypermetabolic state seen in activation of the inflammatory/immune response. MOF may not be manifested until later in the hospitalization. It may be preceded by infection or sepsis and ARDS. Any stimulus that precipitates hypoperfusion or the release of endotoxins can initiate MOF. It is too early to determine if Pam will experience MOF. However, her clinical changes are indicative of ARDS. She may need the addition of PEEP in order to maintain tissue oxygenation and overcome the ventilation-perfusion mismatch. If PEEP is used, a decreased CO may result from the increased intrathoracic pressure decreasing cardiac filling and, thus, ejection.

Expected patient outcomes for Pam would include

1. Improved or clear breath sounds
2. Absence of fever
3. WBC within normal limits (WNL)
4. O_2 saturation greater than 95 percent, ABG WNL
5. GCS score of 15
6. Clear chest film

Additional data clusters pertain to Pam's case. Nursing diagnoses are formulated after data are clustered and patterns are identified.

CLUSTER 2.

Subjective data. As stated in Cluster 1.

Objective data. Responds to painful stimuli by withdrawing. Sinus tachycardia is noted. Decreased blood pressure, and no increase noted with fluid bolus. Presence of fever, hyperglycemia, and elevated WBC. Blood culture pending. Draining wound in right thigh. Negative jugular venous distension (JVD). Hemoglobin 15 g/dL, hematocrit 46 percent.

The same data may support multiple nursing diagnoses. This cluster includes some of the data in the first cluster. The cluster supports the diagnosis of **Fluid volume deficit.** Pam's symptoms are related to an alteration in fluid volume. The fluid volume deficit in Pam's case is probably related to endotoxins released from bacteria secondary to her wound and pulmonary infection. This would account for her tachycardia, fever, and hypotension. Urinary output is adequate, which suggests that CO is within normal limits. Pam's cerebral perfusion may be poor because

of her decreased responsiveness, or her responsiveness level may be related to hypoxia. Since the data are conflicting, direct measurement of Pam's CO is desirable. CO may be decreased from massive vasodilation in response to endotoxins. The physician will most likely insert a pulmonary artery catheter in order to obtain direct CO (and hemodynamic) measurements. However, her hypotension clearly indicates a fluid volume deficit. Pam does appear to have an active infection that will require treatment, but this will be treated in conjunction with her fluid deficit.

Expected patient outcomes for Pam would include

1. Systolic blood pressure greater than 90 mm Hg
2. Decreased wound drainage and size
3. Heart rate 60–100
4. GCS score of 15
5. Urinary output of 30 mL/hour or greater maintained
6. Decreased wound drainage and wound size

Based on the preliminary data already collected on Pam, there are sufficient data to support the following additional nursing diagnoses.

- **Infection** related to aspiration, wounds, and invasive procedures
- **Skin integrity, impaired: actual** related to wound infection right thigh
- **Mobility, impaired, physical** related to

decreased responsiveness, fatigue, and ventilator
- **High risk for altered urinary elimination patterns** related to antibiotic use, decreased renal blood flow

Treatment goals for Pam will focus on increasing her oxygen supply and delivery to the tissue by improving ventilation and perfusion. These goals should be reflected in the nursing diagnoses and expected patient outcomes on the nursing care plan. For example, improving ventilation is addressed in the nursing diagnosis, **Impaired gas exchange.** Accomplishment of this goal will be measured in criteria, such as patient's SaO_2 will be greater than 95 percent.

Development of a Plan of Care

Recall that several collaborative interventions for posttrauma complications were listed on page 345. Additional interventions from this list may be implemented if Pam's status deteriorates further. Thus far, antibiotics and vasopressor therapy have been initiated from this list. Nursing interventions for Pam can be summarized around the goals identified on page 347 for the nursing care of a patient experiencing posttrauma complications.

Independent Nursing Interventions

1. Promote ventilation and oxygenation
   - Suction prn aseptically, hyperoxygenating and hyperventilating before each attempt
   - Pace nursing activities and monitor patient's SaO_2
   - Turn patient at least every 2 hours if SaO_2 does not drop
2. Provide nutritional support
   - Consult with physician concerning preferred nutritional route
   - Administer supplement on time and without interruption
   - Provide oral care at least every shift to promote oral intake as soon as possible
   - Monitor weight daily; maintain intake and output record
3. Prevent increased oxygen demand
   - Promote wound healing by completing dressing changes on time and aseptically
   - Provide pain relief and comfort with backrubs, conversation, and distraction
   - Treat fever with prescribed agent; monitor temperature closely

4. Assess for and prevent bleeding
   - Use gentle force when completing mouth care and dressing changes
   - Monitor for hematuria
   - Monitor laboratory values (PT, platelets)
   - Test all drainage for the presence of blood
5. Prevent infection
   - Monitor for indications of infection (laboratory data, wound drainage, secretions)
   - Administer antibiotics as prescribed
   - Monitor peak and trough antibiotic levels
   - Culture any new drainage per physician order
6. Surveillance
   - Monitor vital sign trends
   - Monitor ventilation trends (ABGs, SaO_2, ventilatory effort in relation to mechanical ventilator)
   - Monitor trends in intake and output, daily weight

Pam's plan of care is now ready to be executed by the intensive care unit nurse. Her progress will be examined at regular intervals to evaluate the effects of various therapeutic actions. If progress is not being noted toward attainment of her expected patient outcomes, Pam's plan of care may need to be revised.

Summary

This module has addressed the nursing care of a patient with traumatic injuries. Concepts from the related modules, *Trauma Assessment and Resuscitation, Wound Management, Responsiveness,* and *Impaired Physical Mobility,* have been applied in a case study approach. It is impossible to address specifically each traumatic injury and associated complication a nurse may encounter in the clinical setting. However, these problems can be managed by applying basic principles. These principles can be classified around assessing and treating the etiology of the patient's altered airway clearance, ineffective breathing patterns, impaired gas exchange, hypotension, distended neck veins, decreased urine output, or change in level of responsiveness. A case study was used to illustrate the relationship between traumatic injury and posttrauma complications. Nursing care responsibilities associated with the initial traumatic injury as well as the development of a posttrauma complication were discussed. Review questions were integrated throughout the module to encourage application of material and assimilation of content. Nursing interventions for a patient with an ICP monitoring device was addressed specifically because of the frequency with which this intervention is used in trauma patients related to the high incidence of head injuries.

REFERENCES

Battistella, F., and Wisner, D. (1991). Combined hemorrhagic shock and head injury: Effects of hypertonic saline (7.5%) resuscitation. *J. Trauma.* 31:182–188.

Bires, B. (1987). Head trauma: Nursing implications from prehospital through emergency department. *Crit. Care Nursing Q.* 10 (1):1–8.

Bruya, M. (1981). Planned periods of rest in the intensive care unit: Nursing care activities and intracranial pressure. *J. Neurosurg. Nursing.* 13:184–194.

Cavallero, D., Mominee, P., Michlin, J., Hillman, J., Grauer, K., and Craver, B. (1988). An algorithm for trauma victim assessment. *J. Emerg. Med. Services.* 13 (2):28–33.

DeLaurier, G., Hawkins, M., Treat, R., and Mansberger, A. (1990). Acute airway management. *Am. Surgeon.* 56:12–15.

Dolan, J.T. (1991). *Critical care nursing: Clinical management through the nursing process.* Philadelphia: F.A. Davis.

Donegan, M., and Bedford, R. (1980). Intravenously administered lidocaine prevents intracranial hypertension during endotracheal suctioning. *Anesthesiology.* 52:516.

Emergency Nurses Association (1991). *Trauma nursing care course instructor manual.* Chicago: The Association.

Epstein, F., and Hamilton, G. (1983). Initial approach to the brain-injured patient. *Crit. Care Q.* 5:13–30.

Gareau, A., Eby, R., McLellan, B., and Williams, D. (1990). Tetanus immunization status and immunological response to a booster in an emergency department geriatric population. *Ann. Emerg. Med.* 19:1377–1381.

Green, B., Eismont, F., and O'Heir, J. (1987). Prehospital management of spinal cord injury. *Paraplegia.* 25:229–238.

Guss, D. (1985). The head-injured patient: Prehospital care. *Trauma Q.* 2 (1):1–7.

Guyton, A. (1986). *Textbook of medical physiology,* 7th ed. Philadelphia: W.B. Saunders Co.

Hendrickson, S. (1987). Intracranial pressure changes and family presence. *J. Neurosci. Nursing* 19(1):14–17.

Hoffman, J., Schriger, D., and Luo, J. (1991). The empiric use of naloxone in patients with altered mental status: A reappraisal. *Ann. Emerg. Med.* 20:246–252.

Jagger, J., and Bobovsky, J. (1983). Nonpharmacologic therapeutic modalities. *Crit. Care Q.* 5(4):31–41.

Kee, J. (1991). *Laboratory and diagnostic tests with nursing implications,* 3rd ed., p. 493. Norwalk, Connecticut: Appleton & Lange.

Kosmos, C. (1989). Emergency nursing management of the multiple trauma patient. *Orthopaed. Nursing.* 6 (1):33–36.

Lehman, L. (1988). Head trauma in the elderly. *Postgrad. Med.* 83 (7):140–147.

LeKander, B., and Cerra, F. (1990). The syndrome of multiple organ failure. *Crit. Care Clin. North Am.* 2:331–342.

Littleton, M. (1989). Complications of multiple trauma. *Crit. Care Clin. North Am.* 1:75–83.

Luce, J. (1987). Septic shock: A threat to the threatened. *Emerg. Med.* Oct 30, 25–33.

Markovchick, V., and Anderson, D. (1988). Initial assessment of chest injury. *Topics Emerg. Med.* 10 (2):11–18.

McQuillan, R. (1987). The effects of the Trendelenberg position for postural drainage on cerebrovascular status in head injured patients. *Heart Lung* 16:327.

Mitchell, P., and Mauss, N. (1978). Relationship of patient-nurse activity to intracranial pressure variations: A pilot study. *Nursing Res.* 27:4–10.

Mitchell, P., Ozuna, J., and Lipe, H. (1981). Moving the patient in bed: Effects on intracranial pressure. *Nursing Res.* 30:212–218.

Moore, F. (1986). *Metabolic care of the surgical patient,* p. 159. London: Saunders.

National Committee for Injury Prevention and Control. (1989). Traffic injuries. In *Injury prevention: Meeting the challenge,* pp. 115–143. New York: Oxford University Press.

Parsons, L., Peard, A., and Page, M. (1985). The effects of hygiene interventions on the cerebrovascular status of closed head injured persons. *Res. Nurs. Health* 8:173–181.

Parsons, L., and Wilson, M. (1984). Cerebrovascular status of severe closed head injured patients following passive position changes. *Nurs. Res.* 33(2):68–75.

Prins, M. (1989). The effect of family visits on intracranial pressure. *West. J. Nursing Res.* 11:281–297.

Reimer, M. (1989). Head injured patients. How to detect early signs of trouble. *Nursing 1989,* 34–41.

Schriger, D., and Baraff, L. (1988). Defining normal capillary refill: Variation with age, sex, and temperature. *Ann. Emerg. Med.* 17:932–935.

Shlafer, M., and Marieb, E. (1989). *The nurse, pharmacology and drug therapy.* Redwood City, California: Addison-Wesley.

Smith, K. (1987). Head trauma: Comparison of infection rates for different methods of intracranial pressure monitoring. *J. Neurosci. Nursing.* 19:310–314.

Snyder, M. (1983). Relation of nursing activities to increase in intracranial pressure. *J. Adv. Nursing.* 8:273–279.

Swain, A., Grundy, D., and Russell, J. (1985). ABCs of spinal cord injury: At the accident. *Br. Med. J.* 291:1558–1560.

Thelan, L., Davie, J., and Urden, L. (1990). *Textbook of critical care nursing,* St. Louis: The C.V. Mosby Co.

Walleck, C. (1989). Controversies in the management of the head injured patient. *Crit. Care Clin. North Am.* 1:67–74.

Wilkinson, H. (1987). Intracranial pressure monitoring: Techniques and pitfalls. In Cooper, P. (ed.) *Head injury,* pp. 197–237. Baltimore: Williams & Wilkins.

Yanno, M., Nishiyama, H., Yokota, H., Kato, K., Yamamoto, Y., and Otsuka, T. (1986). Effect of lidocaine on ICP response to endotracheal suctioning. *Anesthesiology* 65(5):651–653.

PART IV

Metabolism

Module 15

Altered Glucose Metabolism

Kathleen Dorman Wagner and Evelyn Dantzic Geller

The focus of this module, *Altered Glucose Metabolism,* is on physiologic as well as pathophysiologic processes involved in glucose metabolism. Nursing management is addressed primarily in Module 20, *Nursing Care of the Patient with Altered Metabolism.* This module is composed of nine sections. Sections One and Two discuss normal glucose metabolism and the effects of insulin on metabolism. The focus then shifts to abnormal glucose metabolism. Section Three describes the impact of insulin deficit on metabolism. Section Four defines and then differentiates the two major types of diabetes mellitus (type I and type II). Sections Five through Seven discuss the three major diabetes-related crises, including hypoglycemic coma, diabetic ketoacidosis, and hyper-

glycemic hyperosmolar nonketotic coma. Section Eight explains exogenous insulin therapy, focusing on types of insulin therapy used during acute illness. Finally, Section Nine presents an overview of chronic diabetic complications, focusing on how each one alters management of the acutely ill patient. Each section includes a set of review questions to help the learner evaluate understanding of the section content before moving on to the next section. All section reviews and the pretest and posttest in the module include answers. It is suggested that the learner review those concepts that have been missed in the review questions before proceeding to the next section.

Objectives

At the completion of the module, *Altered Glucose Metabolism,* the learner will be able to

1. Discuss normal glucose metabolism
2. Describe the effects of insulin on metabolism
3. Explain the effects of insulin deficit
4. Differentiate the two major types of diabetes mellitus
5. Discuss the diabetic complication, hypoglycemic coma
6. Describe the diabetic complication, diabetic keto-acidosis
7. Discuss the diabetic complication, hyperosmolar hyperglycemic nonketotic coma
8. Explain the use of exogenous insulin in the management of the patient with diabetes mellitus
9. Discuss the acute care implications of chronic diabetic complications

---

Pretest

1. Insulin promotes use of glucose by
   A. breaking down glucose
   B. assisting glucose into the cells
   C. converting glucose to glycogen
   D. transporting glucose in the blood
2. Which of the following is true regarding the effect of insulin on fat metabolism?
   A. inhibits synthesis of fatty acids
   B. inhibits glucose use by tissues
   C. inhibits release of fatty acids
   D. inhibits transport of glucose into fat cells
3. When an insulin deficiency exists, the liver responds by converting
   A. fatty acids to glucose
   B. glycogen to glucose
   C. glucagon to glucose
   D. amino acids to glucose
4. Insulin-dependent cells use which of the following nutritional substances FIRST when insulin is not available?
   A. fatty acids
   B. glycogen
   C. glucagon
   D. amino acids
5. The etiology of type I diabetes is believed to be
   A. obesity
   B. autoimmune reaction
   C. bacterial infection
   D. general pancreatic dysfunction
6. A patient experiencing rapid onset hypoglycemia is most likely to have predominantly _____ symptoms.
   A. cell dysfunction
   B. gastrointestinal
   C. stimulated sympathetic nervous system
   D. stimulated parasympathetic nervous system
7. Central nervous system symptoms associated with hypoglycemia are caused by lack of _____ rather than insulin deficit.
   A. glucose
   B. amino acids
   C. fatty acids
   D. glucagon
8. All of the following are typical clinical manifestations of diabetic ketoacidosis EXCEPT
   A. polydipsia
   B. fluid overload
   C. electrolyte depletion
   D. progressive dehydration
9. Which of the following statements is correct regarding hyperglycemic hyperosmolar nonketotic coma (HHNC)?
   A. it has a high mortality rate
   B. it is most common in type I diabetes
   C. it causes severe fluid volume overload
   D. death occurs from severe metabolic acidosis
10. Which of the following insulin sources is structurally the least like human insulin?
    A. beef
    B. humulin
    C. pork
    D. beef-pork combination
11. All of the following are factors that dictate the type of insulin best suited for a specific person EXCEPT
    A. patient's weight
    B. insulin resistance
    C. patient's allergies
    D. adipose tissue condition
12. Diabetic retinopathy causes blindness by
    A. glucose deposits on the retina
    B. thickening of the retina
    C. destruction of the optic nerve
    D. infarction of retinal tissue
13. Diabetic nephropathy damages the nephrons by causing
    A. glomerulosclerosis
    B. glomerulonephritis
    C. chronic nephritis
    D. renal hypertension

Answers: 1, B. 2, C. 3, B. 4, A. 5, B. 6, C. 7, A. 8, B. 9, A. 10, A. 11, A. 12, D. 13, A.

Glossary

Acetoacetic acid. Produced by fat catabolism, it is one component of ketone bodies

Acetone (dimethyl ketone). Produced by fat catabolism, it is a component of ketone bodies

Acetyl-CoA (acetylcoenzyme A). A product of the reaction between acetic acid and coenzyme A

Aminoacidemia. Amino acids in the blood

Anion gap. A measurement of excessive unmeasurable anions

Atherosclerosis. A form of arteriosclerosis characterized by plaque deposits

β-Hydroxybutyric acid. One component of ketone bodies

Carbohydrate. A nutritional substance composed of complex and simple sugars

Catabolism. Breakdown of a substance

Diabetes mellitus. A complex metabolic disorder in which the person has either an absolute or a relative insulin deficiency; this insulin deficiency results in disordered carbohydrate, protein, and fat metabolism

Diabetic ketoacidosis. A potentially devastating form of metabolic acidosis, characterized by a clinical syndrome of symptoms associated with elevated serum blood sugar and serum ketones and metabolic acidosis

Glucagon. A hormone produced by the alpha cells of the islets of Langerhans of the pancreas

Gluconeogenesis. Formation of glycogen in the liver from a noncarbohydrate substance

Glycogen. The stored form of carbohydrate for conversion into glucose

Glycogenolysis. Conversion of glycogen to glucose

Glycosuria. Excretion of sugar in the urine

Hormone-sensitive lipase. A fat-splitting enzyme

Hyalinization. A degenerative cell process affecting the basement membrane of arteries and arterioles; hyalinized cells take on a glassy appearance

Hyperglycemia. Abnormally high level of glucose in the blood

Hyperglycemic hyperosmolar nonketotic coma (HHNC). A hyperglycemic complication of diabetes mellitus that results from insulin deficiency

Hypoglycemia. Abnormally low level of glucose in the blood

Infarction. Death of tissue

Insulin. An anabolic hormone produced by the beta cells of the islets of Langerhans of the pancreas

Insulin-dependent cells. Cells that require insulin to facilitate diffusion of glucose through the cell membrane

Ketonuria. The presence of ketones in the urine

Ketosis. The presence of ketones in the blood

Lipogenesis. Formation of fat

Lipolysis. Breakdown or splitting of fat

Lipoprotein. A protein that is conjugated (joined) with lipid molecules, such as triglycerides, cholesterol, and phospholipids; lipids exist in the plasma primarily as lipoproteins

Macrovascular disease. Refers to atherosclerosis

Microangiopathy. Small blood vessel disease

Microvascular disease. Disease of the capillaries

Metabolic acidosis. An alteration in acid-base balance characterized by an arterial blood gas pH of <7.35 (normal is 7.35–7.45) with a bicarbonate level of <22 mEq/L (normal is 22 mEq/L–28 mEq/L)

Osmotic diuresis. Excessive urinary excretion caused by osmotic shifting of fluids

Polydipsia. Excessive thirst

Polyuria. Excessive urination

Somogyi effect. A nocturnal hypoglycemia rebound phenomenon

Synthesis. Formation of a substance

Uptake. To take a substance into a cell

Abbreviations

AG. Anion gap

DKA. Diabetic ketoacidosis

HHNC. Hyperglycemic hyperosmolar nonketotic coma

ICA. Islet cell antibodies

IDDM. Insulin-dependent diabetes mellitus

NIDDM. Noninsulin-dependent diabetes mellitus

Section One: Normal Glucose Metabolism

At the completion of this section, the learner will be able to discuss normal glucose metabolism.

Glucose is used by most body cells as an energy source. Some cells (e.g., brain cells) can use only glucose for energy. Glucose, however, does not cross muscle and fat cell membranes using the same mechanisms as do most other molecules. It requires a protein carrier, facilitated by insulin, to transport it into these cells. Fat and muscle cells are, therefore, sometimes referred to as insulin-dependent cells. After combining with the protein carrier in the cell membrane, glucose is able to diffuse across the membrane into the cell, where it is released by the carrier (Guyton, 1987). Supplying the cells with glucose is a complex physiologic task based on important feedback mechanisms for regulating blood glucose levels. This mechanism is primarily controlled by two hormones, insulin and glucagon, with important support by three other hormones, epinephrine, growth hormone, and cortisol.

Insulin

Insulin is a polypeptide (small protein) produced by the beta cells of the islets of Langerhans in the pancreas. Its underlying role is to lower the blood glucose level, and it sometimes is referred to as the *hypoglycemic factor*. Insulin plays a crucial part in regulating carbohydrate, fat, and protein metabolism.

Insulin must bind to special insulin receptor proteins in the cell membrane in order to carry out its functions. Once it is attached to a receptor site, insulin combines with the carrier protein in the cell membrane. The carrier protein, with help from insulin, promotes glucose diffusion across the cell membrane. Insulin's exact role is enhancing the function of the carrier protein.

Glucagon

Glucagon, a small protein, is secreted by alpha cells in the islets of Langerhans in the pancreas. It is the major hormone responsible for raising serum glucose levels and sometimes is referred to as the *hyperglycemic factor*. Its effects are in opposition to those of insulin. The stimulus for glucagon release is a blood glucose level below 70 mg/dL (Guyton, 1987). Glucagon counterbalances the effects of insulin by converting hepatic glycogen (via glycogenolysis) into glucose. Once converted, hepatic glucose rapidly moves into the circulation, increasing blood glucose levels. The reciprocal relationship between insulin and glucagon assists in maintaining homeostatic blood glucose levels.

Epinephrine, Growth Hormone, and Cortisol

When serum glucose drops below normal ranges, the sympathetic nervous system is stimulated. Consequently, the adrenal glands secrete epinephrine. Epinephrine increases serum glucose levels in a manner similar to glucagon but to a lesser extent.

Pituitary growth hormone and cortisol both respond to prolonged periods of hypoglycemia. They help reestablish a more normal glucose level by decreasing the rate of glucose use by the cells. Growth hormone decreases the body's ability to use carbohydrates, sparing them as an energy source. It facilitates the transport of amino acids into the cells. Growth hormone also has a synergistic relationship with insulin in the promotion of growth (Guyton, 1987).

In summary, glucose is the body's main source of fuel. Its control and use are dependent primarily on two hormones, insulin and glucagon. Three other hormones also contribute to regulating serum glucose levels. Epinephrine elevates glucose in response to a hypoglycemic state in a similar manner to glucagon. Growth hormone and cortisol decrease cellular use of glucose, promoting hyperglycemia.

Section One Review

1. Insulin is produced in the
   A. kidneys
   B. pituitary gland
   C. liver
   D. pancreas

2. Insulin promotes use of glucose by
   A. breaking down glucose
   B. assisting glucose into the cells
   C. converting glucose to glycogen
   D. transporting glucose in the blood

3. Glucagon promotes which of the following?
   A. decreased use of glucose
   B. conversion of hepatic glycogen
   C. protein synthesis and transport
   D. transport of glucose into the cells
4. Which of the following is true regarding growth hormone?
   A. it decreases cellular use of glucose
   B. it promotes storage of fat
   C. it decreases blood glucose levels
   D. it increases breakdown of glycogen

5. Release of cortisol
   A. increases mobilization of fats
   B. decreases use of glucose
   C. decreases secretion of insulin
   D. increases breakdown of muscle glycogen

Answers: 1, D. 2, B. 3, B. 4, A. 5, B.

Section Two: The Effects of Insulin on Metabolism

At the completion of this section, the learner will be able to describe the effects of insulin on metabolism.

Carbohydrate Metabolism

The body is dependent on adequate levels of glucose to provide energy for normal functioning. Carbohydrates, a nutritional substance composed of complex and simple sugars, normally provide most of the body's glucose needs. Directly after consumption of carbohydrates, the serum glucose level increases, triggering a rapid increase in insulin secretion. Under the influence of insulin, glucose is moved into cells (cellular uptake) for immediate use or stored for later use. The liver plays a major role in glucose storage, and to a lesser extent fat and muscle tissues also provide glucose storage.

Insulin and the Liver in Glucose Metabolism

Directly after a meal, glucose that is not used immediately by the cells is stored rapidly in the liver as glycogen. In general terms, the glucose storage and release process is as follows.

With the help of insulin, glucose is converted into glycogen, diffusing into the liver cells where it becomes trapped until the serum glucose level becomes low. Insulin levels alter in direct response to glucose levels. Consequently, as serum glucose levels drop (such as between meals) insulin is no longer needed and thus its level rapidly declines. The lack of insulin triggers a reversal of the process, breaking down the liver glycogen into glucose phosphate and releasing it from the liver cells to move back into the circulation. Approximately 60% of glucose is stored in the liver in this manner (Guyton, 1987).

Insulin and Muscle Tissue in Glucose Metabolism

During normal daily activity, muscle tissue uses fatty acids, not glucose, as its major source of energy. This is because the resting membrane of the muscle does not allow glucose into the cell without the presence of insulin. Insulin levels, however, are very low between meals, thereby requiring use of energy sources other than glucose.

Muscle cells use glucose under two circumstances. First, during heavy exercise, muscle cell membranes become highly permeable to glucose. Second, for several hours directly after meals, high levels of insulin in the serum enhances transport of glucose into the muscle cells. Muscle cells store available glucose as muscle glycogen for their own use. They are, however, unable to convert it back into glucose or transport it back out of the muscle tissue into the general circulation. Muscle tissue, therefore, does not contribute to counteracting the effects of insulin because it does not increase serum glucose levels (Guyton, 1987).

Insulin and Fat Metabolism

Insulin also has important effects on fat metabolism. Normal levels of insulin help regulate fat metabolism by

1. Facilitating glucose use by most tissues, thereby sparing fat as the major energy source
2. Promoting synthesis of fatty acids primarily in the liver; fatty acids are then transported to adipose tissue for storage
3. Inhibiting fatty acid release into the circulation
4. Facilitating transport of glucose into fat cells for fatty acid synthesis.

The blood glucose level is the major determining factor as to whether the cells will use carbohydrates or fats for energy. Once the decision is made, the switch from one energy source to the other is done rapidly. When there is a lack of insulin (such as between meals), cells must rely on the use of fat as the primary energy source in insulin-dependent tissues. When insulin is again made available in sufficient quantities, glucose resumes its function as the major energy source. Insulin, then, is a crucial factor in determining which energy source is used (Guyton, 1987).

Insulin and Protein Metabolism

Insulin plays an important part in the storage of protein following ingestion of nutrients. Insulin helps regulate protein metabolism in the following ways.

1. Facilitates transport of amino acids across the cell membrane

2. Promotes protein synthesis
3. Decreases protein catabolism

Amino acids also act as a trigger for insulin secretion (in addition to glucose). Thus, when amino acid levels increase after ingestion of nutrients, insulin is secreted to facilitate cellular uptake, synthesis, and storage of proteins.

In summary, the affects of normal levels of insulin on carbohydrate, fat, and protein metabolism are profound. Insulin helps regulate glucose metabolism in fat and muscle (insulin-dependent) tissues. It plays an important part in the cellular uptake, synthesis, and storage of both amino acids and fatty acids. Blood glucose and amino acid levels are the major triggers of insulin secretion. Blood glucose levels are the decisive factor in the type of food (carbohydrate or fat) used as the energy source for the insulin-dependent cells.

Section Two Review

1. Which of the following substances supplies the primary source of cell energy?
   A. fat
   B. protein
   C. carbohydrate
   D. glucagon
2. Cells requiring insulin to facilitate diffusion of glucose into them are called
   A. insulin-dependent
   B. glucose-dependent
   C. glycogen-dependent
   D. carbohydrate-dependent
3. Excess glucose is stored in the _____ tissues.
   A. pancreas
   B. muscle
   C. adipose
   D. liver

4. During normal daily activities, muscle cells use which of the following as their major energy source?
   A. glucose
   B. fatty acids
   C. amino acids
   D. glucagon
5. Which of the following is true regarding the effect of insulin on fat metabolism?
   A. inhibits synthesis of fatty acids
   B. inhibits glucose use by tissues
   C. inhibits release of fatty acids
   D. inhibits transport of glucose into fat cells

Answers: 1, C. 2, A. 3, D. 4, B. 5, C.

Section Three: The Effects of Insulin Deficit

At the completion of this section, the learner will be able to discuss the effects of insulin deficit.

Insulin deficiency results in disordered carbohydrate, protein, and fat metabolism. In the absence of normal use of carbohydrates as the major glucose energy source, the liver initiates conversion of glycogen to glucose. The principal metabolic altera-

tions associated with insulin deficiency include impaired cellular uptake and use of glucose, increased extracellular (serum) glucose, increased mobilization of fats, and tissue depletion of protein (Figure 15–1).

Movement of glucose into insulin-dependent cells occurs in direct proportion to the amount of insulin available. When insulin-dependent tissues are deprived of glucose as a result of either actual insulin deficiency or the development of insulin re-

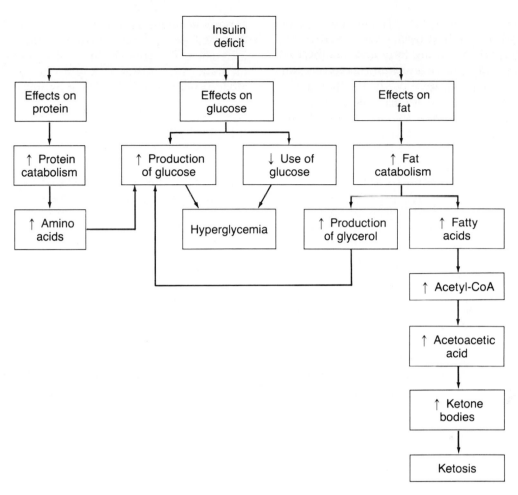

Figure 15–1. Consequences of insulin deficit.

sistance, their functional capacities become restricted. Table 15–1 summarizes the effects of insulin deficiency on insulin-dependent tissues.

Insulin Deficit and Carbohydrate Metabolism

Insulin deficit dramatically alters carbohydrate metabolism. Carbohydrates are the major supplier of simple and complex sugars, producing glucose as the primary energy source. Insulin deficit causes cessation in glucose uptake by insulin-dependent cells and a decrease in glucose use by the cells. The combination of decreased glucose uptake and decreased glucose use causes a rapid buildup of serum glucose, causing hyperglycemia.

In an insulin-poor environment, insulin-dependent cells are actually starving. Though there

TABLE 15–1. EFFECTS OF INSULIN DEFICIT ON INSULIN-DEPENDENT TISSUES

Tissues	Effects
Glucose Transport Problems	
Skeletal muscle	Fatigue; decreased strength
Cardiac muscle	Weaker contractions; decreased cardiac output; decreased peripheral circulation
Smooth muscle	Poor bowel tone; decreased vascular tone
Leukocytes	Depressed leukocyte function; impaired inflammatory response
Crystalline lens of eyes	Opacity/cataracts
Fibroblasts	Impaired healing
Pituitary gland	Retarded growth; impaired regeneration of tissue; other endocrine problems
Insulin Resistance Problem	
Adipose tissue	Lipolysis; lipidemia; elevated serum ketone levels

is abundant potential energy available in the form of glucose, it is of no use to the cells. Other sources of energy are tapped, including fatty acids as the primary backup energy source and amino acids once fat reserves are depleted. Clinically, dysfunctional carbohydrate metabolism is evidenced as hyperglycemia, and if not controlled, ketosis and aminoacidemia may result, each with its own set of complications.

Insulin Deficit and Fat Metabolism

Insulin deficit alters fat metabolism by increasing lipolysis (fat breakdown) and decreasing lipogenesis (fat formation). The decreased availability of intracellular glucose results in increased breakdown of stored triglycerides by hormone-sensitive lipase, causing lipolysis. Free fatty acids become the major energy source for the tissues, with the major exception of the brain. Clinically, this is evidenced as increased blood levels of free fatty acids and glycerol. The liver also converts some of the excess fatty acids into cholesterol and phospholipids. Excess fatty acid breakdown causes increased levels of acetyl-CoA, which either is used by the liver for energy or the excess is converted into acetoacetic acid. Some of the acetoacetic acid is further converted into β-hydroxybutyric acid and acetone. These three substances (acetoacetic acid, β-hydroxybutyric acid, and acetone) move into the circulation as ketone bodies (see Figure 15–1).

Clinically, this sequence of events has both acute and chronic consequences. Acutely, the increased levels of ketone bodies cause ketosis and ketonuria. When ketosis is extreme, severe acidosis and coma result (e.g., diabetic ketoacidosis). The use of fat as energy is evidenced as a significant increase in plasma lipoproteins (as much as three times normal). In the long term, high levels of lipoproteins are associated with the rapid onset of atherosclerosis, especially when high cholesterol levels are present. Many of the complications of diabetes mellitus are secondary to atherosclerotic changes.

Insulin Deficit and Protein Metabolism

Without insulin, the body is unable to store protein. There is an increase in protein catabolism and cessation of protein synthesis. Protein catabolism causes large quantities of amino acids to move into the circulation. The amino acids are then used either directly as an energy source or as part of the gluconeogenesis process.

Clinically, protein catabolism is evidenced by muscle wasting, multiple organ dysfunction, aminoacidemia, and increased urine urea nitrogen. If nitro-

genous wastes accumulate in the body faster than they can be excreted in the urine, the patient exhibits increasing alteration in level of consciousness and mentation. In addition, as gluconeogenesis is initiated, hyperglycemia is further aggravated.

Insulin Deficit and Fluid and Electrolyte Balance

When an insulin deficit exists, the serum glucose level increases, causing plasma osmotic pressure also to increase. The resulting change in pressure produces a shifting of body fluids from the tissues into the intravascular compartment. This shifting of fluids leads to intracellular dehydration.

As the level of hyperglycemia increases beyond the kidney's ability to reabsorb the extra glucose, glycosuria (excretion of sugar in the urine) develops. Urinary excretion of glucose produces an osmotic diuresis evidenced as polyuria (excessive urination). Osmotic diuresis results in excessive loss of water, potassium, sodium, chloride, and phosphate ions. Loss of these ions further increases both extracellular and intracellular dehydration. Deficits in potassium and sodium are manifested by weakness, fatigue, and other signs and symptoms associated with the specific electrolyte imbalances. As fluid is lost, serum osmolality increases. Dehydration stimulates the hypothalamic thirst center, causing excessive thirst (polydipsia). Dehydration also produces hemoconcentration as fluid from the vascular space is lost, causing decreased cardiac output (CO). If the dehydration is allowed to progress, the CO may become critically low, ultimately leading to circulatory failure.

Circulatory failure has two major consequences. First, it causes poor tissue perfusion and tissue hypoxia. Decreased perfusion to the brain results in cerebral hypoxia and the symptoms related to altered cerebral tissue perfusion. Second, it causes severe hypotension, which is responsible for decreased renal perfusion and, ultimately, for acute renal failure. Circulatory failure is fatal if an adequate CO is not reestablished in a timely manner. (Fluid and electrolytes are presented in detail in Module 19, *Fluid and Electrolytes*.)

In summary, insulin deficiency severely alters metabolism of carbohydrates, proteins, and fats. When glucose is unable to move into insulin-dependent cells, cell function becomes rapidly impaired. Fluid and electrolyte balance becomes impaired as plasma osmotic pressure changes due to glycosuria. As fluids shift, the cells become dehydrated, and electrolytes become deranged. Osmotic diuresis, if prolonged, causes hypovolemia and decreased CO, ultimately leading to circulatory failure.

Section Three Review

1. When an insulin deficiency exists, the liver responds by converting
   A. fatty acids to glucose
   B. glycogen to glucose
   C. glucagon to glucose
   D. amino acids to glucose
2. Insulin-dependent cells use which of the following nutritional substances FIRST when insulin is not available?
   A. fatty acids
   B. glycogen
   C. glucagon
   D. amino acids
3. Insulin deficit alters fat metabolism by
   A. increasing lipogenesis
   B. synthesizing triglycerides
   C. increasing lipolysis
   D. synthesizing glycerol

4. When acetoacetic acid combines with acetone and β-hydroxybutyric acid, _____ is/are formed.
   A. amino acids
   B. acetyl-CoA
   C. glycerol
   D. ketone bodies
5. Protein catabolism is evidenced by
   A. muscle wasting
   B. hyperexcitability
   C. decreased urine urea nitrogen
   D. increased triglyceride levels

Answers: 1, B. 2, A. 3, C. 4, D. 5, A.

Section Four: Types of Diabetes Mellitus

At the completion of this section, the learner will be able to differentiate the two major types of diabetes.

Diabetes mellitus is a complex metabolic disorder in which the person has either an absolute or relative insulin deficit. It is divided into two major types: insulin-dependent diabetes mellitus (IDDM) and noninsulin-dependent diabetes mellitus (NIDDM).

Insulin-Dependent Diabetes Mellitus

IDDM, classified as type I diabetes, occurs when there is an absolute lack of endogenous insulin caused by a loss of beta cells in the pancreas. It is diagnosed most commonly in people less than 30 years old, with a peak onset age between 11 and 13 (Gray and Ludwig-Beymer, 1990). Beta cell destruction has been associated with the presence of islet cell antibodies (ICA). Approximately 85 percent of newly diagnosed type I diabetics have ICA present, though the function of these antibodies is yet unknown. A variety of pathologic events have been proposed as being the trigger for development of type I diabetes, including viral infection or immune reaction with an underlying genetic predisposition for type I diabetes. Regardless of the triggering event, it is believed that an autoimmune reaction destroys the beta cells.

Noninsulin-Dependent Diabetes Mellitus

NIDDM, also called type II diabetes, is more common than type I diabetes. It is associated with a relative insulin deficiency (less insulin secretion) rather than a total deficit. The major etiology of type II diabetes is progressive pancreatic dysfunction secondary to hyalinization of the islets of Langerhans. Over the course of the disease, both the pancreas and the liver develop fatty deposits due to high serum lipid levels. They also undergo tissue atrophy, associated with a decrease in size and number of functioning pancreatic and liver cells. Obesity in the presence of hereditary tendencies is considered the major risk factor for development of type II diabetes. It has many different characteristics from type I diabetes. Table 15–2 presents a comparison of type I and type II diabetes as summarized from Gray and Ludwig-Beymer (1990).

Diabetes mellitus is associated with three common complications: hypoglycemic coma, diabetic ketoacidosis (DKA), and hyperosmolar hyperglycemic nonketotic coma (HHNC). Each of these complications is explored in the following sections of this module.

In summary, diabetes mellitus is a complex metabolic disorder associated with an absolute or relative insulin deficit. There are two major types of diabetes mellitus, type I (insulin-dependent diabetes mel-

TABLE 15–2. COMPARISON OF THE TWO TYPES OF DIABETES MELLITUS

Characteristic	Type I (IDDM)	Type II (NIDDM)
Usual age of onset	<30 years of age	>40 years of age
Rate of onset	Rapid	Slow
Weight status	Not associated with obesity	Commonly associated with obesity
Beta cell status/insulin secretion	Total loss of beta cells within 1 year of diagnosis; no insulin secretion	Decrease in size and number of beta cells; decreased insulin secretion
Alpha cell status/glucagon	Abnormal alpha cell function, but relative excess of glucagon in relation to insulin	Decrease in size and number of alpha cells; glucagon and insulin secretion decreased but often balanced (dysfunction of alpha cells may be equal to dysfunction of beta cells)
Islet cell antibodies (ICA)	Common, in approx. 85%	Rare, in approx. 5%
Ketone status	Ketone prone; high risk for ketoacidosis	Not ketone prone unless under stress; low risk for ketoacidosis
Insulin supplement status	Insulin dependent	Usually not insulin dependent
Diabetic crises associated with disorder(s)	Diabetic ketoacidosis (DKA); hypoglycemic coma	Hyperosmolar hyperglycemic nonketotic coma (HHNC); hypoglycemic coma

litus) and type II (noninsulin-dependent diabetes mellitus). Type I is associated with autoimmune destruction of the beta cells in the pancreas. Type II is associated with obesity, insulin resistance, and general dysfunction of the pancreas and the liver. There are many differences between these two types of diabetes. However, both cause progressive deterioration of multiple body systems.

Section Four Review

1. The etiology of type I diabetes is believed to be
   A. obesity
   B. autoimmune reaction
   C. bacterial infection
   D. general pancreatic dysfunction
2. By 1 year after diagnosis of type I diabetes, there is ___ percent of functioning beta cells remaining in the pancreas.
   A. 0
   B. 10
   C. 30
   D. 50
3. Type II diabetes is associated with which of the following major risk factors?
   A. smoking
   B. viral infection
   C. obesity
   D. autoimmune reaction

4. In what way is pancreatic function altered in the type II diabetic?
   A. beta cells become hyalinized
   B. beta cells become overactive
   C. alpha cell activity predominates
   D. alpha cells break down insulin
5. Which of the following statements is true regarding type II diabetes? Type II diabetes _____ than type I diabetes.
   A. is less common
   B. has a slower rate of onset
   C. usually occurs at a younger age
   D. is more commonly associated with ketones

Answers: 1, B. 2, A. 3, C. 4, A. 5, B.

Section Five: Hypoglycemic Coma

At the completion of this section, the learner will be able to discuss the diabetic complication, hypoglycemic coma.

Clinical Presentation

Hypoglycemia often is defined clinically as a blood glucose level of <50 mg/dL in an adult. People do, however, develop initial symptoms of hypoglycemia at levels significantly below or above that point. Therefore, hypoglycemia should be diagnosed on the basis of blood glucose levels in addition to a positive hypoglycemic clinical picture. Hypoglycemia becomes symptomatic when there is insufficient glucose available to meet the energy needs of the central nervous system. The most common precipitating condition for development of hypoglycemia is excessive administration of insulin or oral antidiabetic agent. Other conditions that increase the risk of hypoglycemia include consumption of too little food (fasting), an unusually high activity level, and certain drugs, such as propranolol, which potentiate the effects of insulin.

A patient's clinical presentation reflects two events: sympathetic nervous system stimulation and dysfunction of glucose-starved cells. Patients receiving oral hypoglycemic therapy are at risk for severe and prolonged symptoms of hypoglycemia due to the extended half-life of these agents.

The rate of onset of hypoglycemia influences the type of symptoms that predominate.

Rapid Onset

When the onset of hypoglycemia is rapid, sympathetic nervous system symptoms often predominate for the following reason. A significant, rapid drop of blood glucose level stimulates the sympathetic nervous system, which initiates secretion of epinephrine. Epinephrine causes gluconeogenesis in the liver, thereby increasing the serum glucose level. Concurrently, growth hormone and cortisol also are secreted to assist in increasing glucose levels by decreasing glucose use by the cells. Clinically, sympathetic nervous system symptoms are evidenced as sweating, tachycardia, nervousness, anxiety, weakness, hunger, nausea, and vomiting.

Slow Onset

When the onset of hypoglycemia is slow, the symptoms of central nervous system dysfunction may predominate. Over a period of time, the body is able to adapt to a slow decline in blood glucose. Clinically, the patient initially may have a decreased ability to reason and remember, or a changing mental status may be noted. Other progressive symptoms include emotional lability, headache, thickened speech, loss of coordination, loss of proprioception, drowsiness, convulsions, and coma. Brain cells are not insulin dependent and can take in glucose directly. Central nervous system symptoms, therefore, are caused by lack of available glucose rather than an insulin deficit. The brain is a high-energy tissue, requiring large amounts of glucose to maintain normal functioning. Without glucose, particularly over a prolonged period, the brain can sustain permanent damage that may be either minor or severe (irreversible coma).

Further discussion of the clinical manifestations of hypoglycemia is presented in Module 20, *Nursing Care of the Patient with Altered Metabolism.*

Nocturnal Hypoglycemia

Some patients, particularly those who are acutely ill, have wide swings in serum glucose levels from early morning to postprandial testings caused by an excessive insulin dosage. One explanation of this phenomenon is the *Somogyi effect.* The effect is triggered by nocturnal hypoglycemia. Hypoglycemia causes release of stress hormones, ultimately increasing serum glucose, which, in turn, creates a state of hyperglycemia. Morning urine ketones may be noted as well as an elevated serum glucose caused by catabolic processes. The resulting hyperglycemia, if accompanied by increased insulin dosage, precipitates another episode of hypoglycemia that may be worse than the preceding episode (Figure 15–2).

Recognition of the presence of the Somogyi effect has important treatment implications. Treating this type of rebound phenomenon with increased doses of insulin worsens the level of nocturnal hypoglycemia, further aggravating the problem (McKenna, 1988). When the Somogyi effect is suspected, insulin dosage may actually need to be decreased, or a bedtime snack of protein may be added to the diet to halt the rebound cycle.

Medical Interventions for Severe Hypoglycemia

The major goal of intervention is rapid restoration of normal serum glucose levels. The specific type of intervention is based partially on the patient's level of consciousness.

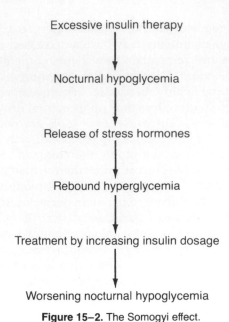

Excessive insulin therapy

↓

Nocturnal hypoglycemia

↓

Release of stress hormones

↓

Rebound hyperglycemia

↓

Treatment by increasing insulin dosage

↓

Worsening nocturnal hypoglycemia

Figure 15–2. The Somogyi effect.

The Conscious Hypoglycemic Patient

McKenna (1988) recommends giving the patient liquids or foods that are absorbed rapidly, such as 6 to 8 ounces of orange juice, 3 tablespoons of raisins, 8 or more Lifesavers, or one can of sugar-containing soft drink.

The Unconscious Hypoglycemic Patient

If a hospitalized diabetic shows evidence of hypoglycemia (confirmed or not confirmed), the following is a suggested regimen (McKenna, 1988; Dolan, 1991).

If a venous excess is unavailable

1. Obtain a blood glucose level
2   Administer glucagon 0.5 to 2 mg (IM) without waiting for laboratory results
3. After 20 minutes, if no response, repeat glucagon administration

If a venous access is available

1. Obtain blood glucose level
2. Administer one ampule of 50 percent glucose (IV) without waiting for laboratory results
3. Administer a continuous 50 percent glucose drip until either blood glucose is over 200 mg/dL or consciousness returns
4. If necessary, maintain a blood glucose level of 100 to 200 mg/dL by using 10 percent dextrose and water until the patient is awake enough to safely consume oral nutrients

In summary, hypoglycemia is a condition in which there is insufficient glucose to meet cellular energy needs. This may be due to fasting, excessive intake of antidiabetic agents, an unusually high level of exercise, or certain insulin-potentiating drugs. Hypoglycemia triggers the sympathetic response, causing secretion of epinephrine, which initiates the conversion of glycogen to glucose. The clinical presentation of hypoglycemia is due to sympathetic nervous system stimulation and starvation of neural cells. The primary goal of treatment is restoration of blood glucose levels to normal.

Section Five Review

1. Which of the following statements is TRUE regarding hypoglycemia?
   A. it is defined only in terms of blood glucose levels
   B. it is defined only in terms of clinical presentation
   C. it becomes symptomatic only when excessive insulin is present
   D. it becomes symptomatic at different blood glucose levels
2. Conditions that increase the risk of hypoglycemia include all of the following EXCEPT
   A. dietary fasting
   B. high fat diet
   C. excessive exercise
   D. excessive insulin dosage

3. Of the following, the clinical presentation of hypoglycemia partially reflects which event?
   A. lack of glucose within the cells
   B. excessive glucose within the cells
   C. stimulation of parasympathetic nervous system
   D. excessive circulating insulin
4. A patient experiencing rapid onset hypoglycemia is most likely to have predominantly _____ symptoms.
   A. cell dysfunction
   B. gastrointestinal
   C. stimulated sympathetic nervous system
   D. stimulated parasympathetic nervous system

5. Central nervous system symptoms associated with hypoglycemia are caused by lack of _____ rather than insulin deficit.
   A. glucose
   B. amino acids
   C. fatty acids
   D. glucagon
6. The Somogyi effect describes a rebound _____ phenomenon.
   A. hyperglycemic
   B. insulin deficit
   C. hypoglycemic
   D. glucagon deficit

7. In the unconscious hypoglycemic patient with a venous access, the treatment of choice is
   A. 50 percent glucose (IV)
   B. 0.5–2 mg glucagon (IM)
   C. 10 percent dextrose and water (IV)
   D. 8 ounces of orange juice (orally)

Answers: 1, D. 2, B. 3, A. 4, C. 5, A. 6, C. 7, A.

Section Six: Diabetic Ketoacidosis

At the completion of this section, the learner will be able to describe the diabetic complication, diabetic ketoacidosis.

Diabetic ketoacidosis (DKA) refers to a type of metabolic acidosis associated with diabetes mellitus produced by excessive levels of ketones in the body. It is a potentially severe, sometimes lethal complication. Annually, the mortality rate from diabetic ketoacidosis is between 5 percent and 10 percent in most institutions (Graves, 1990).

Clinical Presentation

The clinical picture of a patient with DKA is a complex one. In terms of laboratory findings, it can be defined as a pH <7.30 and/or HCO_3 <15 mEq/L, with a blood glucose of >300 mg/dL and positive ketonemia and ketonuria (ketones in the blood and urine, respectively). The clinical manifestations of diabetic ketoacidosis primarily reflect the hyperglycemic state and level of metabolic acidosis. Table 15–3 summarizes the clinical manifestations of DKA.

The clinical presentation of DKA is further discussed in Module 20, *Nursing Care of the Patient with Altered Metabolism*.

Related Pathophysiology

DKA occurs when an insulin deficit results in the mobilization of fat from adipose tissue to be used as the primary cellular energy source. Hepatic biotransformation of free fatty acids releases ketone bodies, creating metabolic acidosis. The learner is referred to Section Three, which details the effects of

TABLE 15–3. SIGNS AND SYMPTOMS OF DIABETIC KETOACIDOSIS

Hyperglycemia
  Blood glucose elevation (>300 mg/dL)
  Urine glucose elevation
Metabolic acidosis
  Elevated serum and urine ketones
  Serum pH <7.30 (acidosis)
  Serum HCO_3 <15 mEq/L (acid)
  Serum Pco_2 <35 mm Hg (alkalotic)
  Anion gap >12 mEq (positive, high)
  Elevated respiratory rate and depth
  Fruity odor to breath
Osmotic diuresis
  Polyuria, polydipsia
  Dehydration
  Hypotension
  Hemoconcentration
  Electrolyte abnormalities
  Azotemia

insulin deficit on fat metabolism and ketone development.

Metabolic acidosis has varied etiologies, DKA being only one of them. Measuring anion gap (AG) is one way to help isolate DKA from some other acidotic conditions. Gaining a basic understanding of the concept of AG may facilitate early diagnosis and treatment of DKA.

Anion Gap

Metabolic acidosis exists either as normal AG acidosis (from loss of bicarbonate ions) or as high AG acidosis (from an accumulation of fixed acids in the serum).

Anions are negatively charged particles (i.e., CO_2^-, HCO_3^-, and Cl^-). They are the opposite of cations, or positively charged particles (i.e., Na^+ or K^+). Normally, cations and anions are in balance with each other. AG "is an expression of the excess unmeasurable anions in the body" (Holloway, 1988, p. 422). Measurement of the anion gap is helpful in differentiating the type of metabolic acidosis present. It is expressed as

$$AG = Na^+ - (HCO_3^- + Cl^-)$$

AG has a normal range of 10 to 12 mEq (Gray and Ludwig-Beymer, 1990). This normal range is a function of such unmeasured serum anions as phosphates, sulfates, ketones, and lactic acid.

High Anion Gap Acidosis

An AG of >12 mEq indicates an accumulation of these unmeasured anions and warrants immediate attention. When metabolic acidosis is caused by elevations in organic acids, the AG increases. Such states as starvation, lactic acidosis, and DKA cause high AG.

Normal Anion Gap Acidosis

When metabolic acidosis is caused by a loss of bicarbonate (buffer), the AG remains normal. This occurs in such states as high chloride intake, renal failure, and diarrhea.

A person admitted with a potential or actual DKA may have an AG determination performed. Although AG alone is inconclusive for DKA, it is used as adjunctive data in clustering critical cues for differential diagnosis.

Causes of Diabetic Ketoacidosis

DKA is seen most commonly in type I diabetics. About one half of diabetic patients requiring hospitalization for DKA develop this complication secondary to an acute infection or failure to follow their prescribed dietary or insulin medical regimen. Sabo and Michael (1989) state that any condition or situation that increases the insulin deficit can precipitate DKA, including previously undiagnosed IDDM, food/insulin imbalance, puberty and adolescence, increased exercise in the uncontrolled diabetic, and stress.

Stress as a Major Precipitating Factor

An increased level of stress causes an outpouring of stress hormones (e.g., epinephrine, growth hor-

mone, and cortisol). As discussed in Section One, when secreted, these hormones increase blood glucose levels by either increasing conversion of glycogen to glucose or decreasing cellular use of glucose. When the stress is severe, as in a severe acute infection, the increase in glucose can be substantial, thus precipitating an imbalance in the glucose/insulin relationship.

Severe infection with systemic involvement also is normally accompanied by hyperthermia (fever). Hyperthermia increases the metabolic rate, greatly increasing cellular need for glucose. Therefore, in the presence of infection, there is both an increased supply and an increased demand for glucose. In such a situation, it would seem that a balance in glucose would exist. However, this is not the case in the insulin-dependent diabetic (type I) patient. A balance can be maintained or regained only when there is sufficient insulin present to meet the increased glucose needs of the cells. DKA is precipitated by a relative insulin deficiency in this situation. If insulin dosage is not increased in response, there is insufficient insulin to meet the increased glucose supply as well as the increased metabolic demand.

A similar situation can occur with a noninsulin-dependent diabetic (type II), who normally is controlled by diet or oral hypoglycemics or both. In situations of high stress (infection, trauma, surgery), the level of insulin secretion in the pancreas often is insufficient to meet the increased supply of and demand for glucose. Thus, this type of patient clinically exhibits hyperglycemia and possibly positive ketones, often requiring temporary exogenous insulin therapy. Insulin is then administered until the level of physiologic stress is sufficiently reduced and balance is regained between the glucose level and the endogenous insulin supply.

Medical and Nursing Management

Module 20, *Nursing Care of the Patient with Altered Metabolism,* describes the medical and nursing management of the patient with DKA.

In summary, DKA is a hyperglycemic complication of diabetes mellitus. It is a type of high AG metabolic acidosis caused by accumulation of ketone bodies. AG is one method of differentiating DKA from several other types of acidosis. DKA may be precipitated by any event that increases the insulin deficit. Physiologic stress and acute infection are two major precipitating conditions.

Section Six Review

1. Which of the following set of laboratory results best reflects diabetic ketoacidosis?
   A. pH 7.28, HCO_3 34 mEq/L, blood glucose 260 mg/dL
   B. pH 7.18, HCO_3 13 mEq/L, blood glucose 120 mg/dL
   C. pH 7.26, HCO_3 14 mEq/L, blood glucose 450 mg/dL
   D. pH 7.38, HCO_3 24 mEq/L, blood glucose 620 mg/dL

2. All of the following are typical clinical manifestations of diabetic ketoacidosis EXCEPT
   A. polydipsia
   B. fluid overload
   C. electrolyte depletion
   D. progressive dehydration

3. Ketosis results from mobilization of
   A. amino acids
   B. glucagon
   C. glucose
   D. fatty acids

4. A high anion gap acidosis is consistent with which of the following problems?
   A. diarrhea
   B. high intake of chloride
   C. starvation
   D. high intake of sodium

5. All of the following are common precipitating factors for development of diabetic ketoacidosis EXCEPT
   A. stress
   B. decreased exercise
   C. puberty
   D. food/insulin imbalance

Answers: 1, C. 2, B. 3, D. 4, C. 5, B.

Section Seven: Hyperglycemic Hyperosmolar Nonketotic Coma

At the completion of this section, the learner will be able to discuss the diabetic complication, hyperglycemic hyperosmolar nonketotic coma (HHNC).

HHNC, also known as hyperglycemic hyperosmolar nonketosis (HHNK), is a hyperglycemic complication of diabetes mellitus that results from insulin deficiency. It is a more catastrophic complication than DKA, though not as common. HHNC has a high mortality rate (>50 percent), partially due to the severe degree of fluid and electrolyte derangements present before initiation of medical intervention. Most patients with HHNC die of concurrent illnesses or complications, such as severe infection or acute myocardial infarction.

Many HHNC-triggering events have been noted in the literature, including acute infection, hyperalimentation therapy, peritoneal dialysis, tube feedings, worsening of an existing chronic illness, and others.

Clinical Presentation

DKA/HHNC Similarities

DKA and HHNC have many similarities, as both are associated with (Graves, 1990)

- An absolute or relative insulin deficit
- Hyperosmolality secondary to hyperglycemia and water loss
- Depletion of volume secondary to osmotic diuresis
- Electrolyte abnormalities secondary to the osmotic diuresis
- Altered mental status from mild to profound coma

DKA/HHNC Differences

One of the major differences between the two hyperglycemic crises is the ketone factor. DKA results in ketonemia and ketonuria, whereas HHNC does not. The following is one possible explanation of why the type II diabetic does not develop significant ketosis.

In type II diabetes, the pancreas has become increasingly dysfunctional, although it still has a certain amount of secreting beta cells (insulin producers) that are able to maintain a balanced glucose state when the body is not experiencing increased stress and carbohydrate intake is controlled. However, if the person experiences increased stress or has an excessive amount of carbohydrate administered (e.g., tube feeding or hyperalimentation), the dysfunctional pancreas is unable to supply more insulin to meet the new glucose load, and hyperglycemia increases. In other words, although there is sufficient insulin being secreted by the beta cells to prevent lipolysis, there is not enough to prevent hyperglycemia. It is the lack of lipolysis that prevents significant ketosis.

There are other significant differences between diabetic ketoacidosis and HHNC, including

- DKA is associated with rapid onset, whereas HHNC develops more slowly and insidiously
- Hyperglycemia is more severe with HHNC (600–2,500 mg/dL)
- Hyperosmolality is more severe in HHNC, causing profound dehydration
- HHNC is associated with other neurologic signs in addition to mental status changes (e.g., seizures and hemiparesis); in addition, mental status changes may occur over a period of days with HHNC

Further description of the clinical manifestations as well as a comparison of HHNC with DKA are presented in Module 20, *Nursing Care of the Patient with Altered Metabolism.*

Medical Interventions

Medical goals for management of the patient with HHNC are essentially the same as for the patient with DKA. In management of HHNC, the first priority is rehydration and restoration of normal electrolyte levels. Other goals include correction of the precipitating event (if possible) and prevention of complications. Fluid replacement needs in the HHNC patient are often greater than in the DKA patient due to the more profound state of dehydration. Careful monitoring is necessary to prevent complications associated with too rapid rehydration, particularly if the patient has renal or cardiovascular dysfunction or both (both are common in this patient population). Because the type II diabetic is very sensitive to exogenous insulin, insulin generally is administered in lower doses in treatment of the HHNC patient than in the DKA patient.

In summary, hyperosmolar hyperglycemic nonketotic coma (HHNC) is a type of hyperglycemic diabetic crisis associated with type II diabetes mellitus. The hallmark of HHNC is a hyperosmolar hyperglycemic state without significant ketosis. The degree of hyperglycemia and dehydration is more severe in HHNC than in DKA. Treatment of DKA and HHNC is similar, although HHNC generally requires higher volumes of fluids and lower doses of insulin.

Section Seven Review

1. Which of the following statements is correct regarding hyperglycemic hyperosmolar nonketotic coma (HHNC)?
   A. it has a high mortality rate
   B. it is most common in type I diabetes
   C. it causes severe fluid volume overload
   D. death occurs from severe metabolic acidosis
2. Common precipitating events causing HHNC include which of the following?
   A. hemodialysis
   B. hyperalimentation
   C. chronic infection
   D. high fat diet
3. HHNC does not cause ketosis because
   A. lipolysis does not occur
   B. protein catabolism is occurring
   C. high glucagon levels prevent it
   D. hyperglycemia is not sufficiently severe

4. Which of the following statements regarding the differences between diabetic ketoacidosis (DKA) and HHNC is correct?
   A. the onset of HHNC is faster
   B. dehydration is less severe in HHNC
   C. hyperosmolality is more severe in HHNC
   D. mental status changes more rapidly in HHNC
5. Which of the following statements is correct regarding insulin management of the patient with HHNC?
   A. insulin management is contraindicated
   B. usually requires low dose insulin management
   C. the type II diabetic is resistant to exogenous insulin
   D. the type I diabetic is resistant to exogenous insulin

Answers: 1, A. 2, B. 3, A. 4, C. 5, B.

Section Eight: Exogenous Insulin Therapy

At the completion of this section, the learner will be able to explain the use of exogenous insulin in the management of the patient with diabetes mellitus.

Type I (insulin-dependent) diabetics require exogenous insulin replacement, without which they would not survive. Type II diabetics do not usually require exogenous insulin. However, during a period of stress, the type II diabetic may experience hyperglycemia, requiring temporary insulin therapy until the stressful condition is resolved and glucose levels return to normal.

Sources of Exogenous Insulin

Insulin is derived from two major sources, either animal pancreas or synthesized in a laboratory. Insulin produced from animal pancreas is further divided into three types: beef, pork, and beef–pork combination. Of all types of exogenous insulin, beef insulin differs most from human insulin and, therefore, generally is not used as commonly as other forms. Pork insulin is structurally similar to human insulin and usually is well accepted by the body. Beef–pork combination insulin also is available as a less expensive insulin alternative.

Synthetic insulin is developed in a laboratory setting and involves structural conversion of a substance into the amino acid chains identical to human insulin. Currently, this is being done either using pork insulin or inducing *Escherichia coli* to manufacture human insulin using recombinant DNA technology (Guthrie et al, 1984).

Certain factors dictate which type of insulin is best suited to a specific person. Some of these factors include the presence of the following.

- Insulin allergy
- Insulin resistance
- Adipose tissue atrophy at injection sites
- Religious restriction against pork
- Cost of insulin

The final choice of insulin often is based on trial and error in finding which product best meets the individual needs of the person. Insulins are not interchangeable, having differing efficacy levels and possible allergy implications. For this reason, it is important for the nurse to be aware of the type of insulin ordered and take precautions that the same type of insulin is being administered. For example, the patient who normally receives synthetic insulin should not be given pork or beef insulin without specific orders to do so.

TABLE 15–4. FACTORS AFFECTING INSULIN DOSAGE

Factor	Effect
Drug interactions	
Beta-adrenergic blocking agents	May mask hypoglycemic symptoms; propranolol is associated with causing hyperglycemia when given concurrently with insulin
Steroids	Use of steroids is associated with increased glucose levels; may require increased dosage of insulin
Oral antidiabetic agents	Enhance hypoglycemic effects; may require reduction in insulin dosage
Other	
Exercise	An unusually high level of exercise may reduce glucose levels, producing hypoglycemia; may require reduction in insulin dosage
Acute illness	Increases blood glucose levels and insulin needs; often requires sliding scale insulin administration
Nutritional support	Elevates blood glucose, increasing insulin need; often requires sliding insulin administration

Factors That Influence Insulin

Many factors have an impact on insulin dosage or effectiveness. Table 15–4 lists some of the major factors and how they influence insulin dosages, as summarized from McHenry and Salerno (1989).

Types of Insulin

Insulin is divided into three major categories according to its duration of action. The three categories include rapid acting, intermediate acting, and long acting. Table 15–5 differentiates the various insulins according to these categories.

Side Effects of Insulin

Administration of too much insulin causes hypoglycemia. The patient is at greatest risk for hypoglycemia during peak action time. It is crucial to be aware of the type of insulin administered (e.g., rapid acting), when the dose was administered, and what type of nutrition has been consumed after administration. A person receiving a rapid acting insulin, such as regular insulin, at 8:00 AM would have a peak within 2 to 4 hours after subcutaneous administra-

TABLE 15–5. CHARACTERISTICS OF INSULIN PREPARATIONS

Insulin[a]	Onset (hours)	Peak Effect (hours)	Duration of Action (hours)
Rapid acting			
Regular	0.5–1	2–4	6–8
Semilente	1	2–6	10–12
Intermediate acting			
Lente	1–3	8–12	18–28
NPH	3–4	6–12	18–28
Novolin 70/30, Mixtard	0.5	4–8	24
Long acting			
Ultralente	4–6	18–24	36
PZI	4–6	14–24	36

Adapted from *Mosby's pharmacology in nursing*, 18th ed., p. 785, by L.M. McKenry and E. Salerno, 1992, St. Louis: C.V. Mosby Co.
[a] Available as beef, pork, beef–pork combination, and human insulins.

tion. This would mean that the risk for hypoglycemia is greatest between the hours of 10:00 AM and 12:00 noon.

A patient receiving an intermediate acting insulin (such as NPH) at 8:00 AM would peak about 6 to 12 hours later, placing him at greatest risk for hypoglycemia between the hours of 2:00 PM and 8:00 PM. Many acutely ill patients require supplemental rapid acting insulin (regular insulin) as well as their usual intermediate or long acting insulin. Mixing types of insulin gives the patient multiple insulin peak periods throughout a 24-hour period. Other factors commonly seen in acutely ill patients, such as prolonged NPO status and nutritional support, all have an impact on glucose levels and insulin needs.

Continuous Low-Dose Intravenous Insulin Infusion

During a hyperglycemic crisis, a continuous infusion of regular insulin may be ordered to provide better control of serum insulin levels. When preparing to administer IV insulin, it is important to remember

- Only regular insulin is administered IV
- Insulin binds to polyvinylchloride in IV bags and tubing, lowering the insulin concentration in the fluid
- Blood glucose levels must be monitored frequently to avoid hypoglycemia

Graves (1990) suggests the following as a low-dose continuous IV insulin protocol for treatment of both DKA and HHNC.

1. 100 units of regular insulin in 500 mL of normal saline (0.2 unit/mL concentration)
2. Run 50 to 100 mL of the infusion through the

tubing before patient administration to minimize further absorption of insulin in the tubing
3. Run the insulin at the initial dose of 0.1 units/kg/hour, which results in a decrease of glucose by 80 to 100 mg/dL/hour
4. Once glucose levels have been stabilized, IV insulin should not be stopped until 1 to 2 hours after initiation of subcutaneous insulin therapy
5. An initial loading dose of 5 to 10 units (IV) is sometimes ordered; a loading dose may not be necessary, since a therapeutic insulin concentration reaches a steady state rapidly when administered IV

Sliding Scale Insulin Administration

During periods of physiologic stress, glucose levels may be very unstable, requiring supplemental insulin in addition to the patient's usual insulin coverage. Consequently, insulin dosage needs to reflect current blood glucose levels. Orders may be written to titrate the insulin dose to specific glucose levels. This type of insulin regimen is called *sliding scale insulin* coverage. Table 15–6 gives an example of a sliding scale insulin order.

It is recommended that sliding scale insulin administration be carried out based on blood glucose rather than urine glucose measurements. Urine glucose does not reflect hour-by-hour changes in glucose levels. Thus, its value for tight glucose control is diminished. Insulin administration for the patient with DKA and HHNC is further described in Module 20, *Nursing Care of the Patient with Altered Metabolism*.

In summary, exogenous insulin therapy is a necessity for the type I diabetic. The type II diabetic may require it, particularly during periods of physiologic stress. Exogenous insulin is available from either animal or synthetic sources. Animal sources of insulin are similar but not identical to human insulin, making them potentially less acceptable to the body. Synthetic insulin is a laboratory duplication of human insulin. Choice of type of insulin based on source usually is decided by trial and error.

TABLE 15–6. EXAMPLE OF SLIDING SCALE INSULIN REGIMEN

Blood Glucose Level (mg/dL)	Regular Insulin Dose (subcutaneously)
200–250	5 units
251–300	10 units
301–350	15 units
351–400	Call physician

Section Eight Review

1. Which of the following situations would be most likely to necessitate exogenous insulin use in the type II diabetic patient?
   A. a mild common cold
   B. a high carbohydrate meal
   C. an abdominal hysterectomy
   D. a localized toe infection
2. All of the following are sources of insulin EXCEPT
   A. pork
   B. beef
   C. *Eschericia coli*
   D. *Staphylococcus aureus*
3. Which of the following insulin sources is structurally the least like human insulin?
   A. beef
   B. Humulin
   C. pork
   D. beef–pork combination

4. All of the following are factors that dictate the type of insulin that is best suited for a specific person EXCEPT
   A. patient's weight
   B. insulin resistance
   C. patient's allergies
   D. adipose tissue condition
5. Which of the following factors would most likely decrease insulin need?
   A. acute illness
   B. steroid therapy
   C. nutritional support
   D. oral antidiabetic agents

Answers: 1, C. 2, D. 3, A. 4, A. 5, D.

Section Nine: Acute Care Implications of Chronic Complications

At the completion of this section, the learner will be able to discuss the acute care implications of chronic diabetic complications.

The acutely ill patient has many factors that influence patient outcome, such as preexisting chronic diseases. Diabetes is a chronic disease that can profoundly affect patient outcome. Though diabetes mellitus is caused by dysfunction of one organ, the pancreas, it causes dysfunction of virtually all organs. This section presents an overview of major long-term complications associated with diabetes mellitus.

The complications of diabetes mellitus can be divided into three types, peripheral neuropathy, microvascular, and macrovascular.

Diabetic Peripheral Neuropathies

Peripheral neuropathies are the most common complication of diabetes mellitus. They begin early in the course of the disease, affecting both type I and type II diabetics. Peripheral neuropathies primarily alter sensory perception. The underlying cause of neuropathies is poorly understood. They may result from thickening of vessel walls that supply peripheral nerves, impairing nutrition to the nerves. They may result from a segmental demyelinization that results in slowed or disrupted conduction. There is also some evidence that sorbitol may accumulate in the nerve cells, impairing conduction. Whatever the cause, the result is an alteration in sensory perception.

Neuropathies initially may cause pain or abnormal sensations or both. As nerve degeneration progresses, the patient may experience loss of the ability to discriminate fine touch, a decrease in proprioception, and local anesthesia.

The autonomic nervous system also may be affected. As the myelin sheath undergoes degenerative changes, functions governed by the autonomic nerves are affected adversely. The patient may experience an increase in gut motility and diarrhea, postural hypotension, or other autonomic nervous system-related complications.

The neuropathies experienced by diabetics vary in type, severity, and clinical manifestations. Because of this diversity, it is not possible to predict which neuropathy any individual will develop.

Acute Care Implications. When feasible, patients with diabetes should be assessed for the presence and degree of peripheral neuropathy. The presence of a diminished sense of touch and pain may mask injury or infection. The patient needs to be protected from injury at all times to prevent damage to affected tissues. The diabetic patient must also be protected from hyperthermic burns. Excessive heat may not be sensed, increasing the risk of burns by heating pads, hyperthermia blankets, and bathing. Some neuropathies are associated with progressive, permanent damage to the neurons. However, others are reversible when good glucose control is maintained.

Microvascular Disease

Microvascular disease is associated with capillary membrane thickening, causing microangiopathy (small blood vessel disease). As the capillary membrane thickens, the tissues become increasingly hypoperfused, and organs become hypoxic and ischemic. Prolonged ischemia eventually causes infarction (death of tissue). The degree of microvascular disease is believed to be influenced most by the duration of diabetes rather than the level of glucose control. Two organs are at particular risk for microvascular disease secondary to diabetes mellitus, the retina and the kidneys.

Retinopathy

Diabetic retinopathy is responsible for a significant portion of newly diagnosed blindness in the United States. It is caused by an underlying microangiopathy of the retina, leading to retina microvascular occlusion. Once occlusion exists, the retina undergoes increasing areas of ischemia and infarction, eventually leading to blindness. Damage occurs in two complex stages. Stage I is associated with increased capillary permeability, aneurysm formation, and hemorrhage. Stage II is associated with increasing retinal ischemia and eventual infarction, causing blindness. Diabetic retinopathy is associated with both type I and type II diabetes.

Acute Care Implications. The acutely ill diabetic patient may have moderate to severe visual impairment. Early assessment of visual status is important, either by questioning the patient directly or by interviewing the family. Medical and nursing management and teaching must be altered to meet the needs of a visually impaired patient. In the high acuity patient, blindness affects pupillary changes and must be taken into consideration when performing a neurologic assessment. A visually impaired patient in a critical care environment may have more difficulty making sense of distracting noises and equipment surrounding the bedside. Frequent explanation and reorientation may be necessary.

Nephropathy

Diabetic nephropathy is a disease of the glomeruli. The glomerular basement membrane becomes thickened, resulting in intracapillary glomerulosclerosis (hardening and thickening of the glomeruli). Glomeruli become enlarged and eventually are destroyed, causing renal failure when sufficient glomeruli are destroyed. As the degree of renal failure increases, the patient may require a decreased insulin dosage to prevent hypoglycemia. Reduced renal function decreases the ability of the kidney to metabolize insulin. Insulin not metabolized remains available to facilitate glucose metabolism.

Acute Care Implications. The acutely ill patient with some degree of preexisting renal impairment is at risk for further impairment from hypotensive episodes, nephrotoxic drug therapy, or the multisystem complications associated with many acute illnesses. Kidney function must be carefully monitored at regular intervals. Drug therapy may need to be altered based on kidney function. Kidney failure, as a disease entity, has its own set of actual and potential complications.

(Refer to Module 18, *Acute Renal Failure,* and Module 20, *Nursing Care of the Patient with Altered Metabolism,* for further information on assessment and complications of renal failure.)

Macrovascular Disease

Macrovascular disease refers to atherosclerosis. Atherosclerosis is a form of arteriosclerosis (thickening and hardening of arterial walls), characterized by plaque deposits of lipids, fibrous connective tissue, calcium deposits, and other blood substances. Atherosclerosis, by definition, affects only large arteries (excluding arterioles). The cause of rapid development of atherosclerosis in the diabetic patient is described in Section Three.

Macrovascular disease is associated with the development of coronary artery disease, peripheral vascular disease, cerebrovascular accidents, and increased risk of infection. Type II diabetes is most associated with macrovascular diseases. Peripheral vascular disease and increased risk of infection have important implications in care of the acutely ill patient.

Peripheral Vascular Disease

Progressive atherosclerotic changes in peripheral arterial circulation lead to decreasing arterial blood flow to peripheral tissues. As the disease progresses, small arteries become occluded precipitating a tissue ischemia/infarction sequence of events. In the type II diabetic, this is typically noted as small isolated patches of gangrene, particularly noted on the feet and toes. As circulation becomes increasingly compromised, areas of gangrene become larger, and amputation may be required. Major amputation is associated with a 10 percent to 23 percent mortality rate, with a survival rate, following amputation surgery, of approximately 40 percent at the end of 5 years (Gray and Ludwig-Beymer, 1990).

Acute Care Implications. The patient with peripheral vascular disease is at increased risk for complications secondary to poor tissue perfusion and loss of skin integrity. Of particular concern in the acutely ill patient is the development of decubitus ulcers and infection. Development of either of these two problems could lead potentially to gangrene and possible amputation. Careful limb positioning, excellent skin hygiene, and close monitoring of skin integrity are extremely important.

Increased Risk of Infection

The diabetic patient is at high risk for development of infection for a variety of reasons (Gray and Ludwig-Beyman, 1990).

1. Diminished early warning system. Impaired vision and peripheral neuropathy contribute to the decreased ability of the diabetic patient to perform self-monitoring. Breaks in skin integrity may not be seen or felt due to the underlying disease process.
2. Tissue hypoxia. Vascular disease causes tissue hypoxia. When skin integrity is broken, there is a decreased ability to heal, secondary to lack of oxygen.

3. Rapid proliferation of pathogens. Once inside the body, pathogens rapidly multiply because of increased glucose in body fluids and a decreased blood supply. Increased glucose acts as an energy source for the pathogens. A decreased blood supply decreases the ability of white blood cells to move into the infected area.
4. Impaired white blood cells. Diabetes is associated with the development of abnormal white blood cells, which interferes with their ability to function normally.

Acute Care Implications. The acutely ill diabetic patient is at increased risk for development of severe, difficult to treat infections. Any infection, no matter how minor it begins, may become life threatening in this patient population. Close monitoring for infection and rapid, aggressive intervention are needed. Decreased kidney function may be a complicating factor in aggressive antibiotic therapy.

Wound healing also is impaired in the diabetic for several reasons. Impaired tissue perfusion, especially in the peripheral body area, interferes with healing in those areas due to lack of circulation and tissue hypoxia. Hyperglycemic states adversely affect wound healing by interfering with collagen concentrations in a wound. Control of blood glucose significantly increases the amount of collagen in the wound, facilitating the healing process and increasing the strength of the healing tissues (Schumann, 1990).

In summary, the multisystem nature of the chronic complications of diabetes strongly influences patient outcome in acute illness. There are three major categories of complications: (1) peripheral neuropathies, (2) microvascular complications, including retinopathy and nephropathy, and (3) macrovascular complications, including coronary artery disease, cerebrovascular accident, peripheral vascular disease, and increased risk of infection.

Section Nine Review

1. Peripheral neuropathies primarily affect
   A. motor functions
   B. sensory functions
   C. optic functions
   D. vascular functions

2. Microvascular diseases are associated with
   A. deposits of lipoproteins
   B. deposits of calcium products
   C. large blood vessel disease
   D. small blood vessel disease

3. Diabetic retinopathy causes blindness by
   A. glucose deposits on the retina
   B. thickening of the retina
   C. destruction of the optic nerve
   D. infarction of retinal tissue
4. Diabetic nephropathy damages the nephrons by causing
   A. glomerulosclerosis
   B. glomerulonephritis
   C. chronic nephritis
   D. renal hypertension
5. Diabetes-induced atherosclerosis is associated with all of the following complications EXCEPT
   A. peripheral vascular disease
   B. cerebrovascular accidents
   C. gastrointestinal ulcers
   D. coronary artery disease

6. Diabetes increases a patient's chance of infection for which of the following reasons?
   A. abnormal white blood cells
   B. abnormal platelet function
   C. slow proliferation of pathogens
   D. decreased body fluid glucose levels

Answers: 1, B. 2, D. 3, D. 4, A. 5, C. 6, A.

Posttest

The following posttest is constructed in a case study format. A patient is presented. Questions are posed based on available data. New data are presented as the case study progresses.

Connie Doolittle is a 44-year-old housewife with a history of diabetes mellitus. She has been admitted to the hospital for reevaluation of insulin dosage. She has been having periods of drowsiness and confusion at home.

1. Connie's brain cells
   A. do not require glucose for energy
   B. require fatty acids as their major energy source
   C. do not require insulin for cellular uptake of glucose
   D. require high levels of insulin for cellular uptake of glucose
2. When Connie's blood glucose drops below normal, the sympathetic nervous system stimulates secretion of
   A. epinephrine
   B. cortisol
   C. glucagon
   D. growth hormone

3. Which of the following statements best reflects the effect of insulin on glucose metabolism in Connie's liver? Insulin facilitates conversion of _____ .
   A. excess amino acids into glucose
   B. excess fatty acids into glycogen
   C. excess glycogen into glucose
   D. excess glucose into glycogen
4. When Connie's blood amino acid levels increase, insulin
   A. facilitates storage of proteins
   B. inhibits synthesis of protein
   C. facilitates protein catabolism
   D. inhibits transport of amino acids into cell

Connie's diabetes is caused by an absolute or relative insulin deficit.

---

5. An absolute insulin deficit would affect carbohydrate metabolism in which of the following ways?
   A. brain cells rapidly become glucose starved
   B. insulin-dependent cells become glucose starved
   C. brain cells convert glycogen to glucose directly
   D. insulin-dependent cells take in glucose directly

6. In which of the following ways does insulin deficit affect Connie's protein metabolism?
   A. protein synthesis is increased
   B. protein catabolism is halted
   C. protein cannot be stored without insulin
   D. protein cannot be used as energy without insulin

Connie's diabetes is characterized by the following. Her mother also had diabetes. Connie was diagnosed with diabetes at the age of 32. She is 5 feet 5 inches tall and weighs 173 pounds. She requires insulin on a daily basis.

7. Which of the preceding data is most diagnostic of type I diabetes?
   A. her mother also had diabetes
   B. she was diagnosed at the age of 32
   C. she is 5 feet 5 inches tall and weighs 173 pounds
   D. she requires insulin on a daily basis

8. If Connie had type II diabetes, the most common etiologic factors include
   A. viral infection and obesity
   B. obesity and genetic predisposition
   C. immune reaction and viral infection
   D. obesity and autoimmune reaction

During her hospitalization, Connie was kept NPO for 8 hours for a particular set of blood tests. She, however, did receive her usual morning insulin dosage. Consequently, Connie experiences symptoms typical of a hypoglycemic episode.

9. Typical clinical manifestations of Connie's hypoglycemia would include all of the following EXCEPT
   A. bradycardia
   B. tremor
   C. diaphoresis
   D. vomiting

10. Common causes of hypoglycemic episodes include
    A. lack of dietary intake
    B. heavy carbohydrate meal
    C. insufficient insulin dose
    D. decreased exercise level

Connie is experiencing large swings in her glucose levels throughout the day. The physi-

cians order a larger insulin dose to better control the hyperglycemia. The next day, her hyperglycemia is worse. It is decided that she may be experiencing the Somogyi effect. Connie is confused but conscious.

11. The Somogyi effect is characterized by a rebound phenomenon caused by release of
    A. glucagon
    B. amino acids
    C. fatty acids
    D. stress hormones

12. Considering her status, which of the following interventions would be most appropriate?
    A. 5 units of regular insulin
    B. glucagon 1.5 mg (IM)
    C. 8 ounces of orange juice
    D. 50 percent dextrose (IV)

Connie has developed an infection from an ingrown toenail. She currently has a temperature of 100F (oral). A rapid assessment showed the following. Opens eyes and groans to mild shaking but closes them immediately after stimulation.

13. What other clinical manifestations would help confirm a diagnosis of diabetic ketoacidosis at this time?
    A. polydipsia
    B. hand tremors
    C. fruity breath odor
    D. shallow respirations

14. Which of the following laboratory results would be most consistent with a diagnosis of diabetic ketoacidosis?
    A. pH 7.34
    B. anion gap 16 mEq
    C. HCO_3 17 mEq/L
    D. $Paco_2$ 28 mg/L

It has been decided that Connie's diabetic ketoacidosis was precipitated by her foot infection.

15. Infection can precipitate a diabetic ketoacidosis episode due to
    A. stress response
    B. increased insulin resistance
    C. increased glucagon levels
    D. diminished cortisol activity

16. Connie's diabetic ketoacidosis can be differentiated best from hyperosmolar hyperglycemic nonketotic coma by measuring
    A. pH
    B. ketones
    C. bicarbonate
    D. blood glucose

During her diabetic ketoacidosis, Connie receives a continuous drip of IV insulin.

_____

17. Important rules to remember in infusing IV insulin include all of the following EXCEPT
    A. only regular insulin is used IV
    B. insulin binds to plastic bags and tubing
    C. obtain urine glucose every hour
    D. IV doses usually are small

On Connie's history, you note that she has a long history of peripheral neuropathy, poor vision, and peripheral vascular disease.

_____

18. Connie's peripheral neuropathy is best controlled by
    A. steroid therapy
    B. good glucose control
    C. vitamin supplementation
    D. nothing; there is no slowing of process
19. Connie's vision has become progressively impaired over the duration of her diabetes. Diabetic retinopathy is due to
    A. glucose deposits on retina
    B. macrovascular occlusion
    C. fatty deposits on retina
    D. microvascular occlusion
20. Connie's peripheral vascular disease may lead to further complications because it causes
    A. tissue ischemia
    B. acute infection
    C. peripheral edema
    D. coronary artery disease

Posttest Answers

Number	Answer	Section	Number	Answer	Section
1	C	One	11	D	Five
2	A	One	12	C	Five
3	D	Two	13	C	Six
4	A	Two	14	B	Six
5	B	Three	15	A	Six
6	C	Three	16	B	Seven
7	D	Four	17	C	Eight
8	B	Four	18	B	Nine
9	A	Five	19	D	Nine
10	A	Five	20	A	Nine

REFERENCES

Dolan, J.T. (1991). *Critical care nursing: Clinical management through the nursing process.* Philadelphia: F.A. Davis.

Graves, L. (1990). Diabetic ketoacidosis and hyperosmolar hyperglycemic nonketotic coma. *Crit. Care Q.* 13(3):50–61.

Gray, D.P., and Ludwig-Beymer, P. (1990). Alterations of hormonal regulation. In K.L. McCance and S.E. Huether (eds). *Pathophysiology: The biologic basis for disease in adults and children,* pp. 594–643. St. Louis: The C.V. Mosby Co.

Guthrie, D.W., Guthrie, R.A., and Walters, J.F. (eds).

(1984). Dealing with diabetes mellitus. In *Nurse's clinical library: Endocrine disorders,* pp. 125–149. Springhouse, Pennsylvania: Nursing84 Books.

Guyton, A.C. (1987). *Human physiology and mechanisms of disease,* 4th ed. Philadelphia: W.B. Saunders Co.

Holloway, N.M. (1988). *Nursing the critically ill adult,* 3rd ed. Reading, Massachusetts: Addison-Wesley Publishing.

McKenna, B.S. (1988). Diabetic disorders and patient care. In M.R. Kinney, D.R. Packa, and S.B. Dunbar (eds). *AACN's clinical reference for critical-care nursing.* New York: McGraw-Hill Book Co.

McKenry, L.M., and Salerno, E. (1989). *Mosby's pharmacology in nursing,* 17th ed. St. Louis: C.V. Mosby.

Michael, S.R., and Sabo, C.E. (1990). Nursing management of the diabetic patient receiving nutritional support. *Focus Crit. Care AACN.* 17(4):331–333.

Sabo, C.E., and Michael, S.R. (1989). Diabetic ketoacidosis: Pathophysiology, nursing diagnosis, and nursing interventions. *Focus Crit. Care.* 16(1):21–28.

Schumann, D. (1990). Postoperative hyperglycemia: Clinical benefits of insulin therapy. *Heart Lung.* 19(2):165–173.

Module 16

Nutrition

Alice Saint MacPhail

The focus of the module, *Nutrition,* is the nutrient alterations that occur in the high acuity or critically ill patient. This module is composed of eight sections. Sections One through Three include the topics alterations in nutrient metabolism during the metabolic stress response, nutritional goals for each phase of the metabolic stress response, and the criteria used in selecting the appropriate nutritional support for each phase of the metabolic stress response. In Sections Four through Seven, the focus of the module changes to various types of nutrition support and their associated complications. The final section, Section Eight,

delves into nutritional alterations in specific disease states. Nursing assessment and management are addressed in Module 20, *Nursing Care of the Patient with Altered Metabolism.* Each section includes a set of review questions to help the reader evaluate understanding of section content before moving on to the next section. All section reviews and the Pretest and Posttest in the module include answers. It is suggested that the learner review those concepts that have been missed in the review questions before proceeding to the next section.

Objectives

Following completion of the module, *Nutrition,* the learner will be able to

1. Describe the characteristic alterations in nutrient metabolism during the metabolic stress response

2. Discuss the nutritional goals for each phase of the metabolic stress response

3. Identify criteria considered when selecting the appropriate nutrition support

4. Explain the advantages of enteral nutrition over total parenteral nutrition (TPN)

5. Discuss the major complications of enteral nutrition

6. Explain the indications for total parenteral nutrition (TPN)

7. Discuss the major complications associated with total parenteral nutrition (TPN)

8. Describe the major nutritional alterations associated with hepatic failure, pulmonary failure, and acute renal failure

Pretest

1. The metabolic stress response is the result of
   A. psychologic stress
   B. overexertion from exercise
   C. injured tissue in the body
   D. hyperventilation
2. The two phases of the metabolic stress response are
   A. ebb phase and catabolic phase
   B. ebb phase and flow phase
   C. ebb phase and recovery phase
   D. flow phase and recovery phase
3. Hypermetabolism refers to
   A. an elevated metabolic rate
   B. the breakdown of total body protein
   C. elevated serum insulin levels
   D. increased immunoglobulins
4. Hypercatabolism refers to
   A. an elevated metabolic rate
   B. the breakdown of total body protein
   C. elevated serum insulin levels
   D. increased immunoglobulins
5. During the flow phase, each of the following nutrients should be administered EXCEPT
   A. immunoglobulins
   B. calories
   C. protein
   D. micronutrients
6. Selection of nutritional support is based on the following criteria EXCEPT
   A. gastrointestinal function
   B. baseline nutritional status
   C. psychologic status
   D. present catabolic state and possible duration
7. A patient has a relatively functional gastrointestinal tract but is unable to take adequate nutrients by mouth. What is the BEST method for administering nutritional support to this patient?
   A. nasoenteric feedings
   B. oral diet
   C. withhold nutrition
   D. total parenteral nutrition (TPN)
8. Enteral nutrition has many advantages over TPN, including each of the following EXCEPT
   A. less risk of bacterial translocation
   B. providing central venous access
   C. maintaining gut morphology and function
   D. less costly

9. Diarrhea is a potential gastrointestinal complication of enteral feedings. The following are possible causes EXCEPT
   A. sudden cessation of feedings
   B. malnutrition/hypoalbuminemia
   C. antibiotics
   D. contaminated solution or infusion set
10. Feeding tube occlusion is a potential mechanical complication of enteral feedings. The following are possible causes EXCEPT
    A. viscous formulas
    B. lack of proper flushing
    C. food coloring
    D. medications
11. A patient has a functioning gastrointestinal tract but is at risk for aspiration pneumonia. What is the BEST location for nutrition to be delivered?
    A. stomach
    B. withhold nutrition
    C. IV
    D. small bowel
12. TPN is indicated when
    A. adequate amounts of nutrients can be delivered through the gastrointestinal tract
    B. adequate amounts of nutrients cannot be delivered through the gastrointestinal tract
    C. a functioning, usable gastrointestinal tract is capable of absorbing of adequate nutrients
    D. aggressive nutritional support is not warranted
13. Highly concentrated TPN should be administered through a
    A. nasoenteric feeding tube
    B. peripheral vein
    C. surgically placed jejunal feeding tube
    D. central vein
14. Catheter-related sepsis (CRS) is a potentially lethal complication of TPN and is primarily caused by
    A. a malpositioned catheter or guidewire during the central line insertion
    B. lack of sterility during central line placement and inadequate maintenance of the line
    C. inadvertent puncture or laceration of the subclavian or carotid artery
    D. puncture or laceration of the vein on insertion of the needle/catheter

15. Hypoglycemia is a potential metabolic complication of TPN and results from
    A. gluconeogenesis
    B. glucose intolerance
    C. sudden cessation of feeding
    D. insulin resistance
16. Mechanical complications of TPN consist of the following EXCEPT
    A. air embolism
    B. hydrothorax
    C. pneumothorax
    D. catheter-related sepsis
17. A high acuity patient with hepatic failure may experience all of the following EXCEPT
    A. breakdown of skeletal muscle protein
    B. diminished fat use
    C. hyponatremia
    D. increased carbon dioxide levels
18. Nutritional goals for the pulmonary failure patient are the following EXCEPT
    A. lower fat content
    B. lower protein content
    C. lower carbohydrate content
    D. higher fat content
19. A high acuity patient with acute renal failure may experience abnormalities in each of the following EXCEPT
    A. protein catabolism
    B. fluid and electrolytes
    C. fat absorption and digestion
    D. increased carbon dioxide levels

Answers: 1, C. 2, B. 3, A. 4, B. 5, A. 6, C. 7, A. 8, B. 9, A. 10, C. 11, D. 12, B. 13, D. 14, B. 15, C. 16, D. 17, D. 18, A. 19, D.

Glossary

Catheter-related sepsis (CRS). A potentially lethal complication of total parenteral nutrition (TPN); microorganisms are introduced through the TPN catheter, eventually causing a systemic infection (sepsis)

Ebb phase. The first phase of the metabolic stress response, characterized by reduced systemic circulation, decreased metabolic rate, gluconeogenesis, glycogenolysis, and hyperglycemia, and persisting for 24 to 48 hours

Energy. Synonymous with calories; most common sources are carbohydrates and fats

Enteral nutrition. Enteral nutrition is delivered into the gastrointestinal tract through a feeding tube; it is a lactose-free, nutritionally complete formula composed of protein, carbohydrates, fats, electrolytes, vitamins, and minerals

Flow phase. The second phase of the metabolic stress response, characterized by hypermetabolism, hypercatabolism, increased nitrogen losses, gluconeogenesis, and hyperglycemia

Gluconeogenesis. Formation of glucose from protein and fat stores in the body; seen in the ebb phase and flow phase

Glycogenolysis. Conversion of glycogen into glucose in the body tissues; seen only in the ebb phase

Harris-Benedict equation. Estimates caloric requirements of a resting, fasting, unstressed individual based on the individual's height, weight, age, and sex; expressed in kilocalories

Hypercatabolism. Breakdown of total body protein; skeletal muscle protein is used initially for conversion to glucose through gluconeogenesis; visceral (organ) protein is used after skeletal muscle protein; occurs in the flow phase of the metabolic stress response

Hypermetabolism. An increased metabolic rate in response to a major bodily insult requiring increased quantities of oxygen and nutrients to meet the increased metabolic needs; occurs in the flow phase of the metabolic stress response

Indirect calorimetry. A technique of estimating an individual's metabolic or energy expenditure through the measurement of oxygen consumed ($\dot{V}o_2$) and carbon dioxide produced ($\dot{V}co_2$); can also calculate respiratory quotient (RQ)

Metabolic stress response. A well-defined pattern of metabolic and physiologic responses that occur as the result of injured tissue in the body

Micronutrients. Electrolytes, vitamins, and trace elements

Nitrogen. A basic unit of protein (amino acid) breakdown; excreted primarily in urine in the form of urea; a 24-hour urinary urea nitrogen (UUN) measures nitrogen losses for a 24-hour period

Respiratory quotient (RQ). A ratio of carbon dioxide ($\dot{V}co_2$) to oxygen consumed ($\dot{V}o_2$); provides information about fuel composition used by the body; $\dot{V}co_2$ and $\dot{V}o_2$ are obtained from an indirect calorimetry study

Total parenteral nutrition (TPN). A nutritionally complete, IV delivered solution composed of protein, carbohydrate, fat, electrolytes, vitamins, and trace elements; highly concentrated TPN is administered through a central vein

Abbreviations

AAA. Aromatic amino acid

BCAA. Branched-chain amino acid

CRS. Catheter-related sepsis

CNS. Central nervous system

kcal. Kilocalories

NPO. Nothing by mouth

RDA. Recommended daily allowances

RQ. Respiratory quotient

UUN. Urine urea nitrogen

Vco_2. Carbon dioxide produced

V̇o_2. Oxygen consumed

Section One: Nutritional Alterations in the Metabolic Stress Response

At the completion of this section, the learner will be able to briefly describe the characteristic alterations in nutrient metabolism during the metabolic stress response.

To understand the need for appropriate nutritional support in the high acuity patient population, one must first have a basic understanding of the concepts of the metabolic stress response. The metabolic stress response refers to a well-defined pattern of metabolic and physiologic responses that occurs as the result of injured tissue in the body. The injured tissue can result from one or a combination of the following causes: hypoxia, inflammation, necrosis, trauma, and infection.

Two phases characterize the metabolic stress response. They are the ebb phase and the flow phase.

Ebb Phase

The ebb phase occurs immediately after the injury and persists for 24 to 48 hours. Reduced systemic circulation occurs initially, with resultant hypoxia and hypovolemia. The body's metabolic rate is decreased. Insufficient insulin is produced in relation to an increased production of glucose. The production of glucose comes from gluconeogenesis (formation of glucose from body protein and fat) and glycogenolysis (conversion of glycogen into glucose in the body tissues). The result is hyperglycemia.

Flow Phase

The flow phase follows the ebb phase. This phase usually lasts 5 to 10 days but may be longer depending on the severity of injury and if such complications as sepsis develop.

The important characteristics of the flow phase are hypermetabolism, hypercatabolism, and increased nitrogen losses.

Hypermetabolism refers to an elevated metabolic rate. Increased amounts of oxygen and nutrients are required in order to meet the energy needs that are expended to maintain the body's increased metabolic needs.

Hypercatabolism refers to the breakdown of total body protein. In an attempt to preserve visceral (organ) protein for host defense and to promote wound healing, the body breaks down its skeletal muscle protein. The skeletal muscle protein is converted to glucose via gluconeogenesis to serve as the major energy source to meet the high energy demand. Liver glycogen is no longer available as an energy source, having been exhausted early in the ebb phase.

Protein is broken down into its basic unit, which contains nitrogen. This is then excreted from the body, and, therefore, a significant amount of nitrogen is lost during the flow phase.

The body becomes more and more dependent on skeletal muscle protein and eventually visceral protein as a source of glucose. Insulin resistance may limit the use of this glucose as an energy source. Serum insulin levels may be normal or elevated, but cellular resistance to its effects results in hyperglycemia. The breakdown of fat stores for an energy source is hindered by the elevated insulin levels.

In summary, the metabolic stress response is a pattern of metabolic and physiologic responses caused by an injury, which produces alterations in nutrient metabolism. The metabolic stress response consists of the ebb phase and flow phase. If the hypermetabolic and hypercatabolic states of the flow phase are not slowed or external nutrients are not provided, the metabolic stress response can progress to multisystem organ failure and eventual death.

Section One Review

1. The metabolic stress response refers to
   A. a well-defined pattern of metabolic and psychologic responses that occurs as the result of injured tissue in the body
   B. a well-defined pattern of metabolic and physiologic responses that occurs as the result of injured tissue in the body
   C. a well-defined pattern of metabolic and physiologic responses that occurs as the result of psychologic stress
   D. a well-defined pattern of metabolic and schizophrenic behavior that occurs as the result of psychologic stress
2. The two phases of the metabolic stress response are
   A. ebb phase and catabolic phase
   B. ebb phase and flow phase
   C. ebb phase and recovery phase
   D. flow phase and recovery phase

3. The characteristic alterations in nutrient metabolism during the first phase of the metabolic stress response are the following EXCEPT
   A. hypermetabolism
   B. hypometabolism
   C. gluconeogenesis
   D. hyperglycemia
4. The three characteristic alterations in nutrient metabolism during the second phase of the metabolic stress response are the following EXCEPT
   A. hypermetabolism
   B. increased nitrogen losses
   C. anabolism
   D. hypercatabolism

Answers: 1, B. 2, B. 3, A. 4, C.

Section Two: Nutritional Goals for the Metabolic Stress Response

At the completion of this section, the learner will be able to discuss the nutritional goals for each phase of the metabolic stress response.

Alterations in nutrient metabolism during the ebb phase and flow phase of the metabolic stress response help determine the nutritional goals for the critically ill patient.

Ebb Phase

Since hemodynamic instability dominates the ebb phase, nutrition plays a secondary role and may be withheld until the patient's circulatory status is stabilized and until electrolyte and acid-base imbalances are corrected. However, recent studies suggest that high acuity patients may benefit from early nutritional support.

Flow Phase

Nutritional support is needed in the high acuity patient during the flow phase to prevent depletion of the skeletal muscle protein stores of the well-nourished patient or to prevent further deterioration of the skeletal muscle protein stores in the malnourished patient. Since hypermetabolism, hypercatabolism, and increased nitrogen losses characterize the flow phase, the body's needs for energy (in the form of carbohydrate and fat) and protein are increased in direct proportion to the severity and duration of the metabolic stress response.

Various methods are used for determining the high acuity patient's calorie, protein, electrolyte, vitamin, and trace element requirements in the flow phase.

Calories

Calories are commonly referred to as energy and expressed as kilocalories (kcal). Most common sources of calories are carbohydrates and fats. Caloric requirements are sometimes estimated using the Harris-Benedict equation (Harris and Benedict, 1919), which is stated as follows.

$$\text{Male: } 66.4 + (13.7 \times \text{weight [kg]}) + (5 \times \text{Height [cm]}) - (6.8 \times \text{age})$$
$$\text{Female: } 65.5 + (9.6 \times \text{weight [kg]}) + (1.7 \times \text{Height [cm]}) - (4.7 \times \text{age})$$

This equation estimates the caloric requirements of a resting, fasting, unstressed individual based on the individual's sex, body size, and age.

TABLE 16–1. HARRIS-BENEDICT EQUATION AND STRESS FACTORS

Clinical Condition	Stress Factor
Well-nourished, unstressed	1.0
Maintenance	1.0–1.2
Surgery	
Minor	1.2
Major	1.2–1.5
Cancer	1.0–1.5
Sepsis (acute phase)	
Hypotensive	0.5
Normotensive	1.2–1.7
Sepsis (recovery)	1.0
Multiple trauma (acute phase)	
Hypotensive	0.8–1.0
Normotensive	1.1–1.5
Multiple trauma (recovery)	1.0–1.2
Burned (before skin graft)	
0–20% BSA	1.2–1.5
20–40% BSA	1.5–2.0
>40% BSA	1.8–2.5
Burned (after graft)	1.0–1.3

From *Nutritional support of the critically ill*, by R. Schlichtig and S. Ayres, 1988, Chicago: Year Book Medical Publishers.

Since most high acuity patients are known to be hypermetabolic, it is necessary to quantify the stress factor if the Harris-Benedict equation is to be used in this patient population. The stress factor accounts for various clinical conditions (such as fever, surgery, infection, trauma, or burns) that are known to increase energy requirements. Table 16–1 contains one such list of stress factors.

A more reliable method of assessing energy requirements for the high acuity patient is to use indirect calorimetry. Indirect calorimetry is a technique of estimating an individual's metabolic or energy expenditure through the measurement of oxygen consumed ($\dot{V}o_2$) and carbon dioxide produced ($\dot{V}co_2$). Using $\dot{V}o_2$ and $\dot{V}co_2$, it is also possible to calculate a respiratory quotient (RQ), which provides information about fuel consumption (the amount of carbohydrate, fat, and protein) by the body. For example, it can be used to determine if a patient is being overfed (high RQ) or underfed carbohydrate (low RQ).

As a general rule, most high acuity patient's energy needs for calories are provided by giving 50 percent to 60 percent carbohydrates and 40 percent to 50 percent fats. Variation in calorie distribution depends on energy use by the body. For example, if the patient is hyperglycemic, he or she may benefit from a reduced carbohydrate intake and slightly increased fat. Insulin also may be added to the total parenteral nutrition (TPN) solution to correct the hyperglycemia.

Protein

Particularly impressive during the flow phase are the protein requirements needed for wound healing, the immune system, and organ function. Protein requirements for the hypercatabolic patient range from 1.5 to 2.0 g/kg/day. (Protein requirements for the healthy, unstressed individual are 0.8 to 1.0 g/kg/day.) Since nitrogen (a by-product of protein breakdown) is excreted primarily in the urine, a 24-hour urinary urea nitrogen (UUN) should be obtained periodically throughout the nutritional therapy to determine if adequate protein is provided. Excessive losses of gastrointestinal contents from vomitus, diarrhea, or nasogastric drainage or from ascites, fistula, or abscess should be accounted for when determining protein requirements.

Micronutrients

The American Medical Association provides guidelines for the micronutrients (electrolytes, vitamins, and trace elements) for the parenterally fed patient. Recommended daily allowances (RDA) exist for the enterally fed patient. Unfortunately, no specific guidelines for micronutrients exist for the high acuity patient. Special considerations should be given to the hypercatabolic patient and patients with healing wounds. Catabolism results in the breakdown of skeletal muscle mass, with subsequent release and urinary excretion of potassium, magnesium, phosphorous, and zinc. Therefore, requirements for these nutrients may be increased in the hypercatabolic patient. Vitamin C, zinc, phosphorous, and magnesium have been shown to promote wound healing. Therefore, increased needs may exist in the patient with open or closed wounds.

In summary, nutritional support may be contraindicated in the ebb phase of the metabolic stress response. However, some form of nutritional support should be initiated during the flow phase. Nutritional goals for the flow phase are to provide appropriate calories based on the individual's estimated caloric requirements by the Harris-Benedict equation or by an indirect calorimetry measurement. Generally, most high acuity patients energy needs for calories are provided by giving 50 percent to 60 percent carbohydrates and 40 percent to 50 percent fats. Protein requirements usually are within the range of 1.5 to 2.0 g/kg/day in the hypercatabolic patient. A 24-hour UUN should be obtained routinely in the high acuity patient to help determine appropriate protein replacement. No specific micronutrient recommendations are given for the high acuity patient. However, certain conditions may require increased supplementation.

Section Two Review

1. Nutritional support is needed during the flow phase of the metabolic stress response for the following reasons EXCEPT
   A. to prevent depletion of skeletal muscle protein of the well-nourished patient
   B. to promote hypercatabolism and hypermetabolism
   C. to prevent further deterioration of the skeletal muscle protein stores in the malnourished patient
   D. to meet the high energy demands

2. Most common sources of calories are carbohydrates and fats. Calories are synonymous with _____ needs.
   A. protein
   B. energy
   C. catabolic
   D. recovery

3. During the flow phase, each of the following nutrients should be administered EXCEPT
   A. immunoglobulins
   B. calories
   C. protein
   D. micronutrients

4. The laboratory test used to determine adequate protein replacement is
   A. serum immunoglobulins
   B. serum glucose
   C. urinary urea nitrogen (UUN)
   D. Harris-Benedict equation

Answers: 1, B. 2, B. 3, A. 4, C.

Section Three: Criteria for Selection of Nutritional Support

At the completion of this section, the learner will be able to identify the criteria to consider when selecting the appropriate nutritional support.

Early initiation of some form of nutritional support is imperative during the flow phase. Selection of the nutritional support is based on the following criteria.

1. Gastrointestinal function
2. Baseline nutritional status
3. Present catabolic state and possible duration
4. Risks associated with the type of nutritional support

Gastrointestinal Function

When determining a patient's gastrointestinal function, first, consider if the patient will be able to eat solid food within 2 to 3 days. If so, nutritional support may not be instituted.

For patients who will be receiving nothing by mouth (NPO) for longer than 2 to 3 days, initiate either TPN or enteral nutrition. If the patient is unable or unwilling to ingest sufficient nutrients normally by mouth and has a relatively functional gastrointestinal tract, the preferred route of nutritional support is enteral. TPN is indicated when adequate amounts of nutrients cannot be delivered through the gastrointestinal tract.

Baseline Nutritional Status

Baseline nutritional status is an important determinant for deciding when and what type of nutritional support to initiate. Clinical studies indicate that severely malnourished patients have a greater risk of developing complications and eventually dying. Therefore, these severely malnourished patients should be fed as early as possible. For the moderately malnourished patient, timing of nutritional support remains uncertain.

Present Catabolic State and Possible Duration

For the high acuity patient who is highly catabolic (nitrogen loss greater than 15 to 20 g/day), nutritional support should be initiated as soon as possible after arrival in the critical care unit. The goal is to minimize further breakdown of the skeletal muscle and visceral protein stores. Attempting to rebuild the protein stores in the skeletal muscles and viscera is considered virtually impossible for these high acuity patients. The cause is unclear but may be related to a resistance of the skeletal muscles to use exogenous protein for protein stores.

Risks Associated with the Type of Nutritional Support

Several complications can occur secondary to nutritional support and to the route of administration. These complications are discussed in Sections Five and Seven.

In summary, there are criteria to consider when selecting nutritional support for the high acuity patient. These criteria consist of gastrointestinal function, baseline nutritional status, present catabolic state and possible duration, and risks associated with the type of nutritional support. TPN is used if the gastrointestinal tract is not functioning, as in acute pancreatitis or a bowel obstruction. Enteral nutrition is the preferred route for nutritional support if the gastrointestinal tract is functioning. Nutritional support should be initiated as early as possible for the severely malnourished patient and the highly catabolic patient. The goal is to prevent further breakdown of the skeletal muscle and visceral (organ) protein stores. The risks associated with the type of nutritional support also should be considered. These possible complications are discussed in detail in Sections Five and Seven.

Section Three Review

1. Criteria to consider when selecting the nutritional support for high acuity patient are the following EXCEPT
   A. gastrointestinal function
   B. baseline nutritional status
   C. psychologic status
   D. present catabolic state and possible duration
2. The severely malnourished patient has a greater risk of developing complications and eventual death. These severely malnourished patients should be fed
   A. whenever oral intake is possible
   B. after recovery from the acute illness
   C. as early as possible
   D. never

3. A patient has a relatively functioning gastrointestinal tract but is unable to take adequate nutrients by mouth. What is the BEST method for administering nutritional support to this patient?
   A. nasoenteric feedings
   B. oral diet
   C. withhold nutrition
   D. total parenteral nutrition (TPN)

Answers: 1, C. 2, C. 3, A.

Section Four: Principles of Enteral Nutrition

At the completion of this section, the learner will be able to explain the advantages of enteral nutrition over total parenteral nutrition (TPN).

Enteral nutrition is indicated for patients who have a relatively functional gastrointestinal tract but are unable or unwilling to ingest sufficient nutrients by mouth. Enteral feedings have many advantages over TPN that are just now beginning to be understood and appreciated.

Advantages of Enteral Feedings

1. Maintenance of gut morphology and function. If the gastrointestinal tract does not receive nutrition for a period of time, atrophy of the microvilli can occur, causing decreased absorptive properties, and peristaltic movement ceases.
2. Maintenance of immunologic function and less risk of bacterial translocation
3. Decreased risk of complications
4. Lower costs

Contraindications to Enteral Feedings

1. Patients with adynamic ileus
2. Patients with intractable vomiting
3. Patients with a proximal high output enterocutaneous fistula
4. Patients who require bowel rest (e.g., acute Crohn's disease and acute pancreatitis)

Numerous enteral formulas are available on the market. Choosing the appropriate formula for the high acuity patient is based on the energy and protein requirements of the patient, the underlying disease state or organ function, intestinal absorptive and digestive function, and fluid requirements. Commonly used are the lactose-free, nutritionally complete formulas that contain a mixture of carbohydrates, fats, protein, trace elements, and vitamins. Feedings are supplied in varying osmolalities and range in caloric density from 1 to 2 kcal/mL.

In high acuity patients, enteral feedings are delivered preferably to the small bowel via a nasoenteric feeding tube to reduce the risk of aspiration. It is believed that despite the presence of gastric dysfunction, the small bowel retains its absorptive properties and peristaltic motility. A number of Silastic or polyurethane, weighted, small-bore (8–12 Fr) feeding tubes are available for enteral feeding. For long-term enteral patients, endoscopic or surgical placement of a gastric or jejunal feeding tube may be preferable.

In summary, enteral feedings are the preferred route of nutritional support in the high acuity patient who cannot or will not ingest sufficient nutrients by mouth but has a functioning gastrointestinal tract. Enteral feedings have many advantages over parenteral feedings. Commonly used enteral feedings are lactose-free, nutritionally complete formulas that contain a mixture of carbohydrates, fats, protein, trace elements, and vitamins. Enteral feedings are delivered preferably to the small bowel via a nasoenteric feeding tube.

Section Four Review

1. Enteral nutrition has many advantages over total parenteral nutrition (TPN), including each of the following EXCEPT
   A. less risk of bacterial translocation
   B. providing central venous access
   C. maintaining gut morphology and function
   D. less costly

2. Enteral feedings are preferably delivered to the _____ via a nasoenteric feeding tube.
   A. oral cavity
   B. gastric mucosa
   C. small bowel
   D. large bowel

Answers: 1, B. 2, C.

Section Five: Complications of Enteral Nutrition

At the completion of this section, the learner will be able to discuss the major complications associated with enteral nutrition.

Complications of enteral feedings are classified under four categories: gastrointestinal, mechanical, metabolic, and infectious. Table 16–2 lists potential enteral complications, possible causes, and suggested treatment.

In summary, potential complications of enteral feedings are categorized under gastrointestinal, mechanical, metabolic, and infectious complications. There are various causes for these potential complications. Diagnostic, pharmacologic, and dietary treatments are suggested for these potential complications.

TABLE 16–2. COMPLICATIONS OF ENTERAL NUTRITION

Complication	Possible Cause	Suggested Treatment
Gastrointestinal		
Nausea/vomiting	Hyperosmolar feeding	Start isotonic feeding
	Rapid infusion rate	Start feedings slowly and advance as tolerated
	Obstruction	Reassess gastrointestinal function
	Delayed gastric emptying	Metaclopramide to increase gastric emptying; feed distal to pylorus
	Contaminated solution or infusion set	Hang formula for no longer than 3–4 hours; change container and infusion set every 24 hours; use good handwashing technique before handling formulas
Diarrhea	Antibiotics may alter intestinal flora causing bacterial overgrowth: *Clostridium difficile* infection and pseudomembranous colitis	Send stool specimens for culture and sensitivity, WBC, ova, parasites and *Clostridium difficile* cytotoxin. Flexible sigmoidoscopy provides a faster and more reliable diagnosis than stool studies; treatment of choice for *Clostridium difficile* toxin is IV/PO Flagyl or IV Vancomycin; hold any antidiarrheal agents until infectious source is ruled out
Nutrition		
Malnutrition	Malnutrition associated with loss of microvilli, villous brush border enzymes, and subsequent reduction in intestinal absorptive surface area	Supply elemental diet to improve absorption; elemental diets are for digestive disorders requiring a more easily digested, absorbed diet
Hypoalbuminemia	Hypoalbuminemia is associated with lack of intravascular osmotic pressure required to draw nutrients across intestinal epithelium, thus compromising absorption	Poor tolerance is evident in patients with serum albumin <2.5 mg/dL; benefit of albumin administration should outweigh cost and potential complications
Mechanical		
Feeding tube occlusion	Medications; lack of proper flushing; viscous formulas	Irrigate feeding tube with 30–50 mL warm water every 4 hours, after medication administration, after checking residuals
		Alternate positive/negative pressure with syringe to dislodge clot
		Meat tenderizer, colas, pancrease/HCO_3 have been cited as agents to dissolve clots.
		Do not attempt to dislodge clots with stylet; may cause esophageal/gastric mucosal perforations; *prevention is key*
Metabolic		
Hypoglycemia	Sudden cessation of feeding	Provide supplemental glucose
Hyperglycemia	Stress response, diabetic or glucose intolerance	Usually resolves as stress is alleviated; initiate feedings slowly; monitor blood glucose every 6 hours
Electrolyte imbalance	Dilutional states (dehydration or fluid overload)	Monitor fluid status; monitor electrolytes and replace as needed
	Excess losses (diarrhea, fistula, NG drainage, ascites)	
	Disease states (renal/liver failure)	Provide appropriate organ failure formula
Infectious		
Aspiration pneumonia	High risk for patients include comatose, weak, debilitated	Elevate head of bed at least 30 degrees; feed into small bowel distal to pylorus
	Patients with tracheostomies or intubated patients; patients with neuromuscular disorders	Add food coloring to feeding to detect for aspiration
		Check residuals every 4 hours if feeding into stomach

Section Five Review

1. The categories of potential complications of enteral feedings are the following EXCEPT
   A. gastrointestinal
   B. mechanical
   C. metabolic
   D. intravenous
2. Diarrhea may occur from enteral feedings, but the more common cause is antibiotics. Antibiotics can alter intestinal flora, causing bacterial overgrowth (*Clostridium difficile* infection and pseudomembranous colitis). The suggested treatment are the following EXCEPT
   A. send stool specimens for testing
   B. perform flexible sigmoidoscopy
   C. administer IV/PO metronidazole (Flagyl) or IV vancomycin
   D. administer antidiarrheal agents

3. Possible causes of an occluded feeding tube are the following EXCEPT
   A. lack of proper flushing
   B. elemental diet
   C. medications
   D. viscous formulas
4. A patient has a functioning gastrointestinal tract but is at risk for aspiration pneumonia. What is the BEST location for nutrition to be delivered?
   A. stomach
   B. withhold nutrition
   C. IV
   D. small bowel

Answers: 1, D. 2, D. 3, B. 4, D.

Section Six: Principles of Total Parenteral Nutrition

At the completion of this section, the learner will be able to explain the indications for total parenteral nutrition (TPN).

TPN is a nutritionally complete, IV delivered solution composed of amino acids (protein), dextrose (carbohydrate), fats, electrolytes, vitamins, and trace elements. Solutions are designed to meet the individual energy and protein needs of a patient based on the clinical condition, underlying disease states, and organ function.

TPN is indicated when adequate amounts of nutrients cannot be delivered through the gastrointestinal tract. These situations include conditions requiring complete bowel rest (e.g., acute pancreatitis, acute Crohn's disease) or disruption of a functional gastrointestinal tract (e.g., bowel obstruction).

TPN is contraindicated in those patients with a functioning, usable gastrointestinal tract capable of absorption of adequate nutrients, when sole dependence is anticipated to be less than 5 days, when aggressive support is not warranted, and when the risks of TPN outweigh the potential benefits.

The irritating effects on peripheral veins by the highly concentrated TPN solutions require that the solutions be administered through a central vein. The central vein of choice is the subclavian because of its large size, turbulent flow, and ability to form an occlusive dressing over catheter and site. The jugular veins are the next alternative, although there is a greater chance of thrombosis with its smaller diameter and increased risk of infection. Maintaining a sterile, occlusive dressing over a jugular catheter for longer than 24 hours is difficult.

Catheters commonly used are multilumen. These catheters allow for one central venous access, with multiple ports for hemodynamic monitoring and fluid/medication delivery without risk of drug incompatibility. However, clinical studies indicate that infectious complications are greater with the multilumen catheter than with the single-lumen catheter. Therefore, single-lumen catheters are a more favorable catheter for delivery of TPN. Standard procedures for aseptic insertion and maintenance of central venous catheters should be developed and implemented in every institution to minimize the risk of infectious complications.

In summary, TPN is a nutritionally complete solution delivered IV to patients when adequate amounts of nutrition cannot be delivered through the gastrointestinal tract. Highly concentrated TPN should be administered through a central vein. The vein of choice is the subclavian vein, followed by the jugular vein. TPN can be administered through different types of catheters. More commonly used are the multilumen catheters and single-lumen catheters. Single-lumen catheters are the preferred catheter for their lesser risk of infection.

Section Six Review

1. Total parenteral nutrition (TPN) is indicated when
   A. adequate amounts of nutrients can be delivered through the gastrointestinal tract
   B. adequate amounts of nutrients cannot be delivered through the gastrointestinal tract
   C. a functioning, usable gastrointestinal tract is capable of absorption of adequate nutrients
   D. aggressive nutritional support is not warranted

2. Highly concentrated TPN should be administered through a
   A. nasoenteric feeding tube
   B. peripheral vein
   C. surgically placed jejunal feeding tube
   D. central vein

Answers: 1, B. 2, D.

Section Seven: Complications of Total Parenteral Nutrition

At the completion of this section, the learner will be able to discuss the major complications associated with total parenteral nutrition (TPN).

Complications from TPN fall under three classifications: septic, metabolic, and mechanical.

Septic Complications

Catheter-related sepsis (CRS) is a potentially lethal complication, particularly in the high acuity population. Review of the literature reveals that the primary causes of CRS are

1. Lack of sterility during placement of central lines
2. Inadequate precautions taken with maintenance of the central line (i.e., changing tubings, dressings, bags)

Clinical signs and symptoms of CRS are

1. Bacteremia/septicemia/septic shock
2. Leukocytosis
3. Sudden temperature elevation that should resolve on removal of catheter
4. Sudden glucose intolerance that may occur up to 12 hours before temperature elevation
5. Erythema, swelling, tenderness, and purulent drainage from the catheter site

Prompt evaluation and identification of the source of septicemia is important. Pancultures (urine, sputum, and two sets of peripheral blood cultures) should be sent. If you are unable to identify a source after 24 hours and CRS is suspected, change the central venous catheter over a guidewire and culture the tip semiquantitatively. If the catheter tip culture results in growth of more than 15 colonies, the catheter should be removed, since this most likely indicates migration of bacteria from a contaminated solution, administration set, catheter, or infected skin tract. Antibiotic therapy should be initiated.

Prevention is the key. In order to avoid contamination of the catheter, maintain dry, sterile, and intact dressings at all times, prepare the junction of administration sets with povidone-iodine, minimize the number of entries into the system, and always use meticulous technique with all aspects of catheter care.

Metabolic Complications

Metabolic complications of TPN are similar to those of enteral nutrition. Refer to Section Five for metabolic complications, possible causes, and suggested treatment.

Other possible metabolic derangements of TPN are prerenal azotemia and hepatic dysfunction.

Prerenal azotemia is caused by overaggressive protein administration and is aggravated by underlying dehydration. Presenting signs and symptoms include an elevated serum blood urea nitrogen (BUN) and clinical signs of dehydration. If the condition is not corrected, the patient may develop progressive lethargy and possible coma. Close monitoring of body weight, fluid balance, and adequate protein intake is important in preventing this complication.

Hepatic dysfunction can occur secondary to long-term TPN administration and usually is considered benign. Serum liver function tests (including SGOT, SGPT, alkaline phosphatase, and rarely, bilirubin levels) become elevated during the course of TPN and usually return to normal spontaneously when the infusion is stopped. Almost all components of the TPN solution have been implicated as the cause of hepatic dysfunction. Excessive glucose administration has been mentioned most frequently as the culprit. While a patient is on TPN, weekly monitoring of serum liver function tests and administration of a balanced TPN solution based on the patient's caloric needs should eliminate problems of hepatic dysfunction.

Mechanical Complications

Mechanical complications include pneumothorax, hydrothorax, subclavian/carotid artery puncture, air embolism, and dysrhythmias. All may be a result of the central venous catheter insertion.

Pneumothorax, the most common mechanical complication, is caused by the puncture or laceration of the vein on insertion of the needle/catheter. Air enters into the pleural space, with partial or complete collapse of the lung. Most pneumothoraces produce symptoms, although some are totally asymptomatic. In general, the larger the collapse, the more pronounced the symptoms. Commonly seen are shortness of breath, restlessness, dyspnea, hypoxia, and chest pain radiating to the back. Treatment depends on the severity of the collapse and respiratory compromise. Moderate to large collapse may require a chest tube.

Hydrothorax occurs when fluid is introduced into the pleural space. Symptoms are similar to those of pneumothorax. A diagnostic tap (thoracentesis) should be performed and eventually may require a chest tube if reaccumulation of fluid occurs.

Inadvertent puncture or laceration of the subclavian or carotid arteries is indicated by a flashback of arterial blood in the syringe, pulsatile blood flow, bleeding from the catheter site or development of a large hematoma, and hypotension. Treatment involves withdrawing the syringe/catheter and applying direct pressure to the site until bleeding ceases.

Air embolism may occur whenever the central venous system is open to air. Signs and symptoms vary with the amount of air pulled into the venous system but may include respiratory distress, tachycardia, hypotension, sudden cardiovascular collapse, neurologic deficits, or cardiac arrest. Immediate action is required. Occlude the catheter nearest to the entry site of the skin. Place the patient on the left side and in the Trendelenburg position. *Prevention is the key.* Always use Luer-Lock connectors and air-eliminating filters on central line tubings.

Dysrhythmias during central venous insertions are the result of a malpositioned catheter or guidewire. The result may be atrial, nodal, or ventricular dysrhythmias, which may cause decreased CO, decreased blood pressure, or loss of consciousness. Appropriate intervention is to withdraw the catheter or guidewire partially. If the dysrhythmia continues, administer lidocaine bolus 1 mg/kg of body weight IV.

In summary, complications from TPN fall under septic, metabolic, and mechanical classifications. Catheter-related sepsis (CRS) is a potentially lethal complication of TPN. It is caused primarily by lack of sterility during central line placement and inadequate maintenance of the line. Again, *prevention is the key.* Metabolic complications of TPN are similar to enteral nutrition. Other metabolic complications include prerenal azotemia and hepatic complications. Prerenal azotemia can be prevented by avoiding dehydration and administering the appropriate level of protein. Hepatic complications can occur secondary to long-term TPN administration and usually are considered benign. Monitor liver function tests routinely while using TPN and provide a balanced caloric mix in the TPN solution. Mechanical complications of TPN occur primarily during the central line placement. These complications include pneumothorax, hydrothorax, puncture or laceration of the subclavian or carotid arteries, air embolism, and dysrhythmias.

Section Seven Review

1. The three classifications of total parenteral nutrition (TPN) complications are the following EXCEPT
   A. gastrointestinal
   B. mechanical
   C. metabolic
   D. septic
2. Catheter-related sepsis (CRS) is a potentially lethal complication of TPN and is caused primarily by
   A. a malpositioned catheter or guidewire during the central line insertion
   B. lack of sterility during central line placement and inadequate maintenance of the line
   C. inadvertent puncture or laceration of the subclavian or carotid artery
   D. puncture or laceration of the vein on insertion of the needle/catheter

3. Hypoglycemia is a potential metabolic complication of TPN and results from
   A. gluconeogenesis
   B. glucose intolerance
   C. sudden cessation of feeding
   D. insulin resistance
4. Mechanical complications of TPN consist of the following EXCEPT
   A. air embolism
   B. hydrothorax
   C. pneumothorax
   D. catheter-related sepsis (CRS)

Answers: 1, A. 2, B. 3, C. 4, D.

Section Eight: Nutritional Alterations in Specific Disease States

At the completion of this section, the learner will be able to describe the major nutritional alterations associated with hepatic, pulmonary, and acute renal failure.

Specific nutritional alterations occur in hepatic failure, pulmonary failure, and acute renal failure requiring more specialized nutritional regimens.

Hepatic Failure

The liver plays a key role in nutrient absorption and metabolism. Disruption of this role creates multiple nutrient alterations. A summary of the nutrient alterations includes the following.

1. Hypercatabolism. Breakdown of skeletal muscle protein occurs at a fairly high rate with the release of amino acids, in particular branched-chain amino acids (BCAA) and aromatic amino acids (AAA). In hepatic failure, AAA can enter the central nervous system (CNS) at an accelerated rate over BCAA and create false neurotransmitters, which may contribute to hepatic encephalopathy.
2. Diminished use of fat as an energy source because the enzyme system that manufac-

tures ketone bodies is less functional and fat metabolism is impaired.
3. Hyperglycemia results from less efficient use of glucose in the peripheral cells, possibly from an inadequate amount of insulin or insulin resistance.
4. Hyponatremia usually is dilutional secondary to reduced renal water excretion.

Nutritional goals in individuals with hepatic failure include the following.

1. Preventing further breakdown of skeletal muscle mass without contributing to hepatic encephalopathy. Since these individuals are highly catabolic, at least 1.1 g/kg/day of protein should be provided to prevent malnutrition unless contraindicated. Specialized parenteral and enteral nutrition containing less AAA and a greater percentage of BCAA is available. Theoretically, this therapeutic approach appears logical, since BCAA are not thought to contribute to hepatic encephalopathy. However, these special hepatic formulations are quite expensive, and their use is controversial.
2. Supplying calories based on the Harris-Benedict equation or indirect calorimetry study. The ratio of carbohydrates/fats is based on patient tolerance, with at least 25 percent to 40 percent of daily calories as fat.

Patient tolerance to fat can be determined by monitoring fasting serum triglyceride levels.

3. Serum glucose levels should be monitored closely to determine carbohydrate use.
4. Restricting fluid to prevent dilutional hyponatremia. Once evidenced, hyponatremia is treated by loop diuretics (e.g., furosemide), which cause water to be lost in greater amounts than sodium.

Pulmonary Failure

A multitude of disorders cause respiratory failure. Malnutrition can contribute to this disease process in the following manner.

1. The respiratory muscles can be catabolized for energy needs.
2. Decreased levels of albumin can cause decreased oncotic pressure, leading to fluid shifts and pulmonary edema. Edema of the capillary and endothelial walls can cause damage to the cells that produce surfactant, leading to alveolar collapse and atelectasis. The end result is inadequate gas exchange.
3. The immune function, itself, may be compromised, increasing the patient's susceptibility to pulmonary infection.

Nutritional alterations to consider in the pulmonary failure patient include the following.

1. Increased respiratory rate, respiratory muscle effort, and respiratory workload from excessive carbohydrate (dextrose) administration. Carbohydrates are oxidized to carbon dioxide, which, in turn, is excreted from the lungs. Administration of excessive exogenous carbohydrates (dextrose) in the pulmonary failure patient may increase carbon dioxide production, thereby increasing the respiratory rate, respiratory muscle effort, and respiratory workload.
2. Low phosphorous levels that can influence respiration in patients receiving nutritional support. Low phosphorous levels can cause decreased 2,3-diphosphoglycerate levels in red blood cells, thereby reducing the delivery of oxygen to the tissues. In addition, low phosphorous levels may cause decreased diaphragmatic muscle contractility.
3. Medications that are commonly used for pulmonary diseases may interfere with nutrient administration.
   - Bronchodilators (aminophylline/theophylline) can cause nausea, vomiting, abdominal cramps, anorexia.

- Adrenergic agonists (terbutaline, albuterol) can cause nausea, vomiting, unusual taste.
- Antibiotics may alter intestinal flora, causing bacterial overgrowth, resulting in diarrhea.

Nutritional goals for the pulmonary failure patient are aimed at the following.

1. Providing calories as 50 percent carbohydrate (dextrose). This decreased carbohydrate content in the nutritional support reduces the production of carbon dioxide levels, which, in turn, decreases respiratory rate, respiratory muscle effort, and respiratory workload.
2. Providing the minimum protein requirements. Protein can stimulate ventilatory drive, it may increase minute ventilation, and it may lead to respiratory muscle fatigue in the respiratory failure patient. Therefore, monitor 24-hour UUN levels closely to determine protein needs so as not to overfeed with protein.
3. Maintaining adequate phosphorous levels.
4. Restricting sodium and fluid intake to prevent pulmonary edema.

Enteral nutrition is usually well tolerated in the respiratory failure patient. Small bowel feeding should be used to avoid the risk of aspiration pneumonia. If enteral nutrition is contraindicated, TPN should be instituted.

Acute Renal Failure

The kidney's major functions are to excrete metabolic waste, regulate electrolytes, and control fluids. When the kidneys fail, these functions are compromised significantly, and dialysis frequently is needed to perform these functions. These patients often are acutely ill, with multisystem organ failure.

Nutritional alterations that may be seen in the individual with acute renal failure include the following.

1. Hypercatabolism. A multitude of factors, such as coexisting catabolic conditions, insufficient nutrition, and loss of nutrients during dialysis, may influence the catabolic response in the acute renal failure patient. The catabolic response in these patients may vary from mild to marked.
2. Hypermetabolism. Hypermetabolism may occur in the acute renal failure patient and is commonly related to the underlying cause of

acute renal failure and other associated diseases.

3. Electrolyte and trace element abnormalities. Initially, levels of serum potassium, serum phosphorous, and serum magnesium can be elevated from the breakdown of skeletal muscle mass, with subsequent cellular release of these micronutrients and, in addition, reduced excretion by the compromised kidney.

4. Fluid retention. Volume overload is a major problem to the individual in the oliguric phase of acute renal failure.

In the acute renal failure patient, controversy exists over whether to withhold appropriate nutrition and risk malnutrition or administer nutritional support to meet calorie and protein needs, thus risking fluid overload and buildup of metabolic waste, requiring dialysis. No data are available currently to determine which situation puts the patient at greater risk. However, the trend is toward supplying the patient with adequate nutritional support and instituting dialysis.

Nutritional goals for the individual with acute renal failure include

1. Administering protein to meet the hypercatabolic state, which usually ranges from 1.5 to 2.0 g/kg/day

2. Supplying fats and carbohydrates to meet the increased metabolic rate

3. Monitoring serum levels of electrolytes and trace elements to prevent abnormalities; removal of specific micronutrients may be necessary if the levels are elevated

In summary, specific disease states require necessary alterations in nutritional support. Hepatic failure can cause hypercatabolism, diminished use of fat as an energy source, hyperglycemia, and sodium and fluid retention. A specialized hepatic formula, containing a greater percentage of BCAA than AAA, is available but expensive.

Malnutrition can contribute to pulmonary disease. Nutritional support should be designed with a lower carbohydrate content to decrease the patient's respiratory rate, thereby decreasing the patient's respiratory workload. Protein supplementation should be based on nitrogen excretion to avoid increasing ventilatory drive. Enteral feedings into the small bowel are preferred to avoid the risk of aspiration pneumonia.

Hypermetabolism, hypercatabolism, electrolyte and trace element abnormalities, and fluid retention occur in acute renal failure. Controversy over whether to feed these patients exists. The trend is toward feeding patients and initiating dialysis. Careful monitoring of electrolytes and trace elements is necessary, since abnormalities occur frequently. Specific micronutrients may need to be withheld initially from the nutritional support.

Section Eight Review

1. A high acuity patient with hepatic failure may experience all of the following EXCEPT
   A. breakdown of skeletal muscle protein
   B. diminished fat use
   C. hyponatremia
   D. increased carbon dioxide levels
2. Nutritional goals for the pulmonary failure patient are the following EXCEPT
   A. lower fat content
   B. lower protein content
   C. lower carbohydrate content
   D. higher fat content

3. A high acuity patient with acute renal failure may experience abnormalities in each of the following EXCEPT
   A. protein catabolism
   B. fluid and electrolytes
   C. metabolic rate
   D. ammonia levels

Answers: 1, D. 2, A. 3, D.

Posttest

1. The metabolic stress response is the result of
   A. psychologic stress
   B. overexertion from exercise
   C. injured tissue in the body
   D. hyperventilation
2. The flow phase consists of the following characteristics EXCEPT
   A. hypermetabolism
   B. increased nitrogen losses
   C. anabolism
   D. hypercatabolism
3. During the flow phase, each of the following nutrients should be administered EXCEPT
   A. immunoglobulins
   B. calories
   C. protein
   D. micronutrients
4. A patient has a functioning gastrointestinal tract but is unable to take adequate nutrients by mouth. What is the BEST method for administering nutritional support to this patient?
   A. nasoenteric feedings
   B. oral diet
   C. withhold nutrition
   D. total parenteral nutrition (TPN)
5. Enteral nutrition has many advantages over TPN. These include each of the following EXCEPT
   A. less risk of bacterial translocation
   B. providing central venous access
   C. maintaining gut morphology and function
   D. less costly
6. A patient has a functioning gastrointestinal tract but is at risk for aspiration pneumonia. What is the BEST location for nutrition to be delivered?
   A. stomach
   B. withhold nutrition
   C. IV
   D. small bowel
7. TPN is indicated when
   A. adequate amounts of nutrients can be delivered through the gastrointestinal tract
   B. adequate amounts of nutrients cannot be delivered through the gastrointestinal tract
   C. a functioning, usable gastrointestinal tract is capable of absorption of adequate nutrients
   D. aggressive nutritional support is not warranted
8. Catheter-related sepsis (CRS) is a potentially lethal complication of TPN and is caused primarily by
   A. a malpositioned catheter or guidewire during the central line insertion
   B. lack of sterility during central line placement and inadequate maintenance of the line
   C. inadvertant puncture or laceration of the subclavian or carotid artery
   D. puncture or laceration of the vein on insertion of the needle/catheter
9. A high acuity patient with hepatic failure may experience all of the following EXCEPT
   A. breakdown of skeletal muscle protein
   B. diminished fat use
   C. hyponatremia
   D. increased carbon dioxide levels
10. Nutritional goals for the pulmonary failure patient are the following EXCEPT
    A. lower fat content
    B. lower protein content
    C. lower carbohydrate content
    D. higher fat content
11. A high acuity patient with acute renal failure may experience abnormalities in each of the following EXCEPT
    A. protein catabolism
    B. fluid and electrolytes
    C. metabolic rate
    D. ammonia levels

Posttest Answers

Question	Answer	Section	Question	Answer	Section
1	C	One	7	B	Six
2	C	One	8	B	Seven
3	A	Two	9	D	Eight
4	A	Three	10	A	Eight
5	B	Four	11	D	Eight
6	D	Four			

REFERENCE

Harris, J.A., and Benedict, F.G. (1919). *A biometric study of basal metabolism in man*, Publ. No. 279. Washington, DC: Carnegie Institute of Washington.

ADDITIONAL READING

Feinstein, E. (1986). Nutrition in acute renal failure. In J.L. Rombeau and M.D. Caldwell (eds). *Parenteral nutrition*, pp. 586–601. Philadelphia: W.B. Saunders Co.

Krey, S., and Murray, R. (1986). *Dynamics of nutrition support: Assessment, implementation, evaluation*. Norwalk, Connecticut: Appleton-Century-Crofts.

Lang, C. (1989). Nutrition support in hepatic failure. In E.P. Schronts (ed). *Nutrition support dietetics*, pp. 155–168. Silver Springs, Maryland: Aspen.

Leupold, C. (1988). Nutritional alterations in illness: Critical care—stress, trauma, burns, and sepsis. In C. Kennedy-Caldwell and P. Guenter (eds). *Nutrition support nursing*, pp. 413–434. Silver Springs, Maryland: Aspen.

Matarese, L. (1989). Nutrition support in renal failure. In E.P. Schronts (ed). *Nutrition support dietetics*, pp. 191–198. Silver Springs, Maryland: Aspen.

Schlichtig, R., and Ayres, S. (1988). *Nutritional support of the critically ill*. Chicago: Year Book Medical Publishers.

Schronts, E. (1989). Nutrition support in metabolic stress. In E. Schronts (ed). *Nutrition support dietetics*, pp. 199–211. Silver Springs, Maryland: Aspen.

Schwartz, D. (1989). Nutrition support in pulmonary failure. In E.P. Schronts (ed). *Nutrition support dietetics*, pp. 183–189. Silver Springs, Maryland: Aspen.

Module 17

Immunocompetence

Helen F. Hodges

With respect to normal physiologic functioning, the immune system serves to protect the body from foreign invaders. These invaders might be disease-producing pathogenic microorganisms (also called pathogens) or abnormal cells, such as cancer cells. However, the immune system is actually the body's third and slowest line of defense against such invasion. An intact skin tissue provides the first line of defense, creating a physical barrier between the internal environment of the body and the external environment surrounding it. If, however, an invading organism or other foreign agent manages to get past this barrier, the inflammatory response is initiated, whereby invading agents are neutralized or destroyed. Failing that mechanism of protection, the immune system is alerted for action. This module is devoted to the structure and function of the immune system, with particular emphasis on the acutely ill adult. Nursing care of the immunosuppressed patient is presented in Module 20, *Nursing Care of the Patient with Altered Metabolism*.

Section One discusses the location and function of the immune system. Particular organs and tissues are described in their relationship to immunity. The emphasis of Section Two is the primary characteristics of active and passive immunity. Section Three presents the learner with characteristics and outcomes of antigen-antibody activity. Section Four addresses with more detail the origin and function of the various cellular components of the immune system, including T cells, B cells, and macrophages. Section Five discusses the nature of immune mechanisms, including cell-mediated and humoral immunity, phagocytosis, and the role of interferon. Section Six explores the pathogenesis of hypersensitivity reactions and the notion of autoimmune disorders. Section Seven discusses the concept of incompatibility and its manifestations as transplant rejection phenomena. Human immunodeficiency virus (HIV) is addressed in Section Eight with regard to the nature of the virus, its transmission and growth, and attempts toward treatment. Section Nine summarizes the impacts of aging, malnutrition, stress, and trauma on the immune system.

Each section includes a set of review questions to help the learner evaluate understanding of the section content. All section reviews and the Pretest and Posttest include answers. It is suggested that the learner review those concepts that have been missed in the review questions before proceeding to the next section.

Objectives

Following completion of the module, *Immunocompetence*, the learner will be able to

1. Cite the location and functional role of organs and tissues primarily involved in the immune response

2. Contrast the nature of natural immunity and acquired (active and passive) immunity

3. Describe the characteristics of antigens and antigen-antibody responses

4. Discuss the nature and primary function of cellular components of the immune system

5. Describe mechanisms of specific immunity (humoral and cell-mediated) and mechanisms of nonspecific immunity

6. Explain the theoretical concepts for the occurrence of types I, II, III, and IV immunoglobulin hypersensitivity and autoimmune disorders

7. Describe the three patterns of transplant rejection as a function of hypersensitivity

8. Characterize the immunodeficiency pattern of HIV, including the mechanism of transmission, viral invasion, growth, antibody formation, treatment approaches, and the ultimate effect of the disease

9. Describe the pathogenesis of aging, malnutrition, trauma, and stress related to the functions of the adult immune system

Pretest

1. Which of the following is primarily responsible for T cell differentiation?
   A. bursa equivalent
   B. thymus
   C. stem cells
   D. lymph nodes

2. The bursa equivalent is thought to be located in the
   A. spleen
   B. Peyer's patches
   C. bone marrow
   D. thymus

3. Nonspecific immune response involves which of the following?
   A. recognition of a particular antigen
   B. production of antibody
   C. recognition of nonself
   D. T cell differentiation

4. A child who first has chickenpox and then is immune from that disease in the future is said to have
   A. active acquired immunity
   B. passive acquired immunity
   C. natural immunity
   D. species-specific immunity

5. An individual whose antibody titer is greater than the preestablished level of immunity is said to
   A. demonstrate immunity from the disease in question
   B. require reimmunization
   C. demonstrate a specific antigen-antibody complex
   D. transmit the disease as a carrier

6. HLA antigen is located on which of the following sites?
   A. gamma globulin protein fraction
   B. erythrocytes
   C. chromosome 6
   D. RNA chains

7. Which of the following is responsible for directing cellular attack and antigen destruction?
   A. helper T cell
   B. killer T cell
   C. suppressor B cell
   D. memory B cell

8. Macrophages are primarily responsible for which of the following?
   A. interfering with the immune response
   B. protecting against local mucosal invasion of bacteria
   C. triggering the complement system
   D. carrying the antigen to B cells and T cells

9. Humoral immunity is best characterized by which of the following?
   A. development of antibodies from B cells
   B. recognition of self and nonself
   C. specific recognition and memory of antigens
   D. differentiation of cellular function known as killer, helper, and suppressor cells

10. Which of the following immunoglobulins comprises about 75 percent of the total immunoglobulins in the healthy human body?
    A. IgA
    B. IgE
    C. IgG
    D. IgM

11. Which of the following immunoglobulins affords the body local protection at the mucosal level against invading organisms?
    A. IgA
    B. IgG
    C. IgD
    D. IgE

12. An example of therapeutically eliciting the primary and secondary response patterns of humoral immunity is
    A. exposure to chickenpox and subsequent immunity
    B. tetanus vaccine and booster vaccines
    C. interferon treatment for malignancy
    D. transference of killer T cells from donor to recipient

13. The results of a true type I hypersensitivity response are due to
    A. a histamine precursor causing anaphylaxis
    B. antigen-IgE-mast cell interaction
    C. antigen-antibody complexes deposited in vessel walls
    D. massive numbers of destroyed RBCs

14. What characterizes the concept of autoimmune disease?
    A. recognition of self as foreign
    B. exacerbation and death
    C. accelerated production of killer T cells
    D. immunosuppression and altered cortisol levels

15. Which immune component creates the greatest destruction in transplant rejection phenomena?
    A. B lymphocytes
    B. killer T cells
    C. helper T cells
    D. IgG immunoglobulins

16. Which of the following best characterizes HIV disease?
    A. symptoms result from opportunistic pathology
    B. clinical manifestation is of a characteristic and predictable sequence
    C. the HIV virus invades cells primarily through the bloodstream
    D. individuals who test positive for the HIV virus are carriers and considered contagious

17. Which of the following fluids is known to be a mode of transmission for the AIDS virus?
    A. tears
    B. perspiration
    C. plasma
    D. saliva

18. What is the function of zinc in the competent immune system?
    A. it is required for normal function of lymphocytes
    B. zinc protects B cells from being destroyed by macrophages
    C. T cells require zinc for production of gamma globulin
    D. macrophages are composed primarily of zinc

19. What effect does the normal aging process have on the immune system?
    A. B cell function in general is particularly depressed
    B. the immune system becomes hypervigilant to invading organisms with increasing age
    C. autoantibodies begin to diminish with increasing age
    D. T cells begin to deteriorate in functioning

20. In the acutely ill adult, which of the following nutritional losses to the body is a critical factor in the immune system integrity?
    A. protein
    B. vitamin C
    C. complex carbohydrate chains
    D. iron

Answers: 1, B. 2, C. 3, C. 4, A. 5, A. 6, C. 7, B. 8, D. 9, A. 10, C. 11, A. 12, B. 13, B. 14, A. 15, B. 16, A. 17, C. 18, A. 19, D. 20, A.

Glossary

Acquired immunity, active. Immunity resulting from exposure to a specific antigen and subsequent formation and programming of antibodies; may be produced from having the disease or by injection of the weakened organism (vaccination)

Acquired immunity, passive. Temporary immunity provided by injection of sera containing antibodies, placental crossover, or mother's milk

Allergy. A hypersensitivity reaction of antigen-antibody activity in response to a specific substance that in nonsensitive people in similar amounts produces no effect

Antigen. A coded material that allows the body to distinguish tissue as nonself or self and that is capable of eliciting the immune response

Antigenic determinant site. Sites on antigens that interact with specific immune cells to bind in lock-and-key fashion; the binding elicits the immune response

Arthus reaction. A severe local inflammatory reaction to an antigen; one example of a type III antigen-antibody hypersensitivity reaction

Autoimmunity. A destructive response in which the immune system recognizes self as foreign and begins to destroy the body's own cells and tissues

B lymphocyte (B cell). A lymphocyte primarily responsible for antibody formation on exposure to a specific antigen; the primary cells in humoral immunity

Bursa equivalent. Tissue thought to be located in the bone marrow primarily responsible for differentiating lymphocytes into B cells for humoral immunity

Cell-mediated immunity. A type of protection against invading antigens characterized by surveillance and direct attack of foreign material; the primary effector cell is the T lymphocyte

Chemotaxis. Attraction of cells to a chemical stimulus, e.g., a mechanism of attracting neutrophils to site of injury is by an eosinophil chemotactic factor

Complement system. A progressive, sequential cascade of events produced by substances found naturally in the circulating sera; components of the system must be triggered individually and cause cellular lysis of antigens

Hapten. A substance with such a low molecular weight that it cannot act as an antigen unless attached to a carrier, such as a protein; examples include dander, dust, and pollen

Histocompatibility antigens (HLA, human leukocyte antigens). Genetically determined surface antigens found in all nucleated cells in the body; one's own HLA antigens are substances that the body recognizes as self

Humoral immunity. The type of protection against foreign antigens provided by antibody formation from B lymphocytes

Hypersensitivity. An exaggerated response of the immune system to an antigen or antigens otherwise considered nonpathogenic; an allergy to a certain substance is an example of a hypersensitivity reaction

Immunity. A normal adaptive response to the external environment; it functions to protect the body from disease by means of both resistance to offending organisms and attack on offending organisms

Immunodeficiency. A general term referring to a state of deficient immune activity

Immunodeficiency, primary. Failure of either T cell or B cell function or both, resulting from embryonic or congenital lack of development of such organs as the thymus

Immunodeficiency, secondary. A deficiency of T cells or B cells or both resulting from illnesses, chemotherapy, radiation therapy, or a direct pathogenic attack on the immune system

Immunoglobulin. The product of plasma cells in the humoral immune response following exposure to a specific antigen; five classes of immunoglobulins are IgG, IgA, IgE, IgM, IgD

Interferon. A family of lymphokines, originating from effector T cells, that are responsible for promoting nonspecific immunity against viruses and other intracellular pathogens

Lymphokines. Substances produced by T cells that influence the function of macrophages and inflammatory cells

Macrophage. A lymphocyte that ingests and digests antigens, then carries the antigen to the T cells and B cells; the link between the immune response and the inflammatory response

Major histocompatibility complex. A group of genes located on the sixth chromosome; responsible for coding histocompatibility antigens

Opsonins. Provide binding sites for attachment of macrophages or neutrophils to the antigen; composed of IgG immunoglobulin and C3b, a fragment of the complement system

Pathogen. A disease-producing microorganism

Plasma cell. The result of transformation of mature B cells in response to exposure to a specific antigen; primary cell to produce or secrete antibodies (immunoglobulins)

Rejection phenomenon. Attempted destruction of transplanted tissue at the cellular level by the host's immune system

Primary response. The initial humoral response to antigen exposure; characterized by a latency period during which the antigen is recognized as nonself and identified specifically, and antibodies are formed in response to the antigen makeup

Secondary response. The humoral response to subsequent exposure to the same antigen; immune response is heightened, and antibody formation is triggered more quickly than in the primary response

T lymphocyte (T cell). A lymphocyte primarily responsible for direct attack and destruction of invading antigens; the primary cell in cell-mediated immunity; killer T cells directly attack invading antigen; helper T cells enhance the action of B lymphocytes; suppressor T cells suppress or inhibit the action of B lymphocytes

Thymus. An organ in the mediastinum primarily responsible for differentiating lymphocytes into various types of T cells for cell-mediated immunity

Abbreviations

AIDS. Acquired immunodeficiency syndrome

AZT. Azidothymidine

B cells. Bursa cells

HIV. Human immunodeficiency virus

HLA. Human leukocyte antigens

HTLV. Human T cell lymphotropic virus

Ig. Immunoglobulin

MHC. Major histocompatibility complex

SCID. Severe combined immune deficiencies

T cells. Thymus cells

Section One: Role of the Immune System in Body Defense

At the completion of this section, the learner will be able to cite the location and functional role of organs and tissues primarily involved in the immune response.

Acting much as a surveillance mechanism, the immune system monitors the internal environment for foreign agents. It is a complex system of organs and cells capable of distinguishing self from nonself, remembering previous invaders, and reacting according to needs as they arise. The primary organs of the immune system are the thymus, lymph nodes,

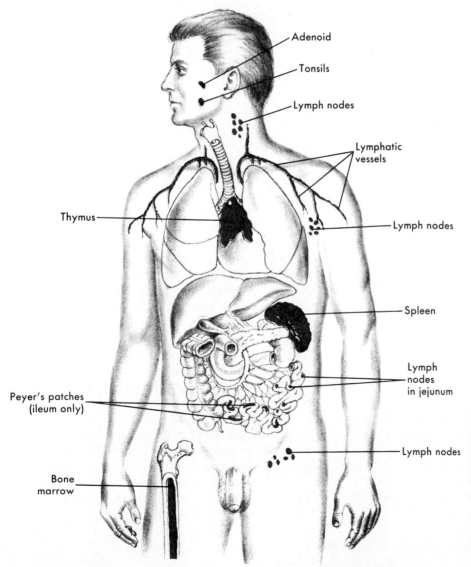

Figure 17–1. Lymphoid tissues: sites of B cell and T cell differentiation. Immature lymphocytes migrate through central lymphoid tissues, the bone marrow and the thymus. Mature lymphocytes later reside in the T and B lymphocyte-rich areas of the peripheral lymphoid tissues. (*From Pathophysiology: The biologic basis for disease in adults and children, p. 196, by K. McCance and S. Huether, 1990, St. Louis: C.V. Mosby Co.*)

Adenoid

Tonsils

Lymph nodes

Lymphatic vessels

Thymus

Lymph nodes

Spleen

Lymph nodes in jejunum

Peyer's patches (ileum only)

Lymph nodes

Bone marrow

spleen, and tonsils. Contributing to the immune response are lymphoid tissues in nonlymphoid organs (such as the intestinal tissue), and circulating immune cells, such as T cells, B cells, and phagocytes. The circulating immune cells are discussed further in Section Four. Figure 17–1 shows primary organs and lymph tissue sites as well as the sites of T cell and B cell differentiation.

The Thymus

The thymus is a flat, lobed organ located in the neck below the thyroid and extending into the upper thorax behind the sternum. Reaching its peak size at puberty, it diminishes in size and composition steadily until it is hardly distinguishable in adulthood. Its lymphoid tissue is gradually replaced by adipose tissue over one's lifetime. The thymus produces a hormone called *thymosin,* thought to be active in the production of lymphocytes and also under investigation as an agent that stimulates the immune function in some immunodeficiency states (Tribett, 1989).

The primary function of the thymus is the development of the immune system. During embryonic life, most lymphocytes develop from stem cells in the bone marrow and travel to the thymus after birth to be marked as T cells (T, of thymus origin). However, there is also evidence to suggest that some lymphocytes are actually in the thymus before birth and, along with other cells, migrate and become the spleen and the lymph nodes (Porth, 1986).

During extrauterine life, the role of the thymus is to differentiate lymphocytes into various types of T cells. In this process, the thymus alters the surface antigens of these cells, which gives them their identity as T cells, a specialized lymphocyte. Mature, differentiated lymphocytes are released into the bloodstream, and they relocate in peripheral lymph tissue, such as lymph nodes, tonsils, intestines, and spleen, where they await a call to action in body defense.

Bursa Equivalent

Much like the thymus in T cell maturation, the bursa equivalent in the bone marrow differentiates lymphocytes into B cells (B, of bursa origin). Once released, these immature B cells migrate to the peripheral lymph tissue (lymph nodes, spleen, tonsils), where they mature and await the body's need for defense against foreign agents.

Lymph System

The blood is filtered continuously by the lymph system. The lymph nodes actually serve two purposes for the body. They act as a filtering system for foreign materials, and they serve as a reservoir for the specialized immunologic T cells and B cells. Peripherally, the serous portion of the bloodstream (excluding platelets, red blood cells, and large proteins) diffuses from the capillaries into the peripheral lymph channels, where it is progressively filtered and then returned to the cardiovascular system. Lymph ducts carry this serous fluid through lymph nodes, where it is filtered. It may be useful to think of a lymph node much as a sponge, where the meshwork serves as a surface on which antigens and other foreign materials are arrested and destroyed or neutralized (Porth, 1986). Large clusters of lymph nodes are found in the axillae, groin, thorax, abdomen, and neck. With many infectious processes, these nodes become enlarged as their activity increases and defense cells proliferate. T cells are most abundant here, although B cells can be found also.

The Spleen

The spleen is a small organ about the size of a fist in the left upper quadrant of the abdomen. It is protected by the 9th, 10th, and 11th ribs and, thus, usually is nonpalpable. The spleen serves three functions, only one of which is actually immune-related. First, it is the site for the destruction of injured and worn-out red blood cells. Second, it is a reservoir for B cells, although T cells also are found there, and third, it serves as a storage site for blood, which it can release from its distended vessels in times of demand. The tonsils, Peyer's patches in the intestine, and the appendix are quite similar in function and structure to the lymph nodes and the spleen. The tonsils, like the thymus, diminish in size after childhood and, unless inflamed, are difficult to distinguish from surrounding tissue in the posterior pharynx.

In summary, the ability to produce and maintain an intact immune system requires the interaction of the thymus, bursa equivalent, lymph nodes, spleen, and tonsils as well as lymphoid tissue in nonlymphoid organs, such as the intestines. Although much of the immune system is well in place before birth, ongoing processes of marking and maturation of cells are critical to adequate functioning for nonspecific immune responses and specific antigen-antibody reactions to occur.

Section One Review

1. Which of the following is primarily responsible for T cell differentiation?
   A. bursa equivalent
   B. thymus gland
   C. stem cells
   D. lymph nodes
2. As a person ages, thymus gland lymphoid tissue is slowly replaced by
   A. Peyer's patches
   B. stem cells
   C. bursa cells
   D. adipose tissue
3. The bursa equivalent is thought to be located in the
   A. spleen
   B. Peyer's patches
   C. bone marrow
   D. thymus

4. A major function of the lymph nodes is to
   A. filter foreign substances
   B. destroy worn-out red blood cells
   C. produce lymphocytes
   D. produce stem cells
5. Which of the following is correct regarding the spleen?
   A. it destroys worn-out white blood cells
   B. it filters out foreign materials
   C. it produces the hormone thymosin
   D. it is a reservoir for B cells

Answers: 1, B. 2, D. 3, C. 4, A. 5, D.

Section Two: Characteristics of the Immune System

At the completion of this section, the learner will be able to contrast the nature of natural immunity and acquired (active and passive) immunity.

Immunity is a normal adaptive response to the external environment. It functions to protect the body from disease by means of both resistance to offending organisms and attack on offending organisms. Immunity can be either natural or acquired. Natural immunity is species-specific; that is, humans are immune to a variety of diseases to which certain animals are susceptible, and vice versa. For example, human beings are not vulnerable to feline leukemia, and cats are not susceptible to human immunodeficiency virus (HIV). Natural immunity is innate, in that we are born with certain immunities. Other immunities are acquired after birth through exposure to an antigen, through transference of antibodies by inoculation, or through such body fluids as mother's milk.

Acquired Immunity

Acquired immunity can be either active or passive. Active immunity is developed on exposure to an antigen, such as the chickenpox virus, during which time antibodies are programmed to protect the body from illness with future exposures. These antibodies are quite specific, often providing lifetime immunity against another attack of the same antigen. Active immunity also can be developed, again with lifetime protection, by exposure to a specific antigen through inoculation. Such vaccines as smallpox and polio vaccines provide a lifetime force of antibody protection without an actual illness occurring. Active immunity following exposure to a specific antigen does not provide immediate protection but develops over a period of days. However, the programming of specific antibodies provides heightened protection with subsequent exposures within a matter of minutes or hours.

Passive immunity is a temporary immunity involving the transference of antibodies from one individual to another or from some other source (laboratory cultures, other animals) to an individual. An infant receives passive immunity both in utero and from breast milk. A neonate does not yet have a mature immune system capable of efficient development of antibodies in response to invading agents. Passive immunity can be transferred also through vaccination either of antiserum such as rabies, an antitoxin such as tetanus, or as gamma globulin, which contains a variety of antibodies.

Both passive and active immunity create levels of antibodies circulating in the body. Many of these levels can be monitored by venipuncture blood tests to determine full immunity to a particular disease. The result of testing the level of a particular antibody is called the antibody titer. The titer of the specific antibody is compared to a preestablished level thought to guarantee immunity. If the individual's titer is found to be lower than the preestablished norm, he or she may require reimmunization with the vaccine. An example of such a process is the increased scrutiny of individuals regarding their immune status to rubella.

In summary, there is ongoing interaction between the body and the environment as substances known as antigens come in contact with the immune system. The body has several avenues by which it might protect itself against foreign antigens. First, a natural immunity occurs normally and is species-specific. Second, the healthy body is able to respond to antigenic stimulation and produce its own antibodies that continue to circulate long after the antigen is destroyed, in some cases for a lifetime. Finally, antibodies may be transferred to the body by injection or through the common maternal–fetal circulation and breast milk.

Section Two Review

1. A child who first had chickenpox and then is immune from that disease in the future is said to have
   A. active acquired immunity
   B. passive acquired immunity
   C. natural immunity
   D. species-specific immunity
2. An infant who receives temporary immunity while being breastfed has which kind of immunity?
   A. active acquired immunity
   B. passive acquired immunity
   C. natural immunity
   D. species-specific immunity

3. An individual whose antibody titer is greater than the preestablished level of immunity is said to
   A. require reimmunization
   B. transmit the disease as a carrier
   C. demonstrate a specific antigen-antibody complex
   D. demonstrate immunity from the disease in question

Answers: 1, A. 2, B. 3, D.

Section Three: Antigens and Antigen-Antibody Response

At the completion of this section, the learner will be able to describe characteristics of antigens and antigen-antibody responses.

Antigens

The immune system responds to foreign material in the body, known as antigens. Some antigens are capable of producing disease and are called *pathogens* or *pathogenic antigens*. Other antigens may be foreign but are not pathogenic microorganisms. An example of a nonpathogenic antigen is a transplanted heart or kidney. The cells making up the tissues of these organs are not disease-producing but are recognized by the body as being nonself and, thus, can precipitate an immune reaction.

Although the immune system is certainly capable of distinguishing self from nonself, in its natural state, it is not able to determine that a foreign material is acceptable even if that material is beneficial to the well-being of the body as a whole. This is the scenario that occurs in organ transplant rejection. The organ is viewed by the immune system as an invading antigen and is then attacked with the intent to destroy. Immunosuppressive drugs are administered to diminish the immune response. At the present time, there is no way to educate the system that an incoming heart, kidney, liver, lung, or other donor tissue must be accepted as self.

Histocompatibility Antigens

In addition to foreign materials being antigens, it is known that all nucleated cells in the body contain surface antigens, proteins found on the surface of a cell. These proteins distinguish an individual's tissue from tissue of other persons. Surface antigens are genetically determined and are referred to as *histo-*

compatibility antigens or human leukocyte antigens (HLA). They were first discovered on leukocytes, thus the label HLA. These surface antigens are similar to ABO antigens found on erythrocytes. Individuals with type A blood type have the A antigen on the surface of their red blood cells. Individuals with type B blood type have B antigens on their red blood cells. Type O blood type individuals have neither A nor B antigens, and type AB blood has both A and B antigens on the red blood cells. Like the ABO antigens, HLA antigens must be matched carefully before transplantation. The HLA antigens are genetically transmitted. The histocompatibility antigens are proteins that are coded by a group of genes called the *major histocompatibility complex* (MHC) located on the sixth chromosome. Five HLA antigen sites have been identified thus far and labeled: HLA-A, HLA-B, HLA-C, HLA-D, HLA-DR. Each of these sites contains varying degrees of information that code the development of the surface antigen. For example, for HLA-A there are approximately 20 pairs of genes carrying information, for HLA-B there are approximately 30, for HLA-C there are approximately 6, and so on. Figure 17–2 represents the relationship of HLA sites to the major histocompatibility complex genes.

Since each offspring receives a pair of genes, one from each parent, the combination of the genes determines the HLA type. There are multiple possibilities of the coding of surface cell antigens for one individual. It is the surface cell antigens in most cases that the immune cells recognize as self. The closer in match of HLA surface cell antigens between two individuals, the less severe the immune response to a transplanted organ or graft.

It is thought that several pathologic disorders may be related to the presence of certain HLA antigens coded by the MHC genes. For example, ankylosing spondylitis appears to have a high correlation with antigen B27 (or HLA-B27), and the presence of psoriasis is highly correlated with the presence of HLA-B17. Clinical interest continues to grow in research efforts in this area.

Antigenic Determinants

Antigens have several specific sites, called *antigenic determinants*, which interact with immune cells to elicit the immune response. These sites are quite specific in configuration, requiring a specific structure of the immunoglobulin molecule or antibody (Figure 17–3). The binding of antigen to antibody is at specific receptor sites and is similar to the notion of a lock and key. Some molecules are so small that they cannot act as antigens until they attach to larger mole-

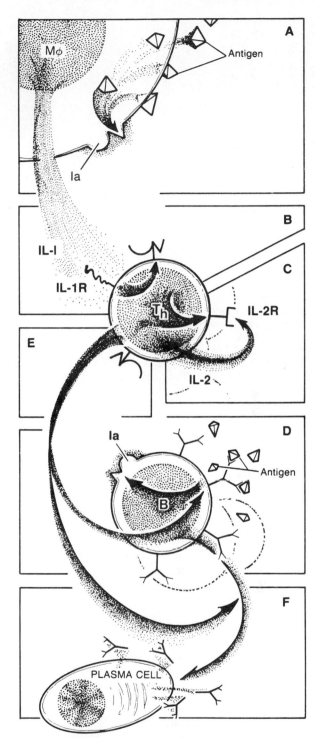

Figure 17–2. Genes for histocompatibility antigens. The human major histocompatibility complex (MHC) known as HLA (human leukocyte antigen) is found on chromosome 6. It consists of five regions. The D region is subdivided into four parts, which code for membrane 1a antigens. Between D and B, there are genes for three proteins of the complement system. B, C, and A (especially A and B) are genes for the serologically defined MHC class I antigens expressed on all nucleated cells and platelets. (*From* Critical care nursing: Clinical management through the nursing process, *p. 1163, by J.T. Dolan, 1991, Philadelphia: F.A. Davis Co.*)

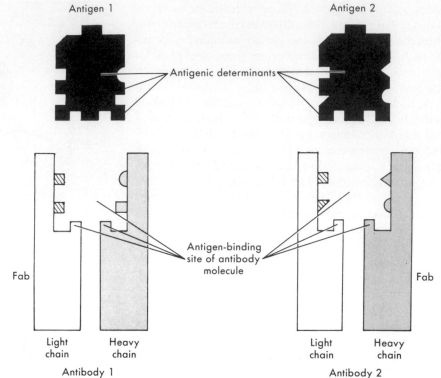

Figure 17–3. Antigenic determinant sites. The specificity required for antibody binding with an antigen is determined by the shape of the combining site on the antibody. (*From* Pathophysiology: The biologic basis for disease in adults and children, *p. 204, by K. Mc-Cance and S. Huether, 1990, St. Louis: C.V. Mosby.*)

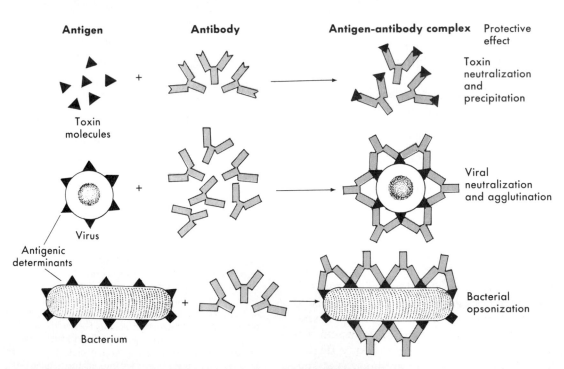

Figure 17–4. Antigen-antibody complex. Protective activities of antibodies: neutralization of bacterial exotoxins, neutralization of viruses and prevention of their interactions with cellular membranes, and opsonization of bacteria. All of these mechanisms are followed by removal of the antigen by phagocytosis, drainage along with body fluid, or both. (*From* Pathophysiology: The biologic basis for disease in adults and children, *p. 204, by K. McCance and S. Huether, 1990, St. Louis: C.V. Mosby Co.*)

MODULE 17 IMMUNOCOMPETENCE

cules or carriers. These substances are called *haptens*. Examples of haptens are house dust, animal hair particles, and pollen.

Immune Responsiveness

Immune responsiveness may be either specific or nonspecific. A specific response requires the recognition of a particular antigen and involves the production and action of a programmed antibody for that antigen. Normally, an antibody circulates in the bloodstream until it encounters an appropriate antigen to which it can bind. Such binding results in antigen-antibody complexes or immune complexes. The process of binding is such that the antibody binds to particularly conformed antigenic determinant sites on the antigen, effectively preventing the antigen from binding with receptors on host cells (Figure 17–4). The overall effect is protection of the host from antigen infection or penetration.

An antigen-antibody reaction can cause several consequences to the invading agent. The reaction can cause agglutination or clumping of the cells, neutralization of the antigen toxin, such as a bacterial toxin, cell lysis or destruction of the antigen, enhanced phagocytosis of the antigen by other cells, or activation of the complement system.

A nonspecific response requires only the recognition of the invader being nonself, or foreign, but does not involve a particular antibody. A nonspecific immunologic response might involve the complement system, interferons, and phagocytosis. These mechanisms of immunity are discussed in Section Five.

Antigen Entry Site

The entry site of an antigen is an important consideration. Many enzymes and other secretions are important components as defense mechanisms. Some antigens are destroyed before they cross into the bloodstream. For example, some antigens are readily destroyed or neutralized by salivary and other digestive enzymes in the gastrointestinal tract and are rendered incapable of causing disease. Other antigens are not affected by these enzymes and can proliferate rapidly, creating pathologic states. The site of entrance also determines the strength or virulence of the antigen. For example, an antigen that is neutralized by digestive enzymes in the gastrointestinal tract might be quite virulent if entering the body through the genitourinary tract or the respiratory tract, where digestive enzymes are not normally found.

In summary, the antigen-antibody phenomenon is the cornerstone for much of the body's protective immune system. Both antigens and antibodies have particular configurations that allow them to bind to one another. Once an antibody binds with an antigen, the antigen is capable of binding with the host cell, causing disease or pathology. The effect of binding may result in either neutralization, precipitation, lysis (destruction), enhanced phagocytosis, or agglutination of the offending antigen. Which effect occurs depends on the class of antibody and the nature of the antigen.

Section Three Review

1. A nonspecific immune response involves
   A. T cell differentiation
   B. production of antibody
   C. recognition of nonself
   D. recognition of a particular antigen
2. HLA antigens are located on which of the following sites?
   A. RNA chains
   B. erythrocytes
   C. chromosome 6
   D. gamma globulin protein fraction
3. Specific sites on antigens that interact with immune cells to elicit the immune response are called
   A. antigenic determinants
   B. surface cells
   C. human leukocyte antigens
   D. histocompatibility complexes
4. Antigens that precipitate disease states are called
   A. immunoglobulins
   B. pathogens
   C. human leukocyte antigens
   D. histocompatibility antigens

5. All of the following statements regarding the entry site of an antigen are correct EXCEPT
   A. saliva in the mouth destroys many antigens
   B. digestive enzymes neutralize many antigens
   C. site of entry helps determine virulence of the antigen
   D. entry location does not determine strength of the antigen

Answers: 1, C. 2, C. 3, A. 4, B. 5, D.

Section Four: Cells of the Immune Response

At the completion of this section, the learner will be able to discuss the nature and primary function of cellular components of the immune system.

There are at least three types of cells involved in the immune response to foreign material: the T cell, the B cell, and the macrophage. Each cell carries a distinct responsibility and contributes to the integrity of the body as a whole. Each set of cells has effector cells and memory cells. The effector cells are those that are capable of attacking and destroying a particular antigen. The memory cells are those that are further imprinted with the antigenic code and are responsible for remembering and recognizing that antigen within minutes of a subsequent exposure.

T Lymphocytes (T Cells)

The T cells provide a type of immunity called cell-mediated immunity, which is discussed in a later section. T cells have a life expectancy of several years. They are marked by the thymus with specific surface antigens that characterize them and distinguish them from B cells. The T cells represent approximately 70 percent to 80 percent of the total lymphocytes. T cells can be further divided into two groups based on their particular functions, effector cells and regulatory cells.

Effector T Cells

These cells directly or indirectly affect immunity. As an indirect effect, they can produce lymphokines, which are substances that influence the function of inflammatory cells and macrophages. Some effector cells directly attack and destroy antigens. The killer T cell, appropriately named, is the effector cell that directly causes cell death of the antigen.

Regulatory T Cells

These are further divided into two groups, helper T cells (T4 cells), which enhance the action of B lymphocytes, and suppressor T cells (T8 cells), which suppress or inhibit the action of B lymphocytes.

B Lymphocytes

The B cells are the larger of the lymphocytes cells and have a much shorter life span than the T cells. They mature with exposure to an antigen. Immature B cells are stored in the bone marrow, the lymph nodes, and other lymphatic tissue. They are also found circulating in the bloodstream. It is the B lymphocytes that are primarily responsible for antibody production. Following exposure to an antigen, mature B cells may be transformed into plasma cells, which then secrete antibodies called *immunoglobulins*. Each plasma cell is specialized to produce only one type of antibody. Several types of antibodies have been identified, and each is active within a given course of events in the immune response. Immunoglobulins are identified as IgA, IgD, IgE, IgG, or IgM. They are discussed in Section Five.

Macrophage

The macrophage participates in the immune response by processing the antigen and presenting it in such a way as to increase its recognition and reaction by the B cells and T cells. By means of phagocytosis, the macrophage ingests and digests the antigen, but in the process, the altered antigen is released through the macrophage cell membrane, where it attaches to receptor sites on the surface of the macrophage (Figure 17–5).

It is at these receptor sites that the interaction

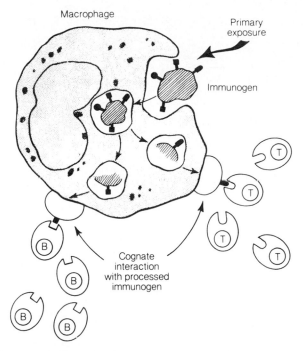

Macrophage

Primary
exposure

Immunogen

Cognate
interaction
with processed
immunogen

Figure 17–5. Macrophage presentation of antigens to B cells and T cells. (*From* Pathophysiology: Concepts of altered health states, 2nd ed., p. 182, by C.M. Porth, 1986, London: J.B. Lippincott Co.)

takes place with the invading antigen and T cells and B cells. Macrophages are primarily responsible for carrying antigens to the lymph tissue, where the B cells and T cells reside. The macrophage is a critical factor in the immune response to both the T cells and the B cells and is considered to be the link between the inflammatory response and the specific resistance of antibody production and cell mediation. In fact, it is also thought that a substance produced by effector T cells (those capable of attacking and destroying antigens) causes migration and activation of the macrophages.

In summary, all three cell types work together to maintain the integrity of the body against invading antigens. It is the macrophage, however, that plays the important role of preparing the antigen for the T lymphocytes and B lymphocytes. Without adequate macrophage support, the remaining cellular components of the immune system would be severely impaired.

Section Four Review

1. Which of the following is responsible for directing cellular attack and antigen destruction?
   A. helper T cell
   B. killer T cell
   C. suppressor B cell
   D. memory B cell
2. A major responsibility of the B lymphocytes is
   A. phagocytosis
   B. direct attack on antigens
   C. helper T cell function
   D. antibody production

3. Macrophages are primarily responsible for which of the following?
   A. interfering with the immune response
   B. protecting against local mucosal invasion of bacteria
   C. triggering the complement system
   D. carrying the antigen to B cells and T cells

Answers: 1, B. 2, D. 3, D.

Section Five: Mechanisms of Immunity

At the completion of this section, the learner will be able to describe mechanisms of specific immunity (humoral and cell-mediated immunity) and mechanisms of nonspecific immunity.

The immune system can be described as providing two types of immunity. Humoral immunity is based on the activity and characteristics of the B cell lymphocyte. Cell-mediated immunity is based on the role of the T cell lymphocyte. Figure 17–6 depicts the differential development of cellular and humoral immunity mechanisms with regard to antigen recognition and memory. In contrast, the nonspecific immune response is initiated solely on the recognition of foreign material being nonself antigens and not on their particular identity.

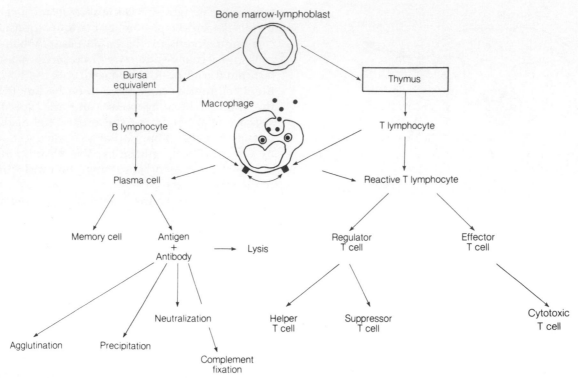

Figure 17–6. Development of cellular and humoral immunity. (*From* Pathophysiology: Concepts of altered health states, *2nd ed.,* p. 180, by C.M. Porth, 1986, London: J.B. Lippincott.)

Specific Immunity

Humoral Immunity

Humoral immunity consists of the activity of the B cell lymphocytes. These lymphocytes mature with exposure to an antigen, develop into plasma cells, and produce specific antibodies or immunoglobulins. Each plasma cell is capable of producing only one type of antibody and thus becomes committed to produce antibody only to a specific antigen. Each plasma cell then produces identical cells capable of continuing production of antibody in response to a particular antigen. Some of the offspring of a particular plasma cell continue to produce antibody, while other cells of that set become memory cells for the particular antigen.

The immunoglobulins are in the globulin fraction of the plasma protein. Each has a distinct amino acid chain that creates its specificity to react with a particular antigen. Because of this basic protein matrix of antibodies, the nutritional status of the individual in general and the protein status in particular are critical to an actively functioning immune system. Five classes of immunoglobulins (Ig) have been identified (Table 17–1). The plasma cell becomes the

TABLE 17–1. CLASSES OF IMMUNOGLOBULINS

Class	Percent of Total	Characteristics
IgG	75.0	Present in majority of B cells; contains antiviral, antitoxin, and antibacterial antibodies; only immunoglobulin that crosses the placenta; responsible for protection of newborn; activates complement and binds to macrophages
IgA	15.0	Predominant immunoglobulin in body secretions, such as saliva, nasal and respiratory secretions, breast milk; protects mucous membranes
IgM	10.0	Forms the natural antibodies, such as those for ABO blood antigens; prominent in early immune responses; activates complement
IgD	0.2	Action is not known; may affect B cell maturation
IgE	0.004	Binds to mast cells and basophils; involved in allergic and hypersensitivity reactions

From *Pathophysiology: Concepts of altered health states,* 2nd ed., p. 181, by C.M. Porth, 1986, London: J.B. Lippincott.

producer of immunoglobulin. Each of the five types plays a particular role in the immune response (Tribett, 1989).

The most common immunoglobulin is called IgG (gamma globulin). It comprises approximately 75 percent of the immunoglobulins and is found circulating in body fluids. It is the only immunoglobulin that is known to cross the placental barrier. IgG contains several types of antibodies, including antiviral, antibacterial, and antitoxin. It also activates the complement system. Gamma globulin can be administered as passive immunity via inoculation.

The immunoglobulin IgA comprises approximately 15 percent of the total immunoglobulins. It is found in large quantities in secretory body fluids, such as tears, saliva, breast milk, and vaginal, bronchial, and intestinal secretions. IgA affords the body a more local protection against invading organisms. The foreign material might well encounter the IgA antibody long before it encounters the IgG antibody. IgA provides protection at the mucosal level of invasion, whereas IgG provides protection more systemically from the position of circulating body fluids.

Smaller amounts of other immunoglobulins play roles in the immunity processes. The immunoglobulin IgM is instrumental in forming such natural antibodies as ABO antigens in the red blood cells. It occurs early in the immune response to most antigens and is also important in activating the complement system. The function of IgE seems to be most prevalent in allergic and hypersensitivity reactions involving the mast cells. The function of IgD is uncertain at the present time.

Humoral Response Patterns. Humoral immunity, the recognition of antigen and the production of specific antibody, occurs with a primary and secondary response pattern (Figure 17–7). During the primary response period, there is a latency period before the antibody can be detected in the serum. This delay or latency period may be 48 to 72 hours after exposure. This represents the time needed for the antigen to be recognized as nonself and identified specifically and for antibodies to be formed in response to the particular molecular makeup. After this latency period, a blood/serum test should reflect the level of antibody to a particular antigen and the degree of immune response. This level of antibody is called the *antibody titer.* The antibody titer normally continues to rise for about 10 days to 2 weeks. At the peak of the titer is generally when recovery is occurring from most infectious diseases.

The secondary response occurs with subsequent exposures to the same antigen. It is during this time that the memory cells of the plasma clones recognize the antigen almost immediately and initiate the immune response with heightened antibody formation. If a titer were to be drawn at this exposure, one would find the antibody titer to be higher than that of the primary exposure. The follow-up booster regimen of many vaccines, such as tetanus, takes advantage of this secondary response and boosts the titer of specific antibodies to a level that will prevent the disease from occurring. This is the rationale for administering a tetanus booster within 24 hours of a new puncture wound.

Cell-Mediated Immunity

Cell-mediated immunity is based on the activity and characteristics of the T cell. During this portion of the immune response, the T cell and macrophage predominate, creating a direct attack on invading antigens. T cell immunity provides protection from intracellular organisms (such as viruses, fungi, and parasites), cancer cells, and foreign tissue. It is the T

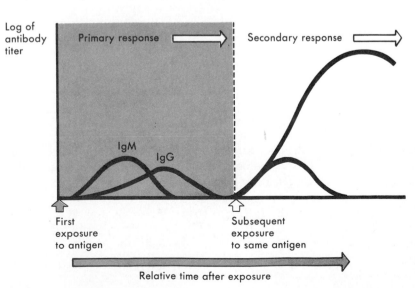

Figure 17–7. Primary and secondary responses of humoral immunity to same antigen. The introduction of antigen induces a response dominated by two classes of immunoglobulins, IgM and IgG. IgM predominates in the primary response, with some IgG appearing later. After the host's immune system is primed, another challenge with the same antigen induces the secondary response, in which some IgM and large amounts of IgG are produced. (*From Pathophysiology: The biologic basis for disease in adults and children, p. 195, by K. McCance and S. Huether, 1990, St. Louis: C.V. Mosby Co.*)

cell that is also responsible for much of the rejection phenomenon of transplanted organs and grafts. It is, however, one of the body's primary surveillance and attack mechanisms for protection from growth of malignant cells.

Unfortunately, T cell protection is not readily transferred from one individual to another, as humoral protection is. Cell immunity depends heavily on thymus and lymph node integrity as well as a nutritionally healthy body.

Complement System

The complement system is an immune mechanism that resembles the blood coagulation cascade, in that, once initiated, it progresses through several sequential stages, each contributing to the immune response and resulting in cellular destruction or cytolysis. The precursors to the complement pathways are normally circulating in the bloodstream. They are only activated by specific agents, such as the immunoglobulins IgG and IgM. The complement system is instrumental in facilitating phagocytosis by making antigens more susceptible to digestion, lysis antigen cell membranes, and attraction of phagocytes to the invading antigen.

Nonspecific Immunity

Phagocytosis

Phagocytosis is a nonspecific immune response whereby invading foreign materials or injured cells are ingested and destroyed by phagocytic cells. Both neutrophils and macrophages are instrumental cellular components to this immune mechanism. Phagocytosis involves chemotaxis, the chemical attraction

of phagocytic cells to antigens, as well as the engulfing of antigens for purposes of destruction or neutralization. A process known as *opsonization* modifies the antigen, making it more susceptible to phagocytosis. Two circulating factors enhance the opsonization process. The IgG immunoglobulin and C3b, a fragment of the complement system, are called opsonins and provide binding sites for attachment of macrophages or neutrophils to the antigen.

Interferons

The interferons also play an important but nonspecific role in the immune response. Interferons serve as the first-line defense in the protection of the body against viruses and other intracellular pathogens. Interferon inhibits the synthesis of viral protein in their reproduction without inhibiting the host's protein synthesis in normal cell reproduction. Interferons are a subfamily of lymphokines originating from effector T cells. Although they are pathogennonspecific, they are species-specific. Thus animal interferons offer little if any protection for human beings as vaccines. However, there is growing interest in the possible role of interferons as cell growth regulators in the study of malignant tumor control.

In summary, to maintain a total surveillance function, the immune system must be diverse enough to provide protection from foreign agents with a variety of immune mechanisms. Specific immune response mechanisms include humoral immunity with the formation of antibodies (immunoglobulins) and cell-mediated immunity with its direct attacking T cells. Nonspecific protection is provided with phagocytes and interferons, which recognize nonself as being foreign but do not specifically program themselves for each individual antigen.

Section Five Review

1. Humoral immunity is best characterized by which of the following?
   A. development of antibodies from B cells
   B. recognition of self and nonself
   C. specific recognition and memory of antigens
   D. differentiation of cellular function known as killer, helper, and suppressor cells

2. The immunoglobulin that comprises about 75 percent of the total immunoglobulin in the healthy human body is
   A. IgA
   B. IgE
   C. IgG
   D. IgM

3. The immunoglobulin that locally protects the body at the mucosal level from invading organisms is
   A. IgA
   B. IgE
   C. IgG
   D. IgM
4. Which of the following statements is correct regarding cell-mediated immunity?
   A. depends on B cell and macrophage activity
   B. part of surveillance mechanism for malignant cells
   C. very easily transferred to an individual
   D. does not protect against invading viruses

5. Interferons act by inhibiting the synthesis of _____, thus limiting abnormal cell growth.
   A. complement
   B. immunoglobulins
   C. lymphokines
   D. viral proteins

Answers: 1, A. 2, C. 3, A. 4, B. 5, D.

Section Six: Pathogenesis of Hypersensitivity

At the completion of this section, the learner will be able to explain the theoretical concepts of the occurrence of types I, II, III, and IV immunoglobulin hypersensitivity and autoimmune diseases.

Although there are several types of hypersensitivity reactions recognized as immune responses, only those particularly associated with the acutely ill adult are discussed here. Of the four recognized categories of hypersensitivity reactions, types I, II, and III involve humoral immunity and specific immunoglobulins. Type IV is a cell-mediated response. Whereas some hypersensitivity responses manifest themselves with uncomfortable symptoms of watery eyes, sneezing, and nasal congestion, other more serious manifestations include the anaphylactic shock response, transfusion reactions with decreased oxygenation to major organs, and allergic asthma responses.

Immunoglobulin Hypersensitivity

Type I Response

One type of hypersensitivity is the allergic response. The true type I allergic response to an antigen results from immunoglobulin IgE activity with mast cells found in the tissues (Figure 17–8). Mast cells, part of the inflammatory process, are known to release histamine and other vasoactive substances when stimulated by immunoglobulin. In addition to histamine, which increases vascular permeability, an eosinophil chemotactic factor is released that attracts eosinophils, an anaphylactic substance causes constriction of smooth muscle (such as in the bronchiole), and a platelet-activating factor causes platelet aggregation

or clumping and lysis. In sensitized individuals, subsequent exposure to an irritating allergen/antigen initiates the antigen-IgE-mast cell interaction, and the immune response and inflammatory response cause symptoms to develop.

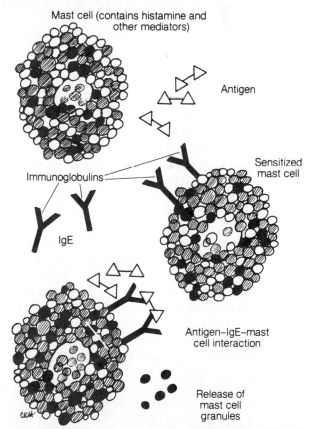

Figure 17–8. Allergen, immunoglobulin, and mast cell interaction, type I. Exposure to the allergen causes sensitization of the mast cell with subsequent binding of the allergen, which causes release of mast cell granules containing inflammatory mediators, such as histamine and SRS-A. (*From* Pathophysiology: Concepts of altered health states, *2nd ed., p. 197, by C.M. Porth, 1986, London: J.B. Lippincott Co.*)

Allergic asthma is an especially noteworthy example of a type I response. The anaphylactic substance causing smooth muscle constriction in the bronchioles as well as the histamine release causing edema of the bronchial tissues warrant close monitoring and often emergency treatment to prevent death by asphyxiation. Antihistamines may block the effect of histamine release, but corticosteroids often are used to suppress the entire immune response. Such an allergic response may be fatal if not interrupted immediately. There is little if any involvement of T lymphocytes in this process.

Type II Response

A type II hypersensitivity response is referred to as a *cytotoxic reaction*. The immunoglobulins or antibodies known as IgM and IgG react directly with cell surface antigens, activate the complement system, and produce direct injury to the cell surface. Transfusion reactions are one example of this type of hypersensitivity. In such reactions, erythrocyte (RBC) surfaces are damaged by antibodies, and the cell is destroyed. Massive numbers of destroyed RBCs not only impair the oxygen-carrying capacity but may obstruct and damage vascular walls and cause kidney damage or failure.

Type III Response

The type III reaction is an example of an immune complex reaction involving antigen-antibody complexes with IgG and IgM immunoglobulins. Type III reactions are characterized by deposits in the epithelial lining of blood vessels. An inflammatory reaction begins as the complement system is initiated by the immune complex, and vessels become occluded with edema, hemorrhage, clotting, and accumulation of neutrophils. One example of the type III reaction is the Arthus reaction. Although it may be considered transient and treatable in some body systems, in the case of a graft tissue rejection, the graft may become necrotic from the vasculitis and fail to recover. The Arthus reaction also may occur in other parts of the body unrelated to graft rejection, such as the alveoli, gastrointestinal tract, and skin from fungal antigens, gluten intolerance, and drug therapy.

Type IV Response

Cell-mediated type IV hypersensitivity responses involve primarily the T lymphocytes and no antibody activity. Tissue destruction is its hallmark, most notably through direct cellular killing by T cell toxins, lysosomal enzymes, or phagocytosis by macrophage

recruiting. Clinical examples include graft or organ transplant rejection in which the HLA antigen is the principal target. Immunosuppressive drugs, such as azathioprine (Imuran) and cyclosporin (Sandimmune) are given to delay or lessen this acute rejection phenomenon.

Autoimmune Disorders

For reasons yet unknown, the immune system occasionally begins to recognize self as foreign. With the usual physiologic actions, the immune system can set out to destroy self. Just as it cannot distinguish beneficial foreign material from destructive foreign material in the transplant phenomenon, the system recognizes self as foreign and initiates a destructive response in autoimmune diseases. Autoimmunity is an intolerance to one's own body tissue and can involve abnormal activity of B cells, T cells, or the complement system. Many diseases are now attributed to such an autoimmune response, and many others are suspected. Table 17–2 provides a partial list of common autoimmune diseases as summarized from McCance and Huether (1990).

Several theories have been postulated to explain the autoimmune phenomenon. Among them are the possibility of alterations of body antigens by chemical or physical means, similarities in exogenous antigens and self-antigens creating a similar immune response to both, mutations of self-antigens to the point where they begin to appear foreign, an abnormal response to HLA antigens on tissue surfaces, and a theory that proposes that certain antigens in

TABLE 17–2. COMMON AUTOIMMUNE DISEASES

Respiratory
    Goodpasture's disease
Gastrointestinal
    Ulcerative colitis
    Crohn's disease
    Pernicious anemia
Endocrine
    Graves' disease
    Insulin-dependent diabetes mellitus
    Addison's disease
Neuromuscular
    Multiple sclerosis
    Cardiomyopathy
    Myasthenia gravis
Connective tissue
    Systemic lupus erythematosus
    Scleroderma
    Rheumatoid arthritis
Hematologic
    Autoimmune hemolytic anemia
    Autoimmune thrombocytopenic purpura

the body were hidden from the immune system over a period of years and on their eventual appearance are recognized as foreign.

In summary, hypersensitivity is an exaggerated or inappropriate immune response to an antigen that results in harm to the body. The allergic response is one type of hypersensitivity reaction and commonly involves an antigen from the environment otherwise considered to be nonpathogenic and not intrinsically harmful to most persons. This section described the four types of hypersensitivity responses, type I, II, III, and IV, and gave examples of each. Finally, the concept of autoimmunity was explored as an altered immunity mechanism.

Section Six Review

1. The results of a true type I hypersensitivity response are due to
   A. a histamine precursor causing anaphylaxis
   B. antigen-IgE-mast cell interaction
   C. antigen-antibody complexes deposited in vessel walls
   D. massive numbers of destroyed red blood cells
2. Which of the following characterizes the concept of autoimmune disease?
   A. recognition of self as foreign
   B. exacerbation and death
   C. accelerated production of killer T cells
   D. immunosuppression and altered cortisol levels
3. Theories of the etiology of the autoimmune phenomenon include all of the following EXCEPT
   A. similarities between self-antigens and non-self antigens
   B. abnormal responses to HLA antigens on tissues
   C. chemical alterations of body antigens
   D. altered mast cell composition

4. Which of the following is correct regarding type IV cell-mediated hypersensitivity responses?
   A. involves primarily antibody activity
   B. does not harm body tissues
   C. T cell activity is responsible
   D. directly interacts with cell surface antigens
5. Disorders thought to be autoimmune in etiology include all of the following EXCEPT
   A. chronic bronchitis
   B. ulcerative colitis
   C. pernicious anemia
   D. diabetes mellitus (insulin-dependent)

Answers: 1, B. 2, A. 3, D. 4, C. 5, A.

Section Seven: Incompatibility as Transplant Rejection Phenomenon

At the completion of this section, the learner will be able to describe the three patterns of transplant rejection as a function of hypersensitivity.

Although an intact immune system is one of our best defenses against the ravages of disease-producing pathogens, sometimes the immune response functions to our disadvantage. In a situation, such as transplant organs and grafts, the immune system cannot distinguish between foreign material that is ultimately to the body's benefit and foreign material that is destructive. For all practical purposes, to the immune cells, any foreign material is detrimental to the host.

Immunologically, tissue of the donor organ (heart, lung, kidney) is different from that of the recipient. The donor antigens that stimulate the immune system attack are primarily those of the ABO blood group found on red blood cells and the HLA antigens found on numerous other tissue surfaces (Muirhead, 1989). After a transplant organ or graft placement, the immune system is activated following its normal mechanisms of B lymphocyte antibody formation, T lymphocyte direct attacks, and macrophage ingestion. Among the most destructive of these processes are the killer T cells, which are able to recognize nonself and act immediately to destroy it. The preexistence of antibodies also can be highly destructive to a new graft. B cell proliferation and subsequent antibody formation play a lesser role in the transplant rejection phenomenon. In transplant rejection, the body recognizes the histocompatibility HLA antigens that reside on the donor's tissue to be foreign, and from there the immune response is initiated.

Transplant rejection can be described using three basic patterns: hyperacute, acute, and chronic.

Hyperacute Rejection

The hyperacute rejection begins almost immediately in some patients, perhaps even during surgery, as the transplanted organ becomes cyanotic and mottled rather than pink and viable. This Arthus III vascular reaction is localized at the new graft by antigen-antibody complex vessel occlusion and vasculitis-induced edema. The transplanted organ may become necrotic within minutes. This hyperacute response is rare and is usually the result of preexisting antibodies from prior blood transfusions, pregnancies, or HLA incompatibility.

Acute Rejection

Acute rejection phenomenon usually occurs within the first 2 weeks posttransplant. Acute rejection involves both humoral immunity and cell-mediated immunity. Patients and donors are matched carefully for tissue HLA antigens and ABO antigens pretransplant. Patients frequently are given immu-nosuppressive drugs preoperatively and postoperatively to minimize transplant rejection phenomena. However, some degree of rejection activity is expected in most recipients of both matched and unmatched tissue. The goal of treatment and care is to minimize the immune response to the degree that the organ or graft is not damaged permanently and rendered useless to the recipient. Based on genetic information, the best possible match for tissue transplantation is an identical twin. Beyond that, siblings and parents are the most likely to be closely matched to the recipient. Unrelated individuals have the least likely chance of offering acceptable organs.

Chronic Rejection

Chronic rejection occurs over a period of months and is characterized by a gradual decline in transplanted organ functioning. The T cell seems to be the most damaging mechanism in these situations. Repeated attacks on the transplanted tissue eventually cause the organ to fail.

In summary, the healthy immune system functions to monitor the body for foreign material, identify such material as nonself, and destroy it. Such a system, however, cannot make judgments about whether foreign material is, in fact, beneficial to the body. The transplant rejection phenomenon is one example of a scenario in which a healthy immune system is following its own mechanisms and cues, yet causing great harm to the body and its new organ. Three basic types of rejection were discussed in terms of immune activity: hyperacute, acute, and chronic.

Section Seven Review

1. Which immune component creates the greatest destruction in transplant rejection phenomena?
   A. B lymphocytes
   B. killer T cells
   C. helper T cells
   D. IgG immunoglobulins
2. Which of the following statements is correct regarding hyperactive transplant rejection?
   A. it is rare
   B. it occurs within a month of transplant
   C. it is primarily a type II immune response
   D. it is characterized by poor oxygenation of transplant tissue

3. To minimize the chance of organ transplant rejection, the best tissue match usually comes from
   A. parents
   B. siblings
   C. identical twins
   D. unrelated individuals

Answers: 1, B. 2, A. 3, C.

Section Eight: HIV Disease: A Manifestation of Immunodeficiency

At the completion of this section, the learner will be able to characterize the immunodeficiency pattern of human immunodeficiency virus (HIV) disease, including the mechanisms of transmission and intracellular extension of the disease.

Assuming that the immune system and its component parts are intact and functioning normally, one might expect reasonable protection against invading microorganisms, pathogens, and foreign material. Even in such a case, the body often cannot overcome a pathogenic process. The immune system can be subject to inadequate development, disease, and injury from illness or treatments that can result in deficient immune activity. Such a situation is called an immunodeficiency state.

Primary Immunodeficiency

Characteristics of immunodeficiency may vary widely depending on the basic etiology. For example, T cells may fail to develop because of some embryonic anomaly or genetic code. DiGeorge syndrome is an example of a congenital thymic aplasia or hypoplasia in which there are greatly decreased levels of T cells because of partial lack of a thymus (McCance and Huether, 1990). B cell deficiency also may develop from embryonic dysfunction or developmental delay of an infant's immune system and results in lowered levels of immunoglobulins. A condition in which immunoglobulins are almost totally absent from the circulation is known as agammaglobulinemia.

In some instances, both B cells and T cells are affected, as in severe combined immune deficiencies (SCID). In SCID, the bone marrow stem cells for lymphocyte development may be absent. Affected children spend a good portion of their short lives in an environment of total protection from any antigen. The child who lived much of his life in a sterile environment is an example of SCID. Most primary states of immunodeficiency are the result of either embryonic anomaly, genetic predisposition, or congenital failure of the system to develop, thus occurring almost exclusively in infants and toddlers.

Secondary Immunodeficiency

Secondary immunodeficiency states can occur in adults but usually are the result of other primary diseases, drug therapy, or irradiation therapy. For example, the patient with Hodgkin's disease, a malignancy of the lymphatic tissue, might well suffer from subsequent immunodeficiency following malignant invasion of that lymph tissue. Prolonged corticosteroid therapy is known to suppress the adrenal glands through the negative feedback loop. Eventually, such a suppression creates a situation of immunodeficiency caused by atrophy of lymphoid tissue, decreased antibody formation, decreased development of cell-mediated immunity, and impaired phagocytosis. Finally, immunosuppressive drugs, such as azathioprine (Imuran) and cyclosporine, are administered for the purpose of suppressing the immune response to transplanted organs and grafts.

Humans can become immunodeficient from a direct attack on the immune system by pathogens. When such a situation exists, it is known as acquired immunodeficiency. Acquired immunodeficiency is not primary in that it is not genetically transmitted, nor is it embryonic in the sense of lymphoid tissue failing to develop adequately. It is secondary in the sense that another disease or therapy caused the deficiency.

Cellular Manifestations Characterizing HIV Disease

The immune deficiency characterizing HIV disease is manifested by markedly depressed T lymphocyte functioning, with a reduction of helper T cells (T4), impaired killer T cell activities, and increased suppressor T cells (T8). By selectively invading and infecting T cells, the virus damages the very cell whose function it is to orchestrate the identification and destruction of the virus as antigen. Other cells with the same molecular makeup might also become infected. Eventually, the individual's supply of functional T cells becomes depleted. In a person with a competent immune system, the number of T4 cells ranges from 600 to 1,200 per mm^3, whereas the patient with HIV might have 0 to 500 per mm^3 T4 cells (Grady, 1988). The humoral response in producing antibodies is less affected by the HIV virus. B cell production does not seem to be decreased, but the induction and regulation of the humoral response may be affected by the lack of T cell regulators (e.g., T4 cell helpers and T8 cell suppressors).

Viral Invasion

The HIV, or human immunodeficiency virus, was known formally as the human T cell lymphotropic virus (HTLV-III). The HIV virus is a retrovirus, carrying genetic information in RNA rather than in DNA. It infects the T cell by binding to it at the CD4 receptor

HIV life cycle

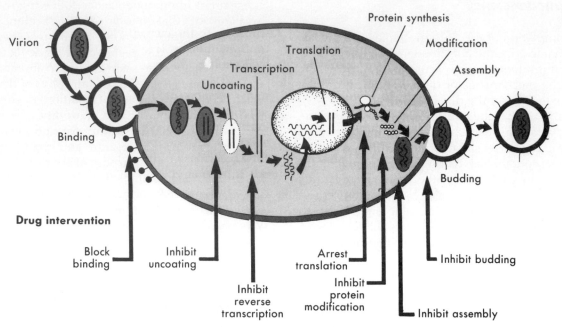

Figure 17–9. HIV life cycle. (*From* Pathophysiology: The biologic basis for disease in adults and children, *p. 273, by K. McCance and S. Huether, 1990, St. Louis: C.V. Mosby Co. [Original but adapted from Yarchoan, Metsurya, and Broder, 1989].*)

site and inserting its RNA into the T cell. Through an enzyme called reverse transcriptase, the HIV RNA is converted to DNA (Figure 17–9). When the T cell is activated to reproduce, its genetic information is now programmed to produce more of the HIV virus, and functional T cells diminish rapidly. Most antiviral drugs now being tested or used in treatment regimens work by inhibiting the action of reverse transcriptase. AZT, or azidothymidine, is one of the few drugs carrying FDA approval for this use (Gee et al, 1989).

HIV Screening

The antibody to this virus has been identified and can be used for screening purposes. However, the latency period, the time the body takes to recognize nonself and program antibodies to the virus, is longer than with many other infectious organisms. The latency period for blood-transmitted HIV infection is thought to be within 4 to 7 weeks, and antibody formation for infection through sexual contact is thought to be from 6 to 14 months. The prolonged latency period thus effectively reduces the accuracy and immediacy of host identification. One of the theories concerning this prolonged latency period is that HIV invades T cells and, in effect, sequesters itself from view of the body's surveillance system, meanwhile multiplying anomalous T cells that are ineffective for purposes of immunity.

Screening for the antibody is helpful only to the extent that individuals can be identified who have been exposed to HIV. However, not all of these individuals actually carry the virus, nor will all of them show signs of illness. Therefore, several situations are possible.

1. Exposure. An individual may be exposed to the virus but neither carry it nor contract the disease.
2. Carrier. The individual may carry the virus with the capability of infecting others but without accompanying signs and symptoms.
3. Terminal disease. The individual may be infectious, symptomatic, and terminal. It is only after signs of opportunistic infections begin to develop that an individual is actually determined to have the disease.

Some suggest that the average incubation period for HIV, that is, from infection to clinical symptoms, is estimated to be from 4 to 6 years (Curran et al, 1986; CDC, 1987). It is also thought that carriers of the virus who test positive for the antibody can remain as carriers for years with the virus in a dormant state. Although approximately one third of those who now test positive for the disease eventually will begin to show clinical manifestations, it is thought by some investigators that the percentage of those who go on to develop the disease will eventually approach 100 percent (Grady, 1988).

Clinical Manifestations

Clinical manifestations of HIV generally are related to opportunistic infections preying on an impaired immune system. These diseases include Kaposi's sarcoma, *Pneumocystis carinii* pneumonia, tuberculosis, and others. The HIV patient commonly succumbs to uncontrollable infection, becoming increasingly debilitated, feverishly ill, malnourished, and often in pain. Lymphadenopathy, pulmonary infiltrates, wasting syndrome, and neurologic abnormalities, such as dementia, tremors, and encephalitis, contribute to the debilitated state. Because the HIV travels from cell to cell rather than through the bloodstream, it is usually not susceptible to circulating antibodies of the body's remaining immune system of B cells. To date, there is no predictable course of curative treatment, and the mortality rate continues to be approximately 60 percent for symptomatic individuals.

Treatment Approaches

Two approaches to treatment have been theorized and tested, both offering little success in curbing the disease. Restoration of immune function may be attempted by bone marrow transplant, transfusions of white blood cells, and interferon treatments. Unfortunately, the newest healthy cells are quickly infected by the virus. Antiviral therapy, such as AZT, has been attempted, but the HIV virus is so variable (much like the variations of flu virus) that a medication formulated against one genetic strain of virus may not provide protection against other strains. Because of the prolonged latency period of HIV, an anti-HIV agent may be required for an individual's protection for up to 9 years or longer to eradicate the virus (Gee et al, 1989). Other treatment approaches are symptomatic, and still others continue to be under experimental investigation.

Epidemiology and Transmission of the Virus

Populations generally thought to be the major contributors to the current HIV epidemic in the United States were first identified as homosexuals and persons using IV drugs while sharing used needles. However, studies now show that the disease has become more widely disseminated to include heterosexual groups and all races and ethnic groups represented in the United States. This pattern of homosexual/bisexual men and IV drug users is particular to advanced or industrialized nations. Heterosexual men and women seem to contract the disease at about an equal rate, however, in African and Caribbean countries (CDC, 1988).

The mode of transmission seems to be blood and body secretions, excluding saliva and tears. The most common modes of transmission seem to be sexual contact, administration of contaminated blood and blood products, contaminated needles, and mother to fetus. Although blood transfusions of whole blood, packed cells, and fresh frozen plasma are most unlikely to be the cause of transmission with the more sophisticated crossmatching and antibody screening measures, individuals needing specific blood components (such as factor VII and frequent plasma replacement) are more at risk because of the large numbers of donors needed to produce adequate quantities of these components. The risk of acquiring the virus increases with the numbers of potential carriers involved, just as multiple sexual contacts create higher risk.

In summary, the basic concept of HIV transmission, cellular transformation, epidemiology, treatment, and outcome has been discussed. Great strides have been made in the last few years in an attempt to understand this disease and to begin to research its detection, treatment, and cure. It is impossible to cover all the aspects of this immunodeficiency disease adequately in such a brief space and to approach currency in information. The learner is encouraged to seek out current information as it becomes available while building on the basic concepts presented in this section.

Section Eight Review

1. Immunodeficiency originating from embryonic anomaly, genetic predisposition, or congenital failure is categorized as
   A. primary
   B. secondary
   C. acute
   D. chronic
2. Which of the following best characterizes HIV disease?
   A. symptoms result from opportunistic pathology
   B. the HIV virus invades cells primarily through the bloodstream
   C. clinical manifestation is a characteristic and predictable sequence
   D. people testing positive for HIV are carriers and contagious

3. Fluids known to be modes of transmission for the HIV virus include
   A. tears
   B. perspiration
   C. plasma
   D. saliva
4. Opportunistic diseases associated with AIDS are all of the following EXCEPT
   A. *Pneumocystis carinii* pneumonia
   B. Kaposi's sarcoma
   C. tuberculosis
   D. acute tubular necrosis

Answers: 1, A. 2, A. 3, C. 4, D.

Section Nine: Aging, Malnutrition, Stress, Trauma, and the Immune System

At the completion of this section, the learner will be able to describe the pathogenesis of aging, malnutrition, trauma, and stress related to the function of the adult immune system.

Aging

The function of the immune system diminishes with increasing age. T lymphocyte function and specific antibody responses are particularly depressed, but in contrast there is an increasing number of autoantibodies (Petrucci et al, 1989). In the older population, the thymus is quite minimal in size and function. T cells, although continuing to be produced and circulated, are deteriorating in function, thus impairing cell-mediated immunity. The very purpose of the immune system as a surveillance system is compromised, as manifested in more frequent infections, diminished capability to overcome infection, and increased evidence of cancer. Whereas helper T cells are less functional, it also seems that suppressor T cells are more active, a major factor in impaired humoral immunity in the elderly. In effect, as the body becomes older, it is less capable of responding to invading antigens and instead turns its immune response more toward self. It is not uncommon to see sharply elevated incidences of diseases thought to be autoimmune in the elderly (Table 17–2).

Malnutrition

Nutritional deficiencies, always a possibility in the acutely ill adult and which should always be a concern to caregivers, can have a profound impact on the immune system. Basic components of calorie and protein intake play key roles in the formation and integrity of T cells. Severe deficits affect both number and function of these cells. The humoral response seems to be less affected by malnutrition, although the activity of macrophages and the complement system is depressed, and more frequent infections occur. Zinc plays a major role in the structure and function of both B cells and T cells and in collagen synthesis for wound healing (Huggins, 1990). As a cofactor, zinc is required for normal function of lymphocytes in their production of enzymes. Although zinc deficiencies do not normally occur with regular eating habits, it can be lost from the body in dangerous amounts through the gastrointestinal tract by malabsorption syndrome or inflammatory bowel disease, characterized by severe diarrhea. It also can be lost through the skin in burn victims. Several vitamins also serve as cofactors in enzyme production and, during deficient states, affect the function of both T cells and B cells. These vitamins include A, E, pyridoxine, folic acid, and pantothenic acid.

Stress

Stress affects the immune system primarily through the effects of cortisol. During periods of stress, either physical or psychologic, the adrenal glands produce more cortisol in response to needs based on increased metabolism, but cortisol has a directly suppressing effect on the immune system. Normally, when an antigen enters the body, a series of reactions takes place. The antigen is recognized as nonself, and it is presented to T cells by macrophages. The macrophages secrete interleukin 1, which activates helper T cells, and these helper T cells produce interleukin 2, which stimulates more T cell production. Finally, B cells may be stimulated to program antibodies to the antigen. Cortisol inhibits the production of interleukin 1 and 2, thus decreasing the T cell response and the subsequent B cell response.

Trauma

Trauma, both intentional (such as surgery) and accidental (such as burns, motor vehicle accidents, and falls) suppresses both T cell and B cell function. Research shows that trauma can cause cellular dysfunction characterized by decreased chemotactic and phagocytic activities and decreased antibody and lymphocyte levels (Barber, 1986; Gann and Amaral, 1985). Although the degree of immunosuppression directly correlates with the severity of the injury, the cause for such changes is unclear (Huggins, 1990). Additionally, several medications can suppress the immune response. Among these are glucocorticoids, general anesthetic agents, and cytotoxic drugs (Tribett, 1989).

The serum of a burn patient contains substances that suppress all immune responses regardless of the origin of the antigen. For the patient with extensive burns, this nonspecific suppression leaves them vulnerable to massive infectious episodes. Most aspects of cell-mediated immunity are depressed following a major thermal injury. Complement component concentrations are reduced by massive activation at the burn site, limiting macrophage activity in preparing antigens for T cell and B cell immune activity (Robins, 1989). Concentrations of lymphokines, derived from T cells, also are decreased, including interleukin 2, which promotes antibody formation by the humoral immune response. Humoral immunity is depressed as IgG (gamma globulin) immunoglobulin is markedly reduced, as are IgA and IgM levels. These immunoglobulins return to normal levels in approximately 2 weeks postburn (Robins, 1989). It is also the burn patient who is likely to become malnourished over time due to pain, immobility, and depression and who might also experience immune suppression related to increased cortisol in response to stress.

In summary, the stressors of illness, age, and trauma play a significant role in immunosuppression, seemingly just when the body is in acute need of protection against invading antigens. The maintenance of one's nutritional status is a common problem in most instances of trauma and illness, as is the excess production of cortisol during periods of psychologic or physical stress. Nutritional deficits of protein, zinc, and calories, along with atrophic changes with aging and the added circulating cortisol during stress, can prove to be devastating to the body's immune system.

Section Nine Review

1. What is the function of zinc in the competent immune system?
   A. it is required for normal lymphocyte function
   B. it protects B cells from being destroyed by macrophages
   C. T cells require zinc for production of gamma globulin
   D. macrophages are composed primarily of zinc

2. What effect does the normal aging process have on the immune system?
   A. B cell function in general is particularly depressed
   B. T cells begin to deteriorate in functioning
   C. autoantibodies begin to diminish with increasing age
   D. immune system becomes hypervigilant to invading organisms

3. In the acutely ill adult, which of the following nutritional losses to the body is a critical factor in the immune system integrity?
   A. iron
   B. vitamin C
   C. complex carbohydrate chains
   D. protein

4. Stress primarily affects the immune system through the effects of
   A. lymphokines
   B. interleukin
   C. cortisol
   D. epinephrine

Answers: 1, A. 2, B. 3, D. 4, C.

Posttest

1. Which of the following is primarily responsible for production of B cells?
   A. bursa equivalent
   B. thymus
   C. stem cells
   D. spleen

2. In defending the body, the immune system is activated after which of the following defenses is unsuccessful?
   A. inflammatory response
   B. skin integrity
   C. phagocytosis
   D. interferons

3. Specific immunity is best described as
   A. antigen-antibody response
   B. foreign material filtration
   C. phagocytosis
   D. interferon antiviral activity

4. By which of the following ways is passive immunity acquired?
   A. exposure to live antigen through inoculation
   B. vaccination with antiserum, such as tetanus toxoid
   C. genetic determination
   D. exposure to IgA antibodies

5. The best definition of antibody titer is
   A. the amount of a specific antibody in a serum
   B. the presentation of processed T lymphocytes
   C. the synthesis of circulating immunoglobulins
   D. the molecular weight of an antigenic determinant

6. Matching of HLA antigens is particularly critical before which of the following?
   A. blood transfusions
   B. factor VIII replacement
   C. organ transplantation
   D. in vitro fertilization

7. Which of the following cells is responsible for the synthesis of circulating immunoglobulins?
   A. suppressor T cells
   B. B cells
   C. macrophages
   D. memory cells

8. The macrophage is primarily responsible for antigen destruction by
   A. lysis
   B. neutralization
   C. differentiation
   D. phagocytosis

9. Cell-mediated immunity is best characterized by
   A. specific recognition and memory of antigen
   B. primary and secondary response patterns
   C. subsets of IgG, IgA, IgE, IgM, IgD
   D. direct attack on invading antigens

10. Which of the following immunoglobulins is found in large quantities in secretory body fluids?
    A. IgA
    B. IgE
    C. IgG
    D. IgM

11. IgG, also known as gamma globulin, is comprised of several types of antibodies and
    A. provides local antibody protection in the mucosa
    B. crosses the placental barrier
    C. can be administered as active acquired immunity
    D. functions with mast cells in hypersensitivity responses

12. The best definition of the complement system is
    A. a nonspecific immune response of engulfing and ingesting foreign antigens by neutrophils
    B. the body's first line of defense against viruses
    C. the body's surveillance system for malignant cells
    D. a progressive, sequential immune response activated by IgG and IgM

13. Which of the following is an example of a type IV hypersensitivity reaction?
    A. blood transfusion reaction
    B. host transplant rejection
    C. allergic asthma
    D. Arthus reaction

14. Which of the following is commonly thought of as being an autoimmune phenomenon?
    A. transplant rejection
    B. polio
    C. *Pneumocystis carinii*
    D. ulcerative colitis

15. What characterizes chronic rejection of transplanted tissue?
    A. visible mottling and cyanosis of tissue
    B. results from preexisting antibodies or HLA incompatibility
    C. commonly seen in most transplant recipients to some degree
    D. gradual decline in transplant function, resulting in eventual organ failure

16. For which of the following has HIV treatment been largely disappointing?
    A. treatment against one genetic strain may not provide protection against other evolving strains
    B. the virus does not attach to immunoglobulin antigenic sites as other antigens do
    C. the HIV virus blocks the complement system
    D. HIV invades B cells and sequesters itself from view of the body's immune system

17. Why are individuals who receive specific blood components more at risk for acquiring HIV than the average person who receives whole blood or packed cell transfusion?
    A. the screening procedures lack the sophistication of whole blood testing
    B. the risk increases with the large numbers of donors required to produce therapeutic amounts
    C. the HIV virus is more difficult to detect in blood components than in whole blood or packed cells
    D. the virus attaches to large amounts of factor VIII and platelets

18. How do increased levels of cortisol released during stress affect the immune system?
    A. increases the production of glycogen
    B. cortisol inhibits the production of interleukin 1 and 2
    C. stimulation of T cell production is enhanced by cortisol
    D. higher levels of cortisol cause accelerated production of immunoglobulins by B cells

19. Zinc plays a major role in B cell and T cell production. For what reasons might an acutely ill adult have a zinc deficiency?
    A. prolonged periods of IV potassium replacement
    B. malabsorption syndromes accompanied by severe diarrhea
    C. third-space fluid deficit
    D. hyperosmolar dehydration

20. In what ways is the immune system thought to be compromised in the patient with extensive burns?
    A. their serum contains substances that suppress all immune responses
    B. zinc levels may become dangerously high, with extensive epidermal loss
    C. T cells are suppressed, but B cell activity and antibody production generally are unaffected
    D. dehydration creates an imbalance between humoral and cell-mediated immunity

Posttest Answers

Question	Answer	Section	Question	Answer	Section
1	A	One	11	B	Five
2	B	Introduction	12	D	Five
3	A	Three	13	B	Six
4	B	Two	14	A	Six
5	A	Two	15	D	Seven
6	C	Three	16	A	Eight
7	B	Four	17	B	Eight
8	D	Four	18	B	Nine
9	D	Five	19	B	Nine
10	A	Five	20	A	Nine

REFERENCES

Barber, J. (1986). Immunological responses to trauma. *Crit. Care Nurse Q.* 9(1):57–67.

CDC. (1987). Human immunodeficiency virus infection in the United States: A review of current knowledge. *MMWR.* 36(6):1–48.

CDC. (1988). Update: AIDS-Worldwide. *MMWR.* 37(18):286–295.

Curran, J., Jaffe, H., Hardy, A., et al. (1986). Epidemiology of HIV infection in the United States. *Science.* 239:610–616.

Dolan, J.T. (1991). *Critical care nursing: Clinical management through the nursing process.* Philadelphia: F.A. Davis Co.

Gann, D., and Amaral, J. (1985). Pathophysiology of trauma and shock. In G. Zuidema, R. Rutherford, and W. Ballinger (eds). *The management of trauma,* 4th ed., pp. 37–103. Philadelphia: W.B. Saunders Co.

Gee, G., Wong, R., and Moran, T. (1989). Current treatment strategies for HIV infection. *Semin. Oncol. Nursing.* 5(4):249–254.

Grady, C. (1988). HIV: Epidemiology, immunopathogenesis, and clinical consequences. *Nursing Clin. North Am.* 23(4):683–696.

Huggins, B. (1990). Trauma physiology. *Nursing Clin. North Am.* 25(1):1–10.

McCance, K., and Huether, S. (1990). *Pathophysiology: The biologic basis for disease in adults and children,* pp. 192–216, 220–225, 249–278. St. Louis: C.V. Mosby Co.

Muirhead, J. (1989). Heart and heart-lung transplantation. *Nursing Clin. North Am.* 24(4):870–880.

Petrucci, K., Booth-Blaemire, E., and Watson, K. (1989). Aging, immunity, and critical care nursing. *Crit. Care Nursing Clin. North Am.* 1(4):787–795.

Porth, C.M. (1986). *Pathophysiology: Concepts of altered health states,* 2nd ed., pp. 130–142, 144–155. London: J.B. Lippincott Co.

Robins, E. (1989). Immunosuppression of the burned patient. *Crit. Care Nursing Clin. North Am.* 1(4):767–774.

Tribett, D. (1989). Immune system function: Implications for critical care nursing practice. *Crit. Care Nursing Clin. North Am.* 1(4):724–740.

ADDITIONAL READING

Warden, G. (1987). Immunologic response to burn injury. In J. Boswick (ed). *The art and science of burn care,* pp. 113–121. Rockville, Maryland: Aspen.

Wright, E.R. (1987). Biological defense mechanisms. In W. Phipps, B. Long, and N. Woods (eds). *Medical surgical nursing: Concepts and clinical practice,* 3rd ed., pp. 1883–1942. St. Louis: C.V. Mosby Co.

Module 18

Acute Renal Failure

Michelle Rountree and Kathleen Dorman Wagner

The focus of the module, *Acute Renal Failure,* is on the physiologic as well as pathophysiologic processes involved in acute renal failure (ARF). Nursing management is addressed primarily in Module 19, *Nursing Care of the Patient with Altered Metabolism.* This module is composed of eight sections. Sections One and Two discuss normal renal function and then shift focus to abnormal kidney function, specifically ARF. Sections Three through Seven present causes, types, and stages of ARF, laboratory tests and procedures used for diagnosing ARF, and the effects of ARF on fluid and electrolyte balance. Section Eight completes the module, with an overview of dialysis concepts. Each section includes a set of review questions to help the learner evaluate understanding of the section content before moving on to the next section. All section reviews and the Pretest and Posttest in the module include answers. It is suggested that the learner review those concepts that have been missed in the review questions before proceeding to the next section.

Objectives

At the completion of the module, *Acute Renal Failure,* the learner will be able to

1. Briefly explain normal kidney function
2. Discuss the influences of selected body systems on renal function
3. Identify the causes of acute renal failure as prerenal, intrarenal, or postrenal
4. Describe the stages of acute renal failure
5. Discuss laboratory tests and procedures used in the diagnosis of acute renal failure
6. Describe the effects of acute renal failure on fluid and electrolyte balance
7. Explain the physiologic implications of acute renal failure
8. Discuss dialysis as a treatment modality for acute renal failure

---

Pretest

1. The functional unit of the kidney is the
   A. nephron
   B. glomerulus
   C. renal tubule
   D. Bowman's capsule

2. Fluid and solutes are moved from the vascular system into the tubular system of the nephron by
   A. tubular reabsorption
   B. glomerular filtration
   C. vascular resistance
   D. tubular secretion

3. A receptor that increases the blood pressure by increasing production of antidiuretic hormone (ADH) is
   A. baroreceptor
   B. chemoreceptor
   C. osmoreceptor
   D. stretch receptor

4. Aldosterone's influence on the maintenance of body fluid levels is based on which of the following principles?
   A. sodium follows water
   B. potassium follows sodium
   C. water follows sodium
   D. sodium follows potassium

5. Approximately ___ percent of patients treated early in the course of acute renal failure have little to no residual loss of renal function.
   A. 10
   B. 25
   C. 50
   D. 75

6. Acute tubular necrosis (ATN) is caused primarily by which of the following two factors?
   A. myoglobin and nephrotoxic drugs
   B. hypoperfusion and myoglobin
   C. myoglobin and hemoglobin
   D. nephrotoxic drugs and hypoperfusion

7. Renal ischemia has which of the following effects on renal blood flow?
   A. vasospasm
   B. vasodilation
   C. vasoconstriction
   D. decreased vascular resistance

8. The early diuretic stage ends when the BUN and creatinine
   A. cease increasing
   B. begin to drop
   C. slow their increase
   D. return to normal

9. Which of the following laboratory values can be used to differentiate acute tubular necrosis from prerenal hypoperfusion?
   A. BUN and chloride
   B. calcium and chloride
   C. sodium and potassium
   D. specific gravity and urine osmolality

10. Renal biopsy would most likely be used to further investigate which of the following?
    A. prerenal failure
    B. intrarenal failure
    C. renal thrombosis
    D. renal calculi obstruction

11. Which of the following imbalances most commonly occur secondary to acute renal failure?
    A. hyperkalemia, hypernatremia, metabolic acidosis
    B. hypokalemia, hyponatremia, hypercalcemia
    C. hyperkalemia, hypocalcemia, metabolic alkalosis
    D. hypernatremia, hypermagnesemia, hypercalcemia

12. Potassium imbalance secondary to acute renal failure is associated with all of the following factors EXCEPT
    A. increased excretion
    B. metabolic acidosis
    C. decreased excretion
    D. increased tissue breakdown

13. Which of the following statements is true regarding the cardiovascular effects of acute renal failure?
    A. it causes hypotension
    B. it causes congestive heart failure
    C. it causes atherosclerosis
    D. it causes increased renal blood flow

14. Acute renal failure can precipitate gastrointestinal bleeding due to increased levels of
    A. uric acid
    B. creatinine
    C. urea
    D. ammonia

15. Common rapid access sites for short-term hemodialysis are
    A. subclavian and femoral veins
    B. femoral and brachial arteries
    C. radial and femoral arteries
    D. internal jugular and subclavian veins

16. Which of the following statements is correct regarding diffusion?
    A. it occurs up a concentration gradient
    B. it moves particles (solute) across a membrane
    C. it occurs down a concentration gradient
    D. it disperses solute within a solution with no membrane

Glossary

Acid-base balance. A stable concentration of hydrogen ions in body fluids

Acidosis. An increased hydrogen ion concentration in the blood or a pH less than 7.35

Active transport. Movement of substances across a membrane without a pressure gradient, using energy

Acute renal failure (ARF). The rapid onset of impaired renal function associated with oliguria/anuria and azotemia

Acute tubular necrosis (ATN). A destructive process of the renal tubules

Aldosterone. A hormone produced by the adrenal cortex, responsible for excretion of potassium and absorption of sodium in the renal tubules, leading to reabsorption of water into the blood volume

Anion. An electrolyte with a negative charge

Antidiuretic hormone (ADH). A hormone produced by the hypothalamus and secreted by the posterior pituitary

Anuria. Cessation of urine production

Autoregulation. A compensatory mechanism that maintains renal blood flow even when there is a great variance in perfusion pressure

Azotemia. The accumulation of uremic toxins (urea, uric acid, and creatinine) in the blood

Bowman's capsule. The initial structure of the tubular system of the nephron

Cardiac output (CO). The amount of blood the heart pumps in 1 minute

Cation. An electron with a positive charge

Dialysis. A process of diffusion by which dissolved particles can be transported across a semipermeable membrane from one fluid compartment to another

Diuretic. Medication that reduces the reabsorption of sodium and water in the kidneys, resulting in an increase in urine excretion

Electrolyte. Element or compound that when dissolved in a fluid, dissociates into ions and can carry an electrical current

Glomerular filtration. The process by which fluid and solutes are moved from the vascular system into the tubular system of the nephron

Glomerular filtration rate (GFR). Measurement of the plasma volume that can be cleared of any given substance within a certain time frame

Glomerulus. A cluster of capillaries located in the nephron; its primary function is to filter solutes

Homeostasis. The normal state of chemical balance within the body

Hydrostatic pressure. Capillary pressure produced by the pumping action of the heart

Hyperkalemia. A greater than normal amount of potassium in the blood

Hypertension. Abnormally elevated blood pressure persistently exceeding 150/90

Hypervolemia. Increase in the amount of fluid in the circulating blood volume

Hypotension. Abnormally low blood pressure, inadequate for normal tissue perfusion and oxygenation

Intrarenal acute renal failure. Kidney dysfunction caused by direct damage to the renal parenchyma

Metabolism. The physical and chemical processes that take place in all living organisms as a means of creating and expending energy necessary in growth and homeostasis

Nephron. The functional unit of the kidney

Oliguric. Excretion or formation of abnormally small amount of urine

Passive transport. Movement of molecules from an area of high concentration to an area of lower concentration; does not require the expenditure of energy

Permeability. The capability of spreading or flowing through small holes or gaps

Postrenal acute renal failure. Kidney dysfunction caused by bilateral obstruction of urine flow distal to the kidney parenchyma

Prerenal acute renal failure. Kidney dysfunction caused by inadequate renal blood flow

Tubular secretion. The process by which substances are secreted into the tubules to be excreted in the final stage of urine formation

Uremia. Clinical symptoms of azotemia

Uremic syndrome. A general term used to describe the clinical manifestations associated with renal failure

Abbreviations

ADH. Antidiuretic hormone

ARF. Acute renal failure

ATN. Acute tubular necrosis

CHF. Congestive heart failure

CO. Cardiac output

CVP. Central venous pressure

GFR. Glomerular filtration rate

Section One: Normal Kidney Function

At the completion of this section, the learner will be able to briefly explain normal kidney function.

The Urinary System

The urinary system, with all of its structures intact, includes two kidneys, two ureters, a urinary bladder, and a urethra (Figure 18–1). This system maintains homeostasis by removing waste products and by either conserving or excreting fluid and electrolytes. An individual requires only one functioning kidney to maintain normal regulatory mechanisms. The kidneys are the only means by which urine is transported and excreted.

The Kidney

A cross-sectional view of the kidney reveals the cortex, medulla, and pelvis (Figure 18–2). The cortex and medulla are called the *renal parenchyma*. The medulla contains the renal pyramids, or collecting ducts. The pyramids house all of the nephrons, which are composed primarily of tubular structures and blood vessels surrounding the nephrons. The nephrons produce urine, which then drains to the papilla, located at the base of the pyramid. The papilla acts as a collecting area, funneling urine to the renal pelvis, where it flows out of the kidney via the ureter. Renal blood supply to the kidney is from

the renal artery, a direct branch of the aorta. The renal artery subdivides further, with some branches nourishing the kidney and others taking part in the filtration process. The majority of the blood being filtered (about 99 percent) returns to the normal circulation via the renal vein (Baer and Reiley, 1984).

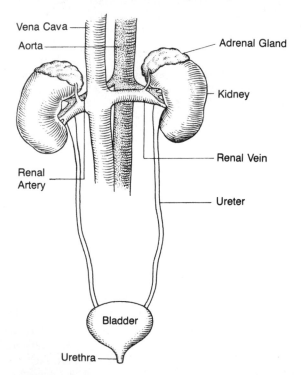

Figure 18–1. Gross anatomy of the renal system. (*From* Nephrology nursing: Concepts and strategies, *p. 2, by B.T. Ulrich, 1989, Norwalk, CT: Appleton & Lange.*)

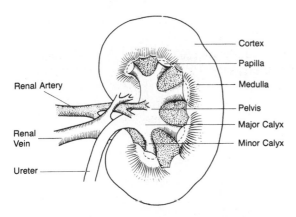

Figure 18–2. Gross anatomy of the kidney. (*From* Nephrology nursing: Concepts and strategies, *p. 3, by B.T. Ulrich, 1989, Norwalk, CT: Appleton & Lange.*)

The Nephron

The nephron is the functional unit of the kidney. Each nephron is composed of three major structures: a glomerulus, tubular apparatus, and collecting duct (Figure 18–3). There are approximately 1.25 million nephrons in each kidney composed of vascular (blood flow) and tubular (urine flow) systems that promote the formation of urine. The vascular system of a nephron includes the glomerulus and vasa recta. The glomerulus is composed of a tight cluster of capillaries, an afferent loop, which becomes the glomerulus, and an efferent loop, which continues on distal to the glomerulus to become the vasa recta, encircling the convoluted tubules and the loops of Henle.

Surrounding each glomerulus is a Bowman's capsule, the initial structure of the tubular system. Connected to the Bowman's capsule is the proximal convoluted tubule which then becomes the loop of Henle. The loop of Henle is a hairpin-shaped section of the tubule. At the distal end of the loop of Henle is the distal convoluted tubule. This section is continuous with a system of collecting ducts that becomes progressively larger, eventually dumping urine into the renal pelvis.

The primary function of the nephron unit is to filter waste products from the blood as it flows through the kidneys. Urine formation is made possible by glomerular filtration and tubular reabsorption and secretion. Figure 18–4 shows nephron transport of substances, as well as their fate in the filtration process.

Glomerular Filtration. Glomerular filtration is the process by which fluid and solutes are moved from the vascular system into the tubular system of the nephron, from an area of relatively high pressure to an area of low pressure. The glomerulus is a high-pressure, semipermeable capillary bed. For filtration

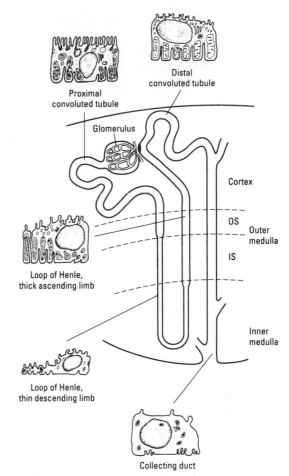

Figure 18–3. The nephron. (*From* Review of medical physiology, *13th ed., p. 581, by W.F. Ganong, 1985, East Norwalk, CT: Appleton & Lange.*)

to occur, there must be adequate blood volume in the intravascular space and adequate hydrostatic pressure from the cardiac output (CO) and vascular resistance. Glomerular filtrate is composed of

- Water (H_2O), hydrogen ions (H^+)
- Electrolytes: sodium (Na^+), potassium (K^+), calcium (Ca^{2+}), magnesium (Mg^{2+}), chloride (Cl^-), bicarbonate (HCO_3^-), phosphate (PO_4^{2-})
- Waste products: urea, creatinine, uric acid
- Metabolic substrates: glucose and amino acids

The glomerular filtration rate (GFR) measures the plasma volume that can be cleared of any given substance within a certain time frame. In a person with normal renal function, the GFR is about 180 L/day. The GFR can be used as an indicator of the adequacy of renal function. The rate of glomerular filtration is altered by any disease condition that alters plasma flow through the glomeruli or the permeability of the cell membrane (Ulrich, 1989).

Tubular Reabsorption. Not all filtrate is excreted. Some is reabsorbed and returned to the blood

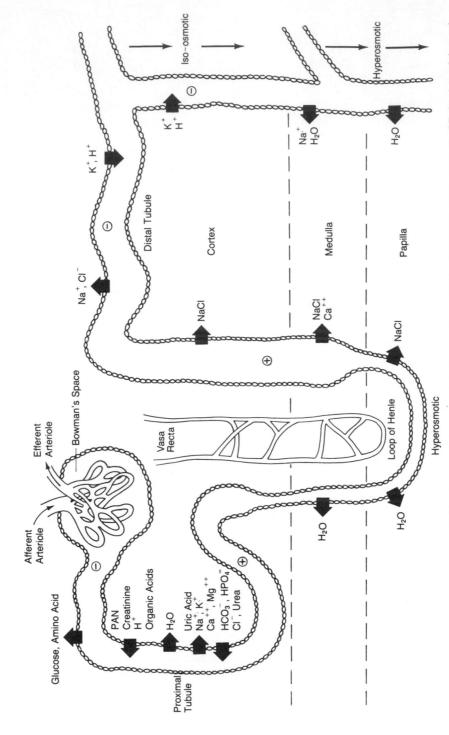

Figure 18–4. Nephron transport. (*From* Nephrology nursing: Concepts and strategies, *p. 15, by B.T. Ulrich, 1989, Norwalk, CT: Appleton & Lange.*)

through tubular reabsorption. Tubular reabsorption is accomplished in the proximal convoluted tubules of the kidneys. Reabsorption occurs due to two transport systems.

1. Active transport. Movement of substances across a membrane without a pressure gradient, using the expenditure of energy. Potassium, sodium, calcium, phosphates, glucose, and amino acids all require active transport (Baer and Reiley, 1984).
2. Passive transport (or diffusion). Movement of molecules from an area of higher concentration to an area of lower concentration. Passive transport does not require an expenditure of energy. Water, chloride, urea, and some phosphate and bicarbonate are reabsorbed by passive transport.

Tubular Secretion. Tubular secretion is the process by which substances, such as potassium, hydrogen, and antibiotics, are secreted into the tubules to be excreted in the final stage of urine formation. The final concentration or dilution of urine occurs in the distal tubules and collecting ducts that lead to the bladder. The volume of urine excreted is about 1,500 mL/day.

In summary, the kidneys are the primary organs responsible for excretion of body wastes and excess fluid, electrolytes, and metabolites. The nephron is the functioning unit of the kidneys and is composed of a glomerulus, Bowman's capsule, and tubular system. Glomerular filtration is the process by which fluid and substances are moved across the nephron vascular cell membrane into the tubular system for either reabsorption or eventual excretion. Glomerular filtration occurs by either an active or a passive transport system. Two hormones, antidiuretic hormone (ADH) and aldosterone play an important part in sodium, potassium, and water regulation.

Section One Review

1. The functional unit of the kidney is the
   A. nephron
   B. ureter
   C. medulla
   D. glomerulus
2. The term renal *purenchyma* refers to
   A. renal pelvis
   B. renal tubules
   C. renal tissue
   D. renal blood supply
3. Fluid and solutes are moved from the vascular system into the tubular system of the nephron by
   A. tubular reabsorption
   B. glomerular filtration
   C. vascular resistance
   D. tubular secretion

4. The movement of substances across a membrane without a pressure gradient using energy is called
   A. active transport
   B. tubular secretion
   C. passive transport
   D. tubular reabsorption
5. The urinary system controls the level of waste products by
   A. excreting hydrogen ions
   B. conserving body water
   C. conserving or excreting excess nutrients
   D. excreting or conserving fluid and electrolytes

Answers: 1, A. 2, C. 3, B. 4, A. 5, D.

Section Two: Influences of Body Systems on Renal Function

At the completion of this section, the learner will be able to discuss the influences of selected body systems on renal function.

Renal function depends on the interrelated functioning of the cardiovascular, nervous, and endocrine systems.

Cardiovascular System

The heart and blood vessels provide the kidneys with sufficient plasma to permit regulation of water and electrolytes in the body fluids. The cardiovascular system delivers blood to be filtered, sustains the blood pressure necessary for filtration to occur, and provides the nephron vascular system. The total renal blood flow is about 180 L/day or about 20 percent of the CO (Baer and Reiley, 1984).

Nervous System

The nervous system helps regulate blood pressure through the sympathetic nervous system. Several types of receptors located in large arteries in the neck and chest help maintain normal arterial blood pressure. Baroreceptors are sensitive to blood pressure changes, activating the hypothalamus when stimulated to alter antidiuretic hormone (ADH) production appropriately.

Chemoreceptors in the carotid and aortic bodies send messages to the vasomotor center to increase blood flow when hydrogen and carbon dioxide content is high and oxygen levels are low. In addition, hypothalamic osmoreceptors are sensitive to changes in water osmolality. As water osmolality changes, the osmoreceptors communicate these changes to the hypothalamus, which results in altered ADH production.

The nervous system influences fluid balance by regulating the thirst mechanism. The thirst center is located in the brain's hypothalamus and is highly sensitive to fluid osmolarity. In circumstances, such as cellular dehydration, the hypothalamus sends impulses to stimulate thirst. Conversely, the drive to drink is diminished when overhydration is present.

Endocrine System

The endocrine system affects renal function directly through secretion of two hormones, ADH and aldosterone. ADH is produced by the hypothalamus and secreted by the posterior pituitary. It is responsible for the ability of water to follow sodium as it is excreted or reabsorbed (Ulrich, 1989). ADH secretion is stimulated by baroreceptors, which are sensitive to changes in arterial blood pressure, and by osmoreceptors, which are sensitive to changes in serum osmolarity. It increases the permeability of the nephron cell membranes to water, allowing more water to be reabsorbed. Urinary output declines in response to the action of ADH.

Aldosterone, produced by the adrenal cortex, is influenced by serum levels of sodium and potassium. Aldosterone causes the kidney tubules to excrete potassium and absorb sodium, leading to a reabsorption of water into the blood volume. Fluid

deficit stimulates production of this hormone. Angiotensin is a major controller of aldosterone secretion and thus is crucial in control of sodium levels. It also is an important part of the renin-angiotensin system, which strongly influences arterial blood pressure, as well as water and sodium regulation.

Compensatory Mechanisms

Compensatory mechanisms for maintaining renal perfusion and prevention of ischemic damage are the renin-angiotensin mechanism and autoregulation.

Renin-Angiotensin System. The renin-angiotensin system is important in control of blood pressure. Renin is an enzyme secreted by the juxtaglomerular apparatus of the kidneys. It is theorized that a decreased blood pressure, low intratubular sodium, or possibly catecholamines may stimulate renin production. Once produced, renin combines with angiotensin I. Ultimately, angiotensin I, originating in the liver, causes peripheral vasoconstriction and also stimulates aldosterone release. Aldosterone stimulates the expansion of the circulatory volume through the reabsorption of sodium and water in the distal tubules. Figure 18–5 shows the sequence of events involved in the renin-angiotensin system.

Autoregulation. Autoregulation maintains renal blood flow by regulating resistance of flow of blood even when there are great variances in perfusion pressure. Through autoregulatory mechanisms, the GFR and renal blood flow remain normal as long as the perfusion pressure remains between 70 mm Hg and 180 mm Hg, a wide variance. Autoregulation is not a well-understood phenomenon. It is known that the kidneys are able to redistribute blood between the cortex and medulla. It is theorized that an increase in pressure causes vasoconstriction of the afferent arterioles, increasing vascular resistance, which makes renal blood flow constant (Ulrich, 1989).

Even with compensatory mechanisms, the GFR is decreased when blood flow in the glomerulus diminishes, passing less water into the filtrate. Thus, with less water being filtered and sodium and water being conserved through compensatory measures, an increase in overall body fluid and hypervolemia can occur (Holloway, 1988).

In summary, renal function is dependent on multiple body systems. The cardiovascular system provides blood to the kidneys for filtering and sufficient blood pressure for perfusion. The nervous system provides special receptors to help control blood pressure and fluid balance. Receptors stimulate the hypothalamus to alter production of ADH to either

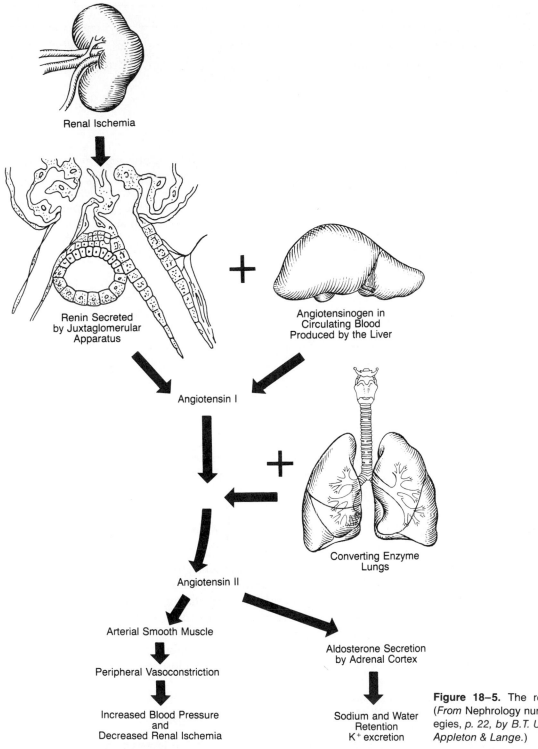

Renal Ischemia

Renin Secreted
by Juxtaglomerular
Apparatus

+

Angiotensinogen in
Circulating Blood
Produced by the Liver

Angiotensin I

+

Converting Enzyme
Lungs

Angiotensin II

Arterial Smooth Muscle

Peripheral Vasoconstriction

Increased Blood Pressure
and
Decreased Renal Ischemia

Aldosterone Secretion
by Adrenal Cortex

Sodium and Water
Retention
K^+ excretion

Figure 18–5. The renin-angiotensin system. (*From* Nephrology nursing: Concepts and strategies, *p. 22, by B.T. Ulrich, 1989, Norwalk, CT: Appleton & Lange.*)

stimulate or inhibit production. The hypothalamus is also responsible for regulation of thirst in response to the level of hydration. The endocrine system in conjunction with the nervous system is responsible for secretion of ADH and aldosterone. ADH alters water reabsorption, and aldosterone alters sodium and potassium serum levels, influencing water balance and arterial blood pressure.

Section Two Review

1. About ____ percent of the cardiac output comprises the total renal blood flow.
   A. 10
   B. 20
   C. 30
   D. 40
2. A receptor that increases the blood pressure by increasing production of antidiuretic hormone (ADH) is
   A. baroreceptor
   B. chemoreceptor
   C. osmoreceptor
   D. ADH receptor
3. Aldosterone's influence on the maintenance of body fluid levels is based on which of the following principles?
   A. sodium follows water
   B. potassium follows sodium
   C. water follows sodium
   D. sodium follows potassium

4. The renin-angiotensin system is important in control of
   A. autoregulation
   B. blood pressure
   C. potassium excretion
   D. ADH production
5. It is theorized that autoregulation works by
   A. vasoconstricting afferent arterioles
   B. vasodilating afferent arterioles
   C. altering basement membrane permeability
   D. altering tubule lumen size

Answers: 1, B. 2, A. 3, C. 4, B. 5, A.

Section Three: Causes of Acute Renal Failure

At the completion of this section, the learner will be able to identify the causes of acute renal failure as prerenal, intrarenal, or postrenal.

Acute renal failure (ARF) is the rapid onset of impaired renal function associated with oliguria/anuria and azotemia. It is associated with loss of renal ability to excrete waste products and loss of the ability to regulate fluid, electrolytes, and acid-base balance. ARF may occur suddenly, within hours, or over a period of days. It is often reversible if diagnosed and treated early. Fifty to sixty percent of patients treated for ARF recover with little to no residual loss of renal function (Baer, 1990). However, if left unrecognized or if inadequately treated, ARF can progress, causing permanent damage of the renal parenchyma.

ARF is categorized on the basis of the location of the insult, being designated as prerenal, intrarenal, or postrenal.

Prerenal Acute Renal Failure

Prerenal failure stems from problems that interfere with renal perfusion, causing renal hypoperfusion.

Underlying conditions that can precipitate prerenal failure include decreased CO and vascular obstruction.

Decreased Cardiac Output

Any problem that significantly diminishes CO can cause prerenal failure (e.g., congestive heart failure, shock, hemorrhage). When CO drops, one of the first compensatory mechanisms to increase CO is vasoconstriction of the kidney capillary beds, to provide more blood to the more critical core organs. Although this serves the immediate needs of the heart and brain, if it is prolonged, renal tissue ischemia results.

Vascular Obstruction

Whereas decreased CO is a systemic cause of ARF, vascular obstruction is a localized cause. When the vessels serving the kidneys suddenly lose their patency, perfusion distal to the obstruction becomes compromised and can precipitate ARF. Examples of obstructions include tumor, embolus, or dissecting aortic aneurysm.

Prerenal failure usually is reversible if the underlying problem is corrected in a timely manner. However, it can progress to intrarenal (commonly acute tubular necrosis) and chronic renal failure if treatment has been initiated too late or has been less than effective.

Intrarenal Acute Renal Failure

Intrarenal failure is caused by problems involving the renal parenchyma (renal tissue). The most common type of intrarenal failure is acute tubular necrosis (ATN), which accounts for about 75 percent of ARF.

Acute Tubular Necrosis

ATN refers to necrosis (death) of renal tubule tissue. It is caused by renal tissue ischemia as a result of inadequate treatment of prerenal failure or by nephrotoxic drugs. Because ATN is associated with tissue destruction, there is a high incidence of permanent renal damage. Tissue ischemia occurs when the mean arterial blood pressure falls below 60 mm Hg and 70 mm Hg (Mars and Treloar, 1984) for more than a 30 minute period (Crandall, 1989).

Drugs commonly associated with nephrotoxicity, a major cause of ATN, include cephalosporin and aminoglycoside antibiotics, nonsteroidal anti-inflammatory drugs, and radiographic contrast dye. Many other agents, such as myoglobin and hemoglobin, also are considered nephrotoxic (Toto, 1990).

Postrenal Acute Renal Failure

Postrenal failure refers to renal dysfunction caused by an obstruction to the outflow of urine from the kidneys. To precipitate renal failure, the obstruction must block urine outflow bilaterally or unilaterally when there is only one operating kidney (Crandall, 1989). Kidney failure is caused by a buildup of pressure caused by the increasing volume of urine proximal to the obstruction. Postrenal failure can be caused by obstruction of the bladder, ureters, or urethra (Jett et al, 1984).

- Bladder, e.g., tumor, infection, anticholinergic drugs, autonomic nerve dysfunction
- Ureters, e.g., renal calculi, tumors, blood clots, edema
- Urethra, e.g., strictures, tumors or prostatic hypertrophy

Section Three Review

1. Congestive heart failure, hemorrhage, and shock are examples of possible etiologic factors for development of which type(s) or renal failure?
   A. prerenal
   B. intrarenal
   C. postrenal
   D. prerenal and postrenal
2. Approximately ____ percent of patients treated early in the course of acute renal failure have little to no residual loss of renal function.
   A. 10
   B. 25
   C. 50
   D. 75
3. Acute tubular necrosis (ATN) is caused primarily by which of the following two factors?
   A. myoglobin and nephrotoxic drugs
   B. hypoperfusion and myoglobin
   C. myoglobin and hemoglobin
   D. nephrotoxic drugs and hypoperfusion

4. Renal tissue ischemia occurs when the mean arterial blood pressure drops to below ____ mm Hg.
   A. 50–60
   B. 60–70
   C. 70–80
   D. 80–90
5. Drugs that are considered highly nephrotoxic include all of the following EXCEPT
   A. cephalosporins
   B. aminoglycosides
   C. cardiac glycosides
   D. nonsteroidal anti-inflammatory drugs

Answers: 1, A. 2, C. 3, D. 4, B. 5, C.

Section Four: The Stages of Acute Renal Failure

At the completion of this section, the learner will be able to explain the stages of ARF.

The progressive course of ARF can be divided into four stages: onset, oliguric-anuric, diuretic (early) and late diuretic (recovery), and convalescent (Baer, 1990; Crandall, 1989). Changes in renal function may be considered on a continuum that ranges from mild renal impairment to complete renal failure. Renal impairment begins when the kidneys are not able to meet the demands of dietary or metabolic stress. Renal impairment may not be discovered until as much as 80 percent of the nephrons have lost nor-

mal functioning. Hypertrophy and hyperplasia of the remaining nephrons permit an increase in their workload and in their ability to maintain function. Table 18–1 presents the major points relevant to each stage, as summarized from Baer and Reiley (1984), Baer (1989) and Crandall (1989).

In summary, there are four stages of acute renal failure, including onset, oliguric/anuric, diuretic (early and late), and convalescent. These stages occur in the same progressive order, though some patients do not experience a distinct oliguric/anuric stage. Fluids and electrolytes must be monitored carefully and controlled during each stage. Early diagnosis and treatment are crucial to prevent or minimize permanent renal damage.

TABLE 18–1. STAGES OF ACUTE RENAL FAILURE

Stage Time Factor	Comments

Onset stage
  Onset: At time of injury
  Duration: Stage ends when
  1. Oliguric/anuric stage begins, or
  2. Azotemia develops in the absence of an oliguric/anuric stage
  Stage lasts about 2 days
	During the onset stage, the acute renal failure patient is acutely ill due to the underlying disorder as well as the rapid onset of acute renal failure
	Rapid, aggressive interventions are needed; urine output is approximately 20% of normal

Oliguric-anuric stage
  Onset: When urine output falls to <400 mL/24 hours (usually by about 48 hours postinjury)
  Duration: Until early diuresis stage begins
  Stage lasts about 1–2 weeks
  [The term *anuria* is used when the urine output falls to <50 mL/24 hours]
  [The longer the patient remains in this stage, the higher the risk of irreversible renal damage and chronic renal failure]
	The pathophysiology of oliguria secondary to ARF is not well understood; Baer (1990) cites the following five interrelated factors as probable contributors to oliguria onset
	1. Renal vasoconstriction secondary to renal ischemia (causing decreased renal blood to glomeruli)
	2. Endothelial cell edema secondary to loss of cell membrane ion pump associated with endothelial cell anoxia (causing decreased renal blood flow)
	3. Decreased glomerular capillary permeability secondary to tissue ischemia; results in decreased GFR and increased dysfunction of renal tubules
	4. Intratubular obstruction secondary to accumulation of cellular debris from tubular damage associated with tissue necrosis (causing decreased GFR)
	5. Back leak of glomerular filtrate secondary to loss of tubular membrane integrity; filtrate is able to leak through the membrane to the plasma

Diuretic stage
  Early
    Onset: When urine output increases to >400 mL/24 hours
    Duration: Continues until BUN and creatinine stabilize (stop increasing); lasts approximately 1–2 weeks
	Early: Renal tubules are beginning to heal, regaining their integrity; as this stage progresses, urine output may be 1–2 L/24 hours due to inability to concentrate urine and diuretic effect of elevated BUN; fluid and electrolyte levels become difficult to manage

Late (recovery)
    Onset: When BUN and creatinine begin to decrease
    Duration: Continues until BUN and creatinine levels return to normal; lasts approximately 10 days
	Late: Renal function continues to improve as nephrons heal; high urine output continues; careful monitoring and control of fluid and electrolytes necessary

Convalescent stage
  Onset: When laboratory values have returned to normal
  Duration: Ends with return of normal renal function; lasts 6 months to 1 year
	Urine output returns to normal with return of ability to concentrate urine; during this stage, it is important to avoid use of nephrotoxic agents; close monitoring and management of fluid and electrolytes crucial; level of permanent renal damage is evaluated

Section Four Review

1. As many as _____ percent of the nephrons may be lost before significant renal dysfunction is noted.
   A. 40
   B. 60
   C. 80
   D. 100

2. The oliguric/anuric stage of acute renal failure begins when urine output falls to below _____ mL/24 hours.
   A. 50
   B. 100
   C. 200
   D. 400

3. Renal ischemia has which of the following effects on renal blood flow?
   A. vasospasm
   B. vasodilation
   C. vasoconstriction
   D. decreased vascular resistance

4. The early diuretic stage ends when the BUN and creatinine
   A. cease increasing
   B. begin to drop
   C. slow their increase
   D. return to normal

5. During the diuretic stage, urine output remains high due to
   A. lack of secretion of antidiuretic hormone
   B. loss of ability to concentrate urine
   C. lack of secretion of aldosterone
   D. loss of ability to reabsorb sodium

Answers: 1, C. 2, D. 3, C. 4, A. 5, B.

Section Five: Diagnostic Aids in Acute Renal Failure

At the completion of this section, the learner will be able to discuss laboratory tests and procedures used in the diagnosis of ARF.

Blood and Urine Tests

The general diagnosis of ARF is made easily with a variety of serum and urine tests. The relationship of urine and blood osmolality is monitored as an indicator of adequate renal function. When renal function is normal, the urine and blood (plasma) osmolality maintain a direct relationship (i.e., as one rises, the other also will increase). Holloway (1988) explains that if renal perfusion becomes diminished, the urine osmolality will be more elevated than the blood osmolality, and urine specific gravity increases. If there is damage to the renal tubules (i.e., ATN), the urine osmolality will be ≤50 mOsm/kg of the blood osmolality. This symptom is accompanied by a low specific gravity due to the lost ability to concentrate urine secondary to nephron damage. Table 18–2 compares key urine and blood laboratory values in differentiating prerenal ARF and ATN. Further discussion of laboratory testing of acute renal failure is presented

TABLE 18–2. DIFFERENTIATING LABORATORY FINDINGS: PRERENAL ARF AND ATN

Test	Prerenal ARF	ATN
Serum urea/creatinine ratio	High	Low
Urine osmolality	High	Low
Urine sodium concentration	Low	High
Urine specific gravity	High	Low
Urine creatinine/plasma creatinine ratio	High	Low

Adapted from *Nephrology nursing: Concepts and strategies*, p. 51, by B.T. Ulrich, 1989, Norwalk, CT: Appleton & Lange.

in Module 20, *Nursing Care of the Patient with Altered Metabolism*.

Special Procedures

Occasionally, the acutely ill patient requires radiographic testing or invasive procedures to help verify the exact etiology of ARF. The following is a brief description of some of the more common tests performed to help make a differential diagnosis.

Renal Biopsy

Renal biopsy is an invasive procedure performed by needle aspiration of renal tissue. Once obtained, the tissue is examined microscopically. Renal biopsy may be used when the exact nature of intrarenal ARF is unknown.

Intravenous Pyelogram

Intravenous pyelogram (IVP) uses a flat plate film of the abdomen before and after injection of a contrast medium into the kidneys via the bloodstream. The IVP is able to outline the kidneys, showing size, shape, and the ability to concentrate and excrete the dye.

Renal Ultrasound

Renal ultrasound uses high frequency soundwaves directed at the kidneys to measure various densities. Ultrasound can distinguish tumors, fluid masses, and obstruction. Major advantages of renal ultrasound are that it is noninvasive, and it can be performed at the bedside with minimal discomfort to the acutely ill patient.

Computed Tomography Scan

The CT scan uses a three-dimensional concept of radiography by taking x-ray slices of an organ. Masses are detected more easily with this method.

Renal Arteriogram

The renal arteriogram requires injection of a contrast dye into the renal artery via the femoral artery. The arteriogram visualizes blood flow through the renal vessels. Prerenal obstruction can be diagnosed using this method.

In summary, early diagnosis of ARF generally is made on the basis of urine and blood chemistry alterations. Certain tests help differentiate the exact nature of the ARF. The acutely ill patient may require a combination of blood, urine, radiographic, or other tests to help differentiate the etiology.

Section Five Review

1. When a patient experiences diminished renal perfusion, how will the urine/plasma osmolality relationship change?
   A. plasma osmolality decreases more than urine osmolality
   B. urine osmolality decreases more than plasma osmolality
   C. plasma osmolality increases more than urine osmolality
   D. urine osmolality increases more than plasma osmolality
2. Which of the following laboratory values can be used to differentiate acute tubular necrosis from prerenal hypoperfusion?
   A. BUN and chloride
   B. calcium and chloride
   C. sodium and potassium
   D. specific gravity and osmolality
3. Renal biopsy would most likely be used to further investigate which of the following?
   A. prerenal failure
   B. intrarenal failure
   C. renal thrombosis
   D. renal calculi obstruction
4. Which of the following tests would most likely be performed to diagnose a prerenal vascular obstruction?
   A. CT scan
   B. intravenous pyelogram
   C. renal biopsy
   D. renal arteriogram
5. A renal diagnostic procedure requiring contrast dye is
   A. arteriogram
   B. biopsy
   C. ultrasound
   D. computed tomography (CT) scan

Answers: 1, D. 2, D. 3, B. 4, D. 5, A.

Section Six: The Effect of Acute Renal Failure on Fluid and Electrolyte Balance

At the completion of this section, the learner will be able to describe the effects of ARF on fluid and electrolyte balance.

When a patient develops ARF, the kidneys are no longer able to function normally, ceasing to regulate reabsorption and excretion of fluids and electrolytes. The body's fluids (primarily composed of water and electrolytes) are found in essentially every organ system. Therefore, because ARF profoundly alters fluid and electrolyte balance, it also has negative influences on all body systems.

Fluid Balance

The importance of fluid regulation is apparent, considering that 60 percent to 70 percent of the body's composition consists of water. Body water is divided into two compartments, intracellular (fluid within the cells) and extracellular (fluid outside the cells). Intracellular fluid can be further subclassified into intravascular fluid within the blood vessels (plasma) and interstitial water in the tissue spaces.

Failure of the kidneys to excrete water unbalances the normal homeostasis of the body, causing serious consequences. Fluid imbalance triggers one of two problems: hypervolemia, an increase in circulatory and body water, or hypovolemia, an inadequate amount of circulating fluid volume. ARF (during the oliguric/anuric stage) is associated with development of an accumulation of fluids (hypervolemia) produced by failure of the kidneys to perfuse and filter fluids properly. Hypervolemia is associated with many complications, including such problems as congestive heart failure, pulmonary edema, and hypertension.

Electrolyte Balance

In addition to the regulatory mechanisms of the endocrine system, the kidneys control the balance of electrolytes within the body fluid. These electrolytes help maintain fluid osmolarity. The major cations regulated by the kidneys are potassium, sodium, calcium, and magnesium. Major anions under renal regulation include chloride and bicarbonate.

Electrolyte imbalance caused by ARF is associated with the following major conditions: hyperkalemia, hypernatremia, hyponatremia, hypocalcemia, hypomagnesemia, and metabolic acidosis.

Potassium Imbalance

ARF is associated most commonly with hyperkalemia. Hyperkalemia is caused by decreased excretion of potassium by the kidneys and increased cellular release of potassium through tissue breakdown and acidosis. Hyperkalemic changes manifest most frequently in cardiac and neuromuscular changes. Occasionally, hypokalemia is associated with ARF as a possible causative factor. Hypokalemia can alter the interstitium of the renal medulla, impairing renal function and precipitating ARF.

Sodium Imbalance

ARF generally causes increased serum sodium. However, this is not always true. Hypernatremia occurs when the GFR is decreased and sodium is unable to be excreted in sufficient amounts. However, since sodium conservation occurs mainly in the renal medulla, any deterioration of this area of the kidney may cause excessive sodium loss (hyponatremia). For these reasons, sodium levels are variable in ARF.

Calcium and Phosphate Imbalances

Calcium follows a similar reabsorption pathway as sodium (Ulrich, 1989), but serum calcium is reduced in ARF due to decreased absorption from the intestine caused by an inability of the kidneys to produce the active component of vitamin D, 1,25-dihydroxycholecalciferol. Lack of active vitamin D results in diminished use of calcium, causing hypocalcemia. Calcium maintains an inverse relationship with phosphate (PO_4^{2-}). Therefore, as calcium levels decrease, phosphate levels increase, causing hyperphosphatemia.

Magnesium Imbalance

Hypermagnesemia occurs because, like potassium, magnesium is excreted primarily by the kidneys. When the kidneys lose their ability to excrete magnesium, serum levels increase. Hypermagnesemia may also result from use of magnesium-containing drugs, such as antacids.

Further discussion of fluid and electrolyte balance is included in Module 19, *Fluid and Electrolyte Balance.*

Metabolic Acidosis

The kidneys play an important role in maintaining normal pH by urinary excretion of excess hydrogen ions. Metabolic acidosis arises as the result of the kidneys' inability to excrete hydrogen ions. As hydrogen ions build up in the body, the pH falls, becoming increasingly acid. ARF also can cause metabolic acidosis by losing its bicarbonate buffering capabilities.

In summary, ARF has a profound impact on fluid and electrolyte balance. Hypervolemia is caused by an inability of the kidneys to excrete adequate volumes of body fluids, which leads to fluid volume excess. ARF causes electrolyte imbalances primarily through loss of the ability to excrete adequate amounts of electrolytes, such as potassium and sodium. This, in turn, interferes with vitamin D production, precipitating hypocalcemia and hypophosphatemia. Thus, the loss of the kidneys' ability to excrete sufficient amounts of hydrogen ions results in metabolic acidosis.

Section Six Review

1. Interstitial fluid is located
   A. inside the cells
   B. inside the blood vessels
   C. within the tissue spaces
   D. within the intracellular compartment
2. Which of the following imbalances most commonly occur secondary to acute renal failure?
   A. hyperkalemia, hypernatremia, metabolic acidosis
   B. hypokalemia, hyponatremia, hypercalcemia
   C. hyperkalemia, hypocalcemia, metabolic alkalosis
   D. hypernatremia, hypermagnesemia, hypercalcemia
3. Potassium imbalance secondary to acute renal failure is associated with all of the following factors EXCEPT
   A. increased excretion
   B. metabolic acidosis
   C. decreased excretion
   D. increased tissue breakdown

4. An inability of the kidneys to produce 1,25-dihydroxycholecalciferol, the active component of vitamin D, lowers the serum levels of which electrolyte?
   A. sodium
   B. magnesium
   C. phosphate
   D. calcium
5. Metabolic acidosis is closely associated with acute renal failure because of the kidneys' inability to
   A. retain sodium ions
   B. excrete hydrogen ions
   C. retain bicarbonate ions
   D. excrete potassium ions

Answers: 1, C. 2, A. 3, A. 4, D. 5, B.

Section Seven: Physiologic Implications of Acute Renal Failure

At the completion of this section, the learner will be able to explain the physiologic implications of ARF.

The onset of symptoms brought about by a decrease in the GFR varies with differences in etiology, course of the disease, and secondary contributing factors. When GFR falls to 5 percent to 10 percent of normal and continues to decline, a catchall term *uremic syndrome* can be used to symptomatically describe the clinical manifestations.

Clinical symptoms of renal secretory and excretory dysfunction are most easily classified into fluid and electrolyte imbalances, as discussed in Section Three, and more specifically, the effects of fluid and electrolyte imbalances on various body systems.

Neurologic Effects

A decrease in alertness, energy, and thought processing is a common manifestation of uremia. Accumulation of nitrogenous waste products from impaired renal excretion and metabolic acidosis contributes to a decrease in mental function. Behavioral changes and a decrease in level of consciousness often are noted. Peripheral neuropathy caused by a slowing of peripheral nerve conduction may be present, causing itching, tingling, numbness, and twitching of the extremities (Roberts, 1985). Headaches due to an increase in cerebral fluid are associated with fluid volume excess. Seizure activity may be present secondary to metabolic imbalances caused by sodium and blood urea nitrogen (BUN) abnormalities.

Cardiovascular and Pulmonary Effects

Hypertension and congestive heart failure are the most common cardiovascular manifestations of ARF. Hypertension secondary to ARF is due to (1) systemic and central fluid volume excess and (2) increased renin production. Renin increases blood pressure as a compensatory mechanism of the juxtaglomerular apparatus as it attempts to increase renal blood flow. The presence of fluid volume excess may cause congestive heart failure accompanied by peripheral and pulmonary edema. Fluid volume excess also contributes to development of possible cerebral edema. The cardiovascular system also responds to imbalances of potassium, sodium, hydrogen, calcium, and magnesium with various arrhythmias.

Hematopoietic Effects

ARF is associated with anemia and bleeding tendencies. Anemia is caused by a decrease in erythropoietin, which is produced by the kidneys. There may be a decrease in the life span of RBCs, an increase in blood loss through gastrointestinal tract irritation, and blood loss from hemodialysis, all contributing to the anemic condition. Bleeding tendencies result from dysfunctional platelets caused by the presence of uremic toxins.

Gastrointestinal Effects

Capillary fragility in the gastrointestinal system caused by an increase in ammonia, may lead to ulcerations of the gastrointestinal tract. Anorexia, nausea, and vomiting are not uncommon in uremic syndrome. An increase in toxins may lead to a marked weight loss if uncorrected. Diarrhea or constipation also may occur because of a hypomotility of the bowel from electrolyte imbalances.

Integumentary Effects

Dry, yellow skin is a common characteristic of ARF. In cases of extreme uremia, uremic frost may be noted on the skin from deposits of uric acid crystals. Increased capillary fragility can lead to excessive bruising. Protein wasting may cause the hair to thin and the nails to become thin and brittle.

Skeletal Effects

Because of the limited ability of the kidneys to metabolize vitamin D in ARF, absorption of calcium in the stomach is increased. In long-term acute renal failure, skeletal disorders become inevitable (Holloway, 1988).

Further discussion of the effects of acute renal failure are presented in Module 20, *Nursing Care of the Patient with Altered Metabolism*.

In summary, the failure of the kidneys to function properly influences virtually every major body system. Fluid volume excess precipitates complications of congestive heart failure. Accumulation of nitrogenous wastes profoundly alters mental function. Accumulation of ammonia in the gastrointestinal tract can lead to gastrointestinal bleeding. Skin becomes fragile and susceptible to bruising associated with the presence of uremic toxins and increase capillary fragility. Bones lose mass due to loss of calcium.

Section Seven Review

1. Alterations in mental function secondary to acute renal failure are caused primarily by which of the following?
    A. uremic toxins
    B. magnesium imbalance
    C. hypoglycemia
    D. fluid overload

2. Peripheral neuropathy can manifest itself in all of the following ways EXCEPT
    A. tingling
    B. numbness
    C. itching
    D. seizures

3. Which of the following statements is true regarding the cardiovascular effects of acute renal failure?
    A. it causes hypotension
    B. it causes congestive heart failure
    C. it causes atherosclerosis
    D. it causes increased renal blood flow
4. Acute renal failure can precipitate gastrointestinal bleeding due to increased levels of
    A. uric acid
    B. creatinine
    C. urea
    D. ammonia

5. Which of the following statements best reflects the effects of acute renal failure on the integumentary system?
    A. thickened hair follicles
    B. excessively oily
    C. excessive bruising
    D. thickened nailbeds

Answers: 1, A. 2, D. 3, B. 4, D. 5, C.

Section Eight: Dialysis, An Acute Renal Failure Treatment Modality

At the completion of this section, the learner will be able to discuss dialysis as a treatment modality for ARF.

A major portion of the management of ARF focuses on maintaining fluid and electrolytes within acceptable limits. During the oliguric/anuric stage, severe kidney dysfunction can cause life-threatening abnormalities in fluid and electrolyte levels. Medical management of ARF varies with the type of failure (prerenal, intrarenal, or postrenal). Module 20, *Nursing Care of the Patient with Altered Metabolism,* presents an overview of the medical management of the patient with ARF. This module focuses on dialysis as one distinct feature in the management of ARF.

Early in the course of the disorder, tests may be performed to define the type of renal failure (e.g., diminished renal function secondary to a postshock state—prerenal—vs parenchymal tubular damage—intrarenal—indicative of ATN. To differentiate between these two etiologies, a diuretic challenge may be given, using either mannitol (an osmotic diuretic) or furosemide (a loop diuretic). If the kidneys are able to respond to the diuretic by increasing urinary output, fluid replacement and additional diuretics are given to treat a prerenal type of problem. If, however, there is no response from the diuretic challenge, ATN is considered seriously, and dialysis may be a viable treatment option. Patients who experience the oliguric/anuric stage for more than 4 to 5 days generally require dialysis. Dialysis has significantly improved the prognosis of patients experiencing ATN (Hudak et al, 1990).

Dialysis

Dialysis is a process of diffusion by which dissolved particles are transported across a semipermeable membrane from one fluid compartment to another. Dialysis does not correct renal dysfunction. It only corrects fluid, electrolyte, and acid-base imbalances. Return of normal renal function is dependent on other treatment modalities used to relieve the underlying problem and the ability of the body to heal the damaged tubules. Hemodialysis, continuous arteriovenous hemofiltration (CAVH), and peritoneal dialysis are three types of dialysis used in the treatment of ARF. Regardless of the type of dialysis used, the major electrolytes manipulated during the procedure include potassium, sodium, calcium, phosphorus, magnesium, chloride, and bicarbonate (Thompson et al, 1989).

Hemodialysis

Hemodialysis requires a direct access into the vascular compartment. For short-term use, as is seen frequently in the high acuity patient, temporary access sites may be used. The two most common sites are the subclavian and femoral veins, using the Seldinger technique (Jett et al, 1984). This technique uses a relatively simple percutaneous venous access, which is effective for hemodialysis on a temporary basis. For long-term use, an internal arteriovenous fistula, shunt, or graft may be formed surgically, usually in the lower arm.

Hemodialysis cleans the blood by pumping it out of the patient via the venous access. The blood then passes through a dialyzer, which removes fluid and solutes, returning the filtered blood back to the patient. The semipermeable membrane necessary for diffusion in hemodialysis is penetrable, thin cellophane. The blood comprises the first fluid compartment, and the dialysate is the second one. The semipermeable membrane pores are large enough to allow small substances to pass across (i.e., creatinine, urea and uric acid, and water molecules) but too small to allow larger particles to diffuse (i.e., proteins, blood cells, and bacteria) (Ceccarelli, 1986).

Diffusion occurs down a concentration gradient because the blood has a higher solute concentration than the dialysate has. This causes the flow of urea, creatinine, and other relatively concentrated solutes to move across the semipermeable membrane (the cellophane) into the dialysate solution.

Continuous Arteriovenous Hemofiltration

CAVH is a relatively new type of dialysis used when hemodialysis is not feasible, often due to hemodynamic instability, or peritoneal dialysis is not tolerated. It also may be used in conjunction with hemodialysis to decrease the number of hemodialysis treatments, using the CAVH to remove fluid and the occasional hemodialysis to remove waste products and excess electrolytes. At this time, CAVH is being used primarily in the critical care setting.

Blood enters the CAVH circuit using the patient's own arterial blood pressure. Therefore, both an arterial and a venous access are necessary. The most common access site is the femoral artery and vein. The volume within the extracorporeal circuit at any one time is small, making it less hemodynamically traumatic than conventional hemodialysis.

Blood in the circuit flows past a hemofilter, which maintains a lower pressure than the blood. This pressure difference facilitates movement of solutes and water across its semipermeable membrane. The resulting ultrafiltrate drains into a collection apparatus. The level at which the collection device is hung determines the ultrafiltration rate. The rate of blood flow through the circuit ranges between 30 and 120 mL/minute, with an ultrafiltration rate of 5 to 16 mL/minute. Once the blood passes the hemofilter, it is rediluted with a predetermined bath of electrolytes, water, and nutrients, based on the patient's fluid, electrolyte, and nutritional status (Thompson et al, 1989).

Peritoneal Dialysis

Peritoneal dialysis uses the patient's own peritoneal lining to serve as the semipermeable membrane through which diffusion, osmosis, and filtration occur. The desired outcome of peritoneal dialysis is the same as other forms of dialysis—to remove meta-

TABLE 18–3. COMPARISON OF HEMODIALYSIS, PERITONEAL DIALYSIS, CAVH: NURSING IMPLICATIONS

Factor	Hemodialysis	CAVH	Peritoneal Dialysis
Complications	Infection; decreased cardiac output; cardiac dysrhythmias; disequilibrium syndrome (disorientation, seizures, headache, agitation, nausea and vomiting); air embolism; shunt thrombosis; disconnection hemorrhage	Infection; bleeding; infiltration; air embolus	Infection; decreased cardiac output; fluid volume overload; hyperglycemia; metabolic alkalosis (prolonged use); respiratory insufficiency; abdominal pain
Nursing goals and care	*Maintain shunt, fistula, or catheter patency* *Prevent complications* Monitor vital signs and hemodynamic status Monitor for signs and symptoms of complications Daily sterile shunt site care Daily fistula care until site is healed No blood pressure cuff, injections, IV insertions, or tourniquets on limb with shunt or fistula Check for presence of thrill and bruit; notify physician if either is absent Keep clamps at bedside at all times Monitor laboratory values for therapeutic effects Weigh before and following dialysis	*Maintain catheter patency* *Prevent complications* Monitor vital signs and hemodynamic status Monitor daily for signs and symptoms of complications Assess for patency (presence of palpable thrill and warmth on both tubings) Hourly intake and output Monitor laboratory values for therapeutic effects Daily weights Daily catheter care Observe color if ultrafiltrate	*Maintain catheter patency* *Prevent complications* *Maintain balanced intake and output* Monitor vital signs and hemodynamic status Weigh daily Monitor laboratory values for therapeutic effects Obtain intermittent cultures of drainage dialysate and catheter tip (if removed) Precise documentation of intake and output with every exchange Turn side to side to facilitate drainage Daily dialysis catheter care Observe color of drainage dialysate

Data from *Critical care certification preparation and review*, 2nd ed., by T. Ahrens, 1991, Norwalk, CT: Appleton & Lange.

TABLE 18–4. COMPOSITION OF DIALYSATE

Component	Dialysate Level	Normal Serum Levels
Sodium	133–142 mEq/L	135–145 mEq/L
Potassium	0.0–4.0 mEq/L	3.5–5.5 mEq/L
Chloride	103–105 mEq/L	96–106 mEq/L
Calcium	2.5–3.5 mEq/L	2.1–2.6 mEq/L
Magnesium	1.0–1.5 mEq/L	1.5–2.5 mEq/L
Glucose	0.0–200 mg/100 mL	70–110 mg/dL
Acetate	33–38 mEq/L	—
Bicarbonate	As ordered	24–28 mEq/L

Adapted from *Nephrology nursing: Concepts and strategies*, p. 130, by B.T. Ulrich, 1989, Norwalk, CT: Appleton & Lange.

bolic wastes and correct fluid and electrolyte imbalances. It can be performed either manually or by use of automatic cycling machines. Dialyzing fluid is introduced into the peritoneal cavity via a peritoneal catheter, which is secured in place. Once in the abdominal cavity, it is held there for a specified period of time, allowing adequate time for the transfer of fluid and solutes across the peritoneal lining. Once the dialyzing pass time is completed, the dialyzing fluid, with its additional fluid and solutes, is drained out of the abdomen. Table 18–3 compares hemodialysis, continuous ultrafiltration, and peritoneal dialysis.

Dialysate Solutions

The exact nature of the dialysate is based on the fluid and electrolyte status of the patient. It consists of a combination of water and variable concentrations of electrolytes. Electrolytes common to dialysate solutions include potassium, sodium, chloride, magnesium, and calcium. Electrolyte concentrations are manipulated carefully depending on whether the serum level of each electrolyte is high, low, or within normal range. Because ARF usually is associated with higher than normal levels of potassium, sodium, magnesium, and phosphate, the electrolyte levels in the dialysate solution will be either within normal range or below normal to pull excess electrolytes out of the blood and into the dialysate solution (down the concentration gradient).

Glucose may be added to the solution to increase filtration of fluid. A buffer is included, either bicarbonate or acetate. Buffers help stabilize any existing metabolic acidosis and also keep electrolytes in solution form. Table 18–4 shows a typical example of the composition of hemodialysis dialysate, including normal serum levels of each component.

Advantages and Disadvantages of Hemodialysis, CAVH, and Peritoneal Dialysis

Each type of dialysis has its own set of advantages, disadvantages, and contraindications. Each is evaluated closely based on the patient's needs and physical status. Table 18–5 compares the three types of dialysis, as summarized from Thompson et al (1989).

Drug Therapy and Dialysis

Administration of drugs requires special consideration when the patient is receiving dialysis. First, between intermittent dialysis treatments, drugs that do not break down fully in the body continue to circulate in active form, since they cannot be excreted via the kidneys. Continuing to deliver the usual normal doses in such a patient can lead to severe toxic effects. Second, during dialysis, many drugs are able to cross the semipermeable membrane to be cleansed from the blood, thereby rendering those drugs as nontherapeutic. This capability makes dialysis a useful option for rapid removal of intentional or accidental overdoses of dialyzable drugs.

Nova (1987) explains that certain properties of

TABLE 18–5. INDICATIONS, DISADVANTAGES, AND CONTRAINDICATIONS OF THREE TYPES OF DIALYSIS

Factor	Hemodialysis	CAVH	Peritoneal Dialysis
Indications	Acute poisoning; acute renal failure; chronic renal failure; severe edema states; extensive burns with prerenal azotemia; metabolic acidosis; transfusion reaction; crush syndrome; hepatic coma	Overhydration; cardiovascular instability; parenteral nutrition; uncomplicated acute renal failure; inability to tolerate hemodialysis or peritoneal dialysis	Used when less rapid treatment is appropriate; inadequate vascular access; hemodialysis not available; severe cardiovascular disease; hemodynamic instability
Disadvantages	Requires vascular access; requires use of heparin during process	Requires vascular access; slow dialyzing process; increased risk of contamination	Slower than hemodialysis; abdominal discomfort; decreased mobility; risk of peritonitis
Contraindications	Coagulopathy; age extremes; hemodynamic instability	Drug or agent poisoning; hyperkalemia; low mean arterial blood pressure; hypercatabolism; congestive heart failure; low colloid oncotic pressure	Adhesions of peritoneum or abdomen; peritonitis; recent abdominal surgery

drugs have an impact on the dialyzability. These properties include the following.

Drug Bioavailability. Drug bioavailability is the amount of drug (in active form) that is able to get into the blood. The administration route is important, since some routes get the drug into the bloodstream more rapidly than others. Having knowledge of the length of time it takes a drug to become bioavailable is important in determining when it needs to be given between dialysis treatments to maximize therapeutic effects.

Distribution Time and Volume. Fat-soluble drugs have a higher distribution time and volume in comparison to water-soluble drugs. This group of drugs has less bioavailability because increased volumes are distributed to the tissues. Thus, lower doses are in the bloodstream to be dialyzed out.

Protein Binding. The amount of a drug that is bound to protein influences how dialyzable it is. Dialysis cannot filter out proteins because they are too large. Drugs that bind themselves to proteins also are not filtered out.

Molecular Weight. Drugs with low molecular weights (<500 Da) are easily dialyzed. However, drugs with heavy molecular weights cannot be dialyzed (>2,000 Da).

The nurse caring for the patient receiving dialysis should be aware of which drugs are dialyzable. Many hospitals have a listing of drugs that will be dialyzed out. These drugs should be scheduled appropriately to avoid undesired dialysis. Table 18–6 is

TABLE 18–6. DIALYZABLE DRUGS

Drugs Dialyzed Out of Blood	Drugs Not Significantly Dialyzed Out of Blood
Acetaminophen	Albumin (large protein molecule)
Aspirin	Diazepam (protein bound, low distribution volume)
Captopril	Digoxin (middle molecular weight, stored in tissues)
Mannitol 25%	
Methyldopa	
Metoclopramide (partially)	Furosemide (protein bound)
Protamine sulfate	Heparin (protein bound)
Pyridoxine	Hydralazine (protein bound, low distribution volume)
Theophylline	Iron products (protein bound)
	Levothyroxine (protein bound)
	Nifedipine (protein bound)
	Prazosin HCl (protein bound)
	Prochlorperazine (protein bound)
	Propranolol HCl (protein bound)
	Quinidine (protein bound)
	Verapamil (protein bound)

a partial listing of some common dialyzable drugs as summarized from Nova (1987).

In summary, when the kidneys are no longer able to adequately cleanse the blood of excess waste products, fluid, and electrolytes, artificial means often are required to correct the imbalances. Three methods were described: hemodialysis, peritoneal dialysis, and continuous arteriovenous hemofiltration (CAVH). Each modality carries with it indications, contraindications, and disadvantages. The nurse needs to be aware of the effect of hemodialysis on drug therapy. Problems of either toxic levels or subtherapeutic levels are associated with acute renal failure and dialysis.

Section Eight Review

1. If the patient responds to a diuretic challenge by increasing urine output, you would anticipate which type of follow-up intervention?
   A. hemodialysis
   B. peritoneal dialysis
   C. large doses of diuretics
   D. fluid replacement and diuretics
2. The major purpose of using dialysis is to
   A. remove proteins from the blood
   B. correct imbalances of fluid and electrolytes
   C. remove drugs from the blood
   D. correct renal dysfunction
3. Common rapid access sites for short-term hemodialysis are
   A. subclavian and femoral veins
   B. femoral and brachial arteries
   C. radial and femoral arteries
   D. internal jugular and subclavian veins

4. Which of the following statements is correct regarding diffusion?
   A. it occurs up a concentration gradient
   B. it moves particles (solute) across a membrane
   C. it occurs down a concentration gradient
   D. it disperses solute within a solution with no membrane
5. Continuous arteriovenous hemofiltration (CAVH) would most likely be used on which of the following patients?
   A. 65-year-old patient diagnosed with prerenal failure
   B. hemodynamically stable, 70-year-old cardiac patient
   C. 24-year-old patient diagnosed with postrenal failure
   D. hemodynamically unstable 40-year-old trauma patient

6. When peritoneal dialysis is performed, the semipermeable membrane is the
   A. peritoneal lining
   B. hemofilter
   C. cellophane membrane
   D. renal lining

7. Assuming that a patient's electrolytes have undergone the typical imbalances associated with acute renal failure, the dialysate solution will contain low levels of which of the following electrolytes?
   A. calcium
   B. chloride
   C. potassium
   D. bicarbonate

Answers: 1, D. 2, B. 3, A. 4, C. 5, D. 6, A. 7, C.

Posttest

The following Posttest is constructed in a case study format. A patient is presented. Questions are posed based on available data. New data are presented as the case study progresses.

Maria Gonzales, a 35-year-old teacher, has been admitted through the emergency department after sustaining multiple injuries in a motor vehicle accident (MVA). The emergency medical team relates that when found at the scene of the accident, she was noted to have an arterial blood pressure of 76/42. It was believed that the ambulance had arrived in 35 to 45 minutes after the accident. In the emergency department, she was found to have a ruptured spleen. She was prepared immediately for surgery. She has no known history.

It has been almost 48 hours since the accident. You note that Ms. Gonzales' urine output has been approximately 25 mL for 2 successive hours.

1. For glomerular filtration to take place, it is important that Ms. Gonzales maintain
   A. a low hydrostatic pressure
   B. an adequate cardiac output
   C. a low renal blood volume
   D. a high renal vascular resistance

2. Certain substances, such as potassium and hydrogen, undergo renal tubular secretion. This term refers to the process by which substances are moved
   A. into the tubules for excretion
   B. back into the vascular system
   C. into the interstitial compartment
   D. back into the glomerulus from Bowman's capsule

3. Assuming Ms. Gonzales' nervous system is intact, it would respond to her low blood pressure in which of the following ways?
   A. osmoreceptors inhibit antidiuretic hormone production
   B. stretch receptors vasoconstrict peripheral arterioles
   C. chemoreceptors stimulate production of aldosterone
   D. baroreceptors stimulate antidiuretic hormone production

4. The renin-angiotensin system assists in increasing Ms. Gonzales' arterial blood pressure by
   A. causing vasoconstriction
   B. decreasing circulatory volume
   C. increasing hydrogen ion concentration
   D. inhibiting reabsorption of sodium

The following data are now available. It is believed that Ms. Gonzales' blood pressure remained low for at least 1 hour directly after the accident. The emergency team had difficulty obtaining a vascular access with which to administer fluids. Her daughter has informed you that

Ms. Gonzales has no known chronic conditions except for mild arthritis, which she controls with aspirin on a daily basis.

_____

5. Considering Ms. Gonzales' recent history, which type of acute renal failure is she initially at most risk of developing?
   A. acute tubular necrosis
   B. postrenal
   C. prerenal
   D. intrarenal

Five days have passed since the accident. Ms. Gonzales' urine output has fallen to 350 mL over the past 24 hours. She has just received a diuretic challenge, to which she had no response. Her blood pressure is now 165/94.

_____

6. Considering the latest changes, what specificially, is Ms. Gonzales most likely developing?
   A. prerenal failure
   B. acute tubular necrosis
   C. postrenal failure
   D. intrarenal failure
7. Ms. Gonzales is at high risk for developing renal failure because ischemia occurs when the mean arterial blood pressure drops to below _____ mm Hg for more than 30 minutes.
   A. 50–60
   B. 60–70
   C. 70–80
   D. 80–90

Ms. Gonzales is now in acute renal failure secondary to acute tubular necrosis. Her urine output has been approximately 350 mL/24 hours and her BUN is now 100 mg/dL. She is confused and drowsy.

_____

8. According to the latest data, Ms. Gonzales is experiencing the _____ stage of acute renal failure.
   A. oliguric/anuric
   B. onset
   C. early diuresis
   D. late diuresis

It has been approximately 12 days since the onset of Ms. Gonzales' acute renal failure. Her urine output is now 450 mL over the past 24 hours, and her BUN and creatinine have both leveled off.

_____

9. According to the latest available data, Ms. Gonzales is in which of the following stages of acute renal failure?
   A. oliguric/anuric
   B. late diuresis
   C. onset
   D. early diuresis

Ms. Gonzales' laboratory values are as follows. *48 hours postinjury:* BUN/creatinine ratio 24:1, urine sodium 38 mEq/L, specific gravity 1.028, serum osmolality 650 mOsm/L.
5 days postinjury: BUN/creatinine ratio 13:1, urine sodium 52 mEq/L, specific gravity 1.008, serum osmolality 285 mOsm/L.

_____

10. Ms. Gonzales' pattern of renal laboratory findings are consistent with an initial _____ failure which became a(n) _____ failure.
    A. postrenal, intrarenal
    B. prerenal, postrenal
    C. prerenal, intrarenal
    D. intrarenal, acute tubular necrosis
11. Ms. Gonzales has a renal ultrasound ordered. Which of the following statements is correct regarding ultrasound?
    A. it is an invasive procedure
    B. it requires use of a contrast dye
    C. it can be performed at the bedside
    D. it requires a local anesthetic
12. Ms. Gonzales' serum phosphate is elevated. Which of the following reasons is most likely the cause?
    A. hypermagnesemia
    B. hypocalcemia
    C. hypomagnesemia
    D. hypercalcemia
13. Ms. Gonzales is at risk for developing metabolic acidosis primarily due to
    A. decreased excretion of potassium
    B. increased excretion of hydrogen ions
    C. increased excretion of potassium
    D. decreased excretion of hydrogen ions

Ms. Gonzales is experiencing some of the clinical manifestations of uremic syndrome. She is complaining of tingling and numbness of her hands and feet. She also has developed skin bruising associated with minimal trauma.

14. Ms. Gonzales' new symptoms of tingling and numbness are most likely caused by
    A. hyperkalemia
    B. hypocalcemia
    C. stimulated stretch receptors
    D. peripheral neuropathy
15. Skin bruising in acute renal failure is secondary to the effects of
    A. increased erythropoietin
    B. decreased ammonia levels
    C. severe hypocalcemia
    D. excessive uremic toxins

It has been decided that Ms. Gonzales needs dialysis. Her present status is as follows. She is hemodynamically stable, and she is 8 days postabdominal surgery. She has generalized edema and severe electrolyte abnormalities.

16. Based only on the available data, which type of dialysis is most likely to be ordered for Ms. Gonzales?
    A. hemodialysis
    B. peritoneal dialysis
    C. continuous ultrafiltration
    D. combination of hemodialysis and peritoneal dialysis
17. Ms. Gonzales is receiving a drug that is highly protein bound while in circulation. What would be the significance of drug protein binding and hemodialysis if this treatment would be ordered?
    A. protein-bound drugs will be released during dialysis
    B. protein-bound drugs break down rapidly in the blood
    C. protein-bound molecules are too large to dialyze out
    D. protein-bound drugs in tissues move into circulation during dialysis

Posttest Answers

Question	Answer	Section	Question	Answer	Section
1	B	One	10	C	Five
2	A	One	11	C	Five
3	D	Two	12	B	Six
4	A	Two	13	D	Six
5	C	Three	14	D	Seven
6	B	Three	15	D	Seven
7	B	Three	16	A	Eight
8	A	Four	17	C	Eight
9	D	Four			

REFERENCES

Baer, C.L. (1990). Acute renal failure: Recognizing and reversing its deadly course. *Nursing90.* 20(6):34–40.

Baer, C.L., and Reiley, P.J. (1984). Reviewing fundamental principles. In Nursing84. *Renal and urologic disorders,* pp. 8–27. Springhouse, Pennsylvania: Springhouse Corp.

Ceccarelli, C.M. (1986). Management modalities: Renal system. In C.M. Hudak, B.M. Gallo, and T. Lohr (eds.) *Critical care nursing: A holistic approach,* 4th ed., pp. 362–375. Philadelphia: J.B. Lippincott.

Crandall, B.I. (1989). Acute renal failure. In B.T. Ulrich (ed.) *Nephrology nursing: Concepts and strategies,* pp. 45–59. E. Norwalk, Connecticut: Appleton & Lange.

Ganong, W.F. (1985). *Review of medical physiology,* 13th ed. E. Norwalk, Connecticut: Appleton & Lange.

Holloway, N.M. (1988). *Nursing the critically ill adult,* 3rd ed. ed. Menlo Park, California: Addison-Wesley Publishing.

Hudak, C.M., Gallo, B.M., and Benz, J.J. (1990). *Critical care nursing: A holistic approach.* Philadelphia: J.B. Lippincott.

Jett, M.F., Lancaster, L.E., and Small, S. (1984). Combating acute renal failure. In Nursing84. *Renal and urologic disorders,* pp. 66–85. Springhouse, Pennsylvania: Springhouse Corp.

Mars, D.R., and Treloar, D. (1984). Acute tubular necrosis: Pathophysiology and treatment. *Heart Lung.* 13(2):194–202.

Nova, G. (1987). Dialysis drugs. *Am. J. Nursing.* 87(7):933–942.

Roberts, S.L. (1985). *Physiological concepts and the critically ill patient.* Englewood Cliffs, NJ: Prentice-Hall.

Thompson, J.M., McFarland, G.K., Hirsch, J.E., Tucker, S.M., and Bowers, A.C. (1989). *Mosby's manual of clinical nursing,* 2nd ed., pp. 1021–1085. St. Louis: C.V. Mosby.

Toto, S.L. (1990). Acute tubular necrosis. In B.C. Mims (ed.) *Case studies in critical care nursing,* pp. 291–302. Baltimore, Maryland: Williams & Wilkins.

Ulrich, B.T. (1989). *Nephrology nursing: Concepts and strategies.* Norwalk, CT: Appleton & Lange.

ADDITIONAL READING

Goldberger, E. (1986). *A primer of water electrolyte and acid-base syndromes.* Philadelphia: Lea & Febiger.

Kee, J.L. (1986). Clinical conditions of fluid and electrolyte imbalance. In: *Fluids and electrolytes with clinical applications.* New York: Wiley.

Methany, N.M. (1987). *Fluid and electrolyte balance: Nursing considerations.* Philadelphia: J. Lippincott.

Price, S.A., and Wilson, L.M. (1986). *Pathophysiology: Clinical concepts of disease processes.* New York: McGraw-Hill.

Module 19

Module **19**

Fluid and Electrolyte Balance

Kathleen Dorman Wagner, Karen L. Johnson, Beatrice DiCostanzo,
and Catherine Paradiso

The focus of the module, *Fluid and Electrolyte Balance* is on the physiologic and pathologic processes involved in fluid and electrolyte balance. Maintenance of fluid and electrolyte balance is a major goal in improving the outcomes of patients with diverse health problems. Therefore, in many of the text's modules, fluid and electrolyte balance is addressed as it applies to specific module topics.

Fluid and Electrolyte Balance is composed of nine distinct sections. Sections One and Two present the concepts of body fluid distribution and fluid balance regulation. Section Three focuses on IV fluid administration, including a discussion of crystalloids, blood and blood products, and colloids. In Sections

Four through Six, specific extracellular electrolytes are presented, including sodium, chloride, and calcium. Sections Seven through Nine address three major intracellular electrolytes, potassium, magnesium, and phosphorus. Discussion of each electrolyte includes major functions and the causes, clinical manifestations, and common treatment of imbalances.

Each section includes a set of review questions to assist the learner in evaluating understanding of the section. All section reviews and the Pretest and Posttest include answers. It is suggested that the learner review those concepts answered incorrectly before proceeding to the next section.

Objectives

At the completion of this module, the learner will be able to

1. Discuss the distribution of body fluid

2. Describe the regulation of fluid balance

3. Identify the clinical use and components of three classifications of IV fluids: crystalloids, blood and blood products, and colloids

4. Discuss the extracellular compartment electrolyte, sodium

5. Describe the extracellular compartment electrolyte, chloride

6. Discuss the extracellular compartment electrolyte, calcium

7. Discuss the intracellular compartment electrolyte, potassium

8. Describe the intracellular compartment electrolyte, magnesium

9. Discuss the intracellular compartment electrolyte, phosphorus (phosphate)

Pretest

1. Two thirds of total body fluid is in which of the following compartments?
   A. intracellular
   B. extracellular
   C. intravascular
   D. interstitial

2. All the following predispose an infant to fluid volume deficit EXCEPT
   A. inability to concentrate urine
   B. low metabolic rate
   C. greater ratio of surface area/volume
   D. high metabolic rate

3. Which of the following electrolytes is found predominantly in the extracellular fluid?
   A. potassium
   B. magnesium
   C. phosphate
   D. sodium

4. Which of the following is the primary regulator of water intake?
   A. nervous system
   B. endocrine system
   C. renal system
   D. hypothalamus

5. The nervous system responds to decreased volume by producing
   A. ADH
   B. ACTH
   C. vasoconstriction
   D. aldosterone

6. All of the following produce increased fluid elimination EXCEPT
   A. fistulas
   B. hypothermia
   C. diabetes insipidus
   D. diabetic ketoacidosis

7. A low serum osmolarity may suggest
   A. fluid volume deficit
   B. fluid volume excess
   C. dehydration
   D. isotonic balance

8. Which of the following solutions closely approximates serum osmolarity?
   A. 0.45 percent normal saline
   B. dextrose 5 percent in normal saline
   C. 3 percent normal saline
   D. lactated Ringer's solution

9. A patient's hematocrit is 25 percent. After 1 unit of whole blood, you could anticipate the hematocrit to be
   A. 26–27 percent
   B. 28–29 percent
   C. 30–31 percent
   D. 32–33 percent

10. Signs and symptoms of hypernatremia include
    A. diarrhea
    B. decreased muscle tone
    C. stomach cramps
    D. muscle twitching

11. Hyponatremia is associated with which of the following symptoms?
    A. edema
    B. lethargy
    C. hyperreflexia
    D. restlessness

12. Chloride levels closely follow the levels of which of the following electrolytes?
    A. potassium
    B. sodium
    C. calcium
    D. magnesium

13. Calcium is absorbed in the intestines under the influence of
    A. phosphorus
    B. vitamin D
    C. sodium
    D. vitamin C

14. Hypocalcemia is associated with which of the following symptoms?
    A. tingling and numbness
    B. constipation
    C. lethargy
    D. shortened QT interval

15. Hypokalemia has what effect on the kidney function?
    A. urine output increases
    B. potassium excretion increases
    C. potassium is reabsorbed
    D. potassium is excreted at same rate

16. The normal range of serum magnesium is
    A. 1.5–2.2 mEq/L
    B. 3.5–5.5 mEq/L
    C. 8.5–10.5 mg/dL
    D. 135–145 mEq/L

17. The symptoms of hypomagnesemia reflect
    A. CNS hypoactivity
    B. fluid compartment shifts
    C. cardiac depressant effects
    D. neuromuscular and CNS hyperactivity

18. Hypophosphatemia is associated with which of the following conditions?
    A. malnourished state
    B. metabolic alkalosis
    C. hypocalcemia
    D. hyperthyroidism

19. Severe hypophosphatemia is associated with which of the following symptoms?
    A. joint pain
    B. muscle cramping
    C. respiratory arrest
    D. peptic ulcer disease

Answers: 1, A. 2, B. 3, D. 4, D. 5, C. 6, B. 7, B. 8, D. 9, A. 10, D. 11, B. 12, B. 13, B. 14, A. 15, D. 16, A. 17, D. 18, A. 19, C.

Glossary

Anions. Negatively charged ions.

Baroreceptors. Pressure receptors located in the arch of the aorta and carotid sinus that detect arterial pressure changes

Cations. Positively charged ions

Colloids. Solutions containing protein or starch molecules

Dilutional effect. Net gain of water in the extracellular spaces

Electrolytes. Electrically charged microsolutes found in body fluids

Extracellular. Fluid compartment within the body composed of plasma and interstitial fluid

Hypertonic. A high osmolarity state in which the particle concentration in a solution is less than exists inside the cell (> 295 mOsm/L)

Hypervolemia. Excess volume of circulating fluids

Hypotonic. A low osmolarity state in which the concentration of particles in a solution is greater than inside the cell (< 285 mOsm/L)

Hypovolemia. Decreased volume of circulating fluids

Intracellular. Fluid compartment within the cells composed of approximately two thirds of the total body water

Intravascular. Fluid compartment in the blood vessels; fluid here is available for exchange of nutrients and oxygen

Isotonic. Concentration of particles in a solution on one side of a membrane is the same as it is on the other side of the membrane; it closely approximates normal serum plasma osmolarity (285 to 295 mOsm/L)

Osmolarity. The solute concentration per volume of a solution

Osmosis. The net diffusion of water from an area of greater concentration to an area of lesser concentration across the cell membrane; this movement occurs as the result of osmotic pressure

Tonicity. Osmolarity of an IV fluid

Abbreviations

ACTH. Adrenocorticotropic hormone

ADH. Antidiuretic hormone

ATN. Acute tubular necrosis

BUN. Blood urea nitrogen

CNS. Central nervous system

CVP. Central venous pressure

DKA. Diabetic ketoacidosis

ECF. Extracellular fluid

HHNC. Hyperglycemic hyperosmolar nonketotic coma

ICF. Intracellular fluid

IV. Intravenous

mOsm. Milliosmols

PAWP. Pulmonary artery wedge pressure

PTH. Parathyroid hormone

SIADH. Syndrome of inappropriate antidiuretic hormone

TPN. Total parenteral nutrition

Section One: Body Fluid Distribution

At the completion of this section, the learner will be able to discuss the distribution of body fluid.

Body fluids compose more than 60 percent of the body weight in the average adult male. The composition of body fluids is primarily water with various electrolytes and dextrose, urea, and creatinine. These fluids provide both an internal and an external environment for the cells. Body fluids provide a medium for metabolic reactions, cushion body parts from injury, and influence regulation of body heat (Groer and Shekleton, 1989). The percentage of body water varies depending on age and body fat content.

Variables Affecting Body Fluid Content

Age and body fat content influence total fluid volume. Greater percentages of body fluids are found in individuals with a small body surface area. Thus, infants have a larger fluid reserve—77 percent greater than adults (Brasfield, 1990). Even though infants have a larger fluid reserve, three factors can predispose the infant to a serious, rapid fluid volume deficit: limited ability to concentrate urine, a proportionately greater ratio of surface area/volume, and higher metabolic rate (Groer and Shekleton, 1989). Fluid balance in individuals over age 65 is influenced by a reduction in total fluid body weight. The elderly patient's fluid balance also is affected by alterations in thirst and nutritional intake, diminished renal function, chronic illness, and medications. Decreased muscle mass, smaller fat stores, and a lesser percentage of body fluids collectively create a greater risk for dehydration in the elderly. Body fat content influences total fluid volume, since fat cells do not contain a significant amount of water. Obese individuals, who have a larger body fat content, actually have a smaller percentage of body fluids.

Fluid Compartments

Body fluids are found primarily in two compartments: the intracellular fluid (ICF) and the extracellular fluid (ECF) spaces. Two thirds of total body fluid is intracellular, and the remaining one third is extracellular. The fluid in each compartment has its own major electrolytes.

Intracellular Fluids

Intracellular fluids are located within the cell. Intracellular fluids contain large amounts of potassium, phosphate, and protein and moderate amounts of magnesium and sulfate ions. Intracellular fluids provide cells with nutrients and assist in cellular metabolism.

Extracellular Fluids

Fluid outside the cell is said to exist in the extracellular compartment. The ECF fluids contain the nutrients needed to maintain cellular functions. The ECF circulates between the cells and contains water, electrolytes (particularly sodium, chloride, and calcium), glucose, fatty acids, and amino acids. The ECF compartment is further divided into the intravascular compartment and the interstitial compartment. The intravascular compartment contains plasma, and the interstitial compartment contains fluid in and around tissues.

Third Spacing. Third spacing is the shift of fluid from the intravascular compartment into a third, or extra, space within the extracellular compartment, often a body cavity. Fluids in the third space tend to accumulate and are unavailable for use by the body (Jones et al, 1991). Third spacing can result from such underlying problems as intestinal obstruction, intestinal surgery, liver or renal failure, peritonitis, or thermal injury. Clinically, third spacing manifests itself as ascites, pleural effusion, peripheral edema, compartment syndrome, and other conditions. As the third space volume increases, intravascular volume decreases. Hypovolemia can occur if a hemodynamically significant volume of fluid is absorbed into the third space.

In summary, body fluids compose more than 60 percent of total body weight. Age and body fat content can influence total fluid volume. Three factors are known to predispose infants to rapid fluid volume deficits. The elderly have reduced total body fluid, which can be further reduced by the presence of the normal aging process and disease states. Body fluids are found in the intracellular fluid and the extracellular fluid compartments. Each compartment has its own functions and major electrolytes. Fluid shifts disrupt homeostasis and can result in decreased circulating volume.

Section One Review

1. Two thirds of total body fluid is in which of the following compartments?
   A. intracellular
   B. extracellular
   C. intravascular
   D. interstitial
2. All of the following predispose an infant to fluid volume deficit EXCEPT
   A. low metabolic rate
   B. high metabolic rate
   C. inability to concentrate urine
   D. greater ratio of surface area/volume
3. Which of the following electrolytes is found predominantly in the extracellular fluid?
   A. potassium
   B. magnesium
   C. phosphate
   D. sodium

4. Examples of third space fluids include all of the following conditions EXCEPT
   A. ascites
   B. pleural effusion
   C. congestive heart failure
   D. peripheral edema
5. Body fluids comprise what percentage of total body weight?
   A. 20
   B. 40
   C. 60
   D. 80

Answers: 1, A. 2, A. 3, D. 4, C. 5, C.

Section Two: Regulation of Fluid Balance

At the completion of this section, the learner will be able to describe the regulation of fluid balance.

Nervous System Regulation

The hypothalamus is the primary regulator of water intake. The thirst center in the hypothalamus is stimulated by changes in quantity or quality of fluids in the body.

Baroreceptors (pressure receptors) located in the arch of the aorta and carotid sinus detect arterial pressure changes. When baroreceptors sense a decrease in arterial blood pressure, they send a message to the autonomic nervous system. The sympathetic nervous system responds to this message by causing peripheral vasoconstriction. Vasoconstriction of renal arteries decreases glomerular filtration, which reduces urine output in an attempt to increase circulating blood volume.

Renal and Endocrine Regulation

The renal and endocrine systems work synergistically to regulate blood volume. When the hypothalamus senses a decrease in serum sodium or an increase in serum potassium, it sends a message to

the pituitary to release adrenocorticotropic hormone (ACTH). ACTH stimulates the adrenal cortex to release aldosterone. Aldosterone is called the *salt-regulating hormone*. It regulates water balance by facilitating sodium reabsorption in the ascending loop of Henle and the distal and collecting tubules. The sodium reabsorption produced by aldosterone can increase circulating blood volume and thus increase blood pressure through the reabsorption of water and sodium.

When the hypothalamus detects changes in concentration of body fluid, it also sends a message to the pituitary to release antidiuretic hormone (ADH). ADH stimulates the distal and collecting tubules to reabsorb water, expand the ECF space, and subsequently improve perfusion. The ADH regulating mechanism is further described in Module 8, *Shock States*.

When sodium concentration in the ECF is decreased or blood flow through the kidneys is diminished, the kidneys release renin. Renin combines with angiotensin I, ultimately converting to angiotensin II, which is a powerful vasoconstrictor, causing an increase in blood pressure and subsequent perfusion. The renin, aldosterone, and ADH mechanisms are three endocrine responses to decreased circulating blood volume. For further discussion of the renin-angiotensin system, refer to Module 18, *Acute Renal Failure*, and Module 8, *Shock States*.

Fluid Intake Regulation

Fluid intake is regulated by the hypothalamic thirst center. Neuron cells located in the hypothalamus are sensitive to body fluid concentration. As body fluids become more concentrated, a sense of thirst is triggered. The conscious person responds to thirst by drinking fluids. Clinical conditions that alter the sense of thirst or the individual's ability to respond to thirst ultimately have an impact on the circulating extracellular volume. The unconscious or high acuity patient often can not respond to the thirst signals from the hypothalamus. In the clinical setting, the nurse uses physical assessment and serum laboratory data to assess the need for fluid intake.

Alteration in Fluid Elimination: Increased

Fluid elimination can be increased enormously in the high acuity patient. Conditions that create increased elimination are summarized in Table 19–1. Patients with excessive fluid elimination require additional fluids to maintain a balanced intake and output.

Alteration in Fluid Elimination: Decreased

A decreased volume of urine excretion (less than 30 mL/hour) may be indicative of dehydration or renal failure. Decreased urinary output in the patient with dehydration is actually a protective mechanism for the body to reserve volume. Decreased urinary output in the patient with renal failure leads to fluid volume excess. (Refer to Module 18, *Acute Renal Failure,* for a detailed discussion.)

Alteration in Fluid Balance

Extracellular fluid volume deficit is identified as hypovolemia or dehydration. Fluid volume deficit oc-

TABLE 19–1. CONDITIONS THAT PRODUCE INCREASED FLUID ELIMINATION

Burns

Gastrointestinal losses: Colostomy, ileostomy, fistulas, diarrhea, vomiting, nasogastric suction

Insensible losses: Hyperventilation, hyperthermia, diaphoresis, tachypnea, mechanical ventilation

Excessive use of diuretics

Syndrome of inappropriate ADH (SIADH)

Diabetes insipidus

Diuretic phase of acute tubular necrosis (ATN)

Diabetic ketoacidosis (DKA)

Hyperglycemic hyperosmolar nonketotic coma (HHNC)

TABLE 19–2. NURSING ASSESSMENT OF PATIENT WITH FLUID VOLUME DEFICIT

Assessment	Data
Physical assessment	Weight loss
	Poor skin turgor
	Dry mucous membranes
	Flattened neck veins
	Mental status changes
Vital signs	Orthostatic changes
	Decreased blood pressure
	Rapid, weak, thready pulse
	Rapid, shallow respirations
	Temperature may be elevated
	Low CVP, PAWP
	Decreased CO
Laboratory data	Elevated hematocrit
	Elevated BUN (normal creatinine)
	Low serum osmolarity
Urine	Increased osmolarity
	Increased specific gravity
	Decreased volume
	Dark color

curs when insufficient amounts of sodium and water exist in the extracellular compartment. Assessment of a patient with hypovolemia, dehydration, or both is summarized in Table 19–2.

Nursing interventions may include further encouragement of oral fluids or administration of IV solutions. The expected patient outcomes will include increased cardiac output, increased blood pressure; improved CVP/PAWP; normal serum osmolarity; and increased urine output with normal specific gravity.

Extracellular fluid volume excess produces a state of overhydration. Fluid volume excess in the high acuity patient often is manifested by weight gain. A 1 kg weight gain may represent the retention of 1 L of fluid. Nursing assessment of the patient with fluid volume excess is summarized in Table 19–3.

TABLE 19–3. NURSING ASSESSMENT OF PATIENT WITH FLUID VOLUME EXCESS

Assessment	Data
Physical assessment	Weight gain
	Distended neck veins
	Periorbital edema; pitting edema over body processes
	Adventitious lung sounds, moist rales
	Shortness of breath
	Mental status changes
Vital signs	Elevated blood pressure
	High CVP/PAWP
	Increased CO
Laboratory data	Decreased hematocrit (dilutional)
	High serum osmolarity
	Chest x-ray: pulmonary vascular congestion, pleural effusions

Nursing interventions may include fluid restriction, administration of diuretics, or dialysis. The expected patient outcomes will include decreased blood pressure, decreased CVP/PAWP, lung sounds clear to auscultation, weight loss, and resolution of edema.

In summary, the nervous, renal, and endocrine systems work synergistically to maintain fluid balance. Aldosterone, ADH, and the renin-angiotensin-aldosterone cycle regulate fluid balance. When these physiologic mechanisms fail or when conditions exist that affect fluid elimination, a fluid volume imbalance occurs. Nursing assessment of the patient should include a physical assessment, vital signs, and laboratory data. Nursing diagnoses for alterations in fluid balance may include alteration in elimination, fluid volume deficit, or fluid volume excess.

Section Two Review

1. Which of the following is the primary regulator of water intake?
   A. nervous system
   B. endocrine system
   C. renal system
   D. hypothalamus
2. The nervous system responds to decreased volume by producing
   A. ADH
   B. ACTH
   C. vasoconstriction
   D. aldosterone
3. All of the following produce increase fluid elimination EXCEPT
   A. fistulas
   B. hypothermia
   C. diabetes insipidus
   D. diabetic ketoacidosis

4. A weight gain of 10 kg indicates what volume of fluid volume excess?
   A. 5 L
   B. 10 L
   C. 15 L
   D. 20 L
5. Nursing assessment of the patient with fluid volume excess would include
   A. moist rales
   B. decreased blood pressure
   C. low PAWP
   D. increased hematocrit

Answers: 1, D. 2, C. 3, B. 4, B. 5, A.

Section Three: Intravenous Fluid Administration

At the completion of this section, the learner will be able to identify clinical use and components of three classifications of IV fluids: crystalloids, blood and blood products, and colloids.

Osmolarity

The osmolarity of a solution is the solute (or particle) concentration per volume of solution. Osmolarity is expressed in milliosmols (mOsm), with normal serum osmolarity being 285 to 295 mOsm/L. Clinically, serum osmolarity can be used to determine fluid replacement in the high acuity patient.

The principle of osmosis explains the net diffusion or movement of water across the cell membrane (Groer and Shekleton, 1989). Water moves across a semipermeable cell membrane from an area of lesser concentration of solutes to an area of greater concentration of solutes. Osmosis is a passive process, requiring no expenditure of energy. The purpose of osmosis is to maintain fluid equilibrium between the compartments. Water moves freely between the various fluid compartments. Therefore, an alteration in one compartment can produce a shift in body fluids to the other compartment (Clement, 1990).

A low serum osmolarity suggests fluid volume excess, meaning there is more fluid than solute. A high serum osmolarity suggests fluid volume deficit, meaning there is less fluid than solute. Osmolarity can be determined by using the following formula (Clement, 1990).

$$Osm/L = (Na \times 2) + \frac{BUN}{2.6} + \frac{Glucose}{18}$$

For example, given that a patient's Na is 140 mEq/L, BUN 20 mg/dL, glucose 250 mg/dL, using the formula, it can be calculated that the serum osmolarity is 302 Osm/L. This indicates that there are more particles than fluid in this patient's serum. Therefore, this patient's osmolarity is slightly high, suggestive of fluid volume deficit.

Serum osmolarity may be increased or decreased in various diseases. For example, diabetes insipidus produces an increased serum osmolarity, whereas carcinoma of the lung can produce a low serum osmolarity due to secretion of an excessive amount of ADH or ADH-like substance (Clement, 1990). Signs of decreased serum osmolarity are similar to those of hyponatremia. Signs of increased serum osmolarity usually occur when the osmolarity is greater than 350 mOsm. Coma can occur when the osmolarity is approximately 400 mOsm or greater (Clement, 1990).

Fluid Tonicity

Serum osmolarity is used to determine the type of IV fluids needed. IV fluids are classified according to their osmolarity or tonicity. Three classifications of IV fluids are available currently for clinical use (Ley et al, 1990): crystalloids (balanced salt solutions), blood and blood products, and colloids (balanced salt solutions that contain albumin or other oncotically active particles).

Crystalloid Solutions

Crystalloid solutions are further classified into isotonic solutions, hypotonic solutions and hypertonic solutions. Table 19–4 summarizes the use of crystalloid solutions.

TABLE 19–4. ADMINISTRATION OF CRYSTALLOID IV SOLUTIONS

Solution Type	Examples	Comments
Isotonic	0.9% normal saline (NS) Lactated Ringer's solution	Osmolarity closely approximates serum osmolarity Expands intravascular volume Used for dehydration, shock states
Hypotonic	NS 0.45% NS 0.2% Dextrose 2.5% Dextrose 5% and water	Have low osmolarity; will shift water to intracellular spaces
Hypertonic	Dextrose 5% in NS Dextrose 10% in NS Dextrose 10% in water Dextrose 5% in 0.45 NS Dextrose 20% in water NS 3%	High osmolarity; shift fluid from intracellular to extracellular spaces

Isotonic Solutions

The term, isotonic, means that the osmolarity of the solution on one side of a membrane is the same as the osmolarity on the other side of the membrane. The osmolarity of isotonic fluid closely approximates normal serum plasma osmolarity (285–295 mOsm/L). Isotonic fluids are used to hydrate the intravascular compartment. A loss of intravascular fluid volume can occur with dehydration, hemorrhage, or a massive gastrointestinal bleed. Administration of an isotonic IV solution can expand the intravascular volume. Frequently used isotonic solutions include 0.9 percent normal saline and lactated Ringer's solution.

Hypotonic Solutions

Hypotonic solutions contain a lower concentration of particles than exists inside the cell. Therefore, hypotonic solutions have a low osmolarity. The low osmolarity of these solutions can shift fluid from the intravascular compartment into the intracellular compartments. Hypotonic solutions include: Half-strength normal saline (0.45 percent), dextrose 2.5 percent, and dextrose 5 percent in water. Hypotonic solutions are useful in hydrating a patient and preventing dehydration, increasing diuresis, and assessing kidney status (McKenry and Salerno, 1989). (Refer to Module 8, *Shock States*, for further discussion of hypotonic solutions.)

Hypertonic Solutions

Hypertonic solutions have a high osmolarity. These fluids have a higher concentration of particles than exists inside the cell. The high osmolarity of the solutions shifts fluids from the intracellular space to the extracellular spaces. Hypertonic solutions include 3 percent normal saline, solutions with dextrose concentration greater than 5 percent, a combination of dextrose and saline, and total parenteral nutrition (TPN) with dextrose concentrations from 20 percent to 70 percent (Kessler, 1991).

Hypertonic solutions are used in the treatment of water intoxication problems. Water intoxication (hypotonic expansion) occurs when there is too much water in the cells. In the high acuity patient, water intoxication can be caused by administration of large amounts of solutions that are free of electrolytes or 5 percent dextrose and water. It also is seen in elderly postoperative patients, associated with the endocrine system's response to stress (McKenry and Salerno, 1989).

Blood and Blood Products

Blood and blood products are substances that have been produced naturally in the body and later do-

TABLE 19–5. REASONS FOR BLOOD AND BLOOD PRODUCTS ADMINISTRATION

Administration of blood and blood products can
  Increase the amount of hemoglobin and red blood cells to carry oxygen to the tissues
  Improve hemoglobin and hematocrit levels during active bleeding
  Increase intravascular volume
  Replace deficient substances (protein, coagulation factors, platelets)

nated for either the patient's own use (autotransfusion) or someone else's use (Mathewson, 1989). Blood and blood products are administered to restore circulating blood volume, replenish the supply of red blood cells, and correct coagulation deficiencies (Sommers, 1990). Reasons for administering blood and blood products are summarized in Table 19–5.

Following the administration of whole blood, 12 to 24 hours should be allowed before assessing for an increased hemoglobin and hematocrit. Twenty-four hours after administration of 1 unit of whole blood,

the patient's hematocrit should have increased 2 percent to 3 percent, and the hemoglobin should have increased 1.0 g% (Jennings, 1985). Administration of 1 unit of packed red blood cells should elevate the hemoglobin 1.3 g%, and the hematocrit should rise 3 percent to 4 percent within 6 hours after administration (Langfitt, 1984). The expected increase in platelet count after a unit of platelets is 10,000 platelets/mm^3 (Langfitt, 1984). Commonly administered blood and blood products are summarized in Table 19–6.

Colloids

Colloids are solutions containing protein or starch molecules. Two colloid solutions frequently administered to high acuity patients are dextran and hetastarch (Hespan). When colloids are administered, the colloid molecules remain in the vascular space and increase the osmotic pressure gradient in the vascular compartment. This increased osmotic

TABLE 19–6. COMMONLY ADMINISTERED BLOOD AND BLOOD PRODUCTS

Blood/Blood Product	Amount Delivered	Contents	Uses
Whole blood (WB)	500 mL	Blood cells, plasma, proteins, nutrients, clotting factors	Hemorrhage Replace intravascular volume Increase oxygen-carrying capacity of blood
Packed blood cells (PRBC)	200–250 mL	Red blood cells	Anemias without blood loss Minimizes fluid volume overload because of its concentration (increases oxygen-carrying capacity with less volume than WB)
Fresh frozen plasma (FFP)	200–250 mL/unit	All clotting factors except platelets; albumin; sodium; potassium	Little/no actual blood loss (i.e., burns) Volume expansion Hypoproteinemia Coagulation disorders Increase serum colloid osmotic pressure
Plasma	200–250 mL	Fluid portion of blood after centrifuging to remove RBCs; contains all clotting factors except platelets	Replace clotting factors Restore plasma volume without increasing hematocrit
Cryoprecipitate	20–30 mL/unit of blood	Contains factors VIII, XIII, and fibrinogen	Disseminated intravascular coagulation (DIC) Hemophilia A Von Willebrand disease
Platelets	20–30 mL per pack	Platelets; lymphocytes; some plasma	Thrombocytopenia Splenomegaly DIC Control of bleeding
Albumin	5%: 250–500 mL 25%: 25, 50, 100 mL	Aqueous fraction of pooled plasma from WB; buffered with normal saline	Increase plasma colloid osmotic pressure Rapidly expand plasma volume

pressure pulls fluids from the interstitial spaces into the vascular compartment. The net effect is expansion of the intravascular volume. Because of the expansion effect, colloids often are referred to as *plasma expanders*. Plasma expanders are inexpensive and readily available, and since the patient does not have to wait for blood typing and matching, they can be administered immediately (Mathewson-Kuhn, 1991).

Dextran

Dextran is made from sucrose. There are two types of dextran available, low molecular weight dextran (Dextran 40) and high molecular weight dextran (Dextran 70). Dextran 40 enhances CO and circulation because it expands intravascular volume and also reduces RBC aggregation. Dextran 70 has a heavier molecular weight and has the ability to increase intravascular oncotic pressure for longer periods of time than does Dextran 40 (Mathewson-Kuhn, 1991). Dextran 40 is used as a plasma expander in shock states and as deep vein thrombosis prophylaxis because it minimizes sludging of blood in the microcirculation and decreases platelet aggregation. Dextran 70 is used primarily as a plasma expander in shock states.

Hetastarch

Hetastarch (Hespan) is a synthetic colloid made from cornstarch and sodium chloride. Hetastarch's colloid oncotic pressure influence remains in the vascular space for 24 to 36 hours, much longer than does dextran (Mathewson-Kuhn, 1991). Hetastarch also can be administered in shock states.

In summary, through osmosis, a state of fluid balance exists between the intracellular and extracellular fluid compartments. Assessment of this fluid balance can be made by determining serum osmolarity. Serum osmolarity is used to determine the type of IV fluid to be administered. The three types of IV fluids are crystalloids, blood and blood products, and colloids. Crystalloids replace intracellular or extracellular volume, depending on their tonicity. Blood and blood products are administered to restore circulating blood volume, replace lost RBCs, and correct coagulation abnormalities. Colloids are plasma expanders, since when administered, they expand intravascular volume. Effective evaluation of the patient's response to IV fluid administration requires knowledge of both the properties and indications for use of all IV fluids.

Section Three Review

1. A low serum osmolarity may suggest
   A. fluid volume deficit
   B. fluid volume excess
   C. dehydration
   D. isotonic balance
2. Which of the following solutions closely approximates serum osmolarity?
   A. 0.45 percent normal saline
   B. dextrose 5 percent in normal saline
   C. 3 percent normal saline
   D. lactated Ringer's solution
3. A patient's hematocrit is 25 mg%. After 1 unit of whole blood, you could anticipate the hematocrit to be
   A. 26–27 mg%
   B. 28–29 mg%
   C. 30–31 mg%
   D. 32–33 mg%

4. A patient's hemoglobin is 9.0. After 1 unit of packed red blood cells, you would anticipate the hemoglobin to be
   A. 9.3
   B. 10
   C. 10.3
   D. 11
5. Dextran 40 is used for all the following situations EXCEPT
   A. to expand blood volume
   B. deep vein thrombosis prophylaxis
   C. to treat shock states
   D. to improve hemoglobin

Answers: 1, B. 2, D. 3, A. 4, C. 5, D.

TABLE 19–7. NORMAL RANGES OF SERUM ELECTROLYTE

Electrolyte	Normal Range
Sodium (Na^+)	135–145 mEq/L
Chloride (Cl^-)	96–106 mEq/L
Calcium (Ca^{2+})	8.5–10.5 mg/dL
Potassium (K^+)	3.5–5.5 mEq/L
Magnesium (Mg^{2+})	1.5–2.2 mEq/L
Phosphate (PO_4^{2-})	3.0–4.5 mg/dL

Section Four: Sodium

At the completion of this section, the learner will be able to discuss the extracellular compartment electrolyte, sodium.

Electrolytes are electrically charged microsolutes found in body fluids. There are two types of electrolytes, cations (positively charged ions) and anions (negatively charged ions). Electrolytes play a vital role in many physiologic activities, including enzyme activities, muscle contraction, and metabolism. Sections Four through Nine present an overview of six major electrolytes commonly monitored by nurses. Table 19–7 lists the normal ranges of frequently monitored serum electrolytes.

The normal serum sodium range is 135 to 145 mEq/L. It is the most abundant cation in the extracellular fluid. Sodium is responsible for shifts in body water and the amount of water retained or excreted by the kidneys. Sodium is required for normal transmission of impulses across muscle and nerve cells, through the sodium pump mechanism. It helps maintain acid-base balance by combining with chloride or bicarbonate to increase or decrease serum pH.

Sodium and Water Balance

Changes in sodium levels alter water balance. Thus, the clinical manifestations of sodium alterations also reflect symptoms of water imbalance. Since water is drawn to sodium, an excess sodium level in the extracellular fluid pulls water from the intracellular spaces. This results in shrinking of the intracellular fluid space and expansion of the extracellular space. Such expansion may precipitate congestive heart failure and pulmonary edema in patients whose renal or cardiovascular system cannot tolerate such fluid shifts.

When serum levels of sodium are low, water moves from an area of low sodium concentration (extracellular) to an area of high sodium concentration (intracellular). This causes excess volume in the intracellular compartment and fluid volume deficit in the extracellular compartment.

The amount of sodium in the diet varies widely, since the supply is large in almost all foods. When sodium intake is excessive, fluid volume in the intravascular space increases. In response, the kidneys increase urinary excretion of sodium through enhanced filtering from the blood, release of ADH prevents reabsorption of sodium by the kidneys, and aldosterone release is suppressed, enhancing urinary excretion of sodium. When sodium intake is excessively low, plasma volume is decreased. The kidneys sense the decreased volume, triggering the renin-angiotensin-aldosterone cycle to increase blood pressure and decrease urine output by reabsorbing more sodium.

Hypernatremia

Serum sodium levels above 145 mEq/L can result from excessive sodium intake or excess water loss. Excessive sodium intake can occur from the administration of hypertonic IV fluid (3 percent normal saline) or excessive sodium bicarbonate administration. A high serum sodium pulls water from the intracellular space into the intravascular space. Although this depletes intracellular fluid, it results in extracellular hypervolemia.

Hypernatremia can be due to defective ADH release, decreased renal responsiveness to ADH, or excessive water loss (Clement, 1990). Acute and chronic renal dysfunction limit the kidneys' ability to respond to ADH. Excessive water loss can occur with such problems as diabetes insipidus, administration of osmotic diuretics that foster water loss, excessive gastrointestinal drainage, or excessive diaphoresis.

Hyponatremia

Hyponatremia occurs when the serum sodium levels falls below 135 mEq/L. It can result from excessive sodium loss or water gain, which produces a dilutional effect.

Excessive Sodium Loss

Sodium loss occurs with administration of diuretics and in the presence of diarrhea, nasogastric suction, or diaphoresis. In the gastrointestinal system, 60 mmol/L of sodium may be lost in gastric juices, 129 mmol/L in diarrhea or intestinal drainage, 80 mmol/L of sodium in fecal fluid, and 45 mmol/L in profuse diaphoresis (Innerarity, 1990). Excessive sodium loss also can occur from osmotic diuresis as a result of hyperglycemia, as in diabetic ketoacidosis (DKA). Persistent sodium excretion can occur with consistent release of ADH from the pituitary or ectopic production of ADH. This unregulated production of ADH causes the syndrome of inappropriate ADH (SIADH). SIADH can result from cerebral disease or trauma, pulmonary diseases (i.e., tuberculosis, malignancy, pneumonia), and such drugs as morphine, tranquilizers, and anesthetics (Clement, 1990).

Dilutional Effect

Under certain circumstances, hyponatremia can result from a net gain of water in the extracellular spaces. For example, excessively high serum levels of glucose can cause a shift of water from the intracellular spaces into the intravascular space to regain equilibrium. During the dilution process, sodium, which is also present in the serum, becomes diluted, lowering the serum sodium levels.

Clinical Manifestations of Sodium Imbalances

The clinical manifestations of hypernatremia are predominantly neurologic because brain cells are especially sensitive to sodium levels. If hypernatremia develops rapidly, cellular shrinkage also contributes to the neurologic symptoms. Hyponatremia is associated with early changes in muscle tone, since sodium plays a role in transmission of neuromuscular impulses. If sodium levels continue to fall (less than 120 mEq), intracellular edema occurs, producing further neurologic deterioration. The clinical manifestations of both hypernatremia and hyponatremia, as well as common treatments to correct these imbalances, are presented in Table 19–8.

In summary, sodium is the major extracellular cation. It is crucial to regulation of body fluids. It also plays an important role in nerve impulse transmission. Hypernatremia results from excessive sodium intake or excess water loss. Hyponatremia results from excessive sodium loss or the dilutional effect. The clinical manifestations of sodium imbalances are predominantly neurologic because of the sodium sensitivity of brain cells.

TABLE 19–8. CLINICAL MANIFESTATIONS AND TREATMENT OF SODIUM IMBALANCES

Imbalance	Clinical Manifestations	Treatment

Hypernatremia (>145 mEq/L)	Early
	  Generalized muscle weakness, faintness, muscle fatigue, headache
	Later
	  Cardiovascular
	    Edema
	  Neurologic
	    Restlessness, thirst, hyperreflexia, muscle twitching, irritability, seizures, possibly coma
		Replacement of lost ECF volume via administration of free water
		Vasopressin if hypernatremia is secondary to pituitary diabetes insipidus (DI); if nephrogenic diabetes insipidus, eliminate cause of DI (hypercalcemia, hypokalemia, lithium) (Clement, 1990)

Hyponatremia (<135 mEq/L)	Neuromuscular
	  Decreased muscle tone
	Cardiovascular
	  Hypotension
	Gastrointestinal
	  Vomiting, diarrhea, stomach cramps
	Neurologic
	  Confusion, headache, lethargy, seizures, coma
		Mild depletion: Treated with water restriction
		Moderate depletion: May be treated with IV 0.9% NaCl or 0.45% NaCl (Innerarity, 1990)
		Severe depletion with life-threatening symptoms: Hypertonic (3%) sodium chloride IV may be given (Clement, 1990)

Section Four Review

1. The normal range of serum sodium is
   A. 1.5–2.2 mEq/L
   B. 3.5–5.5 mEq/L
   C. 8.5–10.5 mg/dl
   D. 135–145 mEq/L

2. Hypernatremia can be caused by which of the following?
   A. SIADH
   B. hyperglycemia
   C. diabetes insipidus
   D. diabetic ketoacidosis

3. Signs and symptoms of hypernatremia include
    A. diarrhea
    B. decreased muscle tone
    C. stomach cramps
    D. muscle twitching
4. Hyponatremia is associated with which of the following symptoms?
    A. edema
    B. lethargy
    C. hyperreflexia
    D. restlessness

5. The major function of sodium is
    A. carbohydrate metabolism
    B. tissue oxygenation
    C. blood coagulation
    D. fluid balance

Answers: 1, D. 2, C. 3, D. 4, B. 5, D.

Section Five: Chloride

At the completion of this section, the learner will be able to describe the extracellular compartment electrolyte, chloride.

Chloride is the most abundant anion in the extracellular fluid. The normal serum chloride range is 96 to 106 mEq/L. Chloride works with sodium in regulation of body fluids by its influence on osmotic pressures within the interstitial and intravascular spaces (Dolan, 1991). Serum chloride levels tend to closely follow sodium levels, since chloride normally follows sodium in the body. Aldosterone regulates chloride levels indirectly by stimulating reabsorption of sodium in the kidney. Chloride assists in maintaining the resting membrane potential of cells and, with sodium, maintains osmolarity of the extracellular fluid space.

The extracellular fluid acid-base status requires a balance between the total number of anions and cations within the fluid. Thus, the major cation (sodium) must be in balance with the two major extracellular anions (chloride and bicarbonate). To regulate this balance, chloride and bicarbonate maintain an inverse relationship, competing for sodium ions. For example, if a patient receives an excessive does of sodium bicarbonate to treat metabolic acidosis, the presence of excess bicarbonate ions in the serum can result in the excretion of chloride ions, precipitating hypochloremia.

Hyperchloremia

Hyperchloremia is defined as a serum chloride of more than 106 mEq/L. Hyperchloremia is associated with excessive loss of bicarbonate and normal anion gap metabolic acidosis. (Refer to Module 15, *Altered Glucose Metabolism.*) Normal anion gap metabolic acidosis most commonly is caused by loss of bicarbonate ions through either renal or gastrointestinal loss (e.g., diarrhea). As bicarbonate is lost, chloride is reabsorbed to maintain acid-base balance.

Hypochloremia

Hypochloremia is defined as a serum chloride of less than 96 mEq/L. Hypochloremia can result from met-

---

TABLE 19–9. CLINICAL MANIFESTATIONS AND TREATMENT OF CHLORIDE IMBALANCES

Imbalance	Clinical Manifestations	Treatment
Hyperchloremia (>106 mEq/L)	Musculoskeletal Muscle weakness Respiratory Rapid, deep respirations Neurologic Headache, lethargy, decreasing level of consciousness Symptoms of hypernatremia and fluid volume deficit	Correct underlying cause Fluid replacement for dilutional effect, possibly with lactated Ringer's solution Sodium bicarbonate to increase pH Diuretic therapy
Hypochloremia (<96 mEq/L)	Neurologic Irritability, tetany, agitation Respiratory Shallow, slow respirations Musculoskeletal Muscle weakness (Baer, 1988) Symptoms of hyponatremia	Correct underlying problem Fluid replacement for dilutional effect; IV sodium chloride or potassium chloride. (Baer, 1988)

abolic alkalosis or hypokalemia. Excessive use of loop diuretics, such as furosemide, enhances the loss of chloride and sodium in the urine. When chloride levels are low, the kidneys sense the need for more anions to maintain electrical neutrality, and bicarbonate is reabsorbed.

Clinical Manifestations of Chloride Imbalances

The signs and symptoms of chloride imbalance reflect the manifestations of the associated acid-base imbalance. Neurologic, musculoskeletal, and respiratory dysfunction and the symptoms of a concurrent sodium imbalance also are associated with chloride imbalances. The clinical manifestations of chloride imbalances and their treatments are listed in Table 19–9.

In summary, chloride is the major extracellular anion. It maintains a direct relationship with sodium and an inverse relationship with bicarbonate. Chloride is important in fluid regulation and acid-base balance. Hyperchloremia is associated with loss of bicarbonate ions and metabolic acidosis (normal anion gap). Hypochloremia is associated with loss of sodium or potassium ions and metabolic alkalosis.

Section Five Review

1. Chloride levels closely follow the levels of which of the following electrolytes?
   A. potassium
   B. sodium
   C. calcium
   D. magnesium
2. Hypochloremia is associated with which of the following symptoms?
   A. tetany
   B. headache
   C. lethargy
   D. rapid, deep respirations
3. The normal serum chloride range is
   A. 3.5–5.5 mEq/L
   B. 8.5–10.5 mg/dl
   C. 96–106 mEq/L
   D. 135–145 mEq/L

4. Hyperchloremia is associated with which of the following problems?
   A. metabolic acidosis (normal anion gap)
   B. metabolic acidosis (high anion gap)
   C. metabolic alkalosis (normal anion gap)
   D. metabolic alkalosis (high anion gap)
5. Which of the following substances indirectly regulates serum chloride levels?
   A. parathyroid hormone
   B. calcitonin
   C. renin
   D. aldosterone

Answers: 1, B. 2, A. 3, C. 4, A. 5, D.

Section Six: Calcium

At the completion of this section, the learner will be able to discuss the extracellular compartment electrolyte, calcium.

The normal serum calcium level is 8.5 to 10.5 mg/dL. Ninety-nine percent of body calcium is located within bone. The remaining 1 percent exists in the extracellular fluid and soft tissues (Graves, 1990). Calcium is required for blood coagulation, neuromuscular contraction, enzymatic activity, and intact bones.

Calcium regulation is under the influence of parathyroid hormone (PTH), calcitonin, and calcitriol.

Serum calcium levels are maintained by (1) calcium excretion from the kidneys, (2) absorption of calcium from the gastrointestinal tract, and (3) mobilization of calcium from the bone (Clement, 1990). Calcium is absorbed in the intestines only under the influence of vitamin D, which is activated in the kidneys. It is reabsorbed in the proximal renal tubules after being filtered by the glomerulus and is excreted by the kidneys. Renal disease prevents activation of vitamin D, thus reducing the body's ability to absorb calcium.

Calcitonin and PTH work in opposition to regulate calcium levels. When calcium levels are low, PTH is released by the parathyroid gland, stimulating the conversion of calcitriol (the active form of vitamin D), which causes the small intestines to absorb more calcium. PTH also stimulates release of calcium from bony tissues into the blood. When calcium levels are high, PTH secretion is suppressed, and calcitonin is secreted by the thyroid, inhibiting the release of calcium from bone into the blood.

Serum calcium can be measured in two different ways, as total calcium and as ionized calcium. These two measurements look at calcium in a slightly different manner.

- Total calcium. Normal levels 4.3 to 5.5 mEq/L or 8.5 to 10.5 mg/dL. Total calcium reflects calcium that is bound to proteins (i.e., albumin) in the serum. Total calcium levels are influenced by the patient's nutritional state.
- Ionized calcium. Normal levels (adult) 4.5 to 5.5 mg/dL. Approximately 50 percent of serum calcium exists in an ionized state. Ionized calcium represents the calcium that is active in physiologic activities and is crucial for neuromuscular activity (Brunner and Suddarth, 1988). Ionized calcium levels may remain normal even when total calcium levels are low.

Hypercalcemia

Hypercalcemia is defined as a serum calcium level above 10.5 mg/dL. Hypercalcemia results from mobilization of calcium from bone. Malignancy is the most common cause of hypercalcemia in the high acuity patient by either destruction of bone (from bone metastasis) or tumor secretion of humoral substances that increase the resorption of bone (Graves, 1990). Other causes of hypercalcemia include hyperparathyroidism, thyrotoxicosis, immobility, and thiazide diuretics. Excessive ingestion of vitamin D or calcium and altered renal tubular absorption of calcium also elevate serum calcium levels. Gastrointestinal and renal absorption of calcium decreases the reabsorption of phosphorous. Therefore, hypercalcemia accompanies hypophosphatemia, as calcium and phosphorous levels shift in opposite directions.

Hypocalcemia

Hypocalcemia is defined as a serum level below 8.5 mg/dL. In the high acuity patient, the most common cause of hypocalcemia is depressed function or surgical removal of the parathyroid gland. It is also associated with hypomagnesemia and hyperphosphatemia, which can cause diminished vitamin D synthesis by the kidneys. It can be induced by the administration of large amounts of stored blood. Stored blood is preserved with citrate, and when administered, the citrate binds with calcium, lowering serum calcium.

Clinical Manifestations of Calcium Imbalances

The signs and symptoms of hypercalcemia primarily reflect dysfunction of the gastrointestinal and mus-

TABLE 19–10. CLINICAL MANIFESTATION AND TREATMENT OF CALCIUM IMBALANCES

Imbalance	Clinical Manifestations	Treatment

Hypercalcemia (>10.5 mg/dL) (severe >14 mg/dL)	Gastrointestinal
	    Anorexia, constipation, peptic ulcer
	        disease
	Neurologic
	    Lethargy, depression, fatigue; if severe,
	        confusion, coma
	Cardiovascular
	    Shortened QT interval, arrhythmias
		Initial use of isotonic saline to expand the
		    ECF (to dilute calcium concentration and
		    increase urinary excretion).
		Loop diuretics (to block renal reabsorption
		    of calcium); in severe hypercalcemia,
		    furosemide 80–100 mg every 1–2 hours
		    with isotonic saline flush
		Possible use of phosphate, calcitonin, or
		    glucocorticoids (Graves, 1990)

Hypocalcemia (<8.5 mg/dL)	Musculoskeletal
	    Cramps: abdominal, extremities; tingling
	        and numbness; severe state, positive
	        Chvostek or Trousseau sign; tetany
	Neurologic
	    Irritability, reduced cognitive ability,
	        seizures
	Cardiovascular
	    ECG changes: prolonged QT interval;
	        decreased blood pressure and
	        myocardial contractility
		IV calcium
		    10% calcium chloride (360 mg elemental
		    Ca/10 mL); 10% calcium gluconate (93
		    mg elemental Ca/10 mL); initial dose of
		    200 mg of elemental calcium over 5–10
		    minutes; if continual replacement is
		    necessary, 1–2 mg/kg/hour of elemental
		    calcium
		Cardiac monitoring
		Close monitoring of serum calcium
		Monitoring of digitalis levels (for possible
		    toxicity) (Graves, 1990)

culoskeletal systems. Hypercalcemia can be accompanied by the signs and symptoms of hypophosphatemia.

Hypocalcemia becomes symptomatic when ionized calcium levels fall to below normal limits. Symptomatic hypocalcemia affects the musculoskeletal, neurologic, and cardiovascular systems. The clinical manifestations and treatment of both hypercalcemia and hypocalcemia are presented in Table 19–10, as summarized from Graves (1990).

In summary, calcium plays an important part in blood coagulation and is the major component of bone tissue. It is regulated by parathyroid hormone, calcitonin, and calcitriol. Calcium is measured in its protein-bound state (total calcium) and its ionized state (ionized calcium). Hypercalcemia results from movement of calcium from the bone. Hypocalcemia is associated with depressed parathyroid function. Calcium imbalances are particularly associated with neuromuscular and cardiac dysfunction.

Section Six Review

1. The normal range of serum calcium is
   A. 1.5–2.2 mEq/L
   B. 3.5–5.5 mEq/L
   C. 8.5–10.5 mg/dl
   D. 135–145 mEq/L
2. Calcium is absorbed in the intestines under the influence of
   A. phosphorus
   B. vitamin D
   C. sodium
   D. vitamin C
3. Hypocalcemia is associated with which of the following symptoms?
   A. tingling and numbness
   B. constipation
   C. lethargy
   D. shortened QT interval

4. Calcium regulation is under the influence of all of the following EXCEPT
   A. calcitriol
   B. calcitonin
   C. parathyroid hormone (PTH)
   D. aldosterone
5. Which of the following statements is correct regarding serum total calcium?
   A. it may remain normal even if ionized calcium is abnormal
   B. it represents calcium that is physiologically active
   C. it is influenced by the patient's nutritional state
   D. it measures calcium that is not bound to protein

Answers: 1, C. 2, B. 3, A. 4, D. 5, C.

Section Seven: Potassium

At the completion of this section, the learner will be able to discuss the intracellular compartment electrolyte, potassium.

Potassium is the major intracellular cation, with most potassium being found within the cells (150 mEq/L, compared to 3.5 to 5.5 mEq/L in the plasma). Although the concentration in plasma is small, serum potassium is very important because the body is intolerant of abnormal serum levels. Potassium is found readily in many foods, and average daily consumption is estimated at 30 to 100 mEq. Excess potassium is eliminated in the urine by the kidneys (McKenry and Salerno, 1989). Normally, about 40 mEq/L of potassium is excreted daily in the urine (Innerarity, 1990).

Potassium is vital in maintaining normal cardiac and neuromuscular function because it affects muscle contraction. (Refer to Module 7, *Cardiac Monitoring and Related Interventions*.) Potassium also influences nerve impulse conduction. Therefore, abnormal serum potassium levels can produce cardiac conduction abnormalities. Potassium has an important role in cell membrane function, being vital to carbohydrate metabolism. It also plays an important part in the maintenance of acid-base balance. The serum pH strongly influences serum potassium levels. A decrease of 0.1 unit of pH raises the serum K^+ level by 0.6 mEq/L (DeAngelis and Lessig, 1991).

Hyperkalemia

Hyperkalemia is defined as a potassium level above 5.5 mEq/L. Hyperkalemia can result from excessive potassium intake, particularly in the presence of renal dysfunction, excessive use of potassium-sparing diuretics (i.e., spironolactone), or release of excessive intracellular potassium. Significant quantities of intracellular potassium are released into the extracellular space in response to injury, stress, acidosis, or a catabolic state. Acidosis contributes to hyperkalemia as potassium moves out of cells in exchange for the hydrogen ions that move into the cells. Additionally, sodium depletion results in hyperkalemia as potassium is exchanged for sodium across the proximal renal tubule. False laboratory readings of hyperkalemia also can result from inaccurate phlebotomy techniques. If the tourniquet is too tight or if blood is withdrawn using a small gauge needle, the RBCs can burst, releasing potassium ions into the serum, potentially resulting in a falsely elevated serum potassium.

Hypokalemia

Hypokalemia is defined as a serum potassium below 3.5 mEq/L. Loss of potassium for any reason can cause hypokalemia. Hypokalemia can result from (1) loss of gastrointestinal secretions (i.e., vomiting, diarrhea, excessive nasogastric loss, fistulas), (2) excessive renal excretion of potassium, (3) movement of potassium into the cells (i.e., diabetic ketoacidosis), or (4) prolonged fluid administration without potassium supplementation.

When hypokalemia occurs, the body does not attempt to retain or reabsorb potassium. The kidneys continue to excrete it regardless of the existing potassium state. If allowed to continue, the hypokalemia becomes increasingly severe, causing a steady deterioration in the patient's condition (McKenry and Salerno, 1989). Since the body does not compensate for potassium loss, it is essential that hypokalemia be detected rapidly and corrected through appropriate potassium supplementation.

Clinical Manifestations of Potassium Imbalances

Since potassium is important in nerve impulse conduction, muscle contraction, and cell membrane function, the signs and symptoms of imbalances reflect interference with these activities. The signs and symptoms of potassium imbalances, as well as their treatments, are listed in Table 19–11.

TABLE 19–11. CLINICAL MANIFESTATIONS AND TREATMENT OF POTASSIUM IMBALANCES

Imbalance	Clinical Manifestations	Treatments

Hyperkalemia (>5.5 mEq/L)	Musculoskeletal
	  Weakness
	Gastrointestinal
	  Nausea, vomiting, intestinal colic, abdominal cramping, diarrhea
	Cardiovascular
	  ECG changes
	    Bradycardia, prolonged PR interval; flat or absent P wave; slurring of QRS; tall peaked T wave; ST segment depression; at K^+ >8 mEq/L, disappearance of P waves; further widening of QRS complexes; cardiac arrhythmias; cardiac arrest can occur (McKenry and Salerno, 1989)
	Acid-base effect
	  Metabolic acidosis
		Measures to decrease serum potassium:
		  10% calcium gluconate: 10–30 mL over 15–30 minutes; administration of calcium counteracts cardiac effects of hyperkalemia
		  Sodium bicarbonate: 50–100 mL (not to be mixed with calcium solution); promotes potassium movement into the cells
		  50% glucose solution (stimulates insulin release, augmenting cellular potassium intake (Shires and Canizaro, 1986)
		  Kayexalate (a cation exchange resin) given PO or rectally; exchanges K^+ for Na^+; rectal 25–100 g in 100 mL of dextrose 10% or sorbitol (McKenry and Salerno, 1989); each gram of kayexalate removes 1 mEq of K^+ (Innerarity, 1990)

Hypokalemia (<3.5 mEq/L)	Musculoskeletal
	  Skeletal muscle weakness; decreased smooth muscle function
	Cardiovascular
	  Hypotension; ECG: ST segment depression; U waves; T wave inversion, flattening, or depression
	Gastrointestinal
	  Nausea and vomiting; paralytic ileus
	Acid-base effect
	  Metabolic alkalosis
		Hydrate patient if low urine output
		Potassium supplementation:
		  Intravenous: For moderate to severe hyperkalemia; dilute K^+ and infuse at rate of no more than 20 mEq/hour; use of hypertonic glucose solution helps drive K^+ back into cells; IV fluid should not contain more than 40 mEq/L (McKenry and Salerno, 1989)
		  Oral: Preferred method of delivery for mild hypokalemia; many preparations available

In summary, potassium is the major intracellular cation. It is vital in maintaining normal cardiac and neuromuscular function. Hyperkalemia results from excessive potassium intake, renal failure, or use of potassium-sparing diuretics. Hypokalemia results from excessive loss of potassium through the gastrointestinal tract or urine, shifting of potassium into the cells, or excessive administration of potassium-free IV fluids. The clinical manifestations of potassium imbalances reflect dysfunctions in nerve impulse conduction, muscle contraction, and cell membrane activities.

Section Seven Review

1. The normal range of serum potassium is
   A. 1.5–2.2 mEq/L
   B. 3.5–5.5 mEq/L
   C. 8.5–10.5 mg/dL
   D. 135–145 mEq/L
2. Hyperkalemia can be caused by which of the following?
   A. renal failure
   B. potassium wasting diuretics
   C. metabolic alkalosis
   D. severe diarrhea
3. Signs and symptoms of hyperkalemia include
   A. muscle weakness, T wave inversion
   B. muscle twitching, ST segment depression
   C. vomiting, peaked T wave
   D. diarrhea, presence of U wave
4. Hypokalemia has what effect on kidney function?
   A. urine output increases
   B. potassium excretion increases
   C. potassium is reabsorbed
   D. potassium excretion does not change
5. In which of the following ways does pH influence serum potassium?
   A. an increase of 0.1 unit of pH increases potassium by 0.5 mEq
   B. an increase of 0.1 unit of pH increases potassium by 0.1 mEq
   C. a decrease of 0.1 unit of pH increases potassium by 0.6 mEq
   D. a decrease of 0.1 unit of pH increases potassium by 0.1 mEq

Answers: 1, B. 2, A. 3, C. 4, D. 5, C.

Section Eight: Magnesium

At the completion of this section, the learner will be able to describe the intracellular compartment electrolyte, magnesium.

Magnesium is an intracellular electrolyte with a distribution similar to that of potassium. The normal serum magnesium level is 1.5 to 2.2 mEq/L. An important function of magnesium is to ensure sodium and potassium transportation across cell membranes (Brasfield, 1990). Magnesium is required in many biochemical reactions and plays a significant role in nerve cell conduction. Magnesium is important in transmitting CNS messages and maintaining neuromuscular activity. Possibly the most important function of magnesium is that of combining with ATP, assisting in transference of energy (Friday and Reinhart, 1991).

Magnesium is excreted predominantly in feces, but a small amount is excreted in urine. The kidneys, however, have a remarkable ability to conserve magnesium. Magnesium balance is closely related to potassium and calcium balance. The signs and symptoms of magnesium and calcium imbalances are similar. Therefore, when assessing magnesium levels, potassium and calcium levels should be assessed simultaneously (Innerarity, 1990).

Hypermagnesemia

Hypermagnesemia results when magnesium levels rise above 2.5 mEq/L. This abnormality is rare, but can occur with diminished renal excretion as seen in renal dysfunction or excessive magnesium intake. Consumption of large quantities of magnesium-containing antacids or laxatives (i.e., milk of magnesia, Gelusil, Maalox) can be a source of excessive intake.

Hypomagnesemia

Hypomagnesemia is defined as serum magnesium of less than 1.5 mEq/L. It can result from decreased intake or decreased absorption of magnesium or excessive loss through urinary or bowel elimination. Magnesium deficiency can be caused by many disorders, including acute pancreatitis, starvation, malabsorption syndrome, chronic alcoholism, burns, and prolonged hyperalimentation without adequate magnesium replacement. Hypoparathyroidism, with resultant hypocalcemia, also can cause hypomagnesemia, since the regulatory mechanisms of magnesium and calcium are closely related.

Clinical Manifestations of Magnesium Imbalances

Since magnesium is important in maintaining normal CNS and neuromuscular function, magnesium imbalances can cause dysfunction of these activities. Hypermagnesemia has a depressant effect, and hypomagnesemia is associated with hyperactivity. The clinical manifestations and treatments of both hypermagnesemia and hypomagnesemia are presented in Table 19–12.

In summary, magnesium is primarily an intracellular cation with a distribution similar to that of potassium. Magnesium has many functions, including assisting in transport of sodium and potassium across the cell membrane and transference of energy. Hypermagnesemia is rare and is caused primarily by either excessive intake of magnesium-containing drugs or renal failure. Hypomagnesemia can result from decreased intake or excessive loss of magnesium. The clinical manifestations of magnesium imbalances primarily reflect CNS and neuromuscular dysfunction.

TABLE 19–12. CLINICAL MANIFESTATIONS AND TREATMENT OF MAGNESIUM IMBALANCES

Imbalance	Clinical Manifestations	Treatment

Hypermagnesemia ($>$2.5 mEq/L)	Neuromuscular
	  Lethargy, drowsiness
	Cardiovascular
	  Hypotension, bradycardia, cardiac arrest;
	  EKG: prolonged PR intervals, complete
	  heart block
		Withhold magnesium-containing products
		Acute symptoms are controlled by slow IV administration of 5–10 mEq of calcium chloride or calcium gluconate (Shires and Canizaro, 1986)
		IV hydration and diuretics can lower magnesium levels if patient has adequate renal function (Innerarity, 1990)

Hypomagnesemia ($<$1.5 mEq/L)	Neuromuscular
	  Tremors; tetany; positive Chvostek and
	  Trousseau signs
	Cardiovascular
	  PVCs; torsades de point; ventricular
	  fibrillation
		Magnesium replacement: IV magnesium can cause venous sclerosis and must be diluted to 1:10, then 40 mEq diluted in 1L of 0.9% NaCl or D_5W, which then can be infused at 0.2 mEq/kg over 6 hours (Innerarity, 1990)
		When given IV, monitor for hypertension secondary to vasodilation (Friday and Reinhart, 1991)
		Oral forms of magnesium can be used but gastrointestinal absorption may vary; the most frequently used oral forms are magnesium oxide [200 mg (9.9 mEq) to 400 mg (19.86 mEq)] daily or magnesium chloride delayed release [128 mg (10.52 mEq)] once or twice daily (Friday and Reinhart, 1991).

Section Eight Review

1. The normal range of serum magnesium is
   A. 1.5–2.2 mEq/L
   B. 3.5–5.5 mEq/L
   C. 8.5–10.5 mg/dL
   D. 135–145 mEq/L
2. Magnesium balance is closely related to which other two electrolytes?
   A. potassium and phosphorous
   B. calcium and sodium
   C. sodium and phosphorous
   D. calcium and potassium balance
3. The symptoms of hypomagnesemia reflect
   A. CNS hypoactivity
   B. fluid compartment shifts
   C. cardiac depressant effects
   D. neuromuscular and CNS hyperactivity

4. Hypermagnesemia is associated with which of the following symptoms?
   A. tetany
   B. lethargy
   C. tremors
   D. ventricular fibrillation
5. Magnesium plays an active part in all of the following physiologic functions EXCEPT
   A. sodium and potassium transport
   B. nerve cell conduction
   C. fluid regulation
   D. transference of energy

Answers: 1, A. 2, D. 3, D. 4, B. 5, C.

Section Nine: Phosphorus/Phosphate

At the completion of this section, the learner will be able to discuss the intracellular compartment of electrolyte, phosphorus/phosphate.

Phosphorus is an intracellular mineral found commonly in many foods. The normal serum level of phosphorus is 3.0 to 4.5 mg/dL. Phosphorus is essential to tissue oxygenation, and it is vital for normal CNS function and movement of glucose into cells. Phosphorus is required for energy in the production of ATP, and it assists in the regulation of calcium and maintenance of acid-base balance (Cella and Watson, 1989).

The serum phosphate level is under the influence of parathyroid hormone (PTH) and maintains an inverse relationship to calcium. The kidneys are essential to phosphorus regulation through reabsorption and excretion. When glomerular filtration is decreased, phosphorus reabsorption increases, causing an elevation in serum levels. As glomerular filtration increases, phosphorus reabsorption diminishes, and more phosphorus is excreted by the kidneys, reducing the serum phosphate level.

Hyperphosphatemia

Hyperphosphatemia is defined as a serum level above 4.5 mg/dl (Baer, 1988). Hyperphosphatemia is not as common in the high acuity patient as hypo-

phosphatemia. It is predominantly associated with chronic renal failure. Other causes include hyperthyroidism, hypoparathyroidism, severe catabolic states, and conditions causing hypocalcemia.

Hypophosphatemia

Hypophosphatemia is defined as a serum phosphorus level below 2.0 mg/dL (Baer, 1988). This condition is associated with malnourished states and is a relatively common imbalance in the high acuity patient. Other conditions that can cause hypophosphatemia include hyperparathyroidism, certain renal tubular defects, metabolic acidosis (including diabetic ketoacidosis), and disorders that cause hypercalcemia.

Clinical Manifestations of Phosphate Imbalances

Hypophosphatemia depresses cellular function, particularly of the hematologic and cardiovascular systems. This results in symptoms of impaired heart function and poor tissue oxygenation. Because phosphorus is essential in providing energy for ATP, muscle fatigue develops. The clinical manifestations and treatment for hyperphosphatemia, as well as hypophosphatemia, are presented in Table 19–13.

In summary, phosphorus, which exists in the

TABLE 19-13. CLINICAL MANIFESTATIONS AND TREATMENT FOR PHOSPHORUS IMBALANCES

Imbalance	Clinical Manifestations	Treatment

Hyperphosphatemia (>4.5 mg/dL)	Musculoskeletal
	    Muscle cramping; joint pain
	    Other symptoms are those of hypocalcemia
		Restriction of phosphorus-containing foods
		Administration of phosphorus-binding
		    agents, e.g., Amphogel
		Correct the underlying cause
		Diuretics
		Possible dialysis (Baer, 1988)

Hypophosphatemia (<2.0 mg/dL)	Neurologic
	    Disorientation; irritability; seizures; coma
	Musculoskeletal
	    Weakness; numbness and tingling;
	      pathologic fractures
	Gastrointestinal
	    Nausea and vomiting; anorexia
	Severe hypophosphatemia (<1.0 mg/dL)
	    Respiratory arrest; nervous system
	      dysfunction; myocardial dysfunction;
	      hemolysis; WBC and platelet
	      dysfunction (Schlichtig and Ayres, 1988)
		Correct underlying cause
		Replacement of phosphate (IV or orally)
		IV replacement for moderate to severe
		    hypophosphatemia: 0.08 to 0.16 mmol/kg
		    over 6 hours; not to be administered in
		    bolus form; available as sodium phosphate
		    or potassium phosphate (Schlichtig and
		    Ayres, 1988)

serum as phosphate, works closely with calcium and is important in tissue oxygenation and energy production. Hyperphosphatemia is most commonly associated with chronic failure. Hypophosphatemia most commonly results from malnourished states. The clinical manifestations of phosphate imbalances primarily reflect dysfunction of the hematologic, cardiovascular, and neuromuscular systems.

Section Nine Review

1. The normal range of serum phosphorus is
   A. 1.5–2.2 mEq/L
   B. 3.5–5.5 mEq/L
   C. 3.0–4.5 mg/dL
   D. 8.5–10.5 mg/dL
2. Hypophosphatemia is associated with which of the following conditions?
   A. malnourished state
   B. metabolic alkalosis
   C. hypocalcemia
   D. hyperthyroidism
3. Severe hypophosphatemia is associated with which of the following symptoms?
   A. joint pain
   B. muscle cramping
   C. respiratory arrest
   D. peptic ulcer disease

4. Phosphorus is important for all of the following functions EXCEPT
   A. tissue oxygenation
   B. sodium transport
   C. calcium regulation
   D. production of ATP
5. The clinical picture of hyperphosphatemia frequently reflects which other electrolyte abnormality?
   A. hypercalcemia
   B. hypochloremia
   C. hypernatremia
   D. hypocalcemia

Answers: 1, C. 2, A. 3, C. 4, B. 5, D.

Posttest

The following Posttest is constructed in a case study format. A patient is presented. Questions are asked based on available data. New data are presented as the case study progresses.

Donald R, 67 years old, was admitted to the hospital with gastrointestinal bleeding. Donald has a history of chronic alcohol abuse and has had one previous bleeding episode. On admission, the nurse assesses the following: Thin, malnourished appearing male. Blood pressure 108/62, pulse 118/minute, respirations 26/minute, temperature 97.8F. You note pitting edema of the lower legs. His abdomen is distended and tight. He complains of shortness of breath.

1. Donald's age and poor physical condition place him at risk for development of
   A. hypertension
   B. dehydration
   C. acute renal failure
   D. congestive heart failure
2. Donald's peripheral edema is an example of fluid located in which space?
   A. intracellular
   B. interstitial
   C. intravascular
   D. interocular
3. Assuming Donald has ascites, the shift of intravascular fluid into a cavity is also referred to as
   A. third spacing
   B. congestive failure
   C. edema
   D. dehydration
4. As Donald's blood pressure decreases, the baroreceptors will trigger
   A. renal vasodilation
   B. increased heart rate
   C. suppression of ACTH release
   D. peripheral vasoconstriction

Donald's urine output has been 25 mL/hour for the past 2 hours. His serum osmolarity is 260 mOsm/L.

5. Based on the available data, his decreased urine output is most likely due to
   A. dehydration
   B. renal failure
   C. peripheral edema
   D. suppressed ADH release
6. The nurse makes the nursing diagnosis of *Fluid volume deficit*. Which of Donald's symptoms are consistent with this diagnosis?
   A. temperature of 97.8F orally
   B. peripheral edema of lower legs
   C. low serum osmolarity
   D. shortness of breath

Donald's physician writes the following orders:

- Stat. CBC
- Type and crossmatch for 2 units of blood

7. The decision of which type of IV fluid is best for Donald is based on osmolarity. Osmolarity refers to a solution's
   A. particle concentration
   B. protein concentration
   C. glucose concentration
   D. anion concentration

The results of the CBC are now available. Hgb 7.2 mg% and Hct 26.3 percent. Two units of whole blood are ordered. It is decided that Donald requires an IV fluid to hydrate the intravascular compartment.

8. Which type of crystalloid solution is best for loss of intravascular volume secondary to hemorrhage?
   A. hypertonic solutions
   B. isotonic solutions
   C. hypotonic solutions
   D. colloid solutions
9. Twenty-four hours after receiving the 2 units of blood, Donald's hemoglobin should have risen to ____ g%.
   A. 7.8
   B. 8.5
   C. 9.8
   D. 11

Over the past 2 days, Donald has received a large volume of IV solutions. He has blood drawn for electrolyte determination. The results are

Sodium	128 mEq/L
Chloride	92 mEq/L
Total calcium	8.0 mg/dL
Potassium	5.4 mEq/L
Magnesium	1.2 mEq/L
Phosphate	1.8 mg/dL

10. Donald's low serum sodium can cause body water to shift from
    A. interstitial into intravascular spaces
    B. extracellular into intravascular spaces
    C. intravascular into interstitial spaces
    D. intracellular into extracellular spaces
11. If Donald's chloride level continues to fall, he will need to be assessed for
    A. rapid, deep respirations
    B. signs of hypercalcemia
    C. depressed breathing
    D. signs of hypernatremia
12. Donald's total calcium level is 8.0 mg/dL. This level is most likely caused by his
    A. renal status
    B. nutritional status
    C. chloride status
    D. immobilized status

13. Should Donald's serum potassium level become too high, the nurse should be MOST concerned about changes in which body system?
    A. cardiovascular
    B. respiratory
    C. neurologic
    D. genitourinary
14. Given that Donald's serum pH was 7.37 and serum potassium was 5.4 mEq/L, if his pH drops to 7.27, you would anticipate that the serum potassium would
    A. decrease to 4.8 mEq/L
    B. remain at 5.4 mEq/L
    C. increase to 6.0 mEq/L
    D. increase to 6.6 mEq/L
15. Hypomagnesemia, such as Donald has, can be caused by all of the following problems EXCEPT
    A. hypercalcemia
    B. chronic alcoholism
    C. starvation
    D. acute pancreatitis
16. Donald's hypophosphatemia can affect his musculoskeletal system in which of the following ways?
    A. muscle spasm
    B. joint pain
    C. muscle weakness
    D. muscle cramping

Posttest Answers

Question	Answer	Section	Question	Answer	Section
1	B	One	9	C	Three
2	B	One	10	B	Four
3	A	One	11	C	Five
4	D	Two	12	B	Six
5	A	Two	13	A	Seven
6	C	Two	14	C	Seven
7	A	Three	15	A	Eight
8	B	Three	16	C	Nine

REFERENCES

Baer, C.L. (1988). Regulation and assessment of fluid and electrolyte balance. In M.R. Kinney, D.R. Packa, and S.B. Dunbar (eds). *AACN's clinical reference for critical-care nursing*, 2nd ed., pp. 193–236. New York: McGraw-Hill.

Brasfield, K. (1990). Renal and fluids anatomy and physiology. In L.A. Thelan, J.K. Davie, and L.D. Urden (eds). *Textbook of critical care nursing: Diagnosis and management*, pp. 609–621. St. Louis: C.V. Mosby Co.

Brunner, L.S., and Suddarth, D.S. (1988). *Textbook of medical-surgical nursing*, 6th ed. Philadelphia: J.B. Lippincott.

Cella, J.H., and Watson, J. (1989). *Nursing manual of laboratory tests*. Philadelphia: F.A. Davis Co.

Clement, J.M. (1990). Assessment: Renal system. In C.M. Hudak, B.M. Gallo, and J.J. Benz (eds). *Critical care nursing: A holistic approach*, pp. 408–426. Philadelphia: J.B. Lippincott.

DeAngelis, R., and Lessig, M.L. (1991). Hypokalemia. *Crit. Care Nurse.* 11(7):71–75.

Dolan, J.T. (1991). Fluid and electrolyte physiology and pathophysiology. In *Critical care nursing: Clinical management through the nursing process*, pp. 431–467. Philadelphia: F.A. Davis Co.

Friday, B.A., and Reinhart, R.A. (1991). Magnesium metabolism: A case report and literature review. In C.M. Hudak, B.M. Gallo, and J.J. Benz (eds). *Critical Care Nursing: A holistic approach*, pp. 62–72. Philadelphia: J.B. Lippincott.

Graves, L. (1990). Disorders of calcium, phosphorus, and magnesium. *Crit. Care Nursing Q.* 13(3):3–13.

Groer, MW, and Shekleton, ME. (1989). *Basic pathophysiology: A holistic approach*, 3rd ed. St. Louis: CV Mosby.

Innerarity, S.A. (1990). Electrolyte emergencies in the critically ill renal patient. *Crit. Care Nursing Clin. North Am.* 2(1):89–99.

Jennings, B.M. (1985). The hematologic system. In J.F. Alspach and S.M. Williams (eds). *Core curriculum for critical care nursing*, 3rd ed., pp. 496–558. Philadelphia: W.B. Saunders.

Jones, A.M., Mosely, M.J., Halfmann, S.J., Heath, A., Henkelman, W.J., Ciaccio, J., and Bolcar, B.S. (1991). Fluid volume dynamics. *Crit. Care Nurse.* 11(4):74–76.

Kessler, C.A. (1991). IV therapy. In D.S. Suddarth (ed). *The Lippincott manual of nursing practice*, 5th ed., pp. 79–94. Philadelphia: J.B. Lippincott.

Langfitt, D. (1984). Blood component therapy. In D. Langfitt (ed). *Critical care: Certification preparation & review*, pp. 403–407. Bowie, Maryland: Brady.

Ley, S.J., Miller, K., Phylita, S., and Preisig, P.L. (1990). Crystalloid versus colloid fluid therapy after cardiac surgery. *Heart Lung.* 19(1):31–40.

Mathewson, M. (1989). Intravenous therapy. *Crit. Care Nurse.* 9(2):21–36.

Mathewson-Kuhn, M.A. (1991). Colloids vs crystalloids. *Crit. Care Nurse.* 11(5):37–51.

McKenry, L.M., and Salerno, E. (1989). Fluid and electrolytes. In *Mosby's pharmacology in nursing*, pp. 1092–1103. St. Louis: C.V. Mosby.

Schlichtig, R., and Ayres, S.M. (1988). Nutrient requirements of critically ill patients: Electrolytes, vitamins, trace elements, and essential fatty acids. In *Nutritional support of the critically ill*, pp. 129–139. Chicago: Year Book Medical Publishers.

Shires, G.T., and Canizaro, P.C. (1986). Fluid and electrolyte management of the surgical patient. In D.C. Sabiston (ed). *Textbook of surgery*, 13th ed., pp. 64–86. Philadelphia: W.B. Saunders.

Sommers, M.S. (1990). Fluid resuscitation following multiple trauma. *Crit. Care Nurse.* 10(10):74–81.

Nursing Care of the Patient with Altered Metabolism

Kathleen Dorman Wagner

Nursing Care of the Patient with Altered Metabolism is designed to integrate the major points discussed in the modules: *Altered Glucose Metabolism, Nutrition, Immunocompetence, Acute Renal Failure,* and *Fluid and Electrolyte Balance*. This module summarizes relationships between key concepts and assists the learner in clustering information to facilitate clinical application. The module is divided into two major parts. The first part discusses assessment data frequently used in deriving appropriate nursing diagnoses and expected patient outcomes for a patient with the following problem(s): diabetic crises, altered nutrition, altered immunocompetence, acute renal failure, and disturbances in electrolyte balance. The second part applies the content in an interactive learning style using a case study format. The learner is encouraged to cluster data and derive as well as prioritize nursing diagnoses. The module ends with a brief summary of major points.

Objectives

At the completion of the self-study module, *Nursing Care of the Patient with Altered Metabolism,* the learner will be able to

1. Describe the assessment of a patient with a selected metabolic disorder

2. Explain the clustering of critical cues in establishing nursing diagnoses appropriate to selected metabolic disorders

3. Discuss development of nursing diagnoses appropriate to the patient with selected metabolic disorders

4. Explain the development of expected patient outcomes based on nursing diagnoses appropriate to the patient with selected metabolic disorders

5. Describe the nursing management of the physiologic needs of the patient with selected metabolic disorders

6. List the common psychosocial nursing diagnoses associated with patients with selected metabolic disorders

7. Briefly describe the management of the patient with HIV

Glossary

Albumin. A plasma protein used as a common measurement of nutritional status

Anthrometric measurements. Physical measurements used to evaluate muscle protein and percent of body fat

Blood urea nitrogen (BUN). The end product of protein metabolism

Creatinine. The end product of muscle metabolism

Diabetes mellitus. A total or relative deficiency of the hormone, insulin

Hyperglycemia. An abnormally high serum glucose

Hypermetabolism. An increased metabolic rate in response to a major bodily insult requiring increased quantities of oxygen and nutrients to meet the increased metabolic needs; occurs in the flow phase of the metabolic stress response

Hyperosmolar hyperglycemic nonketotic coma. A severe form of hyperglycemic crisis associated with very high serum glucose levels and lack of significant ketones

Hypoglycemia. An abnormally low serum glucose

Immunosuppression. Decreased immune function

Leukocytopenia. An abnormally low level of leukocytes

Leukocytosis. An abnormally high level of luekocytes

Transferrin. A protein manufactured in the liver

Uremia. A collective term used to describe the clinical manifestations of renal failure

Uremic encephalopathy. Brain dysfunction caused by the presence of renal toxins

THE NURSING PROCESS

Nursing Assessment

The Focused Nutritional Assessment

Many high acuity patients suffer from some degree of malnutrition either as a preexisting chronic disorder (e.g., general debilitation, cancer, or emphysema) or as an acute problem during hospitalization. Whether the malnutrition is long-standing or of relatively short duration, it profoundly affects the patient's chances for a full recovery.

Hypermetabolism, as discussed in Module 16, *Nutrition,* is a major aspect of the malnutrition problem. Hypermetabolism is an increased metabolic state in which the body's fat and protein stores are depleted in an attempt to meet high energy demands resulting from increased physiologic stress. Hypermetabolism causes an imbalance in energy supply and demand. During the acute phase of the nutritional stress response, nutrients are not well received by the body for metabolism and energy use, as described in the flow phase. Unfortunately, even when nutrients would be well accepted by the body to supply energy, an adequate supply often is not received. Nutritional support may be lacking or it may be insufficient to meet the increased metabolic needs of the patient under stress.

TABLE 20–1. THE VITAL ROLES OF PROTEIN

Muscle tissue synthesis
Healing
Tissue synthesis
Colloid osmotic pressures
Immunocompetence
Hemoglobin synthesis

The signs and symptoms of malnutrition reflect deficiencies in muscle protein, visceral (nonmuscle) proteins, and electrolyte abnormalities. Proteins are essential to many of the body's functions, causing impairment of those functions when protein stores become depleted. Protein losses can be severe and may lead to death of the patient from complications of protein deficiency. Table 20–1 lists some of the vital roles of protein.

The Nutrition History

Gaining information about the patient's preexisting nutritional state establishes possible malnutrition risk factors. In an emergency, certain nutritional data need to be collected as a priority (Table 20–2). Once time allows, a more detailed nutritional history is obtained.

TABLE 20–2. PRIORITY NUTRITIONAL HISTORY DATA

Height and usual weight
Dietary restrictions
Food and drug allergies
Medication history
Recent events
   Weight change
   Appetite change
   Nausea, vomiting
   Constipation or diarrhea
   Difficulty swallowing
(Possible reasons for recent changes should be explored)

Anthrometric Measurements

Anthrometric measurements are used to evaluate muscle protein and percent of body fat. Height and weight are two anthrometric measurements commonly obtained by nurses at admission. Charts are available to compare an individual's height and weight to a standard. Serial weights are of the greatest value, showing weight gains or losses. The changing trends generally represent fluctuations in fluid or decreasing fat or protein stores.

A weight loss of $\geq$10 percent of body mass places the patient at risk for complications of malnutrition. Accurate weight monitoring is crucial if trends are to be valid. It is best to use the same scale every day and to weigh the patient at the same time of day. Monitoring weight is not necessarily an accurate indicator of muscle protein and fat stores status, since such factors as obesity and edema confound the significance of the weight gain or loss.

In addition to measuring height and weight, other less common measurements can be taken. These include midupper arm muscle circumference and triceps skinfold thickness. As with weight, these measurements can be used either as baseline nutritional data or as intermittent measurements to evaluate muscle protein and body fat loss during hospitalization.

Measuring Proteins

The nutritional status of a high acuity patient should be monitored throughout hospitalization by measuring serum albumin, total lymphocyte count (TLC), or serum transferrin. Serum albumin is a plasma protein and is considered an excellent indicator of malnutrition. Unfortunately, albumin does not reflect rapid visceral protein changes because of its long half-life. Transferrin is a protein manufactured in the liver. It is important in the transport and absorption of iron. Transferrin, like albumin, measures the level

of malnutrition. It better reflects the current visceral protein status because of its shorter half-life. TLC measures malnutrition through monitoring the serum lymphocytes, a type of protein. More specifically, TLC gives valuable information regarding immunocompetence, since lymphocytes are an essential part of the immune system. TLC is measured using the following formula (WBC, white blood cell count).

$$TLC = \frac{\% \text{ lymphocytes} \times WBC}{100}$$

Table 20–3 summarizes the significant value ranges of the three protein measurements (Farley, 1991). The clinical significance of these values in predicting level of malnutrition diminishes greatly when the patient has liver or kidney dysfunction.

Nitrogen Excretion

Proteins consumed but not used by the body are excreted through the urine. The balance between protein (nitrogen) intake and nitrogen excretion establishes whether the patient is in positive or negative nitrogen balance. Nitrogen balance is determined by simultaneously performing a 24 hour calorie count and a 24 hour urine urea nitrogen (UUN). Normally, a person excretes less protein than is consumed, indicating a positive nitrogen balance. However, during periods of starvation, muscle and visceral protein stores are used for energy, and urinary excretion of nitrogen (from protein catabolism) is higher than nitrogen consumption, indicating a negative nitrogen balance. The 24 hour calorie count requires accurate documentation of all nutrients consumed or administered during the comparison period. This requires recording all foods and fluids consumed during the period or documentation of exact tube feeding or TPN intake.

TABLE 20–3. SIGNIFICANT VALUE RANGES OF PROTEIN MEASUREMENTS

Albumin
   Normal 3.5–5.5 g/dL
   Severe malnutrition $\leq$2.5 g/dL
Transferrin
   Normal 200–400 mg/dL
   Severe malnutrition <160 mg/dL
Total lymphocyte count
   Mild deficiency 1,200–1,500 mm^3
   Moderate deficiency 800–1,200 mm^3
   Severe deficiency <800 mm^3

TABLE 20-4. EFFECTS OF MALNUTRITION ON BODY SYSTEMS

Integumentary system
    Decreased subcutaneous fat
    Flaky, dry skin
    Hair loss
Musculoskeletal system
    Wasting of muscles
    Edema
    Weight loss of ≥ 10%
Cardiovascular system
    Decreased cardiac output
Immune system
    Impaired healing

The Nutrition Physical Examination

Physical manifestations of malnutrition are assessed primarily by examination of the integumentary and musculoskeletal systems. If malnutrition is severe, the patient's cardiovascular system also may become affected. Patients with malnutrition are at risk for developing the signs and symptoms of specific mineral or electrolyte abnormalities. Electrolyte abnormalities are discussed in detail in Module 19, *Fluid and Electrolyte Balance*. Table 20–4 lists some of the major physical signs of malnutrition.

The Focused Diabetic Crisis Assessment

Diabetes mellitus is a total or relative deficiency in the hormone, insulin. In the well-controlled adult diabetic, clinical manifestations of the disorder primarily focus on the chronic progressive complications that slowly cause deterioration of the neurologic and vascular systems. Diabetics also are at risk for development of three acute complications: diabetic ketoacidosis (DKA), hyperosmolar hyperglycemic nonketotic coma (HHNC), and hypoglycemic coma. DKA and HHNC are produced by an abnormally high blood glucose, hyperglycemia. In contrast, hypoglycemic coma is produced by an abnormally low blood glucose, hypoglycemia. Many diabetic patients are admitted to the hospital for a diagnosis other than their chronic diabetic state. However, the physiologic stress caused by the acute problem may precipitate a diabetic crisis, which further complicates the patient's prognosis. Diabetes mellitus is discussed in detail in Module 15, *Altered Glucose Metabolism*.

The Focused History

When a diabetic crisis is suspected, there are specific parts of the nursing history that should be obtained rapidly.

- Preexisting history of type I or type II diabetes
- Self-maintenance activities
    - Special diet, including compliance with diet
    - Insulin or oral hypoglycemics (type, dosage, compliance to regimen)
    - Glucose testing history (fingersticks, urine testing)
- Usual pattern of glucose control (stable vs occasional-to-frequent loss of glucose control)
- Possible precipitating factors (i.e., infection, presence of other physiologic or psychologic stressors, failure to follow diet or drug therapy)
- Preexisting neurologic or vascular complications of diabetes (i.e., decreased kidney function, peripheral or cardiovascular disease)
- Unexplained weight loss of ≥10%

Focused Assessment: Diabetic Ketoacidosis

A rapid assessment of the severity and state of compensation of DKA helps establish management priorities. The signs and symptoms of DKA are multisystem in nature. Thus, a systematic assessment is necessary. Not every patient exhibits all of the clinical manifestations of DKA, and confirmation is made by evaluation of appropriate laboratory tests. Table 20–5 concisely presents the various signs and symptoms of diabetic ketoacidosis, relating them to underlying pathophysiology as summarized from McCarthy (1985) and Thelan et al (1990).

Focused Assessment of Hyperosmolar Hyperglycemic Nonketotic Coma

HHNC is a less common but more severe hyperglycemic diabetic crisis than DKA. HHNC is associated with significantly higher serum glucose levels than noted in DKA, making dehydration from osmotic diuresis as well as other symptoms. Whereas the patient experiencing HHNC may lose 15 percent to 20 percent of body fluid volume, the patient in DKA loses up to 10 percent of body fluid volume (McKenna, 1988). HHNC is associated with a much higher mortality rate (40–50 percent) than DKA (approximately 9 percent) (Thelan et al, 1990).

The clinical picture of the patient with HHNC is similar to that of the patient with DKA, with several important differences. Symptoms common to both DKA and HHNC are mental confusion, alteration in level of consciousness, polydipsia and polyuria, dehydration (dry mouth and dry skin, hypotension, tachycardia). Table 20–6 presents a concise comparison of DKA and HHNC as summarized from Graves (1990), Thelan et al (1990) and Dolan (1991).

TABLE 20–5. PATHOPHYSIOLOGIC BASIS OF DKA SYMPTOMATOLOGY

Cardinal Signs and Specific Signs and Symptoms	Physiologic Etiology of Signs and Symptoms	Cardinal Signs and Specific Signs and Symptoms	Physiologic Etiology of Signs and Symptoms

Hyperglycemia
  Elevated serum and
  urine glucose
  elevation
	An absolute or relative deficit in insulin causes the inability of glucose to move into cells, increasing serum glucose levels
	Fat from adipose tissue is converted into free fatty acids (FFA); the FFA, in turn, are converted to glucose by gluconeogenesis in the liver
	The liver also causes glycogenolysis which converts glycogen to glucose
	All of these factors contribute to worsening hyperglycemia
			excretion of glucose and urine; this is associated with increased loss of electrolytes, hemoconcentration, and increasing dehydration
			Gastrointestinal symptoms associated with DKA may be related to abnormally low electrolytes
			Elevated BUN and creatinine may be present (azotemia) due to hemoconcentration

Metabolic acidosis
  Elevated serum and
  urine ketones
  Serum pH, acidotic
  Serum HCO_3,
  acidotic
  Serum Pco_2, alkalotic
  Anion gap, positive
  Elevated respiratory
  rate and depth
  (Kussmaul
  breathing)
  Fruity odor to breath
	Free fatty acids are broken down into ketone bodies (which can be used for energy by the central nervous system) faster than they can be converted to glucose
	Due to lack of insulin, muscle cells cannot oxidize the ketone body's sufficiently, causing a buildup of ketone bodies
	Increased levels of circulating ketone bodies decreases the pH; as pH falls below 7.20, the respiratory center is stimulated to excrete carbonic acid via the lungs in the form of CO_2 and water
	Acetone, contained in ketone bodies, is excreted via the lungs (ketone breath) and the kidneys (ketonuria)
	Bicarbonate reserves become overwhelmed and then exhausted by the severity and prolonged state of the acidosis, causing a drop in serum bicarbonate levels
		Compensatory
		  mechanisms
		  Decreased urinary
		  output
		  Increased serum
		  sodium levels
		  Increased blood
		  pressure, pulse,
		  respiration
		  Peripheral
		  vasoconstriction
			The renin-angiotensin-aldosterone system is activated to increase sodium and water reabsorption; ADH is secreted by the posterior pituitary to cause retention of water and sodium
			Urine output also is controlled by compensatory vasoconstriction, which limits renal blood flow
			The autonomic nervous system is stimulated to secrete catecholamines and glucocorticoids; these cause vasoconstriction, which increases the blood pressure and decreases urine output; blood pressure, pulse, and respiration are all increased as a result
			Hormone secretions are associated with further aggravation of hyperglycemia

Osmotic diuresis
  Polyuria, polydipsia
  Dehydration
  Hypotension
  Hemoconcentration
  Electrolyte
  abnormalities
  Azotemia
	Increasing serum glucose levels increase intravascular osmotic pressure; the increased pressure draws extravascular fluids into the intravascular compartment; as glucose levels and intravascular volume increases, the kidneys respond by dramatically increasing	Decompensation
		  Rapid deterioration in
		  level of
		  consciousness
		  progressing to
		  coma
		  Peripheral
		  vasodilation: skin
		  becomes warm,
		  dry, and flushed
		  Shock symptoms
			Exhaustion of compensatory mechanisms precipitate cardiovascular collapse; the level of consciousness deteriorates, blood pressure and pulse can no longer maintain adequate organ perfusion; the supply of catecholamines becomes exhausted, causing loss of the body's ability to maintain peripheral vasoconstriction; urine output decreases and ceases as hypoperfusion to the kidneys causes them to fail

Focused Assessment: Hypoglycemic Crisis

Hypoglycemia, abnormally low blood glucose, is the most common type of diabetic coma. It may occur with any type of diabetes. Hypoglycemia is triggered by an imbalance between exercise, diet, and medica-tion. Onset of symptoms is usually rapid, and if pro-longed, coma may result (McKenna, 1988). The symptoms of hypoglycemia are primarily related to central nervous system (CNS) effects and catechola-mine effects.

TABLE 20–6. DKA AND HHNC IN CONTRAST

Factor	DKA	HHNC
Population affected	Younger population	Elderly population
Diabetic type	Type I: Insulin-dependent diabetes	Type II: Noninsulin-dependent diabetes
At-risk factors/precipitating factors	Undiagnosed DM; neglected treatment; physiologic stress; certain drugs	Infirm; institutionalized; mentally impaired; undiagnosed DM; physiologic stress; certain drugs; certain medical procedures
Previous history of diabetes	Almost always	In about 50%
Underlying renal or cardiovascular disease	In about 15%	In about 85%; renal disease is considered a predisposing condition
Rate of onset	Sudden (hours)	Slow, insidious (days–weeks)
Complications	Rare	Frequent
Symptomatology differences	Ketoacidosis; fruity breath odor; respirations rapid and deep (Kussmaul type)	No to mild ketosis; no acetone breath odor; respirations non-Kussmaul type
Laboratory data		
Anion gap	Positive anion gap (>7 mEq/L)	Negative anion gap (<7 mEq/L)
Serum glucose	>300–800 mg/dL	>1,000 mg/dL
Serum ketones	Positive ketoacids	Absence of significant ketones
Serum osmolality	<330 mOsm/L	>330 mOsm/L
Free fatty acids	Significantly elevated	Not significantly elevated
Serum pH	<7.30; bicarbonate ≤15 mEq/L	≥7.30; bicarbonate ≥15 mEq/L
Urine glucose	Elevated	Elevated
Urine ketones	Positive ketones	Absence of significant ketones

Central Nervous System Effects

The CNS depends on available glucose for its energy source and is sensitive to insufficient levels of glucose. CNS effects reflect the inability of brain cells to function normally without an adequate energy source. Symptoms include

- Altered level of consciousness, confusion
- Changes in personality, nightmares
- Headache, dizziness
- Visual disturbances, staggering gait

Catecholamine Effects

The lack of circulating glucose triggers the secretion of stress hormones, subsequently causing production of glucose from alternate body sources, such as hepatic gluconeogenesis. The presence of increased levels of the hormone epinephrine, a catecholamine, triggers a sympathetic response. This stress response accounts for many of the symptoms of hypoglycemia, such as

- Tremors, nervousness
- Cold, clammy skin
- Tachycardia, diaphoresis

Laboratory Findings

A patient is considered to be hypoglycemic if the serum glucose is less than 50 mg/dL. A glucose level of less than 20 mg/dL is associated with true coma (McCarthy, 1985). Some patients, however, develop symptoms of hypoglycemia even with a serum glucose of over 50 mg/dL or, if the drop in glucose is very rapid, over 100 mg/dL within 1 to 2 hours (Lumley, 1988).

The age of the patient and rate of onset both have an impact on the clinical presentation of hypoglycemia. The elderly tend to have more severe symptoms and may become symptomatic at higher levels of serum glucose. CNS symptoms, particularly those relating to altered levels of consciousness, may be misdiagnosed in chronically ill elderly if the onset is very slow. In this population, the hypoglycemic symptoms may be masked as worsening dementia. Rapid onset of hypoglycemia triggers the sympathetic response. Thus, catecholamine effects may be the strongest under those circumstances. When the hypoglycemia has a slow onset, such as may be seen in chronic illness, the CNS effects may be more prominent.

The Focused Immunocompetence Assessment

The physical examination for level of immunocompetence primarily reflects the patient's nutritional status. The immune system is dependent on nutritional status. Consequently, if the patient is malnourished, immune status will be negatively affected.

Golightly and Dolan (1991) suggest that the physical assessment focus on seeking evidence of infection, either acute or chronic. This includes assessing for skin lesions, open wounds, the presence of adventitious breath sounds and abnormal sputum, enlarged liver or spleen, or palpable lymph nodes or masses.

Nursing History

The patient history gives important clues to possible altered immunocompetence. Golightly and Dolan (1991) suggest obtaining the following historical data.

- Complaints of fever, fatigue, weakness, swollen glands, or abnormal bleeding
- Presence of increased levels of stress, infection, malignancy, or autoimmune disease
- Recent use of immunosuppressant drugs
- Allergy history
- At-risk factors for development of AIDS
  - Homosexual orientation or sexual partner of homosexual
  - Transfusion of blood or blood products
  - IV illegal drug users or sexual partner of drug user
  - Child born of mother with AIDS
- Presence of preexisting autoimmune disorders

Immunocompetence in the High Acuity Patient

The high acuity patient is at high risk for development of immunocompetence problems secondary to prolonged stress, severe infections, malnutrition, diabetes, and other problems. The nurse needs to monitor the patient for critical cues of an underlying immunocompetence problem. Some of these major critical cues include the presence of

- Fever
- Poor wound healing
- Abnormal CBC with differential
- Abnormal coagulation studies
- Recurrent, prolonged, or severe infections
- Secondary infections
- Immunosuppressive drug therapy, such as corticosteroids or cytotoxic drugs
- Other at-risk factors, such as splenectomy, diabetes mellitus, chronic alcohol abuse, malnutrition, renal failure

Laboratory Findings

Laboratory testing is the major diagnostic tool for establishing immune status. Tests may include common ones, such as the WBC with differential and TLC, as well as tests establishing nutritional status, such as serum albumin. These tests are relatively inexpensive and easy to perform and are used as screening tests for general immune status. The nurse should be able to monitor these levels for abnormal trends.

There are a variety of cell-specific laboratory tests available if further evaluation of immunocompetence is necessary. Many of these tests, however, are both time consuming and expensive. Immunoglobulins, T cells and B cells can be measured both quantitatively and functionally. Skin testing may be ordered to evaluate cellular immunocompetence.

WBC with Differential

WBC with differential cell count is a commonly performed nonspecific test. It indicates whether a person has abnormally high numbers of leukocytes (leu-

TABLE 20–7. WBC DIFFERENTIAL CELL SUMMARY

Cell Type Normals (% WBC)	Significance	
	Increased Levels	Decreased Levels
Neutrophils (54–75%)	Stress, infectious diseases, inflammatory disorders, tissue necrosis, metabolic disorders, malignancies	Bone marrow depression (e.g., overwhelming infection), malnutrition
Bands (immature neutrophils) (3–8%)	Infection, any problem causing increased neutrophils	None
Monocytes (2–8%)	Infection, malignancies	Nonspecific
Basophils (0–1%)	Chronic hypersensitivity states, ulcerative colitis, leukemia, nephrosis	None
Eosinophils (1–4%)	Asthma, malignancies, autoimmune diseases, malignancies	Increased steroid levels, stress, congestive heart failure
Lymphocytes (25–40%)	Infection, malnutrition, malignancies	Immune deficiency diseases, bone marrow failure, septicemia, pneumonia, burns, high doses of corticosteroids

kocytosis) or abnormally low numbers of leukocytes (leukocytopenia). The normal white blood cell count is 5,000 to 10,000/mm³. In general, leukocytosis is associated with inflammation, infection, and leukemia, and leukocytopenia is associated with malnutrition, severe infection, autoimmune diseases, malignancies, and bone marrow depression. Table 20–7 is a summary of the components of the differential WBC count (Cella and Watson, 1989). Some of the major problems associated with each cell type are included in the table.

The Focused Renal Dysfunction Assessment

In the acutely ill patient, renal dysfunction often has an insidious onset. It may be suspected first when urine output stays below normal despite attempts to increase it. It also may be detected first when electrolyte or blood urea nitrogen (BUN) values develop abnormal trends.

Nursing History

Important recent history data to be aware of include

- Recent use of nephrotoxic substances (e.g., nephrotoxic antibiotics, particularly aminoglycosides)
- Recent exposure to heavy metals or organic solvents
- Recent hypotensive episode of more than 30 minutes
- Presence of tumor or multiple clots that might cause renovascular or urine outflow obstruction bilaterally

Physical Assessment Findings

Acute renal failure affects multiple body functions and systems. The collective term used to describe the clinical manifestations of renal failure is *uremia*.

Neurologic Findings. As uremic toxins build up in brain tissue, uremic encephalopathy occurs. Uremic encephalopathy refers to dysfunction of the brain caused by uremic toxins. As the encephalopathy worsens, the patient's level of consciousness decreases, progressing from drowsiness to coma. The patient also may develop muscular twitching or seizures.

Cardiovascular Findings. Fluid volume excess and electrolyte imbalances caused by renal failure are the basis of most cardiovascular symptoms. The in-

ability of the kidneys to excrete electrolytes adequately causes them to build up in the body, predisposing the patient to development of cardiac arrhythmias, electrolyte imbalances, and metabolic acidosis. The inability to excrete urine can precipitate hypertension, congestive heart failure, and other symptoms of fluid volume excess.

Respiratory Findings. Fluid volume excess, if it becomes severe, can cause left heart failure and pulmonary edema. As metabolic acidosis develops, the respiratory pattern may become Kussmaul type. As the level of consciousness decreases and the patient becomes weaker, airway clearance can become a problem, increasing the risk of pneumonia.

Gastrointestinal Findings. Electrolyte imbalances and increasing uremic toxins are the main contributors to gastrointestinal manifestations. As urea decomposes in the gastrointestinal tract, it releases ammonia. Ammonia is irritating to gastrointestinal mucosa, and as ammonia levels increase, small mucosal ulcerations may develop, causing gastrointestinal bleeding. Uremic toxins also cause loss of appetite, nausea, and vomiting. Acute renal failure is associated with both constipation and diarrhea depending on the gastrointestinal motility status secondary to electrolyte imbalances.

Genitourinary Findings. The oliguric phase of acute renal failure is associated with decreased urine output that remains less than 25 to 30 mL/hour even after fluid or diuretic management. Other urine features are described under Laboratory Findings.

Integumentary Findings. Because the uremic toxins cannot be excreted via the kidneys, they may build up on the skin surface, causing pruritus and dry skin. The patient may appear pale because of anemia, and bruising may be noted secondary to dysfunctional platelets. Uremic frost, a late-stage phenomenon of renal failure, is not seen often anymore in the acute care setting because of earlier, more aggressive management of renal failure. The term, uremic frost, refers to a fine white layer of urate crystals that develops on the skin.

Hematopoietic Findings. The kidneys produce erythropoietin, which is necessary for normal red blood cell production. When kidney function fails, red blood cell production becomes compromised, and anemia results. Platelet function also is affected by the presence of uremic toxins, causing bleeding problems. Cellular immunity is interfered with, predisposing the patient to infection. Infection is a major cause of death in acute renal failure patients (Griffin, 1986).

General Findings. Acute renal failure causes weakness and fatigue due to anemia and uremic toxin effects.

Laboratory Findings

The diagnosis and management of renal failure are largely dependent on laboratory tests, measuring uremic toxins and renal excretion. BUN and creatinine are the two most important laboratory measurements of renal status. BUN is the end product of protein metabolism. Creatinine is the end product of muscle metabolism. Under normal circumstances, BUN and creatinine maintain a 20:1 ratio to each other. When the kidneys go into failure, the nephrons are unable to cleanse the waste products (e.g., BUN and creatinine) from the blood. This results in increasing levels of serum BUN and creatinine. Creatinine is a more stable indicator of kidney function than BUN because protein metabolism is less stable than muscle metabolism. Table 20–8 summarizes major laboratory values measuring kidney function. Note that serum and urine values have an inverse relationship.

Assessment of Electrolyte Imbalances

Electrolyte imbalances are the result of some body dysfunction or lack of proper nutrition. Electrolyte imbalances cause a wide range of functional problems, particularly in the neurologic, musculoskeletal, cardiovascular, and gastrointestinal systems. The signs and symptoms of imbalances often reflect either hyperactive or hypoactive organ function, depending on the nature of the imbalance. The effects of electrolyte imbalances are discussed in detail in Module 19, *Fluid and Electrolyte Balance,* and Module 18, *Acute Renal Failure.*

TABLE 20–8. MAJOR LABORATORY VALUES MEASURING KIDNEY FUNCTION

Laboratory Test	Normal Values	Abnormal Trend
Serum		
Blood urea nitrogen	9–12 mg/dL	Increased
Creatinine	0.7–1.5 mg/dL	Increased
Uric acid	3.0–8.0 mg/dL	Increased
Potassium	3.5–5.5 mEq/L	Increased
Calcium	8.5–10.5 mg/dL	Decreased
Chloride	98–110 mEq/L	Increased
Phosphorus	2–4.5 mg/dL	Increased
Albumin	3.5–5.5 g/dL	Decreased
Urine		
Protein	Negative	Increased
Creatinine clearance	0.7–1.5 mg/dL	Decreased
Urea clearance	64–100 mL/minute	Decreased

DEVELOPING A PLAN OF CARE

Nursing diagnoses are based primarily on body functions rather than body systems, as is characteristic of medical diagnoses. Therefore, the disorders presented in this module have many nursing diagnoses in common even though they may disturb different body systems. Although the etiologic factors associated with each nursing diagnosis may differ based on the underlying pathophysiologic problem, the expected patient outcomes and nursing management remain essentially the same. The rest of this section presents some of the major nursing diagnoses and expected patient outcomes (evaluative criteria) commonly associated with this group of disorders.

There are only two North American Nursing Diagnosis Association (NANDA)-approved nursing diagnoses that directly reflect metabolic function.

- **Alteration in nutrition: Less than body requirements**
- **Alteration in nutrition: More than body requirements**

The disorders presented in this module are associated primarily with nutritional deficits rather than excesses.

Nursing Diagnoses/Expected Patient Outcomes

Alteration in Nutrition: Less than Body Requirements

Expected patient outcomes are as follows.

1. Serum glucose, albumin, transferrin, hemoglobin and hematocrit, lymphocyte BUN and creatinine within acceptable ranges
2. Weight trends moving toward normal for patient
3. Triceps skinfold measurements within acceptable range
4. Normal activity tolerance for patient

Both diabetes and renal failure affect fluid balance, though in different ways. Two NANDA-approved nursing diagnoses focus on fluids.

- **Fluid volume deficit**
- **Fluid volume excess**

Fluid volume excess is presented in detail in Module 9, *Nursing Care of the Patient with Altered Cardiac Output.* It, therefore, is not presented in this module.

Fluid Volume Deficit Related to (Applicable Etiologies)

Expected patient outcomes. The patient will regain fluid and electrolyte balance as evidenced by

1. Electrolyte levels within normal ranges
2. Absence of cardiac dysrhythmias
3. Normal mental status for patient
4. Blood pressure and pulse within normal range for patient
5. Serum osmolality within normal range
6. Serum BUN, creatinine, glucose, hemoglobin, hematocrit within acceptable ranges
7. Urine output ≥30 mL/hour
8. Moist mucous membranes
9. Intake = output
10. Capillary refill <3 seconds

Electrolyte imbalances are not addressed directly in any NANDA-approved nursing diagnoses. Consequently, the nurse can choose options that best fit the patient's situation. This module uses the diagnosis: Potential for injury-related complications of electrolyte imbalance because it addresses electrolyte problems specifically. Since fluid imbalance is an important cause of many electrolyte imbalances, fluid volume deficit and fluid volume excess also are commonly used to deal with electrolyte problems.

Injury, Potential for, Related to Complications of Electrolyte Imbalance

Expected patient outcomes. The patient will maintain/regain electrolyte balance, as evidenced by

1. Electrolyte levels within normal ranges
2. Absence of cardiac dysrhythmias
3. Normal neurologic status for patient
4. Normal muscle strength and tone for patient
5. Normal neuromuscular status for patient
6. Normal blood pressure, pulse, and respirations for patient
7. Absence of abdominal pain, nausea, or vomiting

Metabolic problems frequently alter immune function. Infection, therefore, is a relatively common complication. The following nursing diagnosis speaks to this problem.

Infection, Potential for, Related to Deficient Immune Protection

Expected patient outcomes: The patient will be free of infection as evidenced by

1. Pulse and temperature within normal range
2. Absence of lesions with redness, swelling, heat, or drainage
3. Absence of chills
4. Negative cultures
5. Skin integrity intact
6. Absence of adventitious breath sounds
7. WBC within acceptable range

There are many other nursing diagnoses that might be included in the plan of care for the patient with a disorder affecting metabolism. Some of these include

- **Alteration in cardiac output: decreased**
- **Activity intolerance**
- **Impaired skin integrity: potential or actual**
- **Knowledge deficit**
- **Self-care deficit**
- **Anxiety**
- **Comfort, alteration in**
- **Impaired gas exchange**
- **Ineffective airway clearance**

Case Study

——— BEATRICE J, A PATIENT WITH COMPLEX METABOLIC DYSFUNCTION ———

Beatrice J, a 53-year-old woman, was brought into the emergency department by her husband, who simply stated that his wife "just looks real bad."

The Initial Appraisal

On approaching Beatrice's stretcher, you make the following rapid assessment.

General Appearance. Beatrice is a moderately obese Caucasian female. Her hair is gray and unkempt, and she is wearing a soiled nightgown.

Signs of Distress. Beatrice's breathing is even but deep. No facial grimacing is noted, and her limbs are outstretched in a relaxed fashion. She does not move at all on the stretcher and does not open her eyes without moderate shaking of her shoulders.

Other. You note a foul odor emanating from Beatrice suggesting infection. She does not have any tubes or IV lines attached at this time. A man is standing beside the stretcher who states that he is Beatrice's husband, George.

Recent History

George gives you the following brief history. Beatrice has a 15-year history of type I (insulin-dependent) diabetes. About 3 weeks ago, she had a left heel spur removed in an outpatient surgery. Four days before this admission, Beatrice began experiencing abdominal pain and nausea, with intermittent periods of vomiting. Her husband relates that for the past 2 days, his wife had omitted her insulin because "she didn't need it since she hadn't been able to eat anything." Though she was complaining of her foot hurting, she adamantly refused to have her husband call the doctor. Over the past week, her foot had become increasingly swollen and red, with a bad odor. For the past 3 days she required frequent assistance into the bathroom to urinate, but she has not urinated in the last 8 hours. George adds that Beatrice has been less responsive today, and her breathing has not appeared "right." Because of these developments, he felt the need to bring her into the hospital.

QUESTION

Based on these preliminary data, what should your assessment first focus on?
1. Renal
2. Diabetes
3. Nutrition
4. Immunocompetence

ANSWER

2. During the initial appraisal, a critical cue was noted: no insulin in 2 days. Based on this single cue, the nurse can quickly cluster other similar critical cues, including history of type I diabetes, recent and acute physiologic stressors (surgery, probable wound infection), abdominal pain, nausea and vomiting, change in level of consciousness, failure to take insulin, no food consumption for several days, and a pattern of polyuria changing to diminished urine output. The exact nature of the diabetic crisis remains uncertain until laboratory results are evaluated. While waiting for laboratory results, the nurse can obtain a urine sample for sugar and acetone, looking for a sugar of 4+ and strong acetone, as an indicator of DKA.

The Focused Diabetic Assessment

Because Beatrice's initial appraisal, brief recent history, and data clustering are suggestive of a diabetic crisis, immediate attention should be focused on obtaining more data to test your hypothesis. The results are as follows. Beatrice is drowsy and responds by momentarily opening her eyes and groaning to moderate shaking. Her respirations are deep and even at 28/minute (Kussmaul type). When bending down to examine her eyes, a fruity odor is noted on her breath. Her blood pressure is now 88/64, pulse 115/minute, and temperature 102F. Her skin is flushed, hot, and dry. Her mucous membranes also are dry. You note that her jugular veins are collapsed when she is lying in a flat position.

Stat. laboratory samples are drawn, and the results come back as follows.

Arterial blood gas
   pH 7.26, Pco_2 = 28 mm Hg, Po_2 = 88 mm Hg, HCO_3 = 14 mEq/L
Serum glucose: 620 mg/dL   (Normal range 70–110 mg/dL; from Cella and Watson, 1989)
Serum ketones: Positive

Serum electrolytes	(Normal ranges are from Stark, 1985)
Na= 110 mEq/L	(Normal range 136–145 mEq/L)
Cl = 95 mEq/L	(Normal range 96–106 mEq/L)
K = 5.8 mEq/L	(Normal range 3.5–5.5 mEq/L)
Ca= 8.3 mg/dL	(Normal range 8.5–10.5 mg/dL)

Anion gap: Positive

Hemoglobin = 15.4 g/dL	(Normal range 11.7–15.7 g/dL in females)
Hematocrit = 48.2%	(Normal range 34.9–46.9% in females)

QUESTION

Based on the data collected thus far, you hypothesize that Beatrice's clinical presentation is most consistent with which type of crisis?
1. Hypoglycemia
2. Somogyi effect
3. Diabetic ketoacidosis
4. Hyperosmolar hyperglycemic nonketotic coma

ANSWER

3. Beatrice's laboratory data are consistent with DKA. The positive anion gap metabolic acidosis, the positive serum ketones, the level of glucose elevation, as well as her presenting history, suggest DKA rather than HHNC.

The Systematic Bedside Assessment

Beatrice has a No. 18 IV catheter inserted, and appropriate medical interventions for DKA are initiated based on her laboratory results. Interventions include an IV insulin drip and fluid and electrolyte replacement. Medical management is discussed in detail in Module 15, *Altered Glucose Metabolism.* She is then moved from the emergency department to an intermediate care unit.

On arrival in the intermediate care unit, Beatrice is transferred to a bed. An updated report from the emergency department nurse is given, and a systematic bedside assessment is performed.

Head and Neck. Beatrice's face appears flushed, and her lips are dry and cracked. She continues to moan and open her eyes when moderately shaken. Her pupils are equal and react briskly to light. Her neck veins are flat. No abnormalities are noted.

Chest

PULMONARY STATUS. Breath sounds are present equal bilaterally. No adventitious breath sounds are auscultated. Rate and quality are the same as previously noted.

CARDIAC STATUS. S_1 and S_2 with no murmur is auscultated. Tachycardia is present at 120/minute. Rhythm is regular.

Abdomen. The abdomen is slightly distended. Hypoactive bowel sounds are auscultated in all quadrants. The abdomen is soft to palpation.

Pelvis. A Foley catheter is in place. The urine output over the past 2 hours is 25 mL. The urine is clear, dark amber, with a specific gravity of 1.045.

Extremities. There is poor skin turgor. The skin is hot and dry. No peripheral edema is noted. The nailbeds are pale. Peripheral pulses are present in all four extremities but weak. The left foot is hot and edematous. You note a 15 cm open wound on the heel, with a moderate amount of green purulent drainage. Touching the foot causes Beatrice to moan and grimace.

Posterior. No skin breakdown is noted and no sacral edema. Posterior breath sounds are clear.

Developing the Plan of Care: Diabetic Ketoacidosis

Beatrice's DKA is brought under control through appropriate medial management.

The nurse writes the following initial list of nursing diagnoses based on Beatrice's current status.

- **Alteration in nutrition: less than body requirements**

- **Alteration in cardiac output: decreased**
- **Alteration in comfort: pain**
- **Alteration in tissue perfusion: peripheral**
- **Fluid volume deficit**
- **Infection**
- **Self-care deficit**

QUESTION

Which of the preceding nursing diagnoses would be considered as top priority during the first 4 hours after admission?
1. **Infection**
2. **Fluid volume deficit**
3. **Alteration in tissue perfusion: peripheral**
4. **Alteration in nutrition: less than body requirements**

ANSWER

2. A second cluster of critical cues is as follows: blood pressure 88/64, pulse 115/minute. Lips and mucous membranes are dry. There is poor skin turgor. Neck veins are collapsed when lying flat. A history is given of elimination pattern change from polyuria to oliguria over the past few days. These critical cues are very suggestive of fluid volume deficit. Correction of the fluid volume deficit is a priority if complications of hypovolemic shock are to be avoided. Correcting the fluid volume deficit also should increase Beatrice's CO, assuming her cardiovascular system remains intact.

The presence of a large-bore IV catheter is necessary to allow rapid IV infusion rates. CVP line placement early in the course of treatment will facilitate appropriate management of fluid rates to meet her needs. If closer monitoring of fluid and cardiac status is considered desirable, a CVP line or a flow-directed pulmonary artery catheter may be inserted.

Nursing Management: Diabetic Ketoacidosis

The DKA-related treatment goals include (1) rehydrate, (2) prevent/treat circulatory collapse, (3) restore insulin/glucagon ratio, (4) correct the underlying cause, and (5) restore electrolyte balance (Thelan et al, 1990). Nursing interventions are based on activities that help Beatrice meet her expected outcomes. They consist of collaborative interventions, activities ordered by the physician but requiring some actions by the nurse, and independent interventions, activities that are within the nursing scope of practice to write and carry out as nursing orders.

Collaborative Interventions: Diabetic Ketoaci- *dosis.* The physician's orders may include the following.

1. IV therapy. Beatrice's initial management requires rapid rehydration. Osmotic diuresis precipitated by elevated glucose levels has severely depleted her body fluids. Table 20–9 describes a typical rehydration IV protocol as suggested by Thelan et al (1990). She will receive nothing by mouth until the crisis state is resolved.
2. Insulin therapy. Correction of the hyperglycemic state is dependent on careful use of insulin. During the crisis state, only

TABLE 20–9. A MEDICAL INTERVENTION PROTOCOL FOR DKA AND HHNC

Treatment Goal	DKA	HHNC
Fluid replacement	Initial hour: 0.9% normal saline (NS) at 1 L/hour	Initial 2 hours: 0.9% NS × 3 L
	Maintenance: 0.45% NS at 300–500 mL/hour	Maintenance: 0.45% NS × 6–10 L as needed for fluid replacement
	When glucose = 250–300 mg/dL, begin 5% dextrose solution	When glucose = 250–300 mg/dL, begin 5% dextrose in 0.9% or 0.45% NS
	If circulatory collapse, may receive plasma expanders	If circulatory collapse, may receive plasma expanders
Insulin (regular)	Initial IV bolus of 0.3 units/kg	Initial IV bolus of 10–15 units
	Maintenance dose: 0.1 units/kg/hour (about 6–10 units/hour) IV or IM	Alternative maintenance doses: (1) 0.1 units/kg/hour IV until serum glucose = 250 mg/dL; (2) single dose of 15 units subcutaneously
		Maintenance doses are discounted when glucose levels = 250 mg/dL

regular insulin is used because of its short duration, which facilitates better control. Insulin management generally is via continuous IV drip, though IM injections may be used. Table 20–9 describes a typical insulin management protocol as suggested by Thelan et al (1990).

3. Sodium bicarbonate therapy. Sodium bicarbonate is the drug of choice for rapid correction of most metabolic acidosis problems. An exception to this use is the correction of DKA. When the ketoacidosis is corrected too rapidly, it can precipitate cerebrospinal fluid (CSF) acidosis, causing potentially severe neurologic complications. CSF acidosis is difficult to correct because sodium bicarbonate does not cross the blood–brain barrier. Consequently, use of sodium bicarbonate may be confined to severe acidosis associated with a life-threateningly low serum pH. DKA often corrects itself with the use of insulin, electrolyte therapy, and IV fluid replacement.

4. Electrolyte replacement. Potassium, sodium, and phosphate are three of the major electrolytes requiring replacement during a DKA episode. Sodium is replaced primarily during the initial rehydration phase of treatment in the 0.9 percent and 0.45 percent normal saline IV solutions. Particular care is taken in managing potassium replacement, since serum levels decrease as the acidotic state is corrected and normal urine output is regained. Unless the serum potassium is low at the time of admission, potassium replacement is contraindicated for the first 3 to 4 hours of management. Once potassium shifts have stabilized (insulin therapy has been instituted and the urine output has been stabilized), potassium replacement is instituted. Phosphate, a buffer, may become depleted during periods of acidosis particularly if the acidosis is prolonged. Adequate levels of phosphate are important in combating the acidosis. When replacement is warranted, it is generally administered IV in the form of potassium phosphate.

5. Correction of underlying problems. A key to successful management of a hyperglycemic crisis is finding and treating successfully the underlying cause. Beatrice's left foot infection is a likely precipitating factor for her DKA episode. Antibiotic therapy is initiated, and the wound is debrided. Her diabetic condition prevents her from healing well, increasing her risk of further infection complications.

6. Laboratory and other tests. Beatrice's status will be closely monitored throughout the DKA period. Initially, close monitoring of serum pH, glucose, ketones, osmolality, and electrolytes is necessary. She may have an ECG ordered to monitor serum potassium effects on the heart. A culture and gram stain of the foot wound confirm the type of organism so that IV antibiotic therapy can be most effective.

Independent Nursing Interventions: Diabetic Ketoacidosis

Fluid volume deficit

1. Assess for signs and symptoms of fluid volume deficit, report abnormals.

2. Monitor hemodynamics as available, report worsening trends: pulmonary artery pressure, pulmonary artery wedge pressure, and central venous pressure.
3. Monitor laboratory and other test results, report abnormals: BUN and creatinine, electrolytes, hemoglobin and hematocrit.
4. Monitor for therapeutic and nontherapeutic effects of fluid replacement therapy, report abnormals.
5. When taking oral fluids, encourage intake to 2500 mL/24 hours if underlying problems permit.

Alteration in nutrition: Less than body requirements

1. Monitor for therapeutic and nontherapeutic effects of insulin therapy, report abnormals.
2. Monitor laboratory and other test results, report abnormals: serum glucose, ketones, albumin, transferrin, CBC with differential.
3. Monitor and document dietary intake.
4. Encourage intake of prescribed diet
   a. Avoid painful procedures immediately before meals or feedings.
   b. Administer pain medications before meals, when needed; assess effectiveness of PRN medications.
5. Implement measures to reduce energy requirements.

Injury, potential for, related to electrolyte imbalances and metabolic acidosis

1. Assess for signs and symptoms of electrolyte imbalances, report abnormals (specify imbalances based on specific disorder).
2. Assess for signs and symptoms of metabolic acidosis, report abnormals.
3. Monitor laboratory and other test results, report abnormals: serum electrolytes.
4. Monitor for therapeutic and nontherapeutic effects of electrolyte and acidosis drug therapy, report abnormals.
5. Monitor ECG for changes consistent with electrolyte imbalance, such as dysrhythmias, T wave changes, ST segment changes.
6. Encourage intake of appropriate nutrients.
7. Restrict intake of undesirable nutrients based on electrolyte levels.

8. Encourage intake of fluids if fluid volume deficit exists.

Case Study Update: 7 Days Postadmission

Beatrice remains in the intermediate care unit. Although her DKA was resolved within the first 48 hours, her glucose levels remain elevated. An updated systematic assessment shows the following.

Head and Neck. Neurologically, Beatrice is confused and drowsy, oriented to name only. A salem sump is in place in her right nostril, and correct placement is confirmed. Mucous membranes are pink and moist. Positive jugular vein distention (JVD) is noted at a 45-degree angle.

Chest. Cardiovascular status: S_1, S_2, and S_3 are present, with no murmurs. Rhythm is regular with a sinus tachycardia at 110 to 115/minute. T waves are peaked on ECG. Blood pressure is 174/92.

Respiratory status: Breath sounds are heard in all lobes. Bases are diminished, with crackles to midfields bilaterally. Occasional nonproductive cough is noted.

Abdomen. Gastrointestinal status: A nasogastric tube is connected to intermittent low wall suction. Nasogastric drainage is dark green and negative for blood. Bowel sounds are hypoactive in all four quadrants. The abdomen is moderately distended and tight.

Pelvis, Genitourinary Status. Foley catheter remains in place. Urine output for the last 24 hours has been a total of 425 mL.

Extremities. Edema 4+ is noted in all extremities. The skin is dry and flaky. Pulses are difficult to palpate secondary to edema.

Left foot wound status: The wound remains open and draining. It appears pale, with large areas of blackened tissue and patches of white. No healthy tissue is evident.

Posterior. The coccyx is reddened, although the skin is still intact. With Beatrice positioned on her right side, crackles are auscultated over the posterior fields (right more than left).

Other. Temperature is 100 to 102F. A 5 pound weight gain is noted over the past 48 hours. Beatrice continues to receive 5 percent dextrose in normal saline at 125 mL/hour. No type of diet or supplement has yet been ordered.

Current Drug Therapy. Current drug therapy includes regular and NPH insulin (SQ), gentamicin (IV), heparin (SQ), and ranitidine (IV).

QUESTION

Of the following, which assessment is most suggestive of the presence of an underlying nutritional problem?
1. Edema
2. Flaky, dry skin
3. Hypoactive bowel sounds
4. Absence of wound healing

ANSWER

4. Following Beatrice's wound debridement and antibiotic therapy, some degree of wound healing would be expected. However, her wound is again deteriorating according to the latest assessment data. Beatrice's ability to heal is further complicated by her long-standing diabetes as well as possible renal failure, since both of these conditions suppress healing.

QUESTION

Besides Beatrice's prolonged hypotensive episode as a major risk factor for acute renal failure, which of the following drugs is particularly associated with nephrotoxicity?
1. Gentamicin
2. Insulin
3. Heparin
4. Ranitidine

ANSWER

1. Aminoglycosides, such as gentamicin, are highly nephrotoxic. Gentamicin peak and trough levels should be drawn routinely to monitor for toxic blood levels. To monitor renal function for development of nephrotoxicity, serum BUN and creatinine also are determined routinely.

Current Serum Laboratory Results (Abnormal Values Only)

Glucose = 320 mg/dL

Albumin = 2.2 g/dL (Normal range 3.5–5.5 g/dL)

Transferrin = 112 mg/dL (Normal range 200–400 mg/dL)

White blood cell count = 4,900/mm^3 (Normal range 5,000–10,000/mm^3)

WBC differential:
  Neutrophils = 75% (Normal range 54–75%)

Bands = 15% (Normal range 3–8%)

Lymphocytes = 20% (Normal range 25–40%)

BUN = 54 mg/dL (Normal range 9–20 mg/dL)

Creatinine = 2.7 mg/dL (Normal range 0.7–1.5 mg/dl)

Electrolytes:
  Na = 162 mEq/L,
  Cl = 115 mEq/L,
  K = 6.0 mEq/L,
  Ca = 11.2 mEq/L

QUESTION

Which of the following statements best reflects the reason that Beatrice's serum creatinine is elevated?
1. Controlled diabetes causes increased breakdown of protein
2. Malnutrition causes increased excretion of creatinine
3. Gluconeogenesis increases the amount of serum creatinine
4. Nephrons are unable to cleanse the waste products from the blood

ANSWER

4. Creatinine is a waste product of muscle metabolism. When the kidneys go into failure, they can no longer perform their normal functions, and creatinine remains in the blood rather than being excreted. While Beatrice is in acute renal failure, you would anticipate that while her serum creatinine and BUN increase, creatinine and urea nitrogen clearance in the urine will decrease.

QUESTION

Beatrice's leukopenia is most likely caused by which combination of physiologic insults?
1. Hyperglycemic crisis and hypotension
2. Malnutrition and overwhelming infection
3. Acute renal failure and hyperglycemia
4. Hypotension and malnutrition

ANSWER

2. Beatrice's malnutrition is a major factor in failure of the immune system. This has been complicated by a severe infection of prolonged duration that may well have exhausted available neutrophils and lymphocytes.

QUESTION

A disadvantage of using serum albumin as an indicator of malnutrition is that it
1. Reflects muscle protein
2. Has a short half-life
3. Reflects plasma protein
4. Has a long half-life

ANSWER

4. Although considered to be a good indicator of nutritional status, the long half-life of serum albumin can make the laboratory values misleading as to current status. Serum transferrin, another indicator, is better at reflecting current status because of its short half-life.

TABLE 20–10. ACUTE RENAL FAILURE: CAUSES AND TREATMENT

Type	Causes	Treatment

Prerenal
Acute renal failure
	Decreased cardiac output:
	  Cardiac arrhythmias
	  Cardiogenic shock
	  Pulmonary embolism
	  Pericardial tamponade
	Vasodilation
	  Anaphylaxis
	  Sepsis
	Decreased circulatory blood volume
	  Peritonitis
	  Third spacing
	  Cirrhosis
	  Burns
	  Dehydration
	  Hemorrhage
	  Vomiting
	  Diarrhea
		Since kidney tissue is normal in prerenal failure, it is often reversible if the underlying problem is corrected in a timely fashion. Reversal requires rapid diagnosis followed by aggressive treatment; treatment may require any combination of the following
		  Drug management
		  Surgical interventions
		  Crystalloid or colloid IV therapy
		Failure to properly diagnose and treat prerenal failure can lead to ischemic damage to the kidneys (intrarenal failure)

Postrenal
Acute renal failure
	Postrenal failure is caused by bilateral obstruction to outflow of urine from the kidneys; obstruction may be either mechanical or functional
	Mechanical causes
	  Blood clots
	  Calculi
	  Tumors
	  Prostatic hypertrophy
	  Urethral strictures
	Functional causes
	  Diabetic neuropathy
	  Neurogenic bladder
	  Certain drugs (i.e., ganglionic
	    blockers)
		Postrenal ARF is frequently reversible. Treatment consists of removal of the mechanical or functional obstruction when feasible (e.g., prostatectomy) or bypassing the obstruction to reestablish a patent urine outflow tract, when necessary (e.g., ileocecal conduit)

Intrarenal
Acute renal failure
	Acute tubular necrosis is the most common cause of ARF in the high acuity patient; it is caused by
	  Ischemia of kidney tissue
	  Nephrotoxicity
	  Combination of ischemia and
	    nephrotoxicity
		Intrarenal ARF is the least desirable of the three types because it is caused by damage to kidney tissue. General treatment is as follows
		1. Diagnosis and aggressive treatment of the cause.
		2. Maintain normal fluid volume
		  Fluid restriction and replacement based on fluid excess or deficit status
		3. Prevent complications
		  Hyperkalemia
		    Drug therapy: Several options may be used. Cation exchange resins may be used either rectally or via gastrointestinal tract to physically remove the potassium from the body; sodium bicarbonate, insulin, or hypertonic glucose may be used to drive potassium back into cells
		  Diet must be high in fats, carbohydrates, and essential amino acids. PO or tube feeding is preferable route to lessen risk of infection. Dialysis commonly is used to control potassium, particularly when accompanied by excessive fluid volume
		  Hypotension
		  Treatment depends on the cause. Fluid replacement or volume expanders may be necessary. Hypotensive pharmacologic agents such as dopamine (Intropin) may be ordered. If hypotension is severe, treatment will be that typical of shock

TABLE 20–10. ACUTE RENAL FAILURE: CAUSES AND TREATMENT (*Continued*)

Type	Causes	Treatment
		Uremia
		Nitrogenous wastes must be controlled. Protein intake is restricted and dialysis may be performed when BUN = >100 or creatinine is >12.
		Metabolic acidosis
		Sodium bicarbonate is used sparingly to minimize hypernatremic effects; dialysis also is used to control acidosis
		Catabolism
		Nutritional support: Diet must be low in protein, sodium, potassium, and fluids; should be high in carbohydrates, fats, and essential amino acids. PO or via tube feeding is preferable to IV supplement to minimize risk of infection
		Infection
		Infection is the major cause of death from acute renal failure due to immunocompromised status. Minimal use of invasive lines and tubes is crucial. Antibiotic tubes protect against infection. Antibiotic therapy requires dose adjustments based on severity of renal impairment

Nursing Management: Acute Renal Failure

Management Goals. Acute renal failure is a complex disorder that affects metabolism and requires management of metabolic dysfunction. It particularly disturbs fluid and electrolyte balance. The general goals of care include

1. Diagnose/treat the underlying cause
2. Maintain normal fluid volume
3. Prevent complications

Collaborative Interventions. Table 20–10 presents each of the three types of acute renal failure, the common causes of each, and a global picture of collaborative management as summarized from Crandall (1989). Dialysis is covered in more depth in Module 18, *Acute Renal Failure.*

QUESTION

Based on available data, which type of acute renal failure is Beatrice most likely experiencing?
1. Prerenal
2. Postrenal
3. Intrarenal
4. Insufficient data to decide

ANSWER

3. Beatrice's clinical picture and laboratory data are most consistent with intrarenal ARF.

Independent Nursing Interventions. There are many nursing diagnoses pertinent to care of the patient with acute renal failure. During the oliguric phase, some of the most important ones include

- **Fluid volume excess**
- **Nutrition, alteration in: less than body requirements**
- **Injury, potential for**
- **Infection, potential for**
- **Self-care deficit**
- **Anxiety**
- **Activity intolerance**

During the diuretic phase, most of the nursing diagnoses remain the same, with the exception of a shift in fluid volume from fluid excess to potential fluid deficit.

Nursing Management: The Malnourished Patient

General Goals. Beatrice's malnourished state is severely hindering her recovery. Goals for managing this problem include

1. Halt the state of catabolism
2. Regain positive nitrogen balance
3. Prevent/treat complications

Collaborative Interventions.

1. Laboratory testing. High acuity patients need to have blood drawn for intermittent laboratory tests that measure various aspects of nutritional status. These tests include CBC with differential, serum albumin (and/or transferrin), BUN, and creatinine. Urine clearance testing of urea and creatinine may be ordered. Clearance testing helps determine the extent of damage to the nephrons, the effectiveness of renal disease treatment, and the baseline function of the kidneys before initiating treatment (Cella and Watson, 1989).
2. Dietary orders. Nutritional support is needed by all patients. The decision of route of intake (oral, gastric tube, IV) and type of support (diet, tube feeding, TPN) may be made on the basis of an educated guess of nutritional need, or it may result from a more complex and thorough assessment of nutritional needs via the various nutrition-related measurements. Generally speaking, the more physiologically compromised the patient is, the more complex the nutritional needs

are. It is essential that Beatrice's nutritional needs be met to facilitate healing and to build up her immune system, which is dangerously compromised. For 7 days, she has had no nutritional supplementation except for fluid and electrolytes. If Beatrice did not have acute renal failure, she would be placed on a high protein diet to facilitate regaining immunocompetence and the healing process.

3. Nutritional supplementation. Various supplements consisting of vitamins and minerals may be ordered to meet Beatrice's current nutritional needs, which are important in healing and blood cell formation. These supplements may include vitamins, iron, zinc, and folic acid.

Nutritional support is presented in depth in Module 16, *Nutrition.*

Independent Nursing Interventions. **Nutrition, alteration in: less than body requirements** is the primary nursing diagnosis that is included on Beatrice's plan of care to address her state of malnutrition. Other significant nursing diagnoses pertinent to care of the malnourished patient include the following.

- **Infection, potential for**
- **Activity intolerance**
- **Self-care deficit**
- **Comfort, alteration in: pain**
- **Injury, potential for electrolyte imbalances**

The nursing diagnoses: Alteration in nutrition: less than body requirements and potential for injury, are both addressed in detail earlier in this module in the discussion of Nursing Management: Diabetic Ketoacidosis.

Nursing Management: The Immunocompromised Patient

General Goals. The goals for care of the immunocompromised patient include the goals appropriate to the malnourished patient. Additional goals include

1. Reestablish immunocompetence
2. Prevent/treat complications

Collaborative Interventions.

1. Laboratory testing. Various tests may be ordered to evaluate immune status, as discussed previously. Since many of the cell-specific blood tests are not commonly performed and are both expensive

and time consuming to obtain or measure, the nurse needs to clarify nursing responsibilities and expectations regarding the tests before drawing samples or having them drawn to prevent nursing error.

2. Drug therapy. Beatrice is not receiving any drugs that directly affect immunocompetence. There are two types of drugs that have a direct impact on the immune system, immunosuppressive therapy agents and agents that enhance immunity. Immunosuppressants decrease immune function. Uses include control of chronic inflammatory problems, prevention of organ transplant rejection, and others. Examples of immunosuppressant drugs are steroids and cyclosporin A. Drugs that enhance immune function in some way include immunotherapy agents, primarily used in cancer therapy; monoclonal antibodies, antibodies that act against specific antigens; and interleukin, a lymphokine used to enhance immune responses.

3. Environmental protection. Severe leukopenia places the patient at risk for infection. The severely immunocompromised patient is placed in a controlled environment. Hospitals have protocols establishing the exact nature of the environment protection. A private room is ordered. Some hospitals have special positive airflow rooms that diminish airflow of possibly contaminated air into the protected patient's room.

Independent Nursing Interventions. In caring for the immunosuppressed patient, the nurse's role centers around monitoring/prevention of infection, regaining or maintaining adequate nutrition, and meeting the psychosocial needs of the patient and family (Griffin, 1986).

There are two physiologically based nursing diagnoses appropriate in meeting the first two goals.

- **Infection, potential for: related to deficient immune protection**
- **Nutrition, alteration in: less than body requirements**

Potential for infection related to deficient immune protection, neutropenia. Expected patient outcomes. The patient will show no evidence of infection.

NURSING INTERVENTIONS (Griffin, 1986)

I. Monitor every 2 to 4 hours for signs and symptoms of infection
  A. Temperature increases (most important sign, may be slight in immunosuppressed patient)
  B. Signs and symptoms of inflammation, such as pain, redness, heat, swelling (some or all of these may be absent if neutrophils are too low)
  C. Skin or mucous membrane lesions
    1. Check all skin folds, mouth, and anal area
  D. Gastrointestinal lesions
    1. Check all stools for guiac
    2. Monitor for diarrhea or constipation
  E. Genitourinary problems
    1. Check urine for color, odor
    2. Monitor patient for pain
  F. Respiratory
    1. Monitor for adventitious breath sounds, cough, dyspnea, pain
  G. Invasive line/tube sites
    1. Observe all sites closely for signs or symptoms of actual or potential infection
II. Institute measures to environmentally protect patient
  A. Place in private room; keep door closed
  B. Screen all persons coming into contact with patient for signs and symptoms of infection
    1. Apply mask if respiratory infection is suspected or confirmed
  C. Excellent handwashing before contact (gloves recommended)
  D. Maintain strict aseptic technique for all sterile procedures
  E. Minimize foods and objects brought into the room from outside environment
III. Provide ongoing protection against development of infection
  A. Monitor hydration status every shift
  B. Turn every 1 to 2 hours
  C. Skin care
    1. Thorough bathing every day
    2. Keep skin clean and lubricated at all times
  D. Keep linens clean
  E. Pulmonary exercises every 4 hours
    1. Incentive spirometry, deep breathing
    2. As ordered: percussion, postural drainage, vibration (percussion is contraindicated if coagulopathy exists)

F. Minimize invasive procedures: no rectal temperatures or enemas and no injections
G. Protect patient against injury
   1. Instruct patient
      a. No straining
      b. Use no sharp objects: use electric razor
      c. Report any infection signs and symptoms
      d. Brush teeth with very soft bristle brush or toothette

Alteration in nutrition: less than body requirements. The plan of care remains essentially the same as previously described. However, immunocompromised patients often also develops stomatitis, which can interfere with consumption of food.

I. Perform actions to minimize stomatitis problems
   A. Mouth care before mealtime
   B. Offer lidocaine viscous immediately before mealtime

There are many other nursing diagnoses that might apply to the immunosuppressed patient based on individual physiologic and psychosocial needs. Some of the more common ones include

- **Injury, potential for**
- **Anxiety**
- **Coping, potential for ineffective**
- **Comfort, alteration in: pain**
- **Knowledge deficit**
- **Powerlessness**
- **Self-concept, alteration in**
- **Activity intolerance**
- **Social isolation**

Evaluation and Revision of the Plan of Care

Evaluation of the effectiveness of Beatrice's plan of care is based on how well she meets the expected patient outcomes within each nursing diagnosis. The care plan is a working document subject to frequent changes. Interventions that have not effective need to be scrutinized as to why they are ineffective. Revision of the plan is then made, removing ineffective actions and adding alternative ones.

Beatrice's problems are complex and require ag-gressive interventions, both collaborative and independent, if she is to regain her prehospitalization state of health.

Ultimately, following failure of her left heel wound to heal and subsequent development of sepsis, Beatrice required amputation of her left leg to below the knee. On removal of this major physiologic stressor, she rapidly recovered and was able to be discharged home.

In summary, this module has attempted to show how one type of metabolic disorder can precipitate an imbalance in another body function. The case study presented a sequence of events that in reality do occur, profoundly affecting the patient's prognosis. Although each disorder had a different etiology, with the exception of immunocompetence and malnutrition, they shared many of the same nursing diagnoses. Major nursing diagnoses presented included: **Fluid volume deficit, Nutrition: less than body requirements, Potential for injury and infection.** Each of these diagnoses has been described using the case study of Beatrice, a patient with complex metabolic problems. Collaborative as well as independent nursing interventions were discussed.

Addendum: The Patient with Human Immunodeficiency Virus (HIV)

The type of nursing management required for care of the patient who tests positive for the human immunodeficiency virus (HIV) is dependent on the stage of the disease. The most commonly recognized manifestation of the virus is acquired immunodeficiency syndrome (AIDS). Nursing management for the patient with AIDS is essentially the same as for all immunosuppressed patients.

HIV is transmittable. Therefore, nursing management also must include protection of the staff. Many persons who are positive for the virus show no signs or symptoms of AIDS, and, therefore, continuous protection from all patients is necessary through strict adherence to the Centers for Disease Control (CDC) universal precautions. Particular care is taken when drawing blood specimens or when performing a procedure that requires direct exposure to blood, since blood is a major transmitter.

Because of the terminal nature of AIDS as well as the social stigma that it carries, Dolan (1991, pp. 1222–1225) suggests the following additional psychosocial nursing diagnoses.

- **Fear of death and dying**
- **Body image, disturbance**
- **Social isolation**
- **Verbal communication, impaired**

REFERENCES

Cella, J.H., and Watson, J. (1989). *Nurse's manual of laboratory tests.* Philadelphia: F.A Davis Company.

Crandall, B.I. (1989). Acute renal failure. In B.T. Ulrich (ed). *Nephrology nursing: Concepts and strategies,* pp. 45–59. E. Norwalk, Connecticut: Appleton & Lange.

Dolan, J.T. (1991). *Critical care nursing: Clinical management through the nursing process.* Philadelphia: F.A. Davis Co.

Dougherty, S. (1988). The malnourished respiratory patient. *Crit. Care Nurse.* 8(4):13–22.

Farley, J.M. (1991). Nutritional support of the critically ill patient. In J.T. Dolan (ed). *Critical care nursing: Clinical management through the nursing process,* pp. 1125–1150. Philadelphia: F.A. Davis Co.

Golightly, M.G., and Dolan, J.T. (1991). Assessment in immunologic function. In J.T. Dolan (ed). *Critical care nursing: Clinical management through the nursing process,* pp. 1176–1180. Philadelphia: F.A. Davis Co.

Griffin, J.P. (1986). *Hematology and immunology: Concepts for nursing.* E. Norwalk, Connecticut: Appleton & Lange.

Lumley, W. (1988). Controlling hypoglycemia and hyperglycemia. *Nursing.* 18(10):34–42.

McCarthy, J.A. (1985). The continuum of diabetic coma. *Am. J. Nursing.* 85(8):878–882.

McKenna, B. (1988). Diabetic disorders and patient care. In M.R. Kinney, D.R. Packa, and S.B. Dunbar (eds). *AACN's clinical reference for critical-care nursing,* pp. 1067–1087. New York: McGraw-Hill Book Co.

Stark, J.L. (1985). The renal system. In J.G. Alspach and S.M. Williams (eds) *Core curriculum for critical care nursing,* pp. 347–450. Philadelphia: W.B. Saunders.

Thelan, L., Davie, J., and Urden, L. (1990). Endocrine disorders and therapeutic management. In *Textbook of critical care nursing: Diagnosis and management.* St. Louis: C.V. Mosby.

ADDITIONAL READING

Carpenito, L.J. (1987). *Nursing diagnosis: Application to clinical practice,* 2nd ed. Philadelphia: J.B. Lippincott.

Fidler, M.R., Sr., and Keen, M.F. (1988). The immunocompromised patient. In M.R. Kinney, D.R. Packa, and S.S. Dunbar (eds). *AACN's clinical reference for critical care nursing,* 2nd ed., pp 1249–1269. New York: McGraw-Hill Book Co.

Hudak, C.M., Gallo, B.M., and Benz, J.J. (1990). *Critical care nursing: A holistic approach,* 5th ed. Philadelphia: J.B. Lippincott Co.

Roberts, S.L. (1985). *Physiological concepts and the critically ill patient.* Englewood Cliffs, New Jersey: Prentice-Hall, Inc.

Ulrich, B.T. (1989). *Nephrology nursing: Concepts and strategies.* E. Norwalk, Connecticut: Appleton & Lange.

Ulrich, S.P., Canale, S.W., and Wendell, S.A. (1986). *Nursing care planning guides: A nursing diagnosis approach.* Philadelphia: W.B. Saunders.

PART V

Psychosocial Concepts

Caring for the Critically Ill Patient: Patient, Family, and Nursing Considerations

Pamela Stinson Kidd

Caring for the Critically Ill Patient: Patient, Family, and Nursing Considerations is written at a core knowledge level for individuals who provide nursing care for critically ill patients regardless of the practice setting. The focus of the module is the nursing role in caring for critically ill patients and the nature of the critical illness/injury event on the patient, family, and nurse. The module is divided into two parts: Patient and Family Considerations and Nursing Considerations. Part One consists of five sections. Section One introduces the critically ill patient. Sections Two and Three address the stages of illness and nursing strategies to assist the patient in coping with being critically ill. Section Four discusses the influence of the environment on the patient's psychologic and physical integrity. The educational needs of critically ill patients and their family are examined in Section Five.

The second part, consisting of five sections, discusses the nursing role in caring for critically ill patients. Section Six examines the educational needs of nurses working with critically ill patients. The interface between technology and caring is discussed in Section Seven. Stressors and satisfying factors associated with nursing the critically ill patient are addressed in Section Eight. Section Nine examines resource allocation issues, and Section Ten encourages the learner to complete a self-assessment in order to identify potential sources of personal conflict in working with the critically ill.

Each section includes a set of review questions to help the learner evaluate understanding of section content before advancing to the next section. All section reviews, and the Pretest and Posttest in the module include answers. It is suggested that the learner review those concepts that have been missed in the review questions before proceeding to the next section.

Objectives

Following completion of the module, *Caring for the Critically Ill Patient*, the learner will be able to

1. Discuss the evolution of the health care system in regard to caring for critically ill patients
2. Discuss stages of illness a critically ill patient may experience
3. Identify ways the nurse can help the critically ill patient to cope with the illness event
4. Identify the influence of environment on the critically ill patient's psychologic and physical responses
5. Discuss the educational needs of critically ill patients and their families
6. Discuss educational issues surrounding nurses who work with critically ill patients
7. Discuss the interface between technology and caring

8. Describe stressful and satisfying aspects in providing nursing care for the critically ill patient

9. Describe resource allocation issues as they relate to the critically ill patient

10. Identify personal values that may contribute to satisfaction or stress in caring for the critically ill patient

Pretest

1. Critically ill patients frequently complain about which of the following when hospitalized?
   A. lack of privacy
   B. hospital food
   C. inadequate nursing staff
   D. lack of blankets

2. Denial during critical illness
   A. can have positive effects on health outcomes
   B. increases oxygen consumption
   C. is a maladaptive coping strategy
   D. promotes false hope

3. Hypohugganemia is
   A. a reduction in red blood cells related to social isolation
   B. desaturation of oxyhemoglobin
   C. an adversity to touch
   D. a state of touch deficiency

4. Who of the following is at greatest risk for developing sensory problems?
   A. adolescent patient
   B. unresponsive patient
   C. female patient
   D. transplant patient

5. A major reason that computers are being tested to use in decision making with critically ill patients is
   A. computers are compact
   B. computers are time efficient
   C. any staff member can input available data
   D. there is a large amount of data that must be processed in order to make a decision

6. Nurses who work with critically ill patients cite which of the following as a major stressor?
   A. overtime work
   B. nurse/patient ratio
   C. constant need to reverify skills and procedures
   D. interpersonal conflict with other health team members

7. Of the following patient populations, which population is the least vulnerable in regard to resource allocation?
   A. neonates
   B. elderly
   C. oncology patients
   D. transplant patients

8. Which of the following factors may inhibit learning in critically ill patients?
   A. medications
   B. previous knowledge of illness
   C. educational level
   D. sex

9. Families of critically ill patients desire which of the following group of needs to be met first by the nurse?
   A. physical
   B. spiritual
   C. cognitive
   D. emotional

10. Mr. Rogers states, "I'm going to have to put up with this scar and make the best of it." This response indicates he is in which of the following states of illness?
    A. awareness
    B. resolution
    C. restitution
    D. denial

11. The purpose of imagery is to
    A. ignore the real situation
    B. replace unpleasant experiences with relaxation
    C. promote use of the senses
    D. increase neurologic stimulation

12. Critically ill patients have which of the following characteristics?
    A. have been hospitalized previously
    B. need extensive rehabilitation
    C. are physically unstable
    D. have chronic illness

13. The use of equipment in the nursing role may
    A. increase the nurse's stress level
    B. decrease nursing surveillance responsibility
    C. decrease the need for patient advocacy
    D. increase patient satisfaction
14. Which of the following is a hazard of technology?
    A. increased fragmentation of care
    B. decreased demand for nursing staff
    C. decreased competition with patient for nursing time
    D. increased patient feeling of independence
15. Which of the following may be a source of burnout?
    A. hourly nursing assessment
    B. nursing care plans
    C. continuing education requirements
    D. primary nursing
16. Which of the following may be a symptom of burnout?
    A. nurse requests to work a holiday
    B. nurse assists co-workers in care
    C. nurse complains of inadequate physician standing orders
    D. nurse states that "females always give in to their pain"
17. Mr. Martin states that he has dreamed of being tortured while in the intensive care unit. The nurse recognizes that this is a symptom of
    A. sensory deprivation
    B. burnout
    C. fatigue
    D. uncontrolled pain

18. ICU psychosis usually is associated with
    A. chemotherapy
    B. surgery
    C. head trauma
    D. psychologic problems
19. Which of the following have nurses identified as increasing their satisfaction with their role?
    A. getting on-call pay
    B. orienting new staff
    C. working multiple shifts
    D. small nurse/patient ratio
20. All of the following have been cited to relieve stress associated with the nursing role EXCEPT
    A. discussion with co-workers
    B. self-assessment of achievements
    C. serving as unit resource person
    D. watching television

Pretest answers: 1, A. 2, A. 3, D. 4, B. 5, D. 6, D. 7, D. 8, A. 9, C. 10, B. 11, B. 12, C. 13, A. 14, A. 15, D. 16, D. 17, A. 18, B. 19, D. 20, C.

Glossary

Burnout. A crisis state evolving from stress; to become exhausted by making excessive demands on energy, strength, or resources

Delusion. Fixed irrational belief not consistent with cultural mores; may include persecutory or grandiose ideas

Hallucination. False sensory perception occurring without any external stimulus; a person can see, feel, hear, smell, or taste things that another person cannot

Hypohugganemia. A state of touch deficiency when a need for physical contact increases or when the need remains the same and the opportunities for physical contact are diminished

Illusion. False interpretation of an external sensory stimulus that is usually visual or auditory in nature

Intensive care psychosis (ICU psychosis). A reversible, confusional state usually noted between the third and seventh days after admission to an intensive care unit

PATIENT AND FAMILY CONSIDERATIONS

Section One: Evolution of Patient Care Areas for Critically Ill Patients

At the completion of this section, the learner will be able to discuss briefly the evolution of the health care system in regard to caring for critically ill patients.

The nurse caring for the critically ill patient must be able to analyze clinical situations, make decisions based on this analysis, and act on the decisions made in a rapid and precise manner. Comfort with uncertainty and patient instability are requirements in this area. The nurse is instrumental in treating the patients' health problems as well as their reactions to the health care environment. The nurse is usually the constant in caring for the critically ill patient. The nurse coordinates the care of the other health team members.

Nurses working in critical care units have received respect both within and outside the nursing profession. This respect is related to social events. World wars produced the need for trauma care and intensive nursing both before and after surgery. Polio epidemics provided the motivation for respiratory care. Traditionally, patients were admitted to the intensive care unit for nursing care in combination with technologic capabilities. The perception evolved that good nursing care could be found only in the intensive care unit (Baggs, 1989).

Intensive care units were first developed in the early 1960s. The reasons for their development were (1) the implementation of cardiopulmonary resuscitation so that people might survive sudden death events, (2) better understanding of the treatment of hypovolemic shock related to recent war experiences, (3) implementation of emergency medical services, resulting in improved transport systems, (4) development of technologic inventions that required close observation for effective use (i.e., ECG monitoring), and (5) initiation of renal transplant surgery.

The first intensive care units were recovery rooms. Patients admitted were still anesthetized. Problems resulted, however, when the amount of surgery increased, and recovery rooms were needed for patients to recover from anesthesia. The more acutely ill patient who required extra equipment and observation was placed in the newly created intensive care unit.

Although critically ill patients are viewed historically as being in a critical care unit, this is no longer true because of the shortage of critical care beds and increased patient acuity. The critically ill patient is physically unstable and at risk of developing life-threatening problems. These patients require continuous, intensive assessment and interventions for restoration of physiologic stability (AACN, 1984). Patients with chronic illnesses who experience an acute exacerbation, as well as patients with a nonsignificant medical history who are involved in a traumatic event or exhibit an acute problem, fall within this definition. The nursing shortage situation (particularly the shortage of critical care nurses), an increase in life expectancy, an increase in number of persons with chronic illness, and the number of uninsured/underinsured patients create a situation of increased demand for services. Therefore, critically ill patients may be in a variety of settings: intensive care units, emergency departments, postanesthesia care units, medical-surgical units, obstetric units, hospice units, and the home.

Regardless of the setting, patients have complained about the helplessness and embarrassment they have felt when they were critically ill. Some patients fear dying, pain, and the uncertainty of their situation. They are fearful of moving in bed because of tubing, attachments, and incisions. They frequently feel frustrated about their inability to communicate when they are endotracheally intubated. Critically ill patients often are left nude or partially exposed. They are powerless and are stripped of their identity.

Nurses caring for the critically ill patient can anticipate patient feelings and support patient independence. Education about the nature of machinery can decrease fears of harming oneself. Nurses can role-model communication skills. Privacy should not be sacrificed, and the lack of it should not be justified by the intensity of the patient situation.

In summary, the nurse must remember the complexity surrounding critical illness. The physiologic needs of the patient take precedence. The rest of the self-study modules in this book have focused on addressing physiologic needs. In reality, physiologic and psychologic factors both must be considered when analyzing patient responses. For example, sensory alterations may occur because of electrolyte imbalances, drug reactions, or stimuli overload. The aim of this module is to support patient adaptation in a holistic manner using a humanistic approach.

Section One Review

1. Which of the following factors contributed to the development of intensive care units?
   A. increased number of patients requiring hospitalization
   B. development of Medicare/Medicaid system
   C. implementation of cardiopulmonary resuscitation
   D. movement of nursing education to the collegiate setting

2. Which of the following characteristics best describes critically ill patients?
   A. physiologically unstable with uncertain health outcomes
   B. volume depleted and edematous
   C. frustrated and demanding
   D. having impaired physical mobility and altered nutritional state

Answers: 1, C. 2, A.

Section Two: Stages of Illness

At the completion of this section, the learner will be able to discuss the stages of illness a critically ill patient may experience.

Critical illness produces a loss of the familiar self-image and has an impact on self-esteem. The patient may need to adapt to loss of health, loss of limb, disfigurement, or a necessary change in lifestyle. Change may precipitate grieving. Critically ill patients may respond to these losses by experiencing certain predictable phases. The first stage is shock and disbelief because the diagnosis does not have an emotional meaning. The patient may be uncooperative because he or she is projecting difficulties onto hospital procedures, equipment, and personnel. In this stage, a patient may worry more about the equipment being used than about the diagnosis, since the diagnosis may be a threat to life. Denial can have positive effects. It may protect the patient against the emotional impact of the illness and conserve energy by removing worry. The nurse should function as a noncritical listener. Patient statements can be clarified, but reality is not stressed (Suchman, 1965).

The awareness stage is characterized by an attempt to regain control. Patients may express guilt about the illness or injury as a gesture of assuming responsibility for events over which they may or may not have actual control. The patient may be demanding or exhibit signs of withdrawal. Both signs are indicative of anger toward either others or the self. The nurse should not argue with the patient. Consistent, dependable nursing care should be provided.

During the next stage, restitution, the patient may verbalize fears about the future. New behaviors are initiated that reflect new limitations. Sadness is experienced, and crying episodes may be frequent. The patient may reorganize relationships with family and friends. The nurse can assist by building communication to assist with problem solving.

Resolution, the final stage, involves identity change. The patient may begin to think of the illness as a growing experience. Limitations are accepted as consequences and not as defects.

These stages are not fixed but reflect a dynamic process of adjusting to an acute situation. The patient may regress to an earlier stage during periods of heightened anxiety. An aim in caring for the critically ill patient is to foster a feeling of security. A patient may feel vulnerable because of physiologic changes, such as paralysis or traction. Emotional vulnerability may be experienced when restraints are applied as a protective mechanism. Several factors may produce anxiety in the patient even if they may mean that the patient is more physiologically stable. The removal of electrodes, weaning from the ventilator, reduction in pain medication, and increasing mobility are among these factors.

In summary, the critically ill patient may progress through a series of emotional stages because of losses experienced during the illness event. The stages are referred to as denial, awareness, restitution, and resolution. The patient's progression through these stages may not be linear. When an additional stressor occurs, the patient may regress to a previous stage where the patient feels more secure.

Section Two Review

1. A major behavior of a patient in the denial stage of illness is
   A. false humor by the patient
   B. crying
   C. anger
   D. projection of difficulties onto objects and staff
2. The awareness stage of illness is characterized by all of the following EXCEPT
   A. increased dependence on others
   B. expression of guilt
   C. withdrawal behavior
   D. being demanding of caregivers
3. Mr. Abe was involved in a motor vehicle crash and sustained multiple lower extremities fractures. He will need additional surgery and prolonged physical therapy. The nurse finds Mr. Abe drawing plans for remodeling his porch in order to accommodate a wheelchair. This behavior reflects which stage of illness?
   A. denial
   B. awareness
   C. restitution
   D. resolution
4. When interacting with a patient in denial, the nurse should
   A. reinforce reality
   B. function as a noncritical listener
   C. explain the current treatment plan
   D. help the patient to recall the injury event

Answers: 1, D. 2, A. 3, D. 4, B.

Section Three: Coping with Critical Illness

At the completion of this section, the learner will be able to identify ways the nurse can help the critically ill patient to cope with the illness event.

Critically ill patients use strategies to maintain or increase their sense of hope during a life-threatening event. They may use pleasant, distracting images of favored activities. A conviction that a positive outcome is possible may be expressed. The belief that growth results from crisis fosters hope. Spiritual practices and beliefs that allow the patient to transcend suffering facilitate coping. Caregivers who convey positive expectations that the patient will be able to cope with the stresses as well as who assist the patient by gentle pushing support the patient's hope (Miller, 1989).

Because of the increased emphasis on manipulating equipment (this is discussed further in Part II of this module), human contact has received decreased emphasis during critical illness. Touching is a form of communication and a behavior of caring. Fear, pain, and acute stress can increase a person's need for touch (Dominion, 1971), and generally, complex technology increases the need for human touch (Kirchhoff et al, 1985). Although sex, ethnicity, and the age of the patient may influence the perception of touch as a caring behavior, most individuals appreciate being touched during a crisis (Clement, 1988). A state of touch deficiency may occur, hypohug-ganemia, when a person's need for physical contact increases or the need remains constant while the opportunities for touch decrease (Clement, 1986). Touch may decrease perceived pain and anxiety.

Self-regulation strategies, such as progressive muscle relaxation, biofeedback, and self-hypnosis, may be used to enhance the patient's feeling of control and to foster pain and anxiety relief. These strategies have an impact on the autonomic, endocrine, immune, and neuropeptide systems (Dossey, 1990). Promoting relaxation decreases sympathetic nervous system activity. This enhances the effect of pain medications, decreases fatigue, anxiety, and muscle tension, increases effective breathing patterns, and helps the patient to dissociate from pain.

Imagery and progressive muscle relaxation are self-regulation responses that involves all of the senses. Imagery can influence both the voluntary and involuntary nervous systems. The nurse must individualize the imagery process. Individualization requires an understanding of physiology of the illness, knowledge of medication, procedures, and diagnostic tests, and an understanding of the patient's beliefs (Dossey, 1990). The goal is to create an image of healing or the peacefulness of moving into death (if this is appropriate). Imagery desensitizes potentially anxiety-producing events by replacing fear or pain with relaxation. The following case study demonstrates the use of imagery. The case study is referred to again in Sections Four and Five.

Mr. T is a 79-year-old man who had an exploratory laparotomy for a perforated duodenal ulcer. He has a history of COPD and is steroid dependent. Mr. T's wound is healing by secondary intention. He has been having a great deal of pain during dressing changes.

The nurse prepares the patient care area by dimming lights and decreasing noise. The nurse can place a sign outside the patient's room indicating that an imagery session is taking place. The nurse promotes relaxation by encouraging Mr. T to start at the top of his head and imagine that each muscle is going limp. She describes it as a heavy good feeling. The nurse will go through each body section separately (neck, shoulders, and so on). Mr. T will close his eyes and concentrate on his body.

Nurse: "As the old dressing is being removed, your new tissue is getting fresh nutrients because dead skin and bacteria are being pulled away with the gauze. Imagine a tiny skin cell with hands that reach out to join another skin cell to make a firm chain. Although you are a little uncomfortable, you want the dressing to be removed because the new skin cells cannot grow underneath the debris from the old cells. As the new cells get nutrients, there is less drainage and less discomfort. Now, imagine that the skin is completely together just like it was before surgery. There is no need for more dressing changes.

"Each time your dressing is changed, concentrate on this image of the skin cells joining hands to make a firm chain that is completely together and healed. Imagine the cells getting fresh air and food that make them strong."

The goal of this session was to describe positive aspects of the dressing change in order to replace Mr. T's fear with a positive image of healing.

In summary, there are several strategies a nurse can use to assist the critically ill patient in coping with the illness event. These strategies include instilling hope, supporting spirituality, using physical touch, promoting relaxation, and using guided imagery with progressive muscle relaxation.

Section Three Review

1. The rationale for using self-regulation techniques with critically ill patients is to
   A. promote feelings of control
   B. decrease parasympathetic nervous system impulses
   C. improve nurse/patient relationships
   D. help the patient associate with personal pain

2. Which of the following factors influences the perception of touch as a caring behavior?
   A. environmental temperature
   B. cultural background
   C. length of the hospitalization
   D. size of caregiver's hands

Answers: 1, A. 2, B.

Section Four: Environmental Stressors

At the completion of this section, the learner will be able to discuss environmental stresses of the critically ill patient.

Sensory input involves all five senses: visual, auditory, olfactory, gustatory, and tactile. Individual perceptions of stimuli to the senses vary. Usually, people select stimuli that are most acceptable to them. However, during critical illness, the patient does not have control over the choice of the environment and its stimuli. The very young, the very old, the postoperative or unresponsive patients are at greatest risk of experiencing sensory problems.

Sensory deprivation may occur because of either impaired use of the senses or inadequate quality and quantity of sensory input. The patient is not able to relate meaningfully to the environment. Symptoms of sensory deprivation include illusions, delusions, hallucinations, restlessness, and loss of sense of time. These symptoms may appear as early as 8 hours after a period of sensory deprivation (Farrimond, 1984). The nurse must assess if the symptoms are related to psychologic reasons or physical reasons, such as hypoxia or increased intracranial pressure. Restricted movement, a windowless patient care area, monotonous light, and lack of stimuli all can produce sensory deprivation.

A combination of sensory overload and deprivation can exist. The patient is deprived of normal sensory stimuli while being exposed to continuous strange stimuli not normally encountered. The nurse should assess what sounds are in the patient's normal environment and expose the patient to these sounds if possible (through tape recordings). Visitors can be effective by discussing familiar topics with the patient (Smith, 1986). Unresponsive patients are particularly challenging, since information about the patient's normal environment must be collected through a third person. It is difficult to assess if unresponsive patients are experiencing sensory alterations, since they cannot communicate symptoms.

Sensory overload may occur when the patient is exposed to noise for continuous periods of time without rest. Noise produces peripheral vasoconstriction, which can cause increased afterload, especially in patients with hypertension. This response does not diminish on repeated exposure (Williams, 1989). Noise has a potentiating effect on ototoxic drugs (i.e., furosemide, aminoglycoside antibiotics, and salicylates) (Williams, 1989). Noise also stimulates the sympathetic nervous system, resulting in increased heart rate and oxygen consumption. Patients cite equipment noise, verbal noise generated by staff, visitors, and other patients, and noise from other patients in pain as being the most annoying sounds they encountered while hospitalized (Gast and Baker, 1989). Staff may become habituated to the noise. Thus, staff may underestimate the noise level in the patient care setting.

A phenomenon called ICU psychosis has been noted to occur in 12 percent to 38 percent of conscious intensive care unit patients between the third and seventh day after admission to the intensive care unit (Easton and MacKenzie, 1988). The highest incidence of this disorder has occurred in surgical intensive care patients, followed by medical intensive care patients. Varying degrees of delirium exist, but usually illusions, delusions, and hallucinations are present. Patients may be experiencing symptoms but are reluctant to share them with the nurse for fear of being labeled crazy. It is important for the nurse to assess if the delirium is related to physiologic reasons. Liver failure, electrolyte abnormalities, septic shock, hypoxia, and drug toxicities can produce these symptoms. Retrospective research studies have revealed that patients frequently feel that they are being held prisoner and that they were repeatedly trying to escape (Schnaper and Cowley, 1976). ICU psychosis occurs more frequently in patients who deny preoperative anxiety and in windowless patient care areas (Easton and MacKenzie, 1988). The increased acuity of patients in medical-surgical floor settings and the need for sophisticated equipment to monitor these critically ill patients may increase the prevalence of ICU psychosis outside of the intensive care unit.

Planned rest periods that allow for 2 hours of uninterrupted sleep are essential. Rapid eye movement (REM) sleep requires a 90 to 100 minute total sleep period for its occurrence. Therefore, 2-hour periods promote REM sleep. REM sleep helps to maintain optimism, attention span, and self-confidence. There is an increased need for REM sleep after periods of worry. Deprivation of REM sleep can impair memory and learning ability and produce hallucinations (Farrimond, 1984). Lack of REM sleep increases adrenal hormone production, which suppresses the immune system (Smith, 1986).

There are several interventions the nurse can implement to prevent sensory alterations in critically ill patients. The audible volume of bedside monitors should be decreased to allow greater patient rest and to deemphasize how ill a patient may be. Phones can be set on low volume. Patient doors can be closed. Posted reminders to speak softly can be placed in high traffic areas and by telephones. Nurses should ask patients if they have experienced any strange sensory experiences. Wall clocks and calendars may help the patient to remain oriented to time. However, clocks are not helpful if the patient's room does not have a window, since day and night cannot be discriminated (Hansell, 1984).

Darkened eyeshades and earplugs can be used to decrease noise and light. Lights can be dimmed to facilitate discrimination of day from night and promote circadian rhythms. Circadian rhythms influence basal metabolic rate, respiratory and heart rates, and body temperature (Barrie-Shelvin, 1987). Circadian rhythms respond to environmental cues, such as light to dark alternation. Interventions can be spaced to allow rest periods, which should be provided with the same emphasis as that placed on hemodynamic measurements and the assessment of vital signs.

Remember Mr. T from Section Three? Although his primary problem was a perforated ulcer, he also had a history of COPD and was steroid dependent. He had an acute exacerbation of respiratory failure. ABGs are pH 7.29, Pco_2 55, Po_2 50. He is transferred to the surgical intensive care unit. Mr. T is intubated and placed on a Bear One ventilator. Tidal volume is 700, Fio_2 is 40 percent, assist/control mode, PEEP is 5, with a rate of 12.

Mr. T is susceptible to sensory problems.

Surgical intensive care unit patients have the highest incidence of ICU psychosis. It is important for the nurse to know his day of admission into the intensive care unit, since psychosis usually occurs between the third and seventh days. He is unable to communicate verbally. Being placed on the ventilator may prevent adequate rest periods due to frequent suctioning and noise.

To summarize, the critically ill patient is at risk for experiencing sensory deprivation, sensory overload, a combination of both sensory overload and deprivation, sleep deprivation, and ICU psychosis. The nurse can diminish patient susceptibility to these conditions by decreasing the amplitude of voices and telephones, closing patient doors, promoting orientation to time and place, and helping to discriminate night from day by changing unit lighting. Communication can be improved by using chalkboards or establishing a system of symbols.

Section Four Review

1. Intensive care unit (ICU) psychosis occurs
   A. only in intensive care units
   B. in patients over 65 years of age
   C. most often in coronary care units
   D. between the third and seventh day of admission

2. The most frequently cited annoying noise among critically ill patients is
   A. ambulance sirens
   B. hospital paging system
   C. television
   D. equipment noise

3. Lack of rapid eye movement (REM) sleep produces
   A. hypertension
   B. immunosuppression
   C. seizures
   D. aggressive behavior

4. Which of the following nursing interventions would support the patient's circadian rhythm cycle?
   A. dimming lights during normal sleep time
   B. putting a wall clock up in the patient's room
   C. encouraging normal bowel habits
   D. decreasing environmental noise

Answers: 1, D. 2, D. 3, B. 4, A.

Section Five: Educational Needs of Patients and Families

At the completion of this section, the learner will be able to identify educational needs of critically ill patients and their families and strategies to meet these needs.

Critically ill patients have a right to know and understand what procedures are being done to and for them. Health care knowledge may decrease the length of the patient's hospitalization or the number of readmissions for the same condition (Bille, 1990). Initially, when teaching critically ill patients, the nurse must aim at decreasing stress and promoting comfort rather than increasing knowledge. The patient and family may not recall what the nurse said 10 minutes later, but the patient's blood pressure may be decreased or the pain lessened (Bille, 1983). As adult learners, critically ill patients focus on learning in order to solve problems. Thus, the nurse must assess what the patient considers to be problematic in order to make learning meaningful. Basic questions about what the patient and family want to know will assist the nurse in focusing content. It is also helpful to identify what the patient already knows. The reduced nurse/patient ratio used in most settings where critically ill patients are placed facilitates teaching. An interpersonal relationship allows for the patient to trust the abilities and knowledge of the nurse. In order for the critically ill patient to learn, he or she must feel secure.

There are several factors that inhibit learning in critically ill patients. Patients may be fatigued due to hypoxia, anemia, and being in a hypermetabolic state. They may have barriers to communication, such as endotracheal tubes. They may have a large number of hourly procedures and diagnostic tests that prevent quality teaching time. Pain will diminish a person's ability to concentrate. Drugs may depress the central nervous system and affect memory. The nurse should assess the patient for the presence of these factors. Physiologic needs take precedence over the need to know and the need to understand (Maslow, 1970). Once the patient's condition has stabilized, however, the patient is able to concentrate on learning.

Research has demonstrated that families also have a need for knowledge. Families have consistently rated cognitive needs more important than emotional or physical needs. In 100 percent of eight research studies designed to identify needs of families of critically ill patients, "to have questions answered honestly" and "to know specific facts regarding what is wrong with the patient and the patient's progress" were listed as the most important needs (Hickey, 1990). The need to know the prognosis and chance for recovery was listed as important in 90 percent of the studies. "To receive information in understandable terms" was identified 80 percent of the time. In addition to the need for knowledge, families indicated needing a mechanism through which they could receive information, such as a consistent nurse who they could contact or who would contact the family. Regardless of whether the family members were blood relatives or significant others, they indicated the same needs (Bouman, 1984). These findings were consistent up to 96 hours after admission. The use of nontechnical terms and written materials may be appropriate, since the family's ability to comprehend and process information may be limited as a result of the crisis of the critical illness.

> Mr. T, discussed in Sections Three and Four, is improving. His blood gases have improved, and he is being weaned from the ventilator. The ventilator is in synchronized intermittent mandatory ventilation (SIMV) mode at a rate of 8.
>
> The nurse has been teaching Mr. T about his wound care, including the chance for infection related to his wound and the use of steroids. Up to this point, Mr. T has been eager to learn and has asked questions using a writing board. This morning he appears anxious.
>
> Before teaching Mr. T, the nurse should assess the cause of Mr. T's anxiety. Is it related to hypoxia secondary to weaning? The nurse draws blood for an ABG, and the findings are within normal limits. Mr. T's anxiety may be related to the fear of not being able to breathe without the machine. Patient teaching should center on decreasing Mr. T's anxiety. On questioning, Mr. T admits he is frightened about getting weaned and moving out of the intensive care unit. The nurse concentrates on explaining how the staff is sure Mr. T will be able to breathe. Next, she explains when he will be transferred to the general floor and how he will continue to be monitored.

In summary, both critically ill patients and their family members want to learn about their illness and the hospital environment. Adults use problem-centered learning. Therefore, they are interested in information that is immediately useful and applicable. A person is unable to learn if her or his stress level is high. Therefore, the next step in teaching critically ill patients is to address the issue that is causing the most anxiety. Information should be given in clear and succinct terms. The nurse should assess what the patient and family member already know in order to build on this foundation. Physiologic factors that can interfere with learning also must be assessed.

Section Five Review

Questions 1 and 2 pertain to Ms. Bee.

Ms. Bee was admitted with a diagnosis of acute myocardial infarction. Her vital signs are: respiratory rate 32, heart rate 100, temperature 102F orally, blood pressure 90/70. She is on a continuous nitroglycerin IV infusion for chest pain.

1. Which of the following factors would NOT interfere with Ms. Bee's ability to learn?
   A. pain
   B. temperature
   C. respiratory rate
   D. heart rate

2. The nurse should focus on teaching Ms. Bee
   A. cardiac rehabilitation plans
   B. how the heart functions
   C. why it is important to state when she is having pain
   D. rationale for the nitroglycerin

3. Families of critically ill patients list which of the following needs as being the most important?
   A. emotional
   B. psychomotor
   C. cognitive
   D. spiritual

Answers: 1, D. 2, C. 3, C.

NURSING CONSIDERATIONS

Section Six: Nursing Educational Issues

At the completion of this section, the learner will be able to identify educational issues surrounding nurses working with critically ill patients.

Nurses willing to work with critically ill patients are a precious commodity. Hospitals are filled with more acutely ill patients, and the percentage of hospital beds devoted to special care units is progressively increasing (Carlson, 1989). Enrollment in nursing programs has decreased, and in addition to this fact, few programs offer critical care content in their curriculum. Because of changing patient acuity and health care system needs, the American Association of Critical Care Nurses (AACN) has supported the integration of critical care concepts in the baccalaureate nursing curriculum (AACN, 1987).

There has been ongoing debate regarding who should be allowed to provide nursing care to critically ill patients. Houser (1977) indicated that previous nursing experience is helpful because of the necessary cognitive abilities and tasks used with a critically ill patient. However, prior nursing experience may be limited and not as useful if the experience has been with patients who have a specific type of health problem.

The current nursing shortage results from an increased demand for nurses. The aging population, an increasing ability to prolong life, and an increasing number of patients who require cardiovascular surgical procedures contribute to this demand (Searle, 1990). Managers are hiring new graduates to work with critically ill patients in order to meet this demand. However, the new graduate may not be better prepared than previous new graduates to care for a critically ill patient. At present, AACN has not identified any specific skill that new graduates must learn before their employment in order to work in settings where critically ill patients are located (Battles-Daake, 1989). Because there is such diversity in undergraduate nursing curricula, employers should tailor applicant interviews to elicit information about the applicant's motivation for working with critically ill patients and an appraisal of the applicant's strengths and weaknesses. Providing applicants with a critically ill patient scenario that requires an analysis and response will allow insight into the applicant's critical thinking abilities.

If the institution cannot rely on the educational background of nurses to prepare them for working with critically ill patients, the institution is responsible for providing the necessary education (Ahrens, 1989). The educational program should include basic content, as identified by national guidelines, in each system area. Education about less common clinical conditions and information specific to a particular patient population should be delayed until after there is understanding of basic concepts. Orientation programs should include coursework as well as a supervised clinical segment.

Extended orientation programs have been used in the past to prepare new graduates. However, demands have made this type of program an expensive luxury. In addition, it is difficult to assimilate large amounts of information at a given time. There is a trend to more self-paced instruction. Self-paced instruction incorporates adult learning principles, provides factual information, saves institutional resources, and allows for differences among learners.

In summary, as the need for nurses to work with critically ill patients continues to increase, a greater number of new graduates will be employed to work with this patient population. It is essential that the institution develop an orientation program that includes core information in addition to specific information about particular patient populations the nurse will encounter. The new graduate should ask questions about the orientation program during the employment interview. It is wise to look for a match between personal learning style and educational methods used in the orientation program. There is no consensus in the literature supporting the need for a special orientation program for new graduates. It is most important that the orientation program is built on adult learning principles.

Section Six Review

1. Previous nursing experience
   A. is a national requirement to work with critically ill patients
   B. has demonstrated more successful integration into nursing role with critically ill patients
   C. may be limited and not useful to care of critically ill patients
   D. promotes nurse retention in critically ill patient care areas

2. An orientation program should include
   A. advanced material specific to patient population
   B. basic content identified by national guidelines
   C. computer simulations
   D. unit leadership program

Answers: 1, C. 2, B.

Section Seven: Interface Between Technology and Caring

At the completion of this section, the learner will be able to describe the interface between technology and caring.

A major criticism of nurses who work with critically ill patients is that they are strictly technologically oriented. This criticism was derived historically. The advances in surgery created a need for an area where the patient could undergo an operation and the anesthetized patient could recover from anesthesia. The nurse in this area functioned in a monitoring role by using instruments and equipment that recorded physiologic responses (Levine, 1989). Patients were not aware of their surroundings, so the areas were designed to facilitate work flow, not for esthetics.

Patients, by signing the operative permit, became dependent on the health care provider, and an attitude of trust—the professionals know best—was created. Nurses working in recovery rooms were exposed to constant stress, since the patients required continuous monitoring, and the nurse was unable to leave the bedside. Patients were not encouraged to participate in their care. Eventually, machinery allowed nurses to care for more than one critically ill patient at a time. It has been suggested that nurses focused on the technology in order to cope with the stress and to exclude their personal feelings (Levine, 1989).

There has been much deliberation over what separates medical from nursing practice. Because of the autonomous use of technology in caring for the critically ill patient, nurses working with this patient population have been referred to as junior physicians or minidoctors. Nurses have used the words technical, curative, and prescribing to describe caring for the critically ill patient (Schultz and Daly, 1989).

There is an inherent hazard to using technology. The use of technology can be so intriguing that the primary purpose for using the technology—to support the well-being of the patient—may be lost (Bandman, 1985). Another hazard is that technology creates demands where no demands existed before by producing patient fragmentation into subpopulations (e.g., bone marrow transplant floor, cardiac surgery unit). Each subpopulation has its own health care staff. Staff begin to compete for the resources within the hospital system (Zwolski, 1989).

Several other problems result from current technology. Existing technology makes it easy to provide services to patients who may not benefit from use of the equipment. Machines compete with the patient for nursing surveillance. It is possible that nurses may become so dependent on monitoring devices that they trust the equipment even when the data conflict with their own clinical assessment of the situation. Having responsibility for multiple pieces of equipment can increase the nurse's stress level. Data from monitoring devices can either support or help to incriminate a nurse in legal proceedings. Technical devices present mechanical impediments to touching. There may be little surface area available for physical contact. The lack of physical contact can lead to a feeling of depersonalization. A patient who has felt depersonalized may be more likely to sue a nurse.

Nurses working with critically ill patients must be capable of making critical decisions. Although decision making has been viewed somewhat as artful and intuitive, computers have used a scientific, programmed approach to decision making. Because of the massive amount of patient information available related to the multiple pieces of machinery, nurses may be reaching a saturation point in data processing. Computers currently are being tested to aid decision making for critically ill patients (Fuerst, 1989). The use of computers as decision makers could either provide the nurse with more time to provide humanistic caring or encourage the role of the nurse as machine controller.

The nurse must be proficient in the use of machinery. Proficiency is fostered by having the opportunity to become familiar with the machinery before use in patient care and by having an available resource person who understands the machine's operation. Once the nurse is proficient, the nurse can encourage the questions of patient and family members about the machinery. Explaining machinery can increase patient and family trust in the nurse. Most nurses think that machines provide reassurance because they can alert the nurse to a problem situation before clinical manifestations occur (McConnell, 1990). It is essential, however, that the nurse validate the machine data with nursing assessment data. In addition, nurses must appreciate the techniques that patients have developed in order to interact with the technology (Zwolski, 1989). This may include denial, humor, and a compulsiveness to learn everything about a machine.

Caring has been described differently depending on the context where the nurse practices. In the intensive care unit, caring has been described as technical. On medical and surgical floors, caring has been described as a team effort. Traditionally, caring has been viewed as humanistic behavior involving spiritual and ethical aspects. The modern health care delivery system has created a form of bureaucratic caring that includes economic, legal, and technical aspects (Ray, 1989). The nurse caring for the critically ill patient has to address all views, even though they may be theoretically contradictory in nature.

In summary, nurses who care for critically ill patients must be able to use technology in the caring process and still recognize the limitations of technology. The nurse's personal knowledge, observation skills, and senses cannot be substituted for equipment and technologic advances. The nurse must be able to integrate complex technology with individualized, humanistic care (Holyfield, 1983).

Section Seven Review

1. The referral to nurses who work with critically ill patients as junior physicians was derived from
   A. the close collaborative relationship between nurse and physician
   B. increased use of advanced technology
   C. the constant stress of continuous monitoring
   D. the decreased nurse/patient ratio

2. The implications of advanced technology for nursing include
   A. decreased likelihood of malpractice and negligence
   B. provision of data to incriminate or support nurses in court proceedings
   C. allowing greater time for patient contact
   D. encouraging greater use of nursing assessment skills

3. The hazards of technology includes all EXCEPT
   A. creates demands for new services
   B. decreases demands for nursing staff
   C. fosters depersonalization of the patient
   D. creates machine competition with patient for nursing time

Answers: 1, B. 2, B. 3, B.

Section Eight: Nursing Critically Ill Patients

At the completion of this section, the learner will be able to discuss stressful and satisfying aspects to caring for critically ill patients.

The term *burnout* has been used to describe a crisis state evolving from stress. It has been defined as "to fail, wear out or become exhausted by making excessive demands on energy, strength, or resource" (Freundenberg, 1974). Burnout is an automatic response that protects the nurse from pain and conflict. In a classic study conducted by Claus and Bailey (1980), 1,794 nurses who work with critically ill patients were surveyed to identify sources of stress. The major sources of stress were interpersonal conflict, management of the patient care area, nature of the direct patient care, and inadequate knowledge. There are several symptoms that indicate burnout (Table 21–1). Although basic nursing programs usually offer structured coursework in meeting the psychosocial needs of patients, few programs offer instruction in meeting the psychosocial needs of nurses (Continenza, 1989).

Primary nursing may be a source of burnout. Nurses who work with critically ill patients usually have responsibility for one or two patients. Primary nursing, although once regarded as the ultimate method of nursing assignment, can be a stressor because of the intensity and intimacy of the nurse/patient relationship. There is a constant threat that the patient may die. The nurse may experience repetitive losses but still has to reinvest energy into a new patient before adequately mourning the loss of the previous patient.

Another source of burnout is the changing patient's condition. Frequently, the aims of the patient's

TABLE 21–1. SYMPTOMS OF BURNOUT

Behavioral
  Withdrawal
  Risk taking and impulsiveness
  Ambivalence
  Decreased productivity
  Contemplating career change
  Increased use of caffeine, alcohol, and nicotine
Physiologic
  Chronic fatigue
  Frequent minor ailments
  Sleep changes
  Appetite change
  Sexual difficulty
Psychologic
  Attempt to blame others
  Stereotype patients
  Nightmares
  Depression
  Hostility and negativism
  Loss of tolerance
Cognitive
  Decreased ability to make decisions
  Poor judgment
  Lack of initiative
  Forgetfulness

treatment will change drastically within the course of a shift, requiring the nurse to be philosophically flexible. A patient with a presumably poor prognosis may have a prolonged stay that involves the use of all available technology, and in the middle of the shift, a decision to cease extraordinary efforts may be made. The patient may then begin to improve, requiring reevaluation and escalation of care. Conversely, the patient may be pronounced brain dead, and the individual becomes a cadaveric donor. The nursing care for the cadaveric donor may detract from the nursing care of other viable patients, producing a nursing conflict (Fitzgerald, 1989). A significant degree of uncertainty is confronted on a daily basis. In addition, the nurse must view the worst of humanity (gunshot wounds and stabbings) and deal with injury in the prime of life.

Noise-induced stress and burnout may be related. Just as the patient may experience problems from the stimulation in the patient care area, nurses also may be affected. The top three disturbing noises identified by nurses were beeping monitors, equipment alarms, and telephones (Topf and Dillion, 1988).

Burnout may be prevented if the nurse exhibits hardiness. Hardiness is comprised of three components: a sense of commitment, a perception of life changes as challenges, and a sense of control over life. Of the three components, less commitment to work has been linked with greater work stress (Topf, 1989).

Nurses must enhance self-awareness of personal sources of tension. Fatigue, frustration, and anxiety have been listed as nurses' most frequent responses to stress (Robinson and Lewis, 1990). Once these sources of tension are identified, strategies for alleviating the stressors can be developed. The use of written protocols to assist in defining practice and clarifying boundaries, regular assessment of staff goals and achievements, and continuing education programs for personal growth are stress-relieving factors noted in the literature (Orlowski and Gulledge, 1986). Discussing problems with co-workers and watching television or reading have been strategies listed by nurses for coping with work-related stress (Robinson and Lewis, 1990). The presence of social support has demonstrated a buffering effect on stress in nurses working with critically ill patients (Spoth and Konewko, 1987; Norbeck, 1985).

There are advantages to working with critically ill patients. Generally, nurses and physicians have better collaboration because the nature of the patient situation requires close communication. Nurses may have greater freedom in implementing medical guidelines, since there is less emphasis on nonclinical maintenance activities (e.g., ordering supplies). Research findings suggest that nurses who work with critically ill patients are more satisfied in their role than nurses who work with less acute patients (Prescott, 1989). Nurses who experience psychologic stress usually are younger and have less experience and less education (Harris, 1989).

Some of the stressors associated with caring for critically ill patients also can produce satisfaction. The fast-paced environment is stimulating to some nurses. The ability to interact with patients and families during a crisis period can be satisfying. Claus and Bailey (1980) discovered that intellectual challenge, opportunities for learning, smaller nurse/patient ratio, and proficient use of skills were the most frequently mentioned motivators for working with critically ill patients.

In summary, nurses who work with critically ill patients do not appear to have greater degrees of work-related stress than nurses working with less acute patient populations. However, nurses working with the critically ill are still susceptible to burnout. The symptoms of burnout are cognitive, psychologic, physiologic, and behavioral in nature (Table 21–1). Strategies useful in limiting or buffering job-related stressors are an available social support system, developing guidelines to delineate practice boundaries, periodic assessment of personal and unit goals, comprehensive unit orientation, and continuing education for stress reduction.

Section Eight Review

1. Primary nursing
   A. produces stress because of the intensity of the nurse/patient relationship
   B. discourages collaboration among health team members
   C. prevents the nurse from reinvesting energy into a new patient after a previous patient is discharged
   D. is the preferred method of patient assignment

2. Nurses who work with critically ill patients as opposed to nurses who work with less acute patients
   A. experience greater stress
   B. have a stronger support system
   C. are more satisfied in their role
   D. are more susceptible to burnout

3. Which of the following components of hardiness has been linked to burnout?
   A. a sense of control over the patient care area
   B. less commitment to work
   C. perception of change as a challenge
   D. sense of control over life

Answers: 1, A. 2, C. 3, B.

Section Nine: Resource Allocation

At the completion of this section, the learner will be able to discuss resource allocation issues as they relate to critically ill patients.

Who is in need of the greatest health care resources when they are critically ill? The criteria for resources may be based on age, diagnosis, physician preference, bed and nursing staff availability, as well as community and hospital standards. One could argue that resources should be used for patients who want to receive extraordinary support, have a better probability of surviving, or have a higher quality of life (Carlon, 1988). If resource allocation was based on these principles, the actual precipitating event that created the need for resources would be irrelevant. Therefore, oncology patients, trauma patients, the young, and the old should be considered equally. It has been suggested that futility of treatment and informed refusal by the patient are acceptable reasons for physicians to limit treatment. However, only the patient or society can make decisions to withhold treatment based on quality of life or cost considerations (Lo and Jonsen, 1980).

There are several vulnerable patient populations, in regard to resource allocation issues, frequently encountered by nurses who work with critically ill patients. Critically ill neonates are considered a vulnerable population. Almost all infants are born in a hospital. Each hospital has policies regarding resuscitation of the newborn. It is almost impossible to differentiate at birth infants who may benefit from lifesaving interventions from those with poor prognoses. Therefore, all neonates usually are resuscitated (Kohrmann, 1985). Issues arise when cessation of life support is considered later in the infant's hospitalization.

Oncology patients often are stereotyped as not being candidates for aggressive treatment. This can result in a self-fulfilling prophecy, since critically ill patients who are denied technical life support eventually will die (Carlon, 1988). However, oncology patients frequently become critically ill from interventions administered by health care providers. Should these patients be denied access to resources when their condition has been induced? Conversely, oncology patients may be kept alive for research purposes to determine the ultimate effects of certain interventions.

Age has been used to justify the withholding of resources from the elderly (Bellamy and Oye, 1987). Interestingly, age has not been solely related to mortality. The severity of the illness episode, admitting diagnosis, and the patient's previous health status have been positively related to health outcomes. The Medicare and Diagnostic Related Grouping systems send strong signals to hospitals to limit resources provided to the elderly. Financial reimbursement is less than the hospital's cost for providing the resources.

Because of the nature of critical illness, it is difficult to remember that the patient's freedom of choice should still be placed above every other value. Patient situations change rapidly, often preventing discussion with the patient about treatment decisions (Cassell, 1986). Health care providers, including nurses, have a tendency to believe that what they think is good for the patient is indeed good for the patient. The underlying reason for this belief may be to rationalize interventions that produce patient pain. The nurse has the responsibility to act as patient advocate because of the vulnerable nature of the critically ill patient.

Technology forces health care providers to make choices about who receives costly resources. Nurses are encouraged to be more cost conscious and frequently are asked what is a reasonable reduction below ideal care for their patients. Making decisions about allocation of resources is a real but usually unspecified aspect of the nursing role with critically ill patients. These decisions force health care providers to make comparisons based on personal beliefs (Veatch, 1986). Technology alone cannot provide information about who may live and die. A patient's intangibles, such as their family support systems, personal value system, and purpose in life, also may contribute to a patient's ability to recover even when technologic data provide no hope (Van Ora, 1989).

Technology is used not only for its original intention, to resuscitate patients who can benefit, but also for patients who have virtually no possibility of recovering. Health care providers appear more comfortable with stopping life support measures than with not starting life support measures, although there is no moral difference between the two (Cassell, 1986). Since the patient may be distracted by pain or unable to communicate verbally because of intubation or altered mental status, each situation is unique. In some situations, however, nurses working with critically ill patients can be proactive in identifying the wishes of the patient before the moment of need, so that patients and families can express coherent desires. Permission for resuscitation can be obtained as an informed consent, like other invasive procedures. As the patient's clinical condition changes, patients and families need to be informed to ensure that consent for resuscitation is still valid.

Cardiopulmonary resuscitation (CPR) is an example of a technique that has been misused. Guidelines for using the technique stated that it was not to be used in cases of terminal irreversible illness where death is expected. Ironically, hospitals now require that every patient be a candidate to receive CPR unless an order is written to withhold it (Bellamy and Oye, 1987). Technology encourages death to be viewed as a symptom to be treated and not as a life event.

Do not resuscitate (DNR) orders were developed to prevent the use of CPR and advanced cardiac life support measures and not to prevent other forms of treatment for the patient, including the use of critical care resources (Edwards, 1990). However, DNR patients consume more resources and have a higher mortality rate than non-DNR patients. DNR orders may be written for reasons other than terminal illness, such as patient request, chronic, irreversible illness, and poor quality of life. Since DNR patients may be able to benefit from receiving care from nurses skilled in working with critically ill patients, is it fair to withhold these resources? Some argue that scarce resources would be redistributed to non-DNR patients and costs would be reduced if resources were not provided to the DNR patient (Edwards, 1990). The immediate needs of the person may be in conflict with the interests of society. Because of limited resources, patients who can be treated successfully may be denied resources because available resources are being used by patients with questionable survival capability.

Health care providers justify not providing services to the critically ill by stating that they are relieving suffering. However, in some situations, it cannot be verified that suffering is being relieved (Levine, 1989). It is not a nursing responsibility to evaluate the social worth of a patient. Whenever possible, decisions to use or not to use technology to sustain life should be made in advance by the patient. In cases where advanced decision making has not taken place, family members and other individuals requested by the patient should be included in decision making. An ethical review committee may be used in some circumstances. It has been stated that it is impossible for caregivers whose philosophy is to protect life and relieve suffering to make these decisions (Levine, 1989). Historically, the public has not wanted to know that there are times when health care providers do not know which action is best. Added to this is the fact that health care providers have not wanted public scrutiny of their actions (Kohrman, 1985). The development of ethical review committees can be viewed as both a curse and a blessing. They can diminish individual considerations of cases in favor of implementing general standards of treatment based on criteria. The positive aspect of these committees is that a decision is made by a group instead of by an individual health care provider.

In summary, technology has produced ethical dilemmas for nurses working with critically ill patients. Recent dilemmas have focused on the use of valuable critical care resources by infants with congenital abnormalities, oncology patients, the elderly, and DNR patients. It is not the nurse's role to solve these dilemmas alone. Rather, the nurse's responsibility is to become involved in establishing guidelines for resource allocation and to represent nursing's viewpoint on ethical review committees.

Section Nine Review

1. Cardiopulmonary resuscitation was developed to be used
   A. for those who experience sudden unexpected death
   B. for every witnessed arrest
   C. for every arrest situation (witnessed or not)
   D. only in the hospital

2. The DNR order was developed to
   A. provide only custodial care to terminal patients
   B. prevent use of CPR
   C. provide greater resources for non-DNR patients
   D. decrease health costs

3. Resource allocation for critically ill patients may be based on all of the following EXCEPT
   A. admitting diagnosis
   B. bed availability
   C. hospital standards
   D. sex of the patient

Answers: 1, A. 2, B. 3, D.

Section Ten: Personal Values

At the completion of this section, the learner will be able to examine personal values as they relate to the nurse's role in working with critically ill patients.

The American Nurses Association (ANA) (1980) states that essential components of professional nursing practice include care, cure, and coordination. The AACN (1984) believes that nurses who work with critically ill patients should base their practice on individual professional accountability, thorough knowledge of the interrelatedness of body systems, recognition and appreciation of person's wholeness, uniqueness, and significant social-environmental relationships, and appreciation of the collaborative role of all health care team members.

Nurses can improve assessment and technical skills by providing nursing care for critically ill patients. The nurse must be able to interpret and anticipate health outcomes that may result from applying patient care protocols. Verbal and nonverbal communication skills can be refined because communication must be precise and perceptive in these settings. The exposure to death and the saving of human life can strengthen one's integrity. Personal values can be identified and clarified by examining bioethical issues encountered when working with critically ill patients.

The value clarification exercise shown in Table 21–2 is designed to help the learner explore personal values in relation to the profession of nursing and bioethical issues.

In summary, the nurse has several different roles when caring for the critically ill patient. These roles include but are not limited to prevention of illness, counselor, teacher, and patient advocate. The ability to interpret multiple clinical data and anticipate events based on knowledge of physiology is an inherent requirement. As technology advances, patient care has the tendency to become fragmented. The nurse glues the pieces together. Nurses need to be aware of personal fears and feelings they experienced when they first began to work with critically ill patients. Once one becomes a native, it is easy to forget and not appreciate or overlook these same feelings and fears in the critically ill patient.

There are many similarities in nursing regardless of practice setting and patient population. Evaluation of one's personal philosophy can improve one's satisfaction in working with critically ill patients. Clarification of one's values helps to anticipate problems that may be encountered in the practice setting and supports development of positive coping strategies. This knowledge can be transferred for use in other health care settings with less acutely ill patients.

TABLE 21-2. VALUE CLARIFICATION EXERCISE

To the left of each statement, place the number that best explains your position: 1 = mostly agree, 2 = somewhat agree, 3 = neutral, 4 = somewhat disagree, 5 = mostly disagree

_____ 1. Infants with severe handicaps ought to be left to die.

_____ 2. Extraordinary medical treatment is always indicated.

_____ 3. My role as a nurse is to always resuscitate patients who could benefit from it, no matter what has been decided previously.

_____ 4. I must follow physician's orders.

_____ 5. Older patients should be allowed to die with dignity.

_____ 6. Medical technology has advanced the quality of life.

_____ 7. Children should not be involved in giving consent for treatments.

_____ 8. Families ought to make decisions about life or death situations without involving the patient.

_____ 9. Children should participate in human experimentation that is not harmful even if it has no benefit to them.

_____ 10. Prisoners should participate in scientific experiments to repay society for their wrongdoings.

_____ 11. Women should seek medical care from female physicians to avoid potential discrimination.

_____ 12. Children whose parents refuse to have them receive medical care should be removed from their families through court action.

_____ 13. Research using fetuses should be pursued vigorously.

_____ 14. Life support systems should be discontinued after several days of flat EEG.

_____ 15. Health professionals are a scarce resource in many parts of the country.

_____ 16. Nursing is a subservient profession, especially to the medical profession.

_____ 17. As a nurse, I must relinquish my personal philosophy to support the philosophies of others.

_____ 18. All patients, regardless of differences, should be treated in a humanistic way.

_____ 19. I should give mouth to mouth resuscitation to a derelict if he needs it.

_____ 20. A child who is disabled has value.

_____ 21. All forms of human life have value.

_____ 22. I should be involved in decision making regarding ethical issues in practice.

_____ 23. Committees should decide who receives scarce resources, such as kidneys.

_____ 24. Patients' individual rights should be more important than the rights of society at large.

_____ 25. A person has the right to make a living will.

_____ 26. Underdeveloped countries should be given health and financial support from developed countries.

_____ 27. I should support all the positions taken on ethical issues taken by my professional association.

_____ 28. I should aggressively support my own values when they conflict with the values of others.

_____ 29. Consideration of the cultural values of patients is a waste of time.

_____ 30. The care component of nursing practice is not as important as the cure component of medical practice.

_____ 31. The nurse's primary role in decision making on ethical issues is to implement the selected alternative.

_____ 32. I feel afraid when caring for a patient who is dying.

_____ 33. Children who have disabilities should be institutionalized.

_____ 34. Patients in mental health institutions and prisons should be given behavior modification therapy to make them conform to society.

_____ 35. Personal possessions of patients should be removed to guarantee safekeeping during hospitalization.

_____ 36. Patients should have access to their own health information.

_____ 37. Withholding health information fosters the patient's recovery.

_____ 38. A patient with kidney failure is always able to get kidney dialysis when needed.

_____ 39. Society should bear the cost of extraordinary medical interventions.

_____ 40. Confidentiality is an important part of the nurse's role.

_____ 41. As a nurse, I should value responsibility.

_____ 42. Nurses have a right to withhold information to facilitate nursing research on human subjects.

_____ 43. The patient who refuses treatment should be dropped from the health supervision of an agency or professional.

_____ 44. Transplantations should be done whenever needed.

Personal Application

1. Add the number of 1s, 2s, 3s, 4s, and 5s that you have.

2. How many statements do you have clear ideas (1s and 5s) about?

3. Do these outweigh the number of ambivalent (neutral) statements you listed?

4. Look at the statements that you agree with (1s and 2s). Is there a relationship between the statements that influenced your responses (e.g., age of patient, patient acuity)?

5. Look at the statements that you disagree with (4s and 5s). Is there a relationship between these statements that influenced your responses?

6. Analyze the cluster of statements below. Is there any consistency in the way that you rated these statements? What variables influenced your decision?

Cluster 5, 8, 14, 25, and 32: Relates to issues pertaining to death

Cluster 3, 4, 16, 17, 22, 27, 30, 31, and 40: Relates to the profession of nursing

Cluster 2, 6, 14, 38, 39, and 44: Relates to issues raised by advanced technology

Cluster 1, 7, 9, 12, 20, and 33: Relates to children

Cluster 9, 10, 13, and 42: Relates to human experimentation

Cluster 3, 7, 8, 11, 12, 18, 19, 24, 25, 29, 35, 36, 37, 40, and 43: Relates to patients' rights

Cluster 9, 10, 24, 26, 28, and 39: Relates to society's rights

Cluster 15, 23, and 38: Relates to allocation of resources

Cluster 3, 4, 17, 18, 19, 22, 27, 28, 31, and 41: Relates to perceptions of obligations

Adapted from Steele, S., and Harmon, V. (1979). _Value clarification in nursing._ New York: Appleton-Century-Crofts.

Section Ten Review

1. Nurses who work with critically ill patients should base their practice on all of the following EXCEPT
   A. delegated responsibility
   B. thorough knowledge of the interrelatedness of body systems
   C. recognition and appreciation of a person's uniqueness and social-environmental relationships
   D. appreciation of the collaborative role of all health team members

2. Common aspects of the critical care nursing role include
   A. community referral
   B. teacher
   C. disaster management
   D. staff liaison

Answers: 1, A. 2, B.

Posttest

1. Which of the following has been identified by nurses who work with critically ill patients as a primary stressor?
   A. lack of pay
   B. interpersonal conflict
   C. overtime
   D. performing complex skills

2. Extended orientation programs for new graduates to prepare them to work with critically ill patients
   A. are more successful
   B. promote nurse retention
   C. decrease the number of incident reports
   D. are expensive

3. Which of the following groups of critically ill patients is at greatest risk for experiencing sensory problems?
   A. middle-aged adults
   B. renal transplant patients
   C. patients in windowless patient care areas
   D. patients who have been hospitalized previously

4. A patient is crying about a below knee amputation (BKA) sustained as a pedestrian in a pedestrian/vehicle crash. She expresses fears about ambulating in physical therapy. This behavior is a sign of which stage of illness?
   A. denial
   B. awareness
   C. restitution
   D. resolution

5. The decision not to use technology to sustain life should be made
   A. by the health care provider
   B. before an emergency situation
   C. by community standards
   D. when the patient is transferred to the intensive care unit

6. In order to relieve stress associated with nursing critically ill patients, the nurse should
   A. request a transfer
   B. drink more decaffeinated beverages
   C. work with less protocols
   D. attend a continuing education program for personal growth

7. The primary purpose of using technology is to
   A. support the patient's well-being
   B. decrease the patient's length of hospitalization
   C. anticipate complications of therapy
   D. decentralize patient care into specialized units

8. Informed refusal by the patient
   A. is an acceptable reason for limiting treatment
   B. jeopardizes the health care provider's legal status
   C. indicates that the patient did not receive adequate explanation of treatment
   D. indicates that the patient is angry

9. Burnout is
   A. the result of sensory overload
   B. associated with ICU psychosis
   C. an automatic protective response
   D. associated with tenure as a nurse

10. Commitment to work
    A. is associated with less burnout
    B. produces greater work stress
    C. results from extensive orientation to the work area
    D. is associated with the number of years the nurse has worked in the area

11. All of the following variables have been associated with health outcomes EXCEPT
    A. severity of illness
    B. age
    C. patient's previous health status
    D. admission diagnosis

12. Burnout may be manifested by all of the following EXCEPT
    A. pessimism
    B. forgetfulness
    C. tolerance
    D. nightmares

13. Mrs. Baker states she has heard her dead mother calling her. The nurse recognizes this as a symptom of
    A. sensory shutdown
    B. sensory deprivation
    C. auditory damage
    D. antibiotic toxicity

14. ICU psychosis is usually associated with
    A. completion of multiple procedures
    B. attempted suicide
    C. inadequate pain relief
    D. surgery

15. Do not resuscitate orders were developed to prevent
    A. treatment for the patient
    B. use of cardiopulmonary resuscitation
    C. use of critical care resources
    D. patient transfer

16. An ethical review committee may
    A. decrease public scrutiny of health care providers' actions
    B. promote implementation of general standards
    C. enhance health care providers liability
    D. increase individual responsibility for decision making

17. The essential components of professional nursing practice are all of the following EXCEPT
    A. care
    B. cure
    C. coordination
    D. culture

18. Clarification of one's values as a nurse may
    A. decrease the nurse's liability
    B. help the nurse anticipate patient care problems
    C. promote burnout
    D. decrease sensory overload

19. A hazard of technology is
    A. not trusting nursing assessment data
    B. too much touching of the patient
    C. increased nursing surveillance of the patient
    D. the demise of nursing speciality practice

20. One of the most disturbing noises listed by nurses working with critically ill patients is
    A. physician yelling
    B. equipment alarms
    C. ventilator cycling
    D. suction equipment

Posttest Answers

Question	Answer	Section	Question	Answer	Section
1	B	Eight	11	B	Nine
2	D	Six	12	C	Eight
3	C	Four	13	B	Four
4	C	Two	14	D	Four
5	B	Nine	15	B	Nine
6	D	Eight	16	B	Nine
7	A	Seven	17	D	Ten
8	A	Nine	18	B	Ten
9	C	Eight	19	A	Seven
10	A	Eight	20	B	Four

REFERENCES

Ahrens, T. (1989). The recruitment, retention, and education of critical care nurses. In B. Heater and B. AuBuchon (eds). *Controversies in critical care nursing*, pp. 37–44. Rockville, Maryland: Aspen.

American Association of Critical Care Nurses. (1984). *Definition of critical care nursing*. Newport Beach, California: AACN.

American Association of Critical Care Nurses. (1987). *Need for critical care content and clinical experiences in baccalaureate nursing curricula*. Newport Beach, California: AACN.

American Nurses Association. (1980). *Nursing: A social policy statement*. Kansas City, Missouri: ANA.

Baggs, J. (1989). Intensive care unit use and collaboration between nurses and physicians. *Heart Lung*. 18:332–338.

Bandman, E. (1985). Our toughest questions: Ethical quandries in high tech nursing. *Nursing Health Care*. 6:483–487.

Barrie-Shevlin, P. (1987). Maintaining sensory balance for the critically ill patient. Balliere Tindall. 16:597–600.

Battles-Daake, C. (1989). Can new graduates become effective ICU nurses? Some recommendations. In B. Heater and B. AuBuchon (eds). *Controversies in critical care nursing*, p. 48. Rockville, Maryland: Aspen.

Bellamy, P., and Oye, R. (1987). Admitting elderly patients into the ICU: Dilemmas and solutions. *Geriatrics*. 42(3):61–68.

Bille, D. (1990). Patient/family teaching. In B. Dossey, C. Guzetta, and C. Kenner (eds). *Essentials of critical care nursing: Body, mind, spirit*, pp. 29–41. Philadelphia: J.B. Lippincott.

Bille, D. (1983). Process-oriented patient education. *Dimensions Crit. Care Nursing*. 2:108.

Bouman, C. (1984). Identifying priority concerns of families of ill patients. *Dimensions Crit. Care Nursing*. 3:313–319.

Carlon, G. (1988). Admitting cancer patients to the ICU. *Crit. Care Clin*. 4:183–192.

Carlson, R. (1989). Seizing the initiative. *Heart Lung*. 18:332–339.

Cassell, E. (1986). Autonomy in the ICU: Refusal of treatment. *Crit. Care Clin*. 2:27–40.

Claus, K., and Bailey, J. (1980). *Living with stress and promoting well-being*. St. Louis: C.V. Mosby.

Clement, J. (1988). The need for and effects of touch in intensive care patients. In B. Heater and B. AuBuchon (eds). *Controversies in critical care nursing*, p.81. Rockville, Maryland: Aspen.

Clement, J. (1986). Caring and touching as nursing interventions. In C. Hudak, B. Gallo, and T. Lohr (eds). *Critical care nursing: A holistic approach*, p. 36. Philadelphia: J.B. Lippincott.

Continenza, K. (1989). Who cares for the care givers? *Focus Critical Care*. 16:435–436.

Dominion, J. (1971). The psychological significance of touch. *Nursing Times*. 67:163–171.

Dossey, B. (1990). Psychophysiologic self-regulation interventions. In B. Dossey, C. Guzzetta, and C. Kenner (eds). *Essentials of critical care nursing: Body, mind, spirit*, Chap. 5. Philadelphia: J.B. Lippincott.

Easton, C., and MacKenzie, F. (1988). Sensory-perceptual alterations: Delirium in the ICU. *Heart Lung*. 17:229–235.

Edwards, B.S. (1990). Does the DNR patient belong in the ICU? *Crit. Care Clin. North Am*. 2:473–480.

Farrimond, P. (1984). Post-cardiotomy delirium. *Nursing Times*. 80(30):39–41.

Fitzgerald, K. (1989). Trauma. In B. Riegel and D. Ehrenreich (eds). *Psychological aspects of critical care nursing*, pp. 210–233. Rockville, Maryland: Aspen.

Freudenberg, H. (1974). Staff burnout. *J. Social Issues*. 30:159–165.

Fuerst, E. (1989). Computerizing the intensive care unit: Current status and future directions. *J. Cardiovasc. Nursing*. 4:68–78.

Gast, P., and Baker, C. (1989). The coronary care unit patient: Anxiety and annoyance to noise. *Crit. Care Nursing Q.* 12:39–54.

Hansell, H. (1984). The behavioral effects of noise on man: The patient with "ICU psychosis." *Heart Lung.* 13:59–65.

Harris, R. (1989). Reviewing nursing stress according to a proposed coping-adaptation framework. *Adv. Nursing Sci.* 11:12–28.

Hickey, M. (1990). What are the needs of families of critically ill patients? A review of the literature since 1976. *Heart Lung.* 19:401–415.

Holyfield, L. (1983). Equipment vs. people. *Dimensions Crit. Care Nursing.* 2:234–236.

Houser, D. (1977). A study of nurses new to special care units. *Supervisor Nurse.* 8(7):15–22.

Kirchhoff, K., Hansen, C., and Fullmer, N. (1985). Open visiting in the intensive care unit: A debate. *Dimension Crit. Care Nursing.* 4:296–304.

Kohrman, A. (1985). Selective non-treatment of handicapped newborns: A critical essay. *Social Sci. Med.* 20:1091–1095.

Levine, M. (1989). Ration or rescue: The elderly patient in critical care. *Crit. Care Nursing Q.* 12:82–89.

Lo, B., and Jonsen, A. (1980). Clinical decisions to limit treatment. *Ann. Intern. Med.* 93:764–768.

Maslow, A. (1970). *Motivation and personality,* New York: Harper & Row.

McConnell, E. (1990). The impact of machines on the work of critical care nurses. *Crit. Care Nursing Q.* 12:45–52.

Miller, J. (1989). Hope-inspiring strategies of the critically ill. *Appl. Nursing Res.* 2:23–29.

Norbeck, J. (1985). Types and sources of social support for managing job stress in critical care nursing. *Nursing Res.* 34:225–230.

Orlowski, J., and Gulledge, A. (1986). Critical care stress: Burnout. *Crit. Care Clin.* 2:173–182.

Prescott, P. (1989). Shortage of professional nursing practice: A reframing of the shortage problem. *Heart Lung.* 18:436–443.

Ray, M. (1989). The theory of bureaucratic caring for nursing practice in the organizational culture. *Nursing Admin. Q.* 13:31–42.

Robinson, J., and Lewis, D. (1990). Coping with ICU work-related stressors: A study. *Crit. Care Nurse.* 10:80–88.

Schnaper, N., and Cowley, R. (1976). Overview: Psychological sequelae to multiple trauma. *Am. J. Psychiatry.* 133:883–890.

Schultz, M., and Daly, B. (1989). Differences and similarities in nurses' perceptions of intensive care nursing and non-intensive care nursing. *Focus Crit. Care.* 16:465–471.

Searle, L. (1990). Implication of the nursing shortage. *Focus Crit. Care.* 17:219–221.

Smith, J. (1986). Patient responses to the critical care setting. In C. Hudak, B. Gallo, and T. Lohr (eds). *Critical care nursing: A holistic approach,* Philadelphia: J.B. Lippincott.

Spoth, R., and Konewko, P. (1987). Intensive care staff stressors and life event changes across multiple settings and work units. *Heart Lung.* 16:278–284.

Steele, S., and Harmon, V. (1979). *Values clarification in nursing.* New York: Appleton-Century-Crofts.

Suchman, E. (1965). Stages of illness and medical care. *J. Health Hum. Behav.* 6:114.

Topf, M. (1989). Personality hardiness, occupational stress, and burnout in critical care nurses. *Res. Nursing Health.* 12:179–186.

Topf, M. and Dillon, E. (1988). Noise-induced stress as a predictor of burnout in critical care nurses. *Heart Lung.* 17:567–574.

Van Ora, L. (1989). Terminal is a relative term. *Nursing Health Care.* 18:97–100.

Veatch, R. (1986). The ethics of resource allocation in critical care. *Crit. Care Clin.* 2:73–90.

Williams, M. (1989). Physical environment of the intensive care unit: Elderly patients. *Crit. Care Nursing Q.* 12:39–54.

Zwolski, K. (1989). Professional nursing in a technical system. *Image.* 21:238–242.

PART VI

Caring for Special Patients

Module 22

Nursing Care of the Acutely Ill Obstetric Patient

Jane G. E. Silver

The self-study module, *Nursing Care of the Acutely Ill Obstetric Patient*, is written for the nurse who has basic knowledge of the care of the critically ill patient. The focus of the module is on the physiologic changes that occur with pregnancy and the unique needs of the acutely ill pregnant woman. The module is composed of six sections. The first three sections focus on the care of the pregnant woman experiencing alterations in ventilation, perfusion, and metabolism. The fourth section examines care of the pregnant trauma patient. The fifth section examines the care of the patient with pregnancy-induced hypertension, and the final section concentrates on the application of a fetal monitor and basic knowledge of fetal heart rate patterns. The module contains a pretest and a posttest to assist the reader to target areas where knowledge is deficient and to evaluate the knowledge learned after completion of the module.

Objectives

Following completion of this module, the learner will be able to

1. List the cardiorespiratory changes that occur with pregnancy
2. List the indications for hemodynamic monitoring in the pregnant patient
3. Differentiate between the classifications of diabetes during pregnancy
4. Identify potential problems that can develop in the pregnant diabetic patient and her fetus
5. Describe the nursing interventions provided for the pregnant trauma patient
6. Identify risk factors associated with preterm labor
7. State the signs and symptoms of preterm labor
8. Define severe pregnancy-induced hypertension and HELLP syndrome
9. Identify an abnormal fetal heart rate
10. Identify when an obstetrician and obstetric nurse should be notified

Pretest

1. Pregnancy is considered a state of chronic
   A. metabolic alkalosis
   B. metabolic acidosis
   C. respiratory alkalosis
   D. respiratory acidosis

2. Which of the following increases in pregnancy?
   A. blood volume
   B. plasma volume
   C. cardiac output
   D. all of the above

3. Maternal blood loss at delivery of the fetus ranges from
   A. 100 to 250 mL
   B. 500 to 1,200 mL
   C. 250 to 500 mL
   D. 1,000 to 1,500 mL

4. To prevent supine hypotensive syndrome
   A. place the woman on her back
   B. place a wedge under the woman's right hip
   C. give oxygen via nasal cannula
   D. place the woman in Trendelenburg position

5. Uterine massage is performed in order to
   A. assess the size of the uterus
   B. assist in delivery of the fetus
   C. control uterine bleeding
   D. eliminate uterine contractions

6. When applying military antishock trousers (MAST) to a pregnant woman
   A. do not inflate the abdominal region
   B. no special considerations are necessary
   C. MAST cannot be used on pregnant women
   D. inflate all regions at one-half that of a non-pregnant woman

7. Pregnancy-induced hypertension (PIH) resolves quickly by
   A. administration of magnesium sulfate (MgSO$_4$)
   B. administration of hydralazine hydrochloride (Apresoline)
   C. delivery of the fetus
   D. administration of methyldopa (Aldomet)

8. In severe pregnancy-induced hypertension (SPIH) patients, magnesium sulfate (MgSO$_4$) is the drug of choice for
   A. decreasing blood pressure
   B. prevention of convulsions
   C. increasing cardiac output
   D. diuresis

9. Marked bradycardia in the fetus is defined as ___ bpm or less.
   A. 40
   B. 60
   C. 99
   D. 120

10. The normal heart rate in the fetus is between
    A. 160 and 180 bpm
    B. 120 and 160 bpm
    C. 90 and 120 bpm
    D. 60 and 80 bpm

11. If the patient who experiences an amniotic fluid embolus survives the initial cardiorespiratory collapse, the patient is at high risk for
    A. disseminated intravascular coagulation
    B. kidney failure
    C. congestive heart failure
    D. transient ischemic attacks

12. Cardiac output increases during pregnancy and peaks at ___ completed weeks gestation
    A. 15–18
    B. 20–24
    C. 30–32
    D. 38–40

13. Pregnancy is considered diabetogenic due to increasing insulin requirements and
    A. placental production of HPL
    B. beta cell hyperplasia
    C. maternal production of progesterone
    D. all of the above

14. All pregnant diabetics should keep their blood glucose levels between ___ and ___ to prevent fetal compromise.
    A. 165, 190 mg/dL
    B. 130, 160 mg/dL
    C. 110, 130 mg/dL
    D. 70, 110 mg/dL

15. If a pregnant woman who just experienced abdominal trauma has an increase in her fundal height of 4 cm in 1 hour, the nurse should expect
    A. uterine rupture at the fundus
    B. placenta previa with bleeding
    C. placenta abruption with bleeding
    D. impending vaginal delivery of the fetus

Pretest answers: 1, C. 2, D. 3, B. 4, B. 5, C. 6, A. 7, C. 8, B. 9, C. 10, B. 11, A. 12, C. 13, D. 14, D. 15, C.

Glossary

Abruptio placentae. Premature separation of the normally implanted placenta; separation may be complete or partial and is considered an obstetric emergency

Acceleration. Transient increases of the fetal heart rate (FHR) > 15 bpm, associated with fetal movement in the healthy fetus and a uniformly good outcome

Accreta (placenta accreta). A condition where one or more of the cotyledons of the placenta abnormally adhere to the uterine wall, making separation of the placenta difficult or impossible

Acme. The peak of the uterine contraction

Amniotic fluid embolism. Blocking of a maternal artery with amniotic fluid, forced into the artery by uterine contractions

Average FHR variability. 6 to 10 beats/minute

Cardiac classifications. Classifications of heart disease (functional) is by the New York Heart Association:

Class I	Asymptomatic at normal levels of activity
Class II	Symptoms with greater than ordinary physical activity
Class III	Symptomatic with ordinary activity
Class IV	Symptomatic at rest

Cesarean section. Delivery of fetus by an incision through the abdominal wall and the wall of the uterus

Deceleration. Fluctuation of the FHR below baseline; all decelerations must be observed closely by a nurse or obstetrician expert in FHR interpretation

Disseminated intravascular coagulation (DIC). Complex disorder of the clotting mechanism in the blood that can lead to overwhelming hemorrhage; may be caused by placental abruption, sepsis, fetal demise, or HELLP syndrome

Dystocia. Prolonged, painful, or otherwise difficult delivery or birth because of mechanical factors relating to either the passage for the fetus, i.e., pelvis of mother or inadequate pushing energy, i.e., uterine contractions

Early deceleration. Repetitive degree of deceleration does not exceed 110 bpm., uniform shape, onset and recovery correspond with contraction; also associated with fetal head compression

Expiratory reserve. Volume of air left in the lungs after normal expiration and forced expiration

Facilitative diffusion. Energy-dependent process where particles move down the concentration gradient

Fetal monitor. Electronic monitor attached to the mother's abdomen to detect fetal heart tones and uterine activity; a printout of the fetal heart rate and uterine activity is obtained from the monitor for evaluation; monitor also can be attached internally for more accurate measurement of beat to beat variability and pressure of uterine activity in mm Hg

Fetal placental unit. The fetus and placenta connected by the umbilical cord

Fetus. The baby in utero from the end of the fifth week of gestation until birth

Functional residual capacity. Volume of air left in the lungs after a forced expiration

Fundus. Top portion of the uterus

Gestational age. The age of the product of conception between the first day of the last normal menstrual period (of the mother) and birth of the baby; the age is determined in weeks

Gravid. The pregnant woman

Gravity. The total number of times pregnant

HELLP. An extension of preeclampsia involving hemolysis, elevated liver enzymes, and low platelets

Hemorrhagic shock. Condition associated with acute blood loss in which the patient's functional intravascular blood volume is below that of the capacity of the body's vascular bed, which results in low blood pressure, decreased tissue perfusion, cellular acidosis, hypoxia, organ tissue dysfunction, and death

Hydramnios (polyhydramnios). Amniotic fluid in excess of 1.5 L; often indicative of fetal anomaly and frequently seen in poorly controlled, insulin-dependent, diabetic pregnant women even if there is no coexisting fetal anomaly

Hypovolemia. An abnormally decreased volume of liquid (plasma) circulating in the body

Late deceleration. Fetal heart rate tracing with uniform shape, late onset, that occurs usually 20 seconds after beginning of contraction; repetitive; ominous sign especially if associated with change in baseline or absence of variability; associated with placental insufficiency (notify obstetrician immediately, change maternal position, apply oxygen via face mask at 8 L/minute)

Macrosomia. Large body size, as seen in neonates of diabetic or prediabetic mothers

Mammary flow murmurs (mammary souffles). Sounds heard over the breasts that result from increased blood flow through the vessels of the breasts

Marked FHR variability. Greater than 25 bpm; a good sign (continue to observe)

Minimal FHR variability. 3 to 5 bpm; this pattern needs to be watched closely (obstetrician should be alerted; maintain a left uterine tilt; fetus may be in a sleep stage or becoming affected by the MgSO₄ if used)

Moderate FHR variability. 11 to 25 bpm; this is a good sign, but continue to observe

No FHR variability. FHR appears to be a flat line, 0–2 bpm; central nervous system of the fetus is decreased (obstetrician needs to be notified; reposition the mother further to her left side if possible)

Obstetric lacerations. Tearing of the vulvar, vaginal, periurethral, or sometimes rectal tissue during childbirth

Parity. Four series of numbers indicating outcome of previous pregnancies; first number represents number of full-term infants delivered; second, the number of premature infants delivered (>20 weeks <37 weeks); third, the number of abortions or deliveries <20 weeks; the fourth, the number of living children today

Parturition. The act or process of giving birth

Placenta previa. A placenta that is implanted in the lower uterine segment so that it ajoins or covers the internal os of the cervix

Postpartum. Referring to the mother after childbirth

Preeclampsia. A triad of hypertension, pathologic edema, and proteinuria after the twentieth week of gestation

Residual capacity. Volume of air left in the lungs after a normal breath

Retained placenta. Pieces of placenta remaining adhered to the wall of the uterus

Stages of labor. Four-stage process

First stage	Time period from the onset of labor (uterine contractions every 5 minutes) to when the cervix is completely dilated to 10 cm
Second stage	Time period from complete dilation to the birth of the baby
Third stage	Time period from birth of the baby to delivery of the placenta
Fourth stage	Usually considered to be from 1 to 4 hours after delivery

Supine hypotensive syndrome. When a pregnant woman is in the supine position, venous return is decreased and can result in decreased cardiac output, a sudden drop in blood pressure, bradycardia, and syncope

Syncytiotrophoblast. The outer syncytial layer of the trophoblast of the early mammalian embryo that erodes the uterine wall during implantation and gives rise to the villi of the placenta

Term. A pregnant woman between 37 and 40 completed weeks of gestation

Tidal volume. Difference between volume of air after inspiration and volume of air after end-expiration (normal breath)

Tocodynamometer (TOCO). Measures uterine activity; pressure transducer that converts pressure to an electrical signal; TOCO is a flat disk with either a protruding or flush plunger; as uterus contracts, abdominal wall rises and presses against the transducer; the movement against the plunger converts to an electrical signal, which is recorded on the monitor paper, recording the frequency and duration of contractions (the reading at the bottom of the monitor paper)

Tocolytic therapy. Use of medications to halt preterm labor

Toxemia. Pregnancy-induced hypertension

Trimester. A 3-month period; a pregnancy contains three trimesters

Tummy grip. An elastic and cloth material used to hold the instruments of the fetal monitor in place on the abdomen

Uterine atony. Loss of tone by the musculature of the uterus (feels soft or boggy to touch); considered an emergency condition after childbirth and can result in hemorrhage

Uterine inversion. The body of the uterus inverts or prolapses through the vaginal canal

Ultrasound transducer. Records FHR; high-frequency sound waves are transmitted from a crystal and are reflected from the moving fetal heart to a receiving crystal; using this method, may also pick up fetal movement and maternal heart rate (to determine if the heart rate is maternal or fetal, listen to the monitor signal and take the maternal pulse; if the signals are the same, readjust the monitor)

Valsalva maneuver. The bearing-down activity performed during a bowel movement and during the second stage of labor when pushing occurs

Variability. Fluctuation of FHR above or below baseline in bpm

Variable deceleration. Fetal heart rate tracing that is variable in shape with a sudden drop in FHR; onset may be at any time and recovery is rapid; baseline FHR and variability remain unchanged; decelerations look like shark teeth; caused by umbilical cord compression (notify obstetrician, change maternal position, and apply oxygen if deceleration is repetitive)

Abbreviations

ABGs. Arterial blood gases

AFE. Amniotic fluid embolus

ARDS. Adult respiratory distress syndrome

BP. Blood pressure

bpm. Beats per minute

CHF. Congestive heart failure

cm H₂O. Centimeters of water

CNS. Central nervous system

DIC. Disseminated intravascular coagulation

FHR. Fetal heart rate

ga. gauge

HELLP. Hemolysis, elevated liver enzymes, low platelets

HPL. Human placental lactogen

IUGR. Intrauterine growth retardation

LLR. Left lateral recumbent

MAST. Military antishock trousers

Pao₂. Partial pressure of oxygen, arterial

Pco₂. Partial pressure of carbon dioxide

PIH. Pregnancy-induced hypertension

SPIH. Severe pregnancy-induced hypertension

SVR. Systemic vascular resistance

TOCO. Tocodynamometer

Section One: Care of the Pregnant Woman Experiencing Alterations in Ventilation

At the completion of this section, the learner will be able to list the cardiorespiratory changes that occur with pregnancy.

The maternal respiratory system is extremely important for the maintenance of fetal oxygenation during pregnancy (Lee and Cotton, 1987). A relative hyperventilation of pregnancy begins in the first trimester and increases 42 percent by term gestation (Dunn, 1990). Other respiratory changes that occur with pregnancy are as follows.

- Pulmonary vascular bed: Pulmonary vascular resistance may be decreased.
- Arterial blood gases: Decreased Pco₂ related to an increased respiratory rate during pregnancy. A slight increase in pH also occurs.
- Oxygen consumption: Consumption increases due to the increase in vital capacity.
- Lung volumes: There is an increased tidal volume. Alveolar ventilation is increased related to an increase in respiratory rate.

Pregnancy has been called a state of chronic respiratory alkalosis because of the increase in oxygen consumption and vital capacity and a fall in Paco₂. Because of the normal respiratory alkalosis associated with pregnancy, the pregnant woman with an alteration in ventilation must have her ABGs carefully monitored for signs of early acidosis. An indication of acidosis in a pregnant woman would be

a pH of 7.35 (Zolli and Neville, 1985). During respiratory embarrassment, the pregnant woman compensates by increasing her respiratory rate rather than the depth of tidal volume, a less efficient mechanism (Gonik, 1987). Table 22–1 (Dunn, 1990) illustrates the changes in ventilation in the pregnant vs nonpregnant woman.

During delivery of the placenta, abruptio placentae, or abdominal trauma where the placenta abrupts, there is a risk of amniotic fluid embolus. As the placenta separates, there is a possibility of amniotic fluid entering the maternal circulation if the uterine musculature does not contract rapidly and well (Campbell, 1989).

TABLE 22–1. VENTILATORY MEASURES: PREGNANT VS NONPREGNANT

	Nonpregnant	Pregnant
Respiratory rate (breaths/minute)	12–20	20–30
Tidal volume (mL/kg)	6–7	8–10
Minute ventilation (mL/minute)	5–10	7–25
Oxygen consumption (mL/minute)	173–311	249–331
Arterial Pao₂ (mm Hg)	90–105	104–108
Venous Pao₂ (mm Hg)	38–40	27–32
Arterial pH	7.35–7.40	7.40–7.45

From Dunn, P. (1990). Assessing a pregnant woman after trauma. *Nursing '90.* 20:53–57.

Amniotic fluid embolism (AFE) is a rare but frequently fatal obstetric emergency clinically recognized in approximately 1 of 30,000 deliveries. The mortality rate of mothers suffering AFE is 50 percent. Clinical presentation of the syndrome is reflected by five signs that usually occur in the following sequence.

1. Respiratory distress
2. Cyanosis
3. Cardiovascular collapse
4. Hemorrhage
5. Coma

In one half of patients surviving the initial cardiovascular crisis, a life-threatening diathesis will develop. If the patient survives the initial cardiorespiratory collapse, there is a 40 percent to 50 percent risk of development of a coagulopathy within 1 to 2 hours (Benedetti, 1986).

Treatment revolves around three goals: oxygenation, maintenance of CO and blood pressure, and combating of what usually is a self-limited albeit severe coagulopathy (Clark, 1987).

Table 22–2 is a sample nursing care plan for amniotic fluid embolus syndrome (Clark, 1987).

Only scanty information is available on which to base treatment of the initial syndrome of AFE. Early airway control usually necessitating endotracheal intubation has been stressed in the few patients surviving the full-blown syndrome (Resnik et al, 1976). Once maximal ventilation and oxygenation have been achieved, attention should be paid to restoration of cardiovascular equilibrium (Benedetti, 1986). Diagnosis is sometimes not proven until pulmonary arterial blood is aspirated and stained for the presence of fetal squames, lanugo hair, and mucin (Benedetti, 1986).

The cardiorespiratory changes associated with pregnancy occur in order to maintain fetal oxygenation and compensate for the expanding uterus. Although AFE is a rare occurrence, it is nonetheless life threatening to both mother and fetus.

TABLE 22–2. NURSING CARE PLAN FOR AMNIOTIC FLUID EMBOLISM SYNDROME

■ Nursing Diagnosis
High-risk for actual alteration in tissue perfusion: cardiopulmonary related to amniotic fluid embolism syndrome

■ Expected Outcomes
1. To maintain systolic blood pressure > 90 mm Hg, urine output > 25 mL/hour, and arterial Po_2 > 70 mm Hg
2. To correct coagulation abnormalities

■ Interventions
1. Initiate cardiopulmonary resuscitation, if indicated
2. Administer O_2 at a high concentration. Assist as per hospital protocol with intubation and ventilate with 100% Fio_2 if the patient is unconscious
3. Monitor fetal heart rate carefully if gestational age is sufficient to warrant intervention for fetal distress
4. Hypotension is usually secondary to cardiogenic shock. Treatment involves optimization of cardiac preload by rapid crystalloid infusion with subsequent dopamine infusion (2–20 mg/kg/minute) if the patient remains hypotensive (as ordered by doctor)
5. After insertion of a flow-directed pulmonary artery catheter, monitor the hemodynamic status. Blood from the distal port should be aspirated in order to perform a buffy coat examination for squamous cells. If squamous cells are present, amniotic fluid has entered the maternal bloodstream
6. In the patient who is not severely hypoxic or hypotensive, incipient congestive heart failure should be anticipated. Rapid digitalization is indicated (0.5–1.0 mg digoxin in divided doses) as ordered by doctor
7. In the absence of hypotension, fluid therapy should be restricted to maintenance levels to minimize pulmonary edema resulting from developing adult respiratory distress syndrome (ARDS). Again hemodynamic assessment with the pulmonary artery catheter may be of tremendous value
8. Administer fresh whole blood or packed red blood cells and fresh frozen plasma to treat bleeding secondary to disseminated intravascular coagulation. There are insufficient data to warrant routine heparinization or administration of E-aminocaproate (Amicar)
9. Obtain critical laboratory tests: arterial blood gas, CBC, platelet count, fibrinogen, fibrin split products, PT, PTT

From Clark, S. (1987). Amniotic fluid embolus. In S. Clark, Phelane, and D. Cotton (eds). *Critical care obstetrics.* Montvale, New Jersey: Medical Economics. Reprinted by permission of Blackwell Scientific Publications, Inc.

Section One Review

1. Increased respiratory rate will affect which component of the arterial blood gases?
   A. Pao_2
   B. HCO_3
   C. bicarbonate level
   D. $Paco_2$
2. During AFE syndrome, cardiogenic shock occurs. What happens to the blood pressure?
   A. decreases
   B. increases
   C. labile
   D. remains the same

3. After the blood pressure is stabilized during AFE syndrome, what will be a complication if fluid therapy is not restricted to maintenance levels?
   A. oliguria
   B. pulmonary edema
   C. severe hypertension
   D. DIC

Answers: 1, D. 2, A. 3, B.

Section Two: Care of the Pregnant Woman Experiencing Alterations in Perfusion

Following the completion of this section, the learner will be able to list the indications for hemodynamic monitoring in the pregnant patient.

Profound cardiovascular and hemodynamic changes occur with pregnancy. Table 22–3 demonstrates how hemodynamic values change in pregnancy (Dunn, 1990).

TABLE 22–3. HEMODYNAMIC VALUES NONPREGNANT VS PREGNANT

Value	Nonpregnant	Pregnant
Cardiac output (L/minute)	4–7	5–10
Stroke volume (mL/beat)	65	75
Heart rate (bpm)	70	80
Central venous pressure (mm Hg)	2–10	Same
Pulmonary artery pressure (mm Hg)	20–30/5–15	Same
Pulmonary capillary wedge pressure (mm Hg)	6–12	Same
Blood pressure/arterial line readings (mm Hg)	120/80	114/65
Systemic vascular resistance (dynes/second/cm^{-5})	800–1,200	600–900
Pulmonary vascular resistance (dynes/second/cm^{-5})	20–120	15–90
Femoral vascular resistance (cm H_2O)	9	24

From Dunn, P. (1990). Assessing a pregnant woman after trauma. *Nursing '90*. 20:53–57.

One of the more striking changes that occurs during pregnancy is the increase in blood volume. The increase in plasma volume at term pregnancy is 45 percent to 50 percent over nonpregnant levels. The physiologic mechanism responsible for the hypervolemia of pregnancy is complex but appears to be related primarily to increasing production of aldosterone under the influence of estrogen (Lee and Cotton, 1987). Placental production of chorionic somatomammotropin, progesterone, and possibly prolactin stimulates erythropoiesis but results in only a 20 percent red cell mass increase. These changes account for the physiologic anemia often observed in pregnant patients despite adequate iron stores (Lee and Cotton, 1987). Cardiovascular alterations that occur in pregnancy are as follows.

Heart

With pregnancy, myocardial hypertrophy is normal. There is an increased end-diastolic volume related to the thickening of the ventricular wall due to the upward pressure from the diaphragm (from the enlarged uterus), and the point of maximal impulse is higher due to the displacement of the heart superiorly, laterally, and anteriorly.

Heart Sounds

There is an increased loudness of the first heart sound. This change occurs between 12 and 20 weeks gestation and is maintained until approximately 2 to 4 weeks postpartum. Systolic murmurs are common. About 90 percent of pregnant women have a systolic murmur secondary to the increase in blood flow. Mammary flow murmurs (mammary souffles) are normal and usually are heard over the breasts. These sounds result from increased blood flow through the vessels of the breast.

Cardiac Output

As shown in Table 22–3, CO increases in pregnancy. The increase is progressive in the first and second trimesters. The increase peaks by the thirty-second week and then slightly decreases at term (38–40 completed weeks). Uterine blood flow increases from approximately 50 mL/minute at 10 weeks gestation to 500 mL/minute at term. Most of the increased blood volume of pregnancy is distributed to the engorged pelvic veins and lower extremities. In the supine position, venous return is decreased and can result in decreased CO, a sudden drop in blood pressure, bradycardia, and syncope (Lee and Cotton, 1987). These clinical changes are termed *supine hypotensive syndrome* (vena cava syndrome). CO during labor and delivery increases by 15 percent in the early first stage. By the late first stage, CO has increased 30 percent. During the second stage, CO has increased 45 percent due to the repeated performance of the Valsalva maneuver during pushing.

After the delivery of the baby, the increased blood volume that circulated to the placenta is now shifted back into the maternal bloodstream. This shifting of blood volume produces a 65 percent increase in CO 5 minutes postpartum. When the woman is 1 hour postpartum, the cardiac output is at a 30 percent to 50 percent increase over nonpregnant values.

Fluid and Electrolyte Changes in Pregnancy

Laboratory values are altered by the pregnant state. Table 22–4 (Dunn, 1990) demonstrates changes in laboratory values during pregnancy.

During parturition, there are various hemodynamic stresses that occur. With pregnancy, there is an increased plasma volume that produces a hypervolemia and a vasodilated state, which protects the woman against precipitous falls in blood pressure. At the time of delivery, maternal blood loss ranges from 500 mL to 1,200 mL. After expulsion of the baby, the contracting uterus essentially transfuses 500 mL of blood back into the circulation.

Hypovolemic Shock in the Pregnant Patient

An alteration in maternal perfusion can greatly affect the fetal-placental unit. During times of maternal insult, such as hypoxia, shock, or acidosis, vasoconstriction occurs. The maternal cardiovascular system automatically shunts blood to the vital organs

TABLE 22–4. CHANGES IN LABORATORY VALUES DURING PREGNANCY

Component	Nonpregnant	Pregnant
Leukocytes (per cm³)	4,500–10,000	5,000–18,000
Hemoglobin (g/dL)	12–16	10–13
Hematocrit (%)	37–47	32–42
Plasma volume (mL)	2,400	3,700
Blood volume (mL)	4,000	5,250
Erythrocyte volume (mL)	1,600	1,900
Platelet (per cm³)	175,000–250,000	200,000–350,000
Fibrinogen, plasma (mg/dL)	100–700	400–500
Sedimentation rate (mm/hour)	0–20	44–114
Blood urea nitrogen (mg/dL)	10–18	4–12
Sodium (mEq/L)	135–145	132–140
Potassium (mEq/L)	4–4.8	3.5–4.5
Chloride (mEq/L)	98–109	90–105
Bicarbonate (mEq/L)	24–30	19–25
Calcium, ionized (mEq/L)	4.5–5.4	4–5

From Dunn, P. (1990). Assessing a pregnant woman after trauma. *Nursing '90.* 20:53–57.

(brain, lungs, heart, and kidneys) and, therefore, decreases perfusion to the uterus and fetus. Displacing the uterus to the left and providing oxygen therapy to the mother can increase transport of oxygen to the fetus. To prevent supine hypotension syndrome, place a roll of blankets or a pillow under the right hip of the patient. This will displace the woman's uterus to the left and thus maintain venus return.

The term *shock* represents a morbid condition in which the patient's functional intravascular blood volume is below that of the capacity of the body's vascular bed. It is a mismatch between oxygen demand and oxygen supply. If left untreated, resulting cellular acidosis and hypoxia lead to end-organ tissue dysfunction and death.

Obstetric hypovolemic shock, arbitrarily defined as an estimated blood loss of greater than 500 mL, is one of the leading causes of maternal mortality postpartum. Table 22–5 lists the incidence of obstetric hemorrhage (Gonik, 1987).

In the case of antepartum hemorrhage, the

TABLE 22–5. INCIDENCE OF OBSTETRIC HEMORRHAGE

Etiology	Incidence per Delivery
Late pregnancy	
Abruptio placentae	1:120[a]
Placenta previa	1:200
Toxemia-associated	1:20
Delivery and postpartum	
Cesarean section	1:6
Obstetric lacerations	1:8
Uterine atony	1:20
Retained placenta	1:160
Uterine inversion	1:2,300
Placenta accreta	1:7,000

[a] The incidence may have increased due to the increase in maternal crack cocaine use in the urban population.
Modified from Gonik, B. (1987). Intensive care monitoring of the critically ill pregnant patient. In R. Creasy and R. Resnik (eds.). *Maternal-fetal medicine.* Philadelphia: W.B. Saunders.

nurse should establish left uterine displacement, notify an obstetrician stat., place the woman in the Trendelenburg position, assess vital signs, color, and amount of vaginal bleeding, and establish fetal well-being (see Section Six). Notifying an obstetric nurse to assist with fetal monitoring can be helpful.

In the case of immediate postpartum hemorrhage, conventional methods to control bleeding should be instituted. Uterine massage is a useful maneuver to control uterine bleeding and atony. Take your gloved hand and compress the lower abdominal area at the pubic hair line. This compression will rotate the fundal region of the uterus anteriorly and out of the pelvis. Maintaining compression as stated, take your other gloved hand and massage the fundus of the uterus, which at this point should be located at the height of the umbilicus. If the fundus is noted to be deviated to either the right or left side of the abdomen or significantly higher than the umbilicus, the bladder is probably full, and a catheterization will have to be performed. Urinary retention may be secondary to a decreased sensation to urinate caused by the trauma of a vaginal delivery. The nurse should continue to massage the fundus until it feels hard. The amount and consistency of the vaginal bleeding (lochia) should be assessed, and a pad count should be started with all pads weighed (1 g = 1 mL fluid). Any clots, placental parts, or retained membranes in the lochia should be noted. Retained particles can cause an increase in the vaginal bleeding.

Contraction of the uterine musculature, after the delivery of the fetus, clamps down on the bleeding arterioles left behind where the placenta adhered. The overstretched uterus during pregnancy (especially with multiple gestations) may need to be stimulated in order to clamp down (contact). Uterine mas-

sage, as stated in the previous paragraph, stimulates the uterus to contract.

Table 22–6 shows the pharmacologic agents useful for controlling uterine atony.

If bleeding cannot be controlled, an obstetrician must be consulted immediately. Close examination of the lower genital tract may reveal vaginal or cervical lacerations that need repair. A surgical approach may be necessary. In some cases, hemodynamic monitoring may be necessary to obtain accurate assessment of bleeding and compensatory efforts.

Indications for the use of invasive hemodynamic monitoring in the obstetric patient are as follows (Koniak-Griffin and Dodgson, 1987).

1. Hypovolemic shock that is unresponsive to fluid therapy
2. Pregnancy-induced hypertension (see Section Five) complicated by oliguria
3. Administration of rapid IV antihypertensive therapy
4. Adult respiratory distress syndrome requiring intubation
5. Cardiac disease, class 3 or 4, in labor or requiring surgery (cesarean section, appendectomy)
6. Amniotic fluid embolism
7. Isolated pulmonary hypertension diagnosed before pregnancy presented in labor or requiring surgery
8. Pulmonary edema from any etiology unresponsive to initial therapy

As stated in Section One (Benedetti, 1986), if the patient survives an initial cardiorespiratory collapse, there is a 40 percent to 50 percent risk of developing a coagulopathy within 1 to 2 hours. Disseminated intravascular coagulation (DIC) results in the depletion of fibrinogen, platelets, and coagulation factors, especially factors V, VIII, and XIII.

TABLE 22–6. PHARMACOLOGIC AGENTS

Agent	Dose	Route
Oxytocin	10–20 units	IV drip,[a] IM, intramyometrial (multiple sites)
Methergonovine (Ergotrate)	0.2 mg	IM
Prostaglandin F$_2$-alpha	1 mg	Intramyometrial
Prostaglandin 15-methyl	0.25 mg	IM, intramyometrial (multiple sites)

[a] IV bolus administration of oxytocin can result in premature ventricular contractions and hypotension.
From Gonik, B. (1987). Intensive care monitoring of the critically ill pregnant patient. In R. Creasy and R. Resnik (eds). *Maternal-fetal medicine.* Philadelphia: W.B. Saunders.

Section Two Review

1. At which point in pregnancy does the maternal cardiac output reach its peak?
   A. 16 weeks
   B. 24 weeks
   C. 32 weeks
   D. 40 weeks
2. The following are indications for hemodynamic monitoring in the pregnant patient EXCEPT
   A. hypovolemic shock responsive to fluid therapy
   B. PIH with oliguria
   C. ARDS with intubation
   D. class 3 or 4 cardiac disease in labor

3. During maternal insult, such as hypoxia, shock, or acidosis, what happens to the maternal cardiovascular system?
   A. vasodilation
   B. vasoconstriction
   C. placental abruption
   D. hypertension

Answers: 1, C. 2, A. 3, B.

Section Three: Care of the Pregnant Woman Experiencing Alterations in Metabolism

Following the completion of this section, the learner will be able to differentiate among the classifications of diabetes during pregnancy.

Diabetes associated with pregnancy is a significant factor contributing to perinatal loss and morbidity. Diabetes, both overt and gestational, is reported to complicate between 2 percent and 3 percent of all pregnancies, with a mortality rate 4 to 5 times higher than that of the normal pregnancy (Gabbe et al, 1978).

The fetus depends on the maternal compartment for an uninterrupted supply of nutrients. Fetal energy requirements are supplied primarily by glucose obtained from the maternal circulation by facilitative diffusion. The placenta is not permeable to maternal insulin. Thus, fetal glucose use is independent of maternal insulin levels (McDonnall et al, 1986).

The following metabolic responses occur in pregnancy: hyperinsulinemia, hypertriglyceridemia, and a decreased sensitivity to insulin. After meals, insulin levels increase, and glucagon levels decrease. A state of facilitated anabolism occurs, characterized by greater carbohydrate-induced hypertriglyceridemia and enhanced suppression of glucagon (McDonnall et al, 1986).

Characteristically, maternal hyperinsulinemia associated with increased insulin resistance occurs in pregnancy. This becomes most marked late in gestation. The decreased tissue responsiveness to insulin, along with increasing insulin requirements, makes up the basis for calling the effects of pregnancy diabetogenic (McDonnall et al, 1986).

There are many hormonal changes that also induce this state of insulin resistance and hyperinsulinemia. The placental syncytiotrophoblast produces human placental lactogen (HPL), a growth hormonelike glycoprotein that causes insulin resistance and augments maternal lipolysis. Levels of

HPL are directly related to placental mass, increasing as pregnancy progresses. Free cortisol also creates a state of insulin resistance, and estrogen and progesterone directly alter maternal pancreatic islet function, producing beta cell hyperplasia and hyperinsulinemia (Beard et al, 1971).

In 1949, Dr. Priscilla White established a classification system for the pregnant diabetic. This classification, which takes into account the time of onset of diabetes, the duration of the disease, and the presence of vascular complications, is useful for determining management, and expected perinatal outcomes (Cohen et al, 1982). Table 22–7 illustrates this classification system.

TABLE 22–7. WHITE'S CLASSIFICATION OF DIABETES IN PREGNANCY

Class	Description	Insulin Requirement
A	Gestational or chemical diabetes (abnormal GTT) Normal fasting glucose (<105 mg/dL)	0
B	Overt diabetes Onset after age 20 Duration less than 10 years No vascular involvement	+
C	Overt diabetes Onset before age 20 Duration 10–20 years No vascular involvement	+
D	Overt diabetes Onset before age 10 Duration more than 20 years Benign retinopathy	+
F	Nephropathy	+
R	Proliferative retinopathy	+
T	Renal transplant	+

From McDonnall, A.-K., et al. (1986). Diabetes in pregnancy. In B. Wesley and S. Hutchinson (eds). *OB Care: Advanced Obstetrical Regional Education*. Camden, New Jersey: Perinatal Cooperative.

Assessment of a Pregnant Diabetic Patient

Assessment of blood glucose levels with visually read strips (Chemstrips) or with electronic devices (Glucometer, Accucheck, Glucoscan II) is required during pregnancy. Patients must be instructed in self glucose monitoring using one of these methods. Blood glucose levels should be assessed daily at the same time, and a record should be maintained by the patient. Generally, blood glucose levels will be assessed in the fasting state, 30 minutes before lunch, 30 minutes before dinner, and before bedtime (McDonnall et al, 1986).

Assessment of signs and symptoms of hypoglycemia and hyperglycemia is paramount when caring for the pregnant diabetic. The fetus is affected directly by both hyperglycemia and hypoglycemia. Recognition of the specific signs and symptoms related to each is paramount for providing prompt treatment.

Tables 22–8 and 22–9 outline how to recognize hypoglycemia and hyperglycemia and what to do for each.

Signs and symptoms for hyperglycemia and hypoglycemia are the same for both pregnant and nonpregnant patients. The only difference is that fetal development may be affected in the pregnant patient.

TABLE 22–8. HYPOGLYCEMIA

Low blood sugar, insulin reaction

Watch for
  Excessive diaphoresis, faintness
  Headache
  Palpitation, pounding heart, trembling
  Impaired vision
  Hunger
  Irritability
  Personality change
  If severe, unconscious, unable to awaken

What to do
  Test blood sugar
  Give milk, juice, or sugar, depending on severity of
    hypoglycemic reaction
  If patient is unconscious, notify physician and give IV glucose
  Do not give insulin
  Monitor fetal activity after reaction has resolved

Causes
  Too much insulin
  Not enough food
  Unusual amount of exercise
  Delayed meal

From McDonnall, A.-K., et al. (1986). Diabetes in pregnancy. In B. Wesley and S. Hutchinson (eds). *OB Care: Advanced Obstetrical Regional Education.* Camden, New Jersey: Perinatal Cooperative.

TABLE 22–9. HYPERGLYCEMIA

High blood sugar, diabetic acidosis

Watch for
  Increased thirst and polyuria
  Large amounts of sugar and ketones in urine
  Weakness, abdominal pains, generalized aches
  Loss of appetite, nausea and vomiting
  Heavy labored breathing

What to do
  Test blood sugar using bG Chemstrips or portable blood
    glucose monitoring device
  Notify physician
  Give patient fluids without sugar if able to swallow
  Administer insulin as ordered

Causes
  Insufficient insulin dosage
  Dietary noncompliance
  Infection, fever
  Emotional stress

From McDonnall, A.-K., et al. (1986). Diabetes in pregnancy. In B. Wesley and S. Hutchinson (eds). *OB Care: Advanced Obstetrical Regional Education.* Camden, New Jersey: Perinatal Cooperative.

Treatment and Management

The management of all pregnant diabetic patients is aimed at the following four goals (McDonnall et al, 1986).

1. Maintaining blood glucose levels between 70 and 110 mg/dL, with fasting blood glucose levels of 90 mg/dL or below
2. Eliminating maternal complications
3. Avoiding premature delivery
4. Early detection and prevention of fetal compromise

All pregnant diabetic patients will be classified into the appropriate category of White's scheme for pregnant diabetic patients. In addition, accurate estimation of gestational age must be made and should include serial ultrasonography. Such assessments as urine cultures, ophthalmoscopic examinations, and renal function studies should be done at intervals throughout the pregnancy (McDonnall et al, 1986).

Maternal Complications

Pregnancy-induced hypertension (refer to Section Five) is seen about four times more often in the preg-

TABLE 22–10. SIGNS AND SYMPTOMS OF HYPOGLYCEMIA AND KETOACIDOSIS

| | Onset | Signs and Symptoms | |
		Early	Late
Hypoglycemia	Rapid, within minutes	Tachycardia	Confusion
		Diaphoresis	Strange behavior
		Tremor	Stupor
		Hunger	Convulsions
		Pallor	Stroke syndrome
		Dizziness	Coma
		Irritability	
		Nausea	
		Headache	
		Paresthesia	
Ketoacidosis	Slow, over hours or days	Polyuria	Rapid, deep breathing
		Polydipsia	Hypothermia
		Malaise	Acetone breath
			Nausea and vomiting
			Abdominal pain
			Coma
			Death

From Sherwen, L., et al. (1991). *Nursing Care of the Childbearing Family*. E. Norwalk, Connecticut: Appleton & Lange.

nant diabetic patient, even when there is no evidence of preexisting vascular disease. However, information on the effects of pregnancy on existing vascular complications of diabetes is limited. Proliferative retinopathy often worsens with pregnancy, and the ultimate course of diabetic nephropathy is unclear. Generally, kidney function deteriorates during pregnancy but returns to prepregnancy functioning after delivery (McDonnall et al, 1986).

Hydramnios is common, and at times the large volume of amniotic fluid, coupled with fetal macrosomia (which is an increase in the size of the fetus due to increase in nutrient supply during times of maternal hyperglycemia), may cause cardiorespiratory symptoms in the mother. Frequently, the fetus is large and may lead to a difficult delivery, with injury to both mother and fetus (maternal lacerations and fetal shoulder dystocia) (McDonnall et al, 1986).

When the diabetic mother has vascular involvement and there is decreased uteroplacental perfusion, the fetus often will be distressed before the onset of labor. Cesarean deliveries are more common due to fetal distress and fetal dystocia (McDonnall et al, 1986). Also, if the diabetic mother has vascular involvement, the fetus may have IUGR rather than macrosomia, thus resulting in possible fetal complications.

Fetal and Neonatal Complications

The pregnant diabetic patient has an increased incidence of congenital anomalies that may possibly lead to neonatal deaths. Caudal regression syndrome and cardiac, renal, and central nervous system anomalies are the most common. These anomalies result during the first 7 weeks of gestation, a time when many women may be unaware that they are pregnant (Fuhrmann et al, 1983).

Neonatal morbidity is attributed most com-

TABLE 22–11. DIABETIC KETOACIDOSIS IN PREGNANCY

■ Goals of Therapy
1. Rehydration
2. Restoration of electrolyte homeostasis
3. Correction of acidemia
4. Normalization of serum glucose
5. Elimination of underlying cause

■ Management Protocol
1. Infuse 0.9 NaCl, 1000 mL over first hour, 1000 mL over subsequent 2 hours, 250 mL/hour thereafter
2. Change IV solution to D_5NS as serum glucose falls below 250 mg/dL
3. Add KCl 20–40 mEq/L to IV fluids after adequate output is established
4. a. Administer regular insulin 0.1 U/kg IV push
   b. Begin an infusion of 5–10 U/hour
   c. Double infusion rate if serum glucose has not decreased by 25% in 2 hours
   d. Reduce infusion to 1–2 U/hour as serum glucose falls below 150 mg/dL
5. Administer $NaHCO_3$ 44 mEq IV in 1000 mL 0.45 NS for arterial pH < 7.10
6. Search for underlying cause, such as infection

■ Critical Laboratory Tests
Serum electrolytes, glucose, arterial blood gas, CBC, bicarbonate, BUN, ketones

■ Consultation
Internal medicine

From Clark, S. et al. (1987). Diabetic ketoacidosis in pregnancy. In S. Clark, Phelan, and D. Colton (eds.). *Critical care obstetrics*. Montvale, New Jersey: Medical Economics. Permission by Blackwell Scientific Publications, Inc.

monly to fetal hyperglycemia and hyperinsulinemia. When the umbilical cord is cut at delivery, hypoglycemia of the neonate will occur within 2 to 4 hours as a result of the elimination of the maternal blood supply and the continued hyperactivity of the neonatal islet cells and their excessive amounts of insulin.

Care of the Pregnant Patient in Diabetic Ketoacidosis

The development of ketoacidosis is associated with a fetal mortality rate of 50 percent to 90 percent. It de-velops over hours or days when insulin levels are inadequate. As fats are metabolized for energy, ketones are produced faster than the body can catabolize them. Metabolic acidosis occurs and, in severe cases, results in diabetic coma. The need for insulin is increased by such factors as pregnancy, trauma, infection, development of insulin resistance, and psychologic stress. Ketoacidosis is a dangerous complication. Signs and symptoms of early and late ketoacidosis are presented in Table 22–10 (Sherwen et al, 1991).

Table 22–11 outlines the management of the pregnant patient in DKA.

Section Three Review

1. At what blood glucose levels should the pregnant diabetic be maintained?
   A. 150–200 mg/dL
   B. 110–150 mg/dL
   C. 70–110 mg/dL
   D. 50–70 mg/dL
2. All of the following are fetal complications that can occur when the mother is a diabetic EXCEPT
   A. neonatal blindness
   B. fetal death
   C. cardiac anomalies
   D. macrosomia

3. What happens to the neonate once the umbilical cord is cut?
   A. maternal hyperglycemia
   B. maternal hypoglycemia
   C. neonatal hypoglycemia
   D. fetal hypoglycemia

Answers: 1, C. 2, A. 3, C.

Section Four: Care of the Obstetric Trauma Patient

Following the completion of this section, the learner will be able to describe the nursing interventions provided for the pregnant trauma patient.

Trauma is the leading cause of death in women of childbearing age. With regard to the types of trauma, motor vehicle crashes are the leading cause of severe maternal trauma and death (Whittaker et al, 1986). This is followed by violent assaults and suicide. When a pregnant woman suffers a traumatic insult, the fetus is unlikely to be affected directly. Fetal well-being depends on the mother's survival. Therefore, the Number one concern is the hemodynamic stability of the mother (Zolli and Neville, 1985).

Anatomy and Physiology

Anatomically, the genitourinary tract is the organ system in pregnancy most significantly affected by trauma. In early pregnancy, the uterus is protected by bony structures, but after 12 weeks gestation, the uterus becomes a prominent abdominal structure. This results in an overall increase in risk of injury to the uterus and fetus as pregnancy advances. As stated in Section Two, there is an increase in blood supply to the pelvic region, thus adding an additional risk of significant hemorrhage in the event of trauma (Koniak-Griffin and Dodgson, 1987).

The enlarging uterus also can compress the ureters, bladder, and urethra, possibly causing dilatation and loss of tone. The bladder is lifted out of the pelvis and into the abdomen, making it more vulnerable to injury (Zolli and Neville, 1985).

During pregnancy, the enlarged uterus pushes the bowel into the upper abdominal cavity. Upper abdominal trauma during pregnancy affects both small and large bowel. Pregnancy also causes a decreased gastrointestinal motility and gastric emptying. Therefore, pregnant patients requiring general anesthesia are more prone to aspirate during intubation.

Hematologically, as stated in Section Two, pregnancy represents a hypercoagulable state, and this may increase the risk of thrombosis after injury. Disseminated intravascular coagulation (DIC), resulting from placental abruption, amniotic fluid embolism, or a ruptured uterus, is a common component of trauma.

Assessment and Management

The nurse should locate the fundus of the uterus by palpating the top portion of the mother's abdomen. Draw a line in ink on the mother's abdomen denoting this landmark (fundus). Also notice rigidity or tenderness when palpating the abdomen. If intrauterine bleeding is present, the fundus will be higher when assessed with the next set of vital signs. If a change in fundal height is noted, notify the obstetrician immediately. An increase in the fundal height could be associated with internal bleeding from a placental abruption, which is considered an obstetric emergency.

Close attention to the patient's coagulation studies is necessary. A fibrinogen that is falling (see normal for pregnant woman in Section Two) and fibrin split products greater than 40 μg/mL are abnormal. These findings are indicative of DIC.

Keep in mind the effects of supine hypotension syndrome on the pregnant woman's cardiac output (see Section Two). Place a wedge under the mother's right hip to displace her uterus to the left and off the vena cava.

Most code protocols are the same as would be followed for an adult who is not pregnant. The number one priority is the hemodynamic stability of the mother. The benefits of certain drugs or x-rays outweigh the risk of adverse fetal effects (if possible, shield the abdomen during radiation exposure). Military antishock trousers (MAST) can be used as long as the abdominal portion is not inflated (Dunn, 1990).

The mother is not the only patient. The fetus needs to be assessed. Section Six concentrates on the use of the fetal monitor. If the nurse feels uncomfortable using the fetal monitor, an obstetric nurse should be called to assist in monitoring. The mother should be attached to the fetal monitor for 4 to 48 hours after traumatic injury to ensure immediate fetal well-being. Pregnant trauma patients have a high incidence of preterm labor. Section Five reviews this high-risk complication and the medications used to control preterm labor. The traumatized pregnant woman may be having contractions that may be reported as menstrual cramps. The fetal monitor should be interpreted for signs of uterine activity (Section Seven).

The obstetrician may order drugs to halt preterm labor (refer to Section Six for use of these drugs). The pregnant trauma patient may also have a clear or greenish brown watery discharge. This may mean that the amniotic sac has ruptured. The obstetrician will want to use a sterile speculum to obtain a sample of the fluid to be tested with nitrazine paper. Amniotic fluid, blood, or sperm will turn the paper blue. For accurate results, the sample can also be examined microscopically (Zolli and Neville, 1985). If the woman's membranes did break, there is an increased risk of infection. Therefore, the woman's temperature must be assessed every hour and fetal heart rate closely observed for tachycardia (>160 bpm). A pad should not be applied to the perineum because the accumulation of amniotic fluid can harbor bacteria.

In summary, trauma during pregnancy can be life threatening. Internal bleeding can be the results of placental abruption or uterine rupture. The maternal hemodynamic status needs to be continually assessed. The fetus should be continually monitored (if >25 weeks gestation) via fetal monitor to ensure fetal well-being.

Section Four Review

1. Which of the following internal organs is compressed by the expanding uterus?
   A. heart
   B. bladder
   C. pancreas
   D. liver
2. After trauma, an increase in the maternal uterine fundal height is a result of which life-threatening complication?
   A. ruptured uterus
   B. placenta previa
   C. ruptured bowel
   D. placental abruption

3. After maternal trauma, a clear, watery, vaginal discharge is most likely a result of
   A. infection
   B. mucous plug
   C. ruptured amniotic sac
   D. semen

Answers: 1, B. 2, D. 3, C.

Section Five: Care of the Critically Ill Pregnant Woman Experiencing Preterm Labor

Following the completion of this module, the learner will be able to identify the risk factors associated with preterm labor/preterm delivery and state the signs and symptoms of preterm labor.

Preterm labor, uterine contractions accompanied by cervical change (effacement or dialation) that occur between 20 and 37 weeks gestation, is noted in 6 percent to 10 percent of all pregnancies. Certain women are more at risk than others. Table 22–12 lists

the major and minor risk factors associated with preterm birth.

Symptoms of preterm labor include uterine contractions (frequently painless) detected either by palpation of the abdomen or by the fetal monitor, menstrual-like cramps, backache, pelvic pressure, increased vaginal discharge, and blood-stained vaginal discharge. If the fetus were to be delivered prematurely, various complications result. Table 22–13 lists the complications of preterm infants.

Tocolytic therapy is the use of medications to halt preterm labor. Certain patients are not eligible for tocolytics. Table 22–14 shows the absolute and relative contraindications for tocolytic therapy. Tocolytic therapy revolves around the administration of medication and the insurance of maternal bedrest in the left lateral recumbent (LLR) position.

TABLE 22–12. RISK FACTORS FOR PRETERM LABOR

- **Major**
  Trauma in pregnancy, hypovolemia
  Multiple gestation
  DES exposure
  Uterine anomaly
  Cervix dialated > 1 cm at 32 weeks
  Second trimester abortion × 2
  Previous preterm delivery
  Previous preterm labor with term delivery
  Abdominal surgery during pregnancy
  History of cone biopsy
  Cervical shortening < 1 cm at 32 weeks
  Uterine irritability

- **Minor**
  Febrille illness
  Bleeding after 12 weeks
  History of pyelonephritis
  Cigarettes more than 10/day
  Second trimester abortion × 1
  More than two first trimester abortions

TABLE 22–13. COMPLICATIONS OF PRETERM INFANTS

Respiratory distress syndrome
Patent ductus arteriosus
Feeding difficulties
Thermoregulation
Infections
Seizures
Intraventricular hemorrhage
Long-term neurodevelopmental disorders
Chronic lung disease

TABLE 22–14. CONTRAINDICATIONS TO USE OF TOCOLYTICS

Absolute contraindications
  Severe PIH
  Severe abruptio placentae
  Severe bleeding from any cause
  Chorioamnionitis
  Fetal death
  Fetal anomaly incompatible with life
  Severe fetal growth retardation
Relative contraindications
  Mild chronic hypertension
  Mild abruptio placentae
  Stable placenta previa
  Maternal cardiac disease
  Hyperthyroidism
  Uncontrolled diabetes mellitus
  Fetal distress
  Fetal anomaly
  Mild fetal growth retardation
  Cervix more than 4–5 cm dialated

Tocolytics

Ritodrine HCl (Yutopar), Terbutaline Sulfate (Brethine)

Action. Sympathomimetic that stimulates beta$_2$-receptors. Stimulation of the beta$_2$-receptors inhibits the contractility of the uterine smooth muscle. This drug has cardiovascular and bronchial effects.

Mode of Administration

1. Ritodrine is administered by IV infusion. The initial dosage is 0.1 mg/min. The IV infusion is continued for at least 12 hours after uterine contractions have stopped. Oral ritodrine is initiated prior to stopping the IV infusion.
2. Refer to the drug insert for administration of terbutaline for the purpose of stopping uterine contractions.

Side Effects

1. a. Maternal. Tachycardia, hypotension, hypokalemia, palpitations, tremors, nausea, vomiting, headache, arrythmia, occasional nervousness, jittering, restlessness, emotional upset, anxiety, and malaise
   b. Fetal. Tachycardia
   c. Neonatal. Occasionally hypoglycemia, hypotension, ileus, CHF
2. Sometimes cardiac symptoms—chest pain, tightness, and arrythmia
3. Circulatory overload is a severe consequence often resulting in CHF, identified as being related to fluid balance
4. Transient elevations of blood glucose and insulin levels
5. Widening pulse pressure

Antidote. Propranolol HCl (Inderal)

Notes. Controlled diabetic patients need close monitoring for elevations in blood glucose levels, which usually necessitate an increase in the dose of exogenous insulin.

Any baby born to a mother who received tocolytics during pregnancy (e.g., from 34 weeks to term) needs to have blood glucose tested at 10 and 40 minutes after birth and should be observed closely for hypoglycemia due to possible transient elevations in maternal blood glucose levels.

Magnesium Sulfate (MgSO$_4$)

Action

1. Neuromuscular blocking agent
2. Anticonvulsant that prevents or controls convulsions by blocking neuromuscular transmission and decreases the amount of acetylcholine liberated by the motor nerve impulse, therefore acting as a CNS depressant
3. MgSO$_4$ is not an antihypertensive but may transiently decrease blood pressure, since it relaxes smooth muscle
4. Its tocolytic effect is mediated through enhancement of uterine blood flow, as well as its direct effect on myometrial contraction
5. Excretion of MgSO$_4$ is exclusively via the kidneys

Mode of Administration

For PIH and preterm labors, MgSO$_4$ 6 g of a 50 percent solution diluted in 50 mL or 100 mL D$_5$W as a loading dose given over 20 minutes, followed by a continuous infusion of MgSO$_4$ 1 to 2 gs/hour piggyback as a maintenance dosage (MgSO$_4$ 40 g in 1000 mL D$_5$LR). MgSO$_4$ must be administered via an infusion pump. The maintenance dosage depends on serum Mg levels or evaluation of deep tendon reflexes (DTRs) and respiration rates. Normal blood values (patient not on MgSO$_4$ therapy) 1.8 to 3.0 mg/dL. Therapeutic Mg values (for PIH therapeutic range): 4.0 to 7.5 mg/dL. Critical level: Patellar reflex is lost; 9.0 to 11.0 mg/dL; 15 to 20 mg/dL, respiratory and cardiac arrest. Levels are assessed more accurately by clinical appearance. Calculations (for IV pump, based on the concentration of MgSO$_4$ 40 gs in 1000 mL D$_5$LR): 1 g = 25 mL; 1 g/hour = 25 mL/hour; 2 g = 50 mL/hour.

Side Effects

1. Maternal. Feelings of drowsiness, flushing, sweating, depressed or no reflexes, oliguria, respiratory paralysis, circulatory collapse,

respiratory/cardiac arrest. Signs mother may experience
Within normal limits
Hot all over
Flushing
Thirsty
Sweating
Abnormal—require further evaluation
Depression of reflexes
Hypotension
Flaccidity
2. Fetal. Fetal monitoring tracing may exhibit decreased variability
3. Neonate. Hypotonia and respiratory depression due to MgSO₄ toxicity

Antidote. Calcium gluconate. If respiratory depression occurs (respirations less than 12 breaths/ minute), Ca gluconate can be given (1 g, which is 10 mL of a 10 percent solution) IV over 3 minutes.

Notes. Contraindications are

■ Renal failure
■ Absence of DTRs

Late signs of hympermagnesemia are

■ CNS depression: lethargy, stupor, coma
■ Respiratory paralysis; respiratory arrest
■ Circulatory collapse

CNS depression is at first characterized by anxiety. This changes to drowsiness, lethargy, slight slurring of speech, staric gait, and a tendency to fall sideward while standing erect. The nurse should constantly evaluate the patient's orientation to person, place and time.

The probability of the delivery of a preterm infant can be very frightening. The nurse caring for the critically ill pregnant woman may not be accustomed to therapies used for preterm labor. Consultation with a perinatal nurse may establish a team that decreases anxiety, maintains good communication, and provides excellent care for both mother and fetus.

Section Five Review

1. Which of the following is a major risk factor for preterm labor?
   A. previous preterm delivery
   B. bleeding after 12 weeks gestation
   C. febrile illness
   D. >2 first trimester abortions
2. Which of the following is NOT a maternal side effect of sympathomimetic tocolytics?
   A. tachycardia
   B. widening pulse pressure
   C. chest pain
   D. depressed reflexes

3. What would be considered a critical magnesium level?
   A. 4.0–7.5 mg/dL
   B. 9.0–11.0 mg/dL
   C. 1.8–3.0 mg/dL
   D. 7.5–8.0 mg/dL

Answers: 1, A. 2, D. 3, B.

Section Six: Care of the Patient with Hypertensive Disorders of Pregnancy

Following the completion of this section, the learner will be able to define severe pregnancy-induced hypertension and HELLP syndrome.

Hypertension during pregnancy complicates 7 percent to 10 percent of all pregnancies. Apart from being the most common medical complication of pregnancy, hypertension is one of the major causes of maternal and perinatal morbidity and mortality in the United States. The two most common forms of hypertension are pregnancy-induced hypertensive disease (PIH), a disorder that appears during preg-nancy and is reversed by delivery, and preexisting chronic hypertension. The latter is unrelated to but coincides with pregnancy and may be detected for the first time in pregnancy. It is not reversed by delivery (Sibai, 1991).

Hypertension in pregnancy can lead to multisystem damage and failure, with pathologic changes noted in the brain, kidney, liver, and cardiovascular system, as well as altered uteroplacental perfusion. Sequelae, such as liver rupture, cerebral edema, amniotic fluid embolism, and disseminated intravascular coagulopathy (DIC) have been described. Perinatal events associated with PIH include placental abruption, hemorrhage, stillbirth, and intrauterine growth retardation (IUGR) (Creasy and Resnick, 1989). HELLP syndrome is a life-threatening complication of PIH and is diagnosed by hemolysis, elevated liver enzymes, and low platelets (Shannon, 1987).

Sibai (1991) lists the terminology of the five classifications of hypertension in pregnancy.

1. Gestational hypertension is defined as hypertension appearing in the second half of pregnancy or in the first 24 hours postpartum, without edema or proteinuria and with a return to normotension within 10 days after delivery. This group constitutes the majority of patients with PIH.
2. Preeclampsia is defined as hypertension (blood pressure of 140/90 mm Hg or greater, a systolic increase of 30 mm Hg or a diastolic increase of 15 mm Hg over baseline values occurring at two readings taken 6 or more hours apart) together with edema or proteinuria. It should be noted, however, that not all three symptoms may be clinically evident.
3. Eclampsia is defined as the development of convulsions or coma in patients with signs and symptoms of preeclampsia in the absence of other causes of convulsions.
4. Chronic hypertensive disease is defined as chronic hypertension of any cause. This group includes patients with preexisting hypertension, patients with persistent elevation of blood pressure to at least 140/90 mm Hg on two occasions before 20 weeks gestation, and patients with hypertension that persists for more than 6 weeks postpartum.
5. Superimposed preeclampsia or eclampsia is defined as the development of either preeclampsia or eclampsia in patients with diagnosed chronic hypertension.

Tables 22–15 and 22–16 indicate the predisposing factors and warning signs of preeclampsia. Preeclampsia usually is characterized as either mild or severe. Table 22–17 outlines clinical signs that necessitate immediate attention. Tables 22–18 and 22–19

TABLE 22–16. WARNING SIGNS OF PREECLAMPSIA

Sudden development of hypertension 30/15 mm Hg rise over baseline; for example, a woman whose blood pressure at her first prenatal visit was 90/60 mm Hg and now is 120/80 mm Hg

Sudden excessive weight gain, which is due to an accumulation of water in the tissues

Protein in the urine (trace to +1 dipstick on two specimens at least 6 hours apart); this sign usually develops late in pregnancy and is always an ominous sign. Normal urine protein in pregnancy is negative to trace by urine dipstick

Hyperreflexia

outline the characteristics of mild and severe PIH (SPIH).

SPIH represents a multisystem disease characterized by systemic vasospasm and arteriolar vasoconstriction. These pathologic changes lead to damage of the microcirculation, arterial hypertension, and increased systemic vascular resistance (SVR) (Koniak-Griffin and Dodgson, 1987). Figure 22–1 diagrams the pathologic alterations occurring in SPIH.

The cure for SPIH is delivery of the fetus, but until the embedded villi are completely sloughed off with the first menstrual period postpartum (which usually occurs at 6 weeks postpartum), some patients may still exhibit signs and symptoms of SPIH. Although with most patients, the symptoms of SPIH usually revolve within 48 hours, the hematopoietic and hepatic complications of HELLP syndrome may persist for several more days. These findings are often mistaken for symptoms of other conditions, such as DIC.

The immediate postpartum period is considered critical in terms of management. Marked shifts in intravascular and extravascular volume lead to changes in fluid and electrolyte balance. These adaptations may be influenced by compromised renal functioning and bleeding. Convulsions occur in about one third of the patients during the first 24 hours after delivery because of vasoconstriction and cerebral ischemia (Koniak-Griffin and Dodgson, 1987).

The aims of postpartum care are to reverse or reduce the hypertensive process, to prevent life-threatening complications of the disease, such as

TABLE 22–15. PREDISPOSING FACTORS FOR DEVELOPMENT OF PREECLAMPSIA

Multiple gestation
Nulliparity
Previous history of preeclampsia/eclampsia
Family history of preeclampsia/eclampsia
Hydatidiform mole
Preexisting hypertension or renal disease
Poor (or no) prenatal care

TABLE 22–17. CLINICAL SIGNS THAT NECESSITATE IMMEDIATE ATTENTION

Severe, continuous headache, often frontal or occipital
Swelling of the hands, feet, or face
Dimness or blurring of vision
Persistent vomiting
Decrease in amount of urine excreted
Epigastric pain (a late sign)

TABLE 22–18. CHARACTERISTICS OF MILD PIH

Parameter	Value
Blood pressure	> 140/90 mm Hg
Systolic increase	30 mm Hg over baseline
Diastolic increase	15 mm Hg over baseline
Proteinuria	> 1+ or > 300 mg/24 hours
Nondependent edema	Weight gain > 5 pounds in 1 week or 1+ pitting edema after 12 hours of bedrest

TABLE 22–19. CHARACTERISTICS OF SEVERE PIH

Parameter	Value
Blood pressure	160/110 on two occasions at least 6 hours apart
Proteinuria	3+ or 4+ on semiquantitative assay or > 500 mg/24 hours
Oliguria	< 400 mL/24 hours or < 30 mL/hour for 3 hours
Cerebral edema	Visual disturbances, such as altered consciousness, headache, scotoma, or blurred vision
Epigastric or right upper quadrant pain	
Elevated liver function tests	
Pulmonary edema or cyanosis	
Thrombocytopenia	
IUGR	

convulsions and cerebrovascular accidents, and to prevent ischemia to vital organs.

SPIH may be complicated even further with a syndrome of coagulopathies and hepatic failure. HELLP syndrome is potentially fatal. The clinical findings may appear as thrombocytopenia, changes in liver enzymes and hyperbilirubinemia, which is a reflection of red blood cell destruction (Whittaker et al, 1986).

Vasospasm is considered the underlying factor in the development of microangiopathic hemolytic

anemia seen in the HELLP syndrome. As a result of vasospasms, lesions develop in the endothelial layer of the small blood vessels. Platelets aggregate at the site of the lesion, and a fibrin network is established. Red blood cells are forced through the sievelike struc-

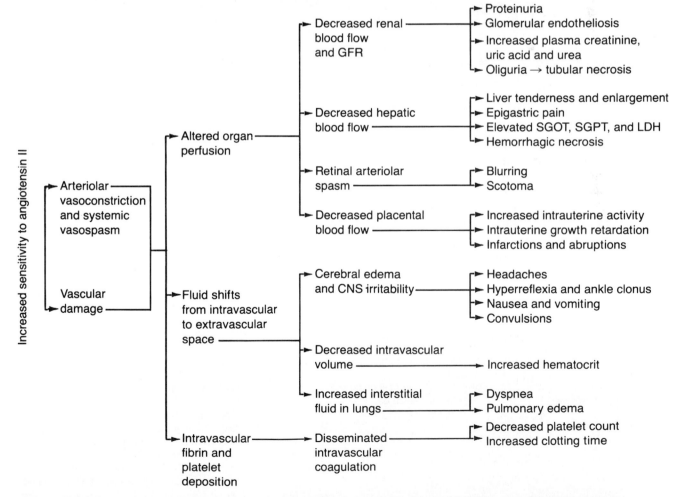

Figure 22–1. Pathophysiologic alterations occurring in SPIH. GRF, glomerular filtration rate; SGOT, serum glutamic-oxaloacetic transaminase; SGPT, serum glutamic-pyruvic transaminase; LDH, lactate dehydrogenase. (*From Severe pregnancy-induced hypertension: Postpartum care of the critically ill patient*, by D. Koniak-Griffin and J. Dodgson, 1987. Heart Lung. 16:661–669.)

ture under high pressure, and many are lysed. As hemolysis continues, the hematocrit level falls. Hyperbilirubinemia occurs as a result. Thrombocytopenia is seen as platelets are consumed in the microcirculation. Transfused platelets may continue to be consumed rapidly in the microvasculature until vasospasm is controlled (Whittaker et al, 1986).

Shannon (1987) outlined the nursing interventions for the care of the SPIH and HELLP syndrome patient (Table 22–20).

TABLE 22–20. NURSING CARE PLAN FOR THE PATIENT WITH PREGNANCY-INDUCED HYPERTENSION AND HELLP SYNDROME

Problem	Goal	Intervention
Alteration in vascular integrity	Blood pressure will remain ≤140/90 Systolic pressure will not increase >30 mm Hg and diastolic pressure will not increase >15 mm Hg over baseline	1. Observe blood pressure every 1 minute 2. Assess and report complaints of headache, visual disturbances, behavior changes, nausea/vomiting, and epigastric pain 3. Strict bedrest in left lateral position 4. Administer antihypertensive medications as ordered. Assess blood pressure every 5 minutes until stable, then every 15–30 minutes after administration of antihypertensive medication. Note adverse reactions and effectiveness of medication
Alteration in health maintenance secondary to impaired renal function	Prevention of permanent renal compromise	1. Test midstream or Foley catheter specimen of urine for protein. Vaginal discharge, blood, or amniotic fluid may cause proteinuria. Proteinuria is defined as the presence of 2+ protein or greater in urine by dipstick or by 0.3 g/L or greater in a 24-hour urine collection 2. Measure hourly intake and output 3. Check specific gravity 4. Maintain bedrest in left lateral position

Fluid volume deficit secondary to vasospasm and extravascular displacement of plasma volume	Maintenance of adequate fluid volume as evident by hemodynamic monitoring and clinical evaluation	1. Assess extent of edema.
		  +1—slight edema of pedal and pretibial areas
		  +2—marked edema of lower extremities
		  +3—edema of hands, face, lower abdominal wall, and sacrum
		  +4—anasarca with ascites
		2. Maintain strict bedrest in left lateral position
		3. Remove all constrictive clothing and jewelry
		4. Monitor hemodynamics with Swan-Ganz catheter and/or central venous pressure line
		  Normal values:
		  Right atrial pressure: 5–15 mm Hg
		  Pulmonary artery pressures (PAP)
		    Systolic: 15–30 mm Hg
		    Diastolic: 5–15 mm Hg
		    Wedge: 8–12 mm Hg
		5. Assess need tor fluid replacement by specific gravity, hematocrit, pulmonary artery pressures, intake and output measurements, and decreasing central venous pressure values
		6. Assess breath sounds and respiratory status every 4 hours and as necessary for signs of pulmonary edema

Alteration in neuromuscular irritability
Potential for injury secondary to eclamptic seizures
	Prevention of eclamptic seizures
	Prevention of injury secondary to eclamptic seizures
		1. Assess deep tendon reflexes (DTR)
		  0—No response
		  +1—Diminished response
		  +2—Normal
		  +3—More brisk than normal
		  +4—Very brisk; clonus present
		2. Decrease sensory stimulation: dim lights, ensure quiet atmosphere, and restrict visitation
		3. Administer magnesium sulfate as ordered. Instruct patient about possible side effects, such as nausea/vomiting and feelings of warmth
		4. Insert Foley catheter. Monitor hourly urine output. Magnesium sulfate is excreted via the kidneys

TABLE 22–20. NURSING CARE PLAN FOR THE PATIENT WITH PREGNANCY-INDUCED HYPERTENSION AND HELLP SYNDROME (*Continued*)

Problem	Goal	Intervention
		5. Monitor cardiac and respiratory functions. Be especially aware of rate and depth of respirations
		6. Check serum magnesium level 6–8 mg/100 mL: therapeutic level 10 mg/100 mL: pateller reflexes disappear 15 mg/100 mL: respiratory depression
		7. Keep calcium gluconate at the bedside for emergency use. Calcium gluconate reverses respiratory depression caused by magnesium sulfate
		8. Keep airway at bedside
		9. Maintain strict bedrest. Pad siderails of bed
Alteration in health maintenance secondary to impaired liver function	Prevention of permanent liver compromise	1. Check serial measurements of alkaline phosphatase, SGOT, SGPT, prothrombin time, and bilirubin 2. Assess and report symptoms of malaise, anorexia, nausea, vomiting, right upper quadrant or epigastric pain, hypoglycemia, and jaundice 3. Be alert for signs and symptoms of hepatic rupture: shock, oliguria, fever, and leukocytosis 4. Keep dextrose 50% at bedside 5. Avoid administration of sedatives
Alteration in hemostasis (hemolysis and thrombocytopenia)	Maintain hemostasis	1. Assess clinical manifestations of bleeding: petechiae, easy bruising, epistaxis, gingival bleeding, hematuria, gastrointestinal bleeding, hemorrhages in conjunctiva and retina, and intracranial bleeding 2. Check laboratory test values: hemoglobin, hematocrit, platelets, and coagulation factors 3. Treat all fevers because fever reduces platelet survival. Acetaminophen does not impair platelet function 4. Avoid thromboytopenic medications, such as aspirin and hydralazine 5. Treat infections, since infection reduces platelet lifespan. Report all signs and symptoms of infection 6. Administer postpartum oxytocin as ordered, which ensures uterine contraction to provide hemostasis 7. Avoid trauma. Bleeding increases platelet consumption 8. Closely monitor lochia. Be alert for postpartum hemorrhage 9. Closely monitor lacerations and episiotomy site 10. Replace blood products and coagulation factors as ordered
Potential for alterations in fetal well-being secondary to vasospasm and decreased placental perfusion Potential for alterations in fetal well-being secondary to abruptio placentae	Prevention of fetal compromise	1. Maintain bedrest in left lateral position 2. Be alert for meconium staining 3. Assess for vaginal bleeding, uterine tenderness, sustained abdominal pain, tetanic contractions, and increasing fundal height 4. Be aware of serial fetal status studies: nonstress test, oxytocin challenge, and biophysical profile 5. Continue electronic fetal monitoring during labor and delivery. Be alert for changes in heart rate baseline, variability, and deceleration patterns
Anxiety	Patient's anxiety will be minimized	1. Encourage patient to verbalize anxiety, fear, and concerns 2. Establish trusting relationship 3. Explain all procedures and equipment 4. Note coping mechanisms 5. Assess support system 6. Encourage participation of support system 7. Offer diversion as appropriate 8. Avoid sleep deprivation by maintaining environment conducive to rest 9. Schedule meeting for family and patient with obstetricians, neonatologists, nurses, and social workers

From Shannon, D. (1987). HELLP syndrome: A severe consequence of PIH. *J. Obstet. Gynecol. Neonatal Nursing.* 16:395–402.

Eclampsia differs from the previous conditions due to the presence of seizures. It is a very frightening and life-threatening condition. Nursing management should center around the following interventions (Sibai, 1991).

1. Prevent the patient from injury (this is the most important nursing intervention).
2. Do not stop the convulsion. It will stop on its own.
3. Ensure adequate maternal oxygenation.
4. Minimize aspiration.
5. Ensure adequate infusion of $MgSO_4$ to prevent future convulsions (6 g load/IV followed by a maintenance of 2 g/hour as per M.D. order).
6. Obtain arterial blood gases and correct acidemia.

7. FHR will demonstrate signs of decreased variability and possible decelerations. Although not healthy for the fetus, it is to be expected. The obstetrician needs to be notified immediately. Maternal stability is paramount and needs to be ensured before cesarean section.

Hypertension is diagnosed in a wide spectrum of patients, from those who have minimal elevation in blood pressure only to those who experience severe hypertension with multiple organ dysfunction. The manifestations in these patients are clinically similar, but they result from several different pathologic processes with many different underlying causes (Sibai, 1991).

Section Six Review

1. All of the following are predisposing factors for the development of PIH EXCEPT
   A. multiple gestation
   B. nulliparity
   C. no prenatal care
   D. preterm labor
2. Headache, hyperreflexia, clonus, convulsions, nausea, and vomiting are the symptoms of what pathophysiologic alteration of SPIH?
   A. cerebral edema
   B. DIC
   C. decreased hepatic blood flow
   D. decreased intravascular volume

3. What is the most important nursing intervention that can be provided for the eclampic patient during a convulsion?
   A. attain the FHR
   B. prevent the patient from injury
   C. IV push $MgSO_4$
   D. IV push diazepam (Valium)

Answers: 1, D. 2, A. 3, B.

Section Seven: Care of the Critically III Patient Requiring Fetal Monitoring

Following the completion of this section, the learner will be familiar with application of the fetal monitor and identify an abnormal fetal heart rate (FHR).

The fetus is a patient. Any pregnant woman needs to have her fetus assessed. Continuous fetal monitoring is necessary for a woman of 25 weeks gestation or greater (the fetus is considered viable at this time, but this can differ from state to state). Be-

fore 25 weeks, intermittent auscultation can be performed as ordered by the obstetrician. Keep in mind that whatever alteration the mother is having, the fetus will be affected. This section focuses on the fundamentals of external fetal monitoring, application of the monitor, and basic evaluation of FHR patterns. Application of internal monitoring and the process of obtaining fetal scalp pH are not discussed. If internal monitoring is to be used, an obstetric nurse should be consulted. The fetal monitor also detects uterine contractions. Section Five examines

TABLE 22-21. APPLICATION OF THE FETAL MONITOR

Equipment Needed	Preparation of Equipment	Nursing Interventions
Fetal monitor Monitor paper Ultrasound transducer Tocodynamometer 2 monitor straps or tummy grip Conductive jelly	Plug fetal monitor into wall outlet Plug ultrasound transducer into outlet on front of monitor Plug tocodynamometer into outlet in front of monitor Turn monitor on and press record button	Explain importance of fetal monitoring to patient Elevate head of bed 15–30° if possible Establish left uterine displacement by placing a wedge under the patient's right hip Apply conductive jelly to ultrasound transducer and place transducer on abdomen; move transducer around until a strong FHR is heard and is recording on the monitor strip Maintain ultrasound in place by straps or cover with tummy grip Locate the fundus of the uterus (the top of the uterus) Place the TOCO on that portion and secure with straps or cover with tummy grip Zero the TOCO for patient by pressing the zero button (varies depending on type of machine) Adjust sound as desired Record on the monitor strip patient's name, hospital number, age, gravity, parity, date, time, and RN signature; this is a legal document and part of the medical records

the care of the critically ill pregnant woman in pre-term labor.

Table 22–21 describes proper application of the fetal monitor. Refer to the glossary for definition of terms.

The nurse assessing the FHR needs to be familiar with certain parameters and recognize possible pathologies when interpreting fetal monitor strips. Various alterations in the FHR can occur. Knowing the language of FHR monitoring will ease communication among intensive care nurses, obstetric nurses, and the obstetrician.

The FHR has variability, or fluctuations, after the 28th week of gestation when the fetal brainstem function has matured (if the fetus has normal neurologic functioning). Fluctuations from the baseline FHR (beat to beat or long-term variability) can range between 6 and 25 bpm. The FHR may fall below the baseline in response to uterine contractions. This is referred to as FHR decelerations. Table 22–22 illustrates the range of various FHR, and Table 22–23 illustrates various patterns of FHR as well as their possible pathologies.

TABLE 22-22. VARIOUS RANGES OF FETAL HEART RATES

FHR Name	Range
Normal FHR	120–160 bpm
Mild bradycardia	100–119 bpm
Marked bradycardia	99 bpm (or less)
Mild tachycardia	161–180 bpm
Marked tachycardia	180 bpm (or greater)

Figure 22–2 demonstrates FHR accelerations. In this figure, the baseline FHR is 140 to 155 bpm, with accelerations to 160 to 170 bpm at the acme of the contraction. This tracing is termed reactive and is very reassuring.

Figure 22–3 illustrates early FHR decelerations. In this figure, the baseline FHR is 125 to 130 bpm. The deceleration starts early in the contraction and fully recovers after the contraction ends (it mirrors the contraction).

Figure 22–4 illustrates variable FHR decelerations. The baseline FHR is 140 to 150 bpm. The deceleration starts as the contraction approaches the acme and is fully recovered to baseline after the contraction is over.

Figure 22–5 illustrates late FHR decelerations. The baseline FHR is 150 to 160 bpm. The deceleration starts at the acme of the contraction and slowly returns to baseline.

Figure 22–6 illustrates decreased FHR baseline variability. The baseline FHR is 140 to 145 bpm. Minimal to no decelerations or accelerations are noted.

Various alterations may occur with the FHR. Knowing the language of FHR monitoring will ease communication among health care providers.

One of the most perplexing problems the critical care nurse encounters when caring for a pregnant patient is providing adequate care for her unborn child. Both mother and fetus are patients, and what affects the mother usually will affect the fetus also. The key in the care of the critically ill pregnant woman is to develop and sustain close communication with the perinatal nurses and obstetricians.

TABLE 22–23. FHR PATTERNS, PATHOLOGIES, AND NURSING INTERVENTIONS

Pattern	Pathology	Nursing Interventions
FHR accelerations above baseline in response to fetal movement	No pathology Referred to as restrictive pattern Indicates fetal well-being	Continue with present plan of care
Lack of FHR variability	Fetal sleep state Fetal distress	Place woman in left lateral recumbant (LLR) position Apply oxygen via face mask or nasal canula at 8 L/minute Increase IV fluids Continue to observe and notify obstetrician if condition persists
Early FHR deceleration	Occurs early in the contraction, usually in the later stages of labor in response to pressure on the fetal skull as it decends into the vaginal canal Usually transient and not necessarily a response to fetal distress	Obstetrician or perinatal nurse should be notified to perform vaginal examination to evaluate fetal station and cervical dilation Delivery of fetus may be imminent, and nurse should prepare for possible delivery Observe FHR pattern for worsening decelerations Apply oxygen at 8 L/minute via face mask or nasal cannula
Variable FHR deceleration	Occurring any time during a contraction Usually associated with unbilical cord compression in uterus	Turn the mother from her back to LLR or from side to side to relieve umbilical cord compression Apply oxygen at 8 L/minute via face mask or nasal cannula Obstetrician should be notified of FHR pattern, especially if decleration is not relieved
Late FHR deceleration	Ocurs late in the contraction after the acme Sometimes decelerations linger after the contraction is over Sign of uteroplacental insufficiency Very ominous sign Can proceed to bradycardia and fetal death Associated with neonatal cerebral palsy if allowed to continue	Notify obstetrician stat. Apply oxygen at 8 L/minute via face mask or nasal cannula Position mother in LLR Increase IV fluids Halt uterine contractions If repetitious, prepare for emergency cesarean delivery

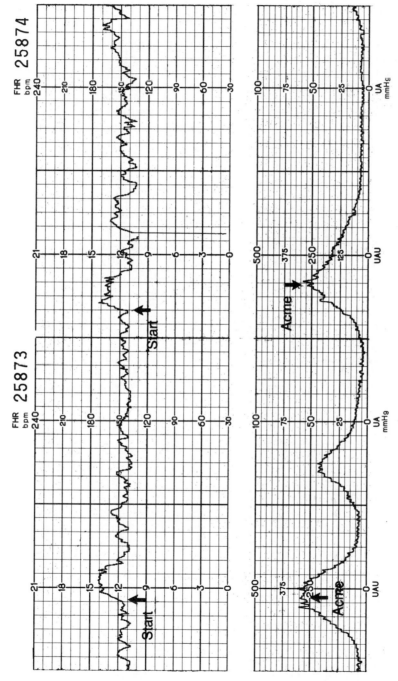

Figure 22–2. FHR accelerations. The baseline FHR is 140 to 155 bpm, with accelerations to 160 to 170 bpm at the acme of the contraction. This tracing is termed reactive and is very reassuring.

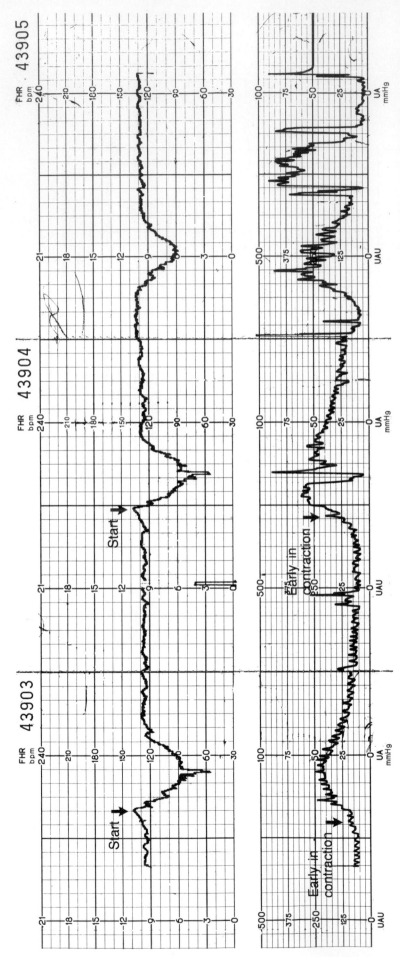

Figure 22–3. Early FHR decelerations. The baseline FHR is 125 to 130 bpm. The deceleration starts early in the contraction and fully recovers after the contraction ends (it mirrors the contraction).

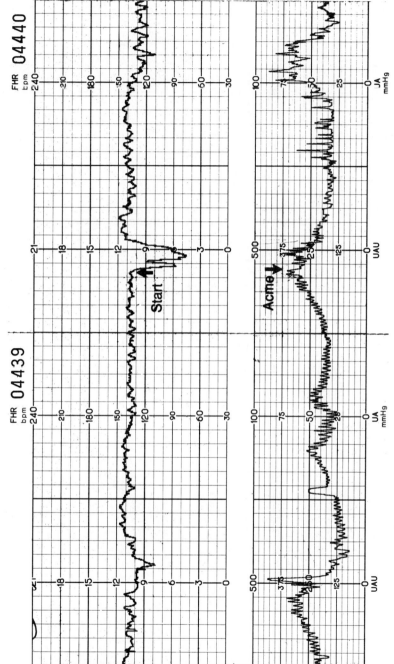

Figure 22–4. Variable FHR decelerations. The baseline FHR is 140 to 150 bpm. The deceleration starts as the contraction approaches the acme and is fully recovered to baseline after the contraction is over.

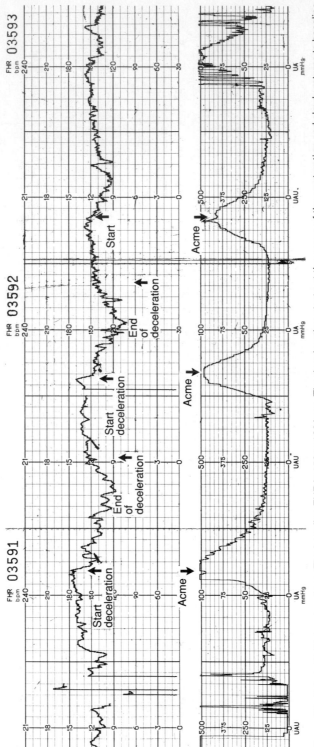

Figure 22–5. Late FHR decelerations. The baseline FHR is 150 to 160 bpm. The deceleration starts at the acme of the contraction and slowly returns to baseline.

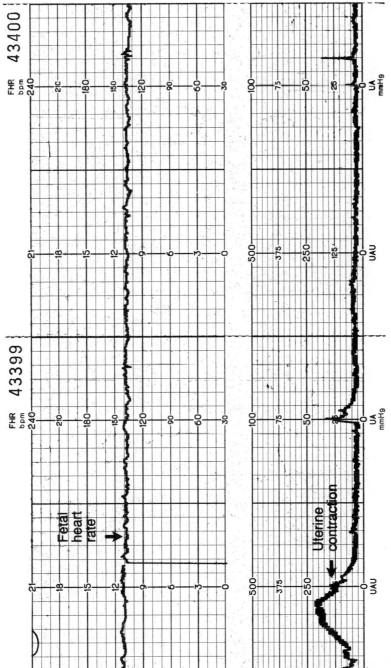

Figure 22–6. Decreased FHR baseline variability. The baseline FHR is 140 to 145 bpm. Minimal to no decelerations or accelerations are noted.

Section Seven Review

1. At what gestational age does the pregnant woman require continuous fetal monitoring during times of maternal stress?
   A. 16–20 weeks
   B. 20–25 weeks
   C. >25 weeks
   D. all of the above
2. What is a normal FHR?
   A. 100–120 bpm
   B. 120–160 bpm
   C. 160–180 bpm
   D. 180–200 bpm

3. What is considered a bradycardic FHR?
   A. 60–90 bpm
   B. 120–160 bpm
   C. 140–160 bpm
   D. 150–180 bpm
4. What is considered a tachycardic FHR?
   A. 60–90 bpm
   B. 90–120 bpm
   C. 120–150 bpm
   D. 180–200 bpm

Answers: 1, C. 2, B. 3, A. 4, D.

Posttest

1. A pH of _____ would be considered acidotic in a pregnant woman.
   A. 7.35
   B. 7.40
   C. 7.45
   D. 7.50
2. The largest increase in cardiac output occurs during which stage of labor?
   A. first
   B. second
   C. third
   D. 5 minutes postpartum
3. The most common form of shock seen in the obstetric patient is
   A. hemorrhagic
   B. cardiogenic
   C. neurogenic
   D. septic
4. Indications for the use of hemodynamic monitoring in the pregnant woman are all of the following EXCEPT
   A. hypovolemic shock unresponsive to fluid therapy
   B. advanced preterm labor resulting in the delivery of a preterm infant
   C. severe pregnancy-induced hypertension
   D. cardiac disease class 3 or 4
5. A pregnant woman with upper abdominal trauma could have damage to the following organs EXCEPT
   A. small intestine
   B. large intestine
   C. bladder
   D. uterus

6. Severe pregnancy-induced hypertension (SPIH) is defined as a combination of the following EXCEPT
   A. macrosomia of the developing fetus
   B. blood pressure > or = 160/110
   C. hypertension with visual disturbances
   D. hypertension with oliguria
7. Plasma volume in the pregnant patient at term has increased _____ percent over nonpregnant levels.
   A. 100
   B. 20
   C. 45–50
   D. 65
8. Which of the following is an absolute contra-indication for the use of tocolytics?
   A. cervical dilation of 5 cm
   B. uncontrolled diabetes mellitus
   C. mild abruptio placentae
   D. SPIH
9. HELLP syndrome commonly may be confused with
   A. chronic hypertension
   B. DIC
   C. hypovolemic shock
   D. sepsis
10. Continuous fetal monitoring in critically ill pregnant patients should be performed after _____ weeks gestation.
    A. 16
    B. 20
    C. 25
    D. 32

11. Mild tachycardia in the fetus is between
   A. 70 and 90 bpm
   B. 90 and 120 bpm
   C. 120 and 160 bpm
   D. 160 and 180 bpm
12. Which type of FHR deceleration is most ominous and indicates placental insufficiency?
   A. early
   B. late
   C. variable
   D. all the above
13. Approximately one third of SPIH patients experience convulsions
   A. before labor
   B. during labor
   C. at delivery
   D. during the first 24 hours after delivery
14. Eclampsia is defined as
   A. HELLP syndrome
   B. preeclampsia with convulsions or coma
   C. preeclampsia with a severe headache
   D. always fatal
15. What is the most important nursing intervention provided for the patient during an eclamptic seizure?
   A. stop the seizure with diazepam (Valium)
   B. obtain FHR immediately
   C. obtain arterial blood gases
   D. keep the patient from injury

16. Cardiovascular changes that occur during pregnancy include
   A. myocardial hypertrophy
   B. flattened T waves in lead 3
   C. PMI located higher
   D. all the above
17. The neonate of a diabetic mother is at highest risk for hypoglycemia
   A. at 25–28 weeks
   B. at 30–32 weeks
   C. at 34–40 weeks
   D. when the umbilical cord is cut
18. _____ is seen more frequently in pregnant diabetics, even when there is no evidence of pre-existing vascular disease.
   A. renal disease
   B. pregnancy-induced hypertension
   C. retinopathy
   D. intrauterine growth retardation
19. The pregnant trauma patient in preterm labor might exhibit
   A. constant backache
   B. pelvic pressure
   C. increased vaginal discharge
   D. all the above
20. The antidote given to a pregnant patient exhibiting side effects from Ritodrine (Yutopar) is
   A. calcium gluconate
   B. digoxin
   C. propranolol
   D. diazepam

Posttest Answers

Question	Answer	Section	Question	Answer	Section
1	A	One	11	D	Seven
2	D	Two	12	B	Seven
3	A	Two	13	D	Six
4	B	Two	14	B	Six
5	C	Four	15	D	Six
6	A	Six	16	D	Two
7	C	Two	17	D	Three
8	D	Five	18	B	Three
9	B	Six	19	D	Five
10	C	Seven	20	C	Five

REFERENCES

Beard, R.W., Turner, R.C., and Oakely, N.W. (1971). Fetal response to glucose loading. *Postgrad. Med.* 47:68.

Benedetti, T. (1986). Obstetric hemorrhage. In F. Grabbe, J. Niebyl, and J.L. Simpson (eds). *Obstetrics: Normal and problem pregnancies*, Chap. 16. New York: Churchill-Livingstone.

Bobak, I.M., Jensen, M.D., and Zalar, M.K. (1989). *Maternity and gynecologic care—The nurse and the family.* St. Louis: C.V. Mosby.

Bremer, C., and Cassata, L. (1986). Trauma in pregnancy. *Nursing Clin. North Am.* 21:705.

Campbell, I. (1989). Second and third stages of labor. In I.M. Bobak, M.D. Jensen, and M.R. Zalar (eds). *Maternity and gynecologic care: The nurse and the family,* Chap. 19. St. Louis: C.V. Mosby.

Clark, S. (1987). Amniotic fluid embolus. In S. Clark, Phelan, and D. Cotton (eds). *Critical care obstetrics.* Montvale, New Jersey: Medical Economics.

Cohen, A.W., Liston, R.M., Mennuti, M.T., and Gabbe, S.G. (1982). Glucemic control in pregnant diabetic women using a continuous subcutaneous insulin infusion pump. *J. Reprod. Med.* 27:6.

Cotton, D. (1987). Cardiovascular alterations in severe PIH. *Critical care obstetrics.* Lake Buena Vista, Florida: Society of Perinatal Obstetricians Annual Meeting.

Creasy, R., and Resnick, R. (1989). *Maternal-fetal medicine: Principles and practice.* Philadelphia: W.B. Saunders Co.

Dunn, P. (1990). Assessing a pregnant woman after trauma. *Nursing '90.* 20:53–57.

Easterling, T., and Benedetti, T. (1989). Preeclampsia: A hyperdynamic disease model. *Am. J. Obstet. Gynecol.* 160:1447–1453.

Fuhrmann, K., Reiher, H., Semmler, K., Fisher, F., and Fisher, M. (1983). Prevention of congenital malformations in infants of insulin-dependent diabetic mothers. *Diabetic Care.* 6:121–123.

Gabbe, S.G. (1986). Definition, detection and management of gestional diabetes. *Obstet. Gynecol.* 67:121–125.

Gonik, B. (1987). Intensive care monitoring of the critically ill pregnant patient. In *Maternal fetal medicine,* Chap. 43.

Koniak-Griffin, D., and Dodgson, J. (1987). Severe pregnancy-induced hypertension: Postpartum care of the critically ill patient. *Heart Lung.* 16:661–669.

Lee, W., and Cotton, D. (1987). Cardiorespiratory changes in pregnancy. In B. Gonik (ed). *Critical care obstetrics,* Chap. 4. Montvale, New Jersey: Medical Economics.

Longo, L., and Hardsky, J. (1984). Maternal blood volume: Measurement, hypothesis of control and clinical considerations. *Rev. Perinatal Med.* 5:35.

McDonnall, A.K., Landon, M., and Gabbe, S. (1986). Diabetes in pregnancy. In B. Wesley and S. Hutchinson (eds). *OB care: Advanced obstetrical regional education.* Camden, New Jersey: Perinatal Cooperative.

Odds, S.B., London, M.L., and Ladewig, P.A. (1988). *Maternal newborn nursing—A family centered approach,* 3rd ed. Redwood City, California: Addison-Wesley.

Reeder, S., and Martin, L. (1987). *Maternity nursing family.* Philadelphia: J.B. Lippincott.

Resnik, R., Swartz, W., Plummer, M., et al. (1976). Amniotic fluid embolism with survival. *Obstet. Gynecol.* 47: 295.

Shannon, D. (1987). HELLP syndrome: A severe consequence of PIH. *J. Obstet. Gynecol. Neonatal Nursing.* 16:395–402.

Sherwen, L., Scoloveno, M., and Weingarten, C. (1991). *Nursing care of the childbearing family.* Norwalk, Connecticut: Appleton & Lange.

Sibai, B. (1991). Lecture given at Pennsylvania Perinatal Association October 8, 1991. Harrisburg.

Whittaker, A., Hull, B., and Clochesy, J. (1986). Hemolysis, elevated liver enzymes, and low platelet count syndrome: Nursing care of the critically ill obstetric patient. *Heart Lung.* 15:402–410.

Zolli, A., and Neville, W. (1985). Chest trauma in pregnancy. In *Trauma and pregnancy,* Chap. 11. Littleton, Massachusetts: PSG Publishing Company.

Module **23**

Nursing Care of the Acutely Ill Pediatric Patient

Paula Vernon-Levett

The self-study module, *Nursing Care of the Acutely Ill Pediatric Patient*, is written at the core knowledge level for the novice nurse who is caring for acutely ill patients. This module is designed to apply and supplement pathophysiologic concepts already discussed in previous modules in relation to the pediatric patient. The focus of the module is on maturational aspects of the child's anatomy and physiology that not only predispose them to certain pathophysiologic disorders but are responsible for the way children respond to illness. The module is composed of six parts, with related sections under each part. In the first part, Sections One through Four discuss four topics related to ventilation: maturational anatomy and physiology, etiology of acute respiratory failure, assessment of respiratory function, and nursing management. The second and third parts cover perfusion and cognition/perception, respectively. They also each contain four related sections covering the same topics as in Sections One through Four. In the next part, there are three sections that highlight maturational aspects and nursing management of fluid and electrolyte homeostasis, of nutrition, and of thermoregulation. The two sections in the fifth part discuss topics related to immunocompetence: risk factors in the critically ill pediatric patient and nursing management to support the immunocompromised patient. The last part has two sections. The first discusses the impact of hospitalization on the acutely ill child, and the last section discusses nursing management to minimize the stress of hospitalization. Each part includes a set of review questions to help the learner evaluate understanding of section content before moving on to the next part. All part reviews and the Pretest and Posttest in the module include answers. It is suggested that the learner review those concepts that have been missed in the review questions before proceeding to the next part.

Objectives

Following the completion of the module, the learner will be able to

1. Describe the unique anatomic and physiologic characteristics of the child's respiratory system

2. Classify the most common etiologies of respiratory failure during infancy and childhood according to the dominant functional abnormality

3. Identify clinical manifestations of acute respiratory failure observed in the infant and child

4. Describe the nursing management of a child with acute respiratory failure

5. Discuss the unique characteristics of the immature cardiovascular system

6. Describe the most common etiologies of circulatory failure in the child

7. List the clinical manifestations of circulatory failure in children

8. Describe specific interventions used to manage a child with circulatory failure

563

9. Discuss the unique anatomic and physiologic characteristics of the immature central nervous system

10. List the most common types of neurologic dysfunction in children

11. Describe the key components of the neurologic examination of the child with altered mental status

12. Discuss the nursing management of the neurologically impaired child

13. Describe the nursing management of a child with alteration in fluid and electrolytes

14. Discuss the nursing management of a child with alteration in nutritional status

15. Identify regulatory mechanisms of heat balance

16. Discuss the nursing management of alteration in heat balance

17. Identify age-related factors and situational stressors that alter the immune response of the acutely ill child

18. State treatment strategies to prevent infection and augment host defenses in the child

19. Discuss age-related stressors and reactions to hospitalization

20. List specific methods to reduce the negative effects of hospitalization

Pretest

Refer to the following case study to answer Questions 1 through 7.

Amanda is a 4-year-old girl brought to the emergency room after aspirating a piece of hot dog in her trachea. She has a respiratory rate of 60, decreased breath sounds in her lower lobes, inspiratory stridor, use of accessory muscles, and supraclavicular retractions. Her mucous membranes, nailbeds, and sclera are bluish in color.

1. What is the underlying dominant functional respiratory abnormality?
   A. obstructive lung disease
   B. restrictive lung disease
   C. ineffective gas transfer from decreased alveoli
   D. ineffective gas transfer from central nervous system depression

2. Amanda's cyanosis is best defined as
   A. central cyanosis from poor perfusion
   B. peripheral cyanosis from poor perfusion
   C. central cyanosis from hypoxemia
   D. peripheral cyanosis from hypoxemia

3. Based on the above data, which of the following nursing diagnoses would you select as being appropriate in Amanda's care?
   A. Ineffective breathing patterns
   B. Alteration in cardiac output: decreased
   C. Potential for infection
   D. Altered tissue perfusion: cerebral

Noninvasive efforts to remove the hot dog were unsuccessful. A bronchoscopy was ordered. During the procedure, Amanda's arterial oxygen saturation decreased acutely to 40 percent, her heart rate dropped to 60, and she had a respiratory arrest. The hot dog piece was removed.

4. What intervention should be performed first?
   A. intubation
   B. bag-valve-mask ventilation with F_{IO_2} 1.0
   C. passive flow of oxygen
   D. chest compressions

5. If Amanda requires chest compressions, what is the correct compression/ventilation ratio?
   A. 5:1
   B. 10:1
   C. 15:2
   D. 10:2

Amanda's cardiopulmonary status is stabilized. ABG results are: pH 7.32, Pao_2 80, $Paco_2$ 30, Sao_2 78 percent.

6. Amanda's ABG results can best be described as
   A. normal for a preschooler
   B. normal for a 6-month-old
   C. normal for an adult
   D. normal for a neonate

Later in the day, Amanda's parents have to leave the hospital. Amanda becomes very upset, crying and yelling for her parents.

7. What nursing intervention would most likely reduce Amanda's anxiety?
   A. use a clock to explain when her parents will return
   B. bring her favorite teddy bear to the bedside
   C. develop a contract with Amanda to negotiate visitation
   D. explain to Amanda she will have no play time if she continues crying

Refer to the following case study to answer Questions 8 through 13.

Johnny is a 2-month-old, 5 kg baby boy admitted to the intensive care unit with a 3-day history of fever. On admission, he is lethargic and minimally responsive to noxious stimuli. Vital signs are: temperature 103.1F (39.5C), heart rate 180, respiratory rate 80, blood pressure 50 by palpation. Extremities are cool and pale in color. Lungs are clear to auscultation.

8. What patient order should be initiated first by the nurse?
   A. IV line insertion
   B. supplemental oxygen
   C. synchronized cardioversion
   D. acetaminophen administration
9. Based on the above data, which of the following nursing diagnoses would you select as being appropriate in Johnny's plan of care?
   A. Ineffective airway breathing
   B. Altered nutrition: less than body requirements
   C. Fluid volume deficit
   D. Self-care deficit

Peripheral IV line insertion has been attempted for 10 minutes without success.

10. Access to the circulation should be attempted by which of the following routes?
    A. central cannulation
    B. cutdown cannulation
    C. intraosseous cannulation
    D. arterial cannulation

Access to the circulation is successful. The patient becomes unresponsive. The heart rate is 190, and the blood pressure is no longer palpable. Femoral pulses are faint.

11. How much fluid should Johnny receive as a bolus?
    A. 50 mL
    B. 150 mL
    C. 500 mL
    D. 100 mL
12. What type of IV solution should you prepare for fluid resuscitation?
    A. lactated Ringer's solution
    B. 5% dextrose in water
    C. 5% dextrose in 0.2 normal saline
    D. albumin

Another bolus of fluid is given. Johnny's vital signs are stabilized. A Foley catheter is inserted for urine output monitoring.

13. What should be the normal urine output per hour for Johnny?
    A. 20 mL
    B. 30 mL
    C. 10 mL
    D. 2 mL

Refer to the following case study to answer Questions 14 through 17.

Ricky, an 18-month-old child, is brought to the intensive care unit with a history of fever for 2 days, irritability, loss of appetite, and lethargy. Vital signs are: temperature 101.3F (38.5 C), heart rate 120, respiratory rate 50, and blood pressure 80/60. Breath sounds are clear, urine culture is negative, white blood count (WBC) is 20,000. A lumbar puncture is performed. Results are: cloudy appearance, WBC 604 mm^3, protein 110 mg/100 mL, gram stain positive for gram-negative rods.

14. If Ricky is not treated quickly, which of the following pathophysiologic processes is most likely to develop?
    A. decreased perfusion from cardiogenic shock
    B. decreased perfusion from hypovolemic shock
    C. increased intracranial pressure (IICP)
    D. hypoxemia from CNS-induced pulmonary edema

Ricky is diagnosed with bacterial meningitis.

---

15. Which of the following pathogens is most likely the cause?
    A. *Escherichia coli*
    B. *Haemophilus influenzae*
    C. respiratory syncytial virus
    D. *Pseudomonas aeruginosa*
16. Which of the following nursing interventions has the highest priority?
    A. administer broad-spectrum antibiotics
    B. assess airway and breathing
    C. administer medications to prevent hypotension
    D. hyperventilate with an Ambubag
17. Which of the following interventions would most likely be needed following the administration of diazepam (Valium) for status epilepticus?
    A. bag-valve-mask ventilation
    B. isotonic fluid bolus 20 mL/kg
    C. naloxone (Narcan) administration
    D. dopamine (Intropin) administration

Refer to the following case study to answer Questions 18 through 21.

Christine is a 3-year-old girl admitted to the intensive care unit with a 3-day history of vomiting and diarrhea. Vital signs are: temperature 102.2F (39C), respiratory rate 40, heart rate 110, blood pressure 74/40. Additional clinical symptoms include grayish skin color, loss of skin elasticity, dry mucous membranes, and irritability. She has not voided for 7 hours. Prehospital weight is not known. Present weight is 17 kg. CBC is normal, glucose normal, serum electrolytes are Na+ 138, K+ 3.4, Cl−102.

---

18. Which type of dehydration does Christine have?
    A. hypertonic
    B. hypotonic
    C. hyponatremic
    D. isotonic
19. Based on clinical symptoms, what degree of dehydration does Christine have?
    A. mild
    B. moderate
    C. severe
    D. none
20. The hourly maintenance fluid requirement for Christine is (based on hospital weight)?
    A. 26 mL
    B. 56 mL
    C. 10 mL
    D. 88 mL
21. If Christine normally weights 19 kg, what percentage of weight loss does she have?
    A. 8
    B. 2
    C. 20
    D. 10

Questions 22 and 23 do not refer to Christine.

22. The infant's level of immunoglobulins is lowest between
    A. 4 and 6 years of age
    B. 4 and 5 months of age
    C. 2 and 3 weeks of age
    D. 2 and 5 years of age
23. Low levels of IgE place the young child at increased risk for
    A. pyogenic infections
    B. bacterial respiratory infection
    C. parasitic infection
    D. overwhelming sepsis

Refer to the following case study to answer Questions 24 through 26.

Cathy is a 2½-year-old girl admitted to the intensive care unit with epiglottitis. She is intubated and started on antibiotics. Restraints are necessary to prevent Cathy from extubating herself. Her parents are allowed to visit her every hour for 5 minutes.

---

24. What reaction is Cathy most likely to have to separation from her parents?
    A. withdrawal from staff
    B. complaints of boredom and loneliness
    C. temper tantrums
    D. repeated requests for parents

Cathy's IV catheter needs to be changed.

_____

25. When preparing Cathy for the procedure, which technique would be most helpful?
    A. demonstrating an IV insertion on a doll
    B. explaining the procedure in a group with other children
    C. sedating her with diazepam (Valium)
    D. restraining her
26. What nursing intervention would be most helpful to prevent feelings of loss of control?
    A. maintain a clock at the bedside
    B. encourage her to make her own bed
    C. minimize change in normal daily routines
    D. obtain a psychiatric consult

27. Which of the following nursing interventions is most effective in lowering IICP acutely?
    A. suctioning the airway
    B. placing patient in Trendelenburg position
    C. elevating the head of bed 25 degrees
    D. applying hypothermia mattress

_____

Pretest answers: 1, A. 2, C. 3, A. 4, B. 5, A. 6, D. 7, B. 8, B. 9, C. 10, C. 11, D. 12, A. 13, C. 14, C. 15, B. 16, B. 17, A. 18, D. 19, B. 20, B. 21, D. 22, B. 23, C. 24, A. 25, A. 26, C. 27, C.

Glossary

Agenesis/hypoplasia of the lung. Varying degrees of absence of pulmonary tissue

Arterial oxygen content. The amount of oxygen in volume percent present in arterial blood

Bradycardia. An abnormally slow heart rate

Choanal atresia. Narrowing of the posterior nares from bony or membranous obstructive tissue or from stenosis

Cystic fibrosis. An inherited disease of exocrine gland dysfunction involving multiple organs; pulmonary disease is the primary cause of morbidity and mortality

Diaphragmatic hernia. Maldevelopment of the diaphragm, with possible herniation of abdominal organs into the thorax; herniation of abdominal organs in utero may prevent or limit lung development

Ductus arteriosus. A fetal cardiovascular shunt that allows blood from the pulmonary artery to be diverted into the descending aorta

Ductus venosus. A fetal cardiovascular shunt that is a pathway for oxygenated blood from the umbilical vein through the liver to the inferior vena cava

Eventration. Partial protrusion of the abdominal contents through an opening in the abdominal wall

Foramen ovale. A fetal cardiovascular shunt from an opening in the atrial septum; it allows blood to shunt from the right atrium to the left atrium

Hyaline membrane disease. A disease of the premature infant's lungs from insufficient development of the pulmonary surfactant system

Kyphoscoliosis. Lateral curvature of the spine

Methemoglobinemia. A condition in which more than 1 percent of circulating hemoglobin has been oxidized to the ferric form

Myasthenia gravis. A disease characterized by muscle weakness due to a lack of acetylcholine or excess of cholinesterase at the myoneural junction

Partial pressure of oxygen (Pao₂). The partial pressure of dissolved gas in the plasma of arterial blood due to oxygen; oxygen tension

Partial pressure of carbon dioxide (Paco₂). The partial pressure of dissolved gas in the plasma of arterial blood due to carbon dioxide; carbon dioxide tension

Pierre-Robin syndrome. Severe mandibular hypoplasia with associated cleft or highly arched palate

Pleural effusion. Excess liquid accumulation in the pleural cavity

Pneumopericardium. Air or gas in the pericardial sac

Pneumothorax. A collection of air or gas in the pleural cavity

Pulmonary sequestration. A condition where pulmonary tissue is embryonic and cystic, nonfunctional, isolated from normal lung tissue, and perfused by systemic arteries

Sarcoidosis. A multisystem granulomatous disease of unknown etiology

Tachycardia. An abnormally high heart rate

Tidal volume. Volume of air that is inhaled and exhaled during normal breathing

Tracheomalacia. Softening of the cartilage of the trachea

Ventilation-perfusion mismatch. An abnormality in the distribution of the ventilation and perfusion of the gas-exchanging units

Wilson-Mikity syndrome. A condition of prolonged respiratory distress in premature infants that is accompanied by characteristic changes in the chest radiograph

Abbreviations

ABG. Arterial blood gas

BMR. Basal metabolic rate

CBF. Cerebral blood flow

CNS. Central nervous system

CO. Cardiac output

CPP. Cerebral perfusion pressure

CSF. Cerebrospinal fluid

CT. Computed tomography

CVP. Central venous pressure

EEG. Electroencephalogram

GCS. Glasgow Coma Scale

Hct. Hematocrit

Hgb. Hemoglobin

ICP. Intracranial pressure

IICP. Increased intracranial pressure

kcal. Kilocalorie

LOC. Loss of consciousness

PaCO_2. Partial pressure of carbon dioxide

PaO_2. Partial pressure of oxygen

PCWP. Pulmonary capillary wedge pressure

PVR. Pulmonary vascular resistance

RDA. Recommended dietary allowances

SaO_2. Arterial saturation of oxygen

SBP. Systolic blood pressure

TBI. Traumatic brain injury

VENTILATION

Section One: Maturational Anatomy and Physiology

At the completion of this section, the learner will be able to describe unique anatomic and physiologic characteristics of the child's respiratory system.

Respiratory disorders producing respiratory distress or failure are the most common admitting diagnoses in the pediatric intensive care unit. To understand the nursing assessment and the nursing care of a pediatric patient with acute respiratory failure, one must first have a basic understanding of the unique anatomic and physiologic characteristics of the immature respiratory system. The focus of this section is to discuss briefly developmental aspects of the respiratory system.

Even though the term newborn's lungs are capable of immediate function at birth, growth of the lungs continues for several years. Growth occurs primarily from an increase in the size of the conducting airways and from an increase in the number of bronchioles and alveoli. The newborn has approximately one-eighth to one-sixth the number of adult alveoli, and the full adult complement of alveoli is not present until about the eighth year of life (Moore, 1988). There also are a number of other significant anatomic and physiologic differences in the immature respiratory system (Table 23–1). Consequently, the young child has a predisposition to respiratory dysfunction, as well as limited respiratory reserve.

In summary, the child's respiratory system is not only quantitatively different but also is qualitatively different, predisposing children to acute respiratory failure. Knowledge of the anatomic and physiologic differences can assist in early recognition and management of acute respiratory failure.

Section Two: Etiologies

At the completion of this section, the learner will be able to classify the most common etiologies of respiratory failure during infancy and childhood according to the dominant functional abnormality.

TABLE 23–1. ANATOMIC AND PHYSIOLOGIC CONSIDERATIONS OF THE IMMATURE RESPIRATORY SYSTEM

Anatomy	Clinical Significance
Small airway diameter	Airway obstruction increases airway resistance in infant to a greater degree than in adult: resistance is inversely proportional to the 4th power of the radius; predisposition to obstruction
Larynx relatively cephalad	Difficult to make a single, visual plan from the pharynx to the glottis for endotracheal intubation
Epiglottis is U-shaped, large	
Vocal cords short	
Large tongue	Predisposition to airway obstruction
Cricoid cartilage narrowest portion of the airway	Uncuffed E-T tubes used, E-T tube less secure
Small lower airways	Predisposition to obstruction and atelectasis from mucus, blood, pus, edema
Decreased number of alveoli and surface area	Decreased diffusion and increased shunting
Cartilaginous thoracic cage	Offers less support during inspiration; predisposition to sternal and intercostal retractions with a decrease in tidal volume
Diaphragm primary muscle of respiration	Respiratory function compromised with gastric distention or pulmonary trypennflation

Physiology	Clinical Significance
Large body surface area, immature thermostatic control	Predisposition to hypothermia causing decreased oxygen consumption and metabolic rate
Metabolic rate twice the adult rate	Predisposition to hypoxemia with altered respiratory function

Respiratory failure is a state in which the respiratory system is unable to deliver adequate oxygen to or remove carbon dioxide from the circulation in order to meet the demands of the body. As noted previously, children are predisposed to respiratory failure because of the unique anatomic and physiologic features of their immature respiratory system. In addition, there are a number of respiratory disorders that can impair the child's ability to adequately oxygenate or ventilate or both. The purpose of this section is to describe common etiologies of acute respiratory failure in children.

The number of potential etiologies producing respiratory failure is vast, but the underlying dominant functional abnormality can assist in classifying etiologies into one of three groups.

1. Obstructive lung disease
2. Restrictive lung disease
3. Primary ineffective gas transfer

All three functional derangements may be present in isolation or in combination. However, all three groups have a common final pathway of the mismatching of ventilation and perfusion in the lung. Consequently, hypoxemia, hypercarbia, and acidosis develop.

Obstructive Lung Disease

Airway obstruction is a common cause of respiratory failure in children. Whether the obstruction is acute or chronic, partial or complete, there is increased resistance to flow. If the obstruction is complete or if the child cannot compensate for a partial obstruction, a ventilation-perfusion ($\dot{V}/\dot{Q}$) mismatch develops, resulting in hypoxemia and hypercarbia. Table 23–2

TABLE 23–2. CAUSES OF OBSTRUCTIVE RESPIRATORY DISEASE

Site of Disturbance	Specific Disease Conditions	
	Newborn and Early Infancy	Late Infancy and Childhood
Upper airway Anomalies	Choanal atresia, Pierre-Robin syndrome, laryngeal web, tracheal stenosis, tracheomalacia, vascular ring	Tracheal stenosis, vocal cord paralysis, vascular ring, laryngotracheomalacia
Lower airway Anomalies	Bronchostenosis, bronchomalacia, lobar emphysema	Bronchostenosis, lobar emphysema, aberrant vessels
Aspiration	Meconium, mucus, vomitus	Foreign body, vomitus
Infection	Pneumonia, pertussis	Laryngotracheitis, epiglottis, peritonsillar or retropharyngneal abscess, bronchiolitis, pneumonia
Tumors	Hemangioma, cystic hygroma, teratoma	Hemangioma, teratoma, hypertrophy of tonsils and adenoids
Allergic or reflex	Larynogospasm from local irritation (intubation) or tetany	Laryngospasm from local irritation (aspiration, intubation, drowning) or tetany, allergy, smoke inhalation, asthma, bronchospasm

TABLE 23–3. CAUSES OF RESTRICTIVE RESPIRATORY DISEASE

Site of Disturbance	Specific Disease Conditions	
	Newborn and Early Infancy	Late Infancy and Childhood
Parenchymal		
Anomalies	Agenesis, hypoplasia, lobar emphysema, congenital cyst, pulmonary sequestration	Congenital cyst
Atelectasis	Hyaline membrane disease	Thick secretions, foreign body
Infection	Pneumonia	Pneumonia, cystic fibrosis, bronchiectasis
Alveolar rupture	Pneumothorax (spontaneous or iatrogenic), interstitial emphysema	Trauma, asthma
Others	Pulmonary hemorrhage, pulmonary edema, Wilson-Mikity syndrome	Pulmonary edema, lobectomy, chemical pneumonitis, pleural effusion, near-drowning
Chest Wall		
Muscular	Diaphragmatic hernia, eventration, edema	Muscular dystrophy, botulism
Skeletal malformations	Hemivertebrae, absence of ribs	Kyphoscoliosis, hemivertebrae, absence of ribs
Others	Abdominal distention	Obesity, flail chest

lists the most common causes of obstructive lung disease during infancy and childhood.

Restrictive Lung Disease

Restrictive lung disease also can cause respiratory failure in children. The main functional alteration with this category of altered respiratory function is impaired lung expansion from loss of lung volume, decreased distensibility of lung tissue, and chest wall disturbance. Regardless of the cause, there is inadequate aeration of the alveoli, where as pulmonary blood flow is normal (intrapulmonary shunt). Table 23–3 lists the most common causes of restrictive lung disease during infancy and childhood.

Ineffective Gas Transfer

The last functional group of respiratory dysfunction producing respiratory failure is primary ineffective gas transfer. Specific disease conditions resulting in ineffective gas transfer can result from pulmonary diffusion defects or from CNS respiratory depression. With pulmonary diffusion defects, gas transfer between alveoli and pulmonary capillaries is blocked by abnormal tissue. Respiratory depression produces a decrease in total minute ventilation, i.e., a reduction in respiratory rate, tidal volume, or both. Table 23–4 lists the most common causes of primary inefficient gas transfer during childhood.

In summary, any condition that impairs oxygenation or ventilation when compensatory mechanisms are inadequate will result in respiratory failure.

TABLE 23–4. CAUSES OF PRIMARY INEFFICIENT GAS TRANSFER

Site of Disturbance	Specific Disease Conditions
Pulmonary diffusion defect	
Increased diffusion path between alveoli and capillaries	Pulmonary edema, pulmonary fibrosis, collagen disorders, *Pneumocystis carinii* infection, sarcoidosis
Decreased alveolocapillary surface area	Pulmonary embolism, sarcoidosis, pulmonary hypertension, mitral stenosis, fibrosing alveolitis
Inadequate erythrocytes and hemoglobin	Anemia, hemorrhage
Respiratory center depression	
Increased cerebrospinal fluid pressure	Cerebral trauma (birth injuries), intracranial tumors, central nervous system infection (meningitis, encephalitis, sepsis)
Excess central nervous system depressant drugs	Maternal oversedation, overdosage with barbiturates, morphine, or diazepam
Excessive chemical changes in arterial blood	Severe asphyxia (hypercapnia, hypoxemia)
Toxic	Tetanus

From *Disorders of the respiratory tract in children*, p. 207, by V. Chernick and E.L. Kendig, 1990, Philadelphia: W.B. Saunders Co.

Section Three: Clinical Manifestations

At the completion of this section, the learner will be able to identify clinical manifestations of acute respiratory failure observed in the infant and child.

Clinical manifestations of acute respiratory failure in children are extremely variable and nonspecific. Consequently, clinical findings must be correlated with diagnostic findings. To be able to recognize signs and symptoms of impending respiratory failure, one must first have an understanding of normal respiratory parameters during childhood. This section compares and contrasts normal and abnormal findings of the respiratory examination.

Respiratory Rate

Respiratory rate normally decreases with age, with the greatest normal variation during the first 2 years of life (Kendig and Chernick, 1990). Approximate averages of breaths per minute during infancy and childhood are

Newborn	<40
1 year old	24
18 year old	18

An abnormally fast respiratory rate (tachypnea) can be seen in children with increased anxiety, fever, anemia, exertion, and conditions producing decreased lung compliance.

Tachypnea is often the first sign of respiratory distress in the young child, especially when it is associated with increased work of breathing (Table 23–5). Tachypnea is the body's attempt to maintain a normal pH by eliminating excess carbon dioxide via the lungs. Tachypnea without associated signs of respiratory distress (Table 23–7), *quiet tachypnea*, usually is due to nonrespiratory causes, e.g., disorders producing metabolic acidosis.

TABLE 23–5. SIGNS AND SYMPTOMS OF INCREASED WORK OF BREATHING

Clinical Finding	Clinical Significance
Inspiratory stridor	Upper airway obstruction between the supraglottic space and lower trachea
Prolonged expiration with wheezing	Bronchial and bronchiolar obstruction
Grunting	Premature glottic closure during expiration, an attempt to increase FRC[a]
Nasal flaring	Enlarges anterior nasal passages and reduces upper and total airway resistance
Chest wall retractions (intracostal, subcostal, suprasternal)	Increased negative intrapleural pressure during inspiration with high airway resistance
Use of accessory muscles (older child), head bobbing (infant)	Upper airway obstruction
Paradoxical breathing	Premature/newborn: extremely compliant rib cage; infant/toddler: respiratory muscle fatigue and impending respiratory arrest

[a]FRC, functional residual capacity.

An abnormally slow respiratory rate (bradypnea) or absent respiratory rate (apnea) can occur with CNS depression, extreme fatigue, and hypothermia. Bradypnea is often a very ominous sign in a child who is acutely ill and usually hallmarks an impending respiratory arrest.

Respiratory Mechanics

After assessing the rate and rhythm of breathing, one should look at respiratory mechanics to determine if there is increased work of breathing. Specific signs and symptoms of increased work of breathing in the child and their clinical significance are listed in Table 23–5.

Color

Cyanosis is a very late and insensitive indicator of acute respiratory failure. It refers to a bluish color, which is due to an absolute amount of reduced hemoglobin (Hgb) in capillary blood. There are two types of cyanosis that may be present. The first is peripheral cyanosis, which is a bluish discoloration of the extremities and nailbeds. It occurs when there is normal arterial saturation but increased extraction of oxygen at the tissue level related to decreased perfusion. The second type of cyanosis is central, which is a bluish discoloration of the mucous membranes, tongue, sclera, extremities, and nailbeds. It results from inadequate oxygenation of the central systemic arterial blood.

Clinically detectable cyanosis is dependent on arterial oxygen saturation (Sao_2) and total circulating hemoglobin concentration. Depending on the amount of hemoglobin, clinical cyanosis will occur at different levels of arterial oxygen saturation. For example, a child with polycythemia (hematocrit of > 60 percent) will show clinical signs of cyanosis before a child with anemia because of an increase in the number of unsaturated red blood cells. In addition, recognition of cyanosis in the newborn is more difficult to observe due to the presence of fetal hemoglobin, which has a higher affinity for oxygen. The newborn's blood may be well saturated even with an arterial partial pressure of oxygen (Pao_2) as low as 40 mm Hg.

Arterial Blood Gases

Arterial blood gases (ABG) are the most widely used clinical method to evaluate acute respiratory failure in children. Normal ABG values for the child are the same as for the adult. ABG values are slightly different for the neonate. Table 23–6 lists the normal ABG values for the neonate and child.

TABLE 23–6. NORMAL ARTERIAL BLOOD GAS VALUES

	Neonate[a]	Child[a]
pH	7.32–7.42	7.35–7.45
Pco_2	30–40 mm Hg	35–45 mm Hg
HCO_3	20–26 mEq/L	22–28 mEq/L
Po_2	60–80 mm Hg	80–100 mm Hg

From *Nursing care of the critically ill child*, by M. F. Hazincki, 1984, St. Louis: C. V. Mosby.

[a] The neonatal values represent normals for neonates between a few hours after birth and 4 weeks of age. Values for the child are the same as for the adult.

Once ABGs are obtained, the degree and type of respiratory failure can be determined. A general guideline for determining the type of respiratory failure is:

Type I   Low partial pressure of oxygen (Pao_2) Low/normal partial pressure of carbon dioxide ($Paco_2$)

Type II   Low Pao_2 High $Paco_2$

Type I patients usually have a significant $\dot{V}/\dot{Q}$ mismatch (e.g., atelectasis, pulmonary edema). Type II patients usually have relative hypoventilation superimposed on $\dot{V}/\dot{Q}$ mismatch (e.g., CNS respiratory depression, oversedation). The degree of respiratory distress is determined by how low the Pao_2 is and how high the $Paco_2$ is on room air.

In summary, a key factor in reducing mortality and morbidity from a respiratory arrest is early recognition of signs and symptoms of respiratory failure. Table 23–7 summarizes the early signs and symp-

TABLE 23–7. RESPIRATORY DISTRESS CLINICAL DATA

Heart rate	Tachycardia
	Bradycardia (infant)
	Tachycardia leading to bradycardia (child)
Respiratory rate	Tachypnea
	Newborn > 60 bpm
	2 months–2 years > 30 bpm
	2–12 years > 30 bpm
	> 12 years > 20 bpm
Respiratory effort	Nasal flaring, expiratory grunt, paradoxial breathing, chest retractions, inspiratory stridor, wheezing
Color	Pale, dusky leading to cyanotic
Auscultatory finds	Variable: absent or diminished breath sounds, adventitious breath sounds
Level of consciousness	Altered or depressed
Arterial blood gases	With loss of compensation: decreased Pao_2[a] and/or increased $Paco_2$

[a] Pao_2, partial pressure of oxygen; $Paco_2$, partial pressure of carbon dioxide.

toms of respiratory compromise. These signs and symptoms coupled with diagnostic information provide the database to guide respiratory management.

Section Four: Nursing Management

At the completion of this section, the learner will be able to describe the specific steps in managing a child with acute respiratory failure.

The specific interventions needed to manage a child with altered respiratory function are based on clinical data. For the child with mild respiratory distress, only comfort measures may be required. At the opposite end of the continuum with total respiratory arrest, complete cardiopulmonary resuscitation may be required. This section presents guidelines for managing a child with altered respiratory function.

On the basis of a rapid respiratory assessment, the child should be categorized into one of three groups.

1. Mild respiratory distress (stable)
2. Impending respiratory failure (unstable)
3. Respiratory arrest

The goal in treating the child with respiratory distress is to minimize oxygen demand while correcting the underlying disease process. The first nursing intervention to implement is opening the airway. Infants should be placed in a sniffing position, and older children should be allowed to determine their own position of comfort. Second, maximize tidal volume by elevating the head of bed. This position prevents abdominal organs from impinging on the diaphragm and the thoracic cavity. Third, maximize oxygenation by administering supplemental oxygen via an age-appropriate delivery system. Finally, provide interventions to minimize oxygen demand. For example, withhold feedings or administer them through a nasogastric tube, minimize environmental stress, and maintain normothermia.

In patients with respiratory failure or arrest, more aggressive management is required to stabilize the patient. The goal is to restore ventilation and oxygenation to prevent ensuing cardiac asystole. Figure 23–1 outlines a systematic approach to the emergent management of respiratory failure or arrest.

There are a number of oxygen delivery systems that can be used in children. The selection of a system is based on patient tolerance of the device, patient minute ventilation, and oxygen concentration needed. In general, a patient with acute respiratory failure or impending respiratory arrest requires the highest concentration of oxygen available. There-

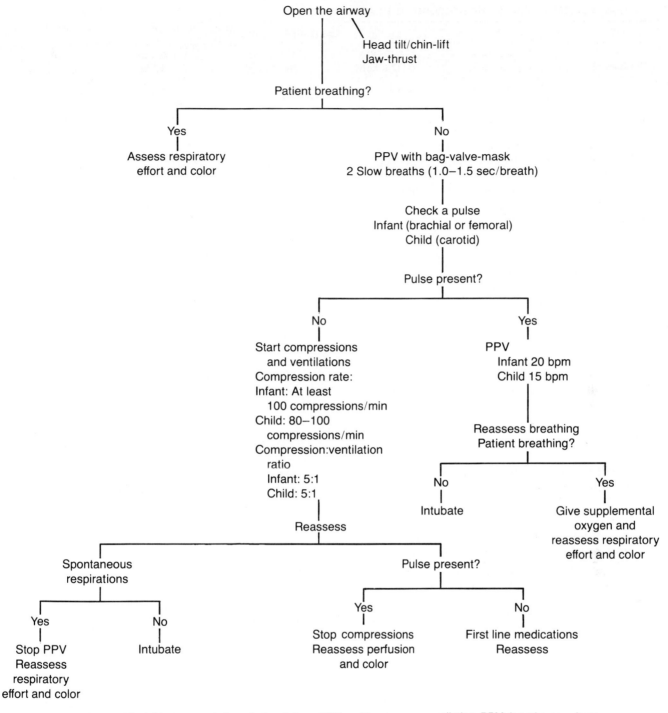

Figure 23–1. Management of respiratory failure. PPV, positive pressure ventilation; BPM, breaths per minute.

fore, high-flow oxygen masks that can reliably deliver high oxygen concentrations should be used. Table 23–8 provides equipment guidelines for airway resuscitation in the infant and child.

In summary, regardless of the cause of a respiratory failure or arrest and the age of the child, the management steps are the same: (1) airway, (2) breathing, and (3) circulation. Attention to these basic steps can significantly improve survival and minimize hypoxic brain damage.

TABLE 23–8. EQUIPMENT GUIDELINES ACCORDING TO AGE AND WEIGHT

Equipment	Age (50th Percentile Weight)				
	Neonate (2.5–4.0 kg)	6 Months (7.0 kg)	1–2 Years (10–12 kg)	5 Years (16–18 kg)	8–10 Years (24–30 kg)
Airway–oral	Infant/small (0)	Small (1)	Small (2)	Medium (3)	Medium/large (4/5)
Breathing Self-inflating bag	Infant	Child	Child	Child	Child/adult
O$_2$ ventilation mask	Newborn	Infant/child	Child	Child	Small adult
Endotracheal tube	3.0–3.5 (uncuffed)	3.5–4.0 (uncuffed)	4.0–4.5 (uncuffed)	5.0–5.5 (uncuffed)	5.5–6.5 (cuffed)
Laryngoscope blade	1 (straight)	1 (straight)	1–2 (straight)	2 (straight or curved)	2–3 (straight or curved)
Suction/stylet (F)	8/6	8–10/6	10/6	14/14	14/14
Orogastric tube (F)	5–8	8	10	10–12	14–18

Adapted from *Textbook of pediatric advanced life support*, p. 105, by L. Chameides, 1988, Dallas: American Heart Association.

Ventilation Review

1. The infant is predisposed to upper airway obstruction because of
   A. decreased number of alveoli
   B. immature thermostatic control
   C. increased metabolic rate
   D. small airway diameter
2. The dominant functional disturbance with obstructive lung disease is
   A. increased resistance to airflow
   B. impaired lung expansion
   C. a primary diffusion defect
   D. impaired respiratory control mechanism
3. Clinically detectable central cyanosis is dependent on
   A. arterial oxygen saturation and blood pressure
   B. arterial oxygen saturation and hemoglobin concentration
   C. partial pressure of oxygen and hemoglobin concentration
   D. partial pressure of carbon dioxide and hemoglobin concentration
4. Chest wall retractions in the young child are produced from
   A. premature glottic closure during expiration
   B. constriction of the anterior nasal passages
   C. increased negative intrapleural pressure during inspiration
   D. diaphragmatic muscular spasms
5. An initial intervention for a child experiencing mild respiratory distress is
   A. endotracheal intubation
   B. elevating the head of bed
   C. positive pressure ventilation
   D. administration of a mild sedative

Refer to the following case study to answer Questions 6 through 10.

Amanda is a 4-year-old girl brought to the emergency room after aspirating a piece of hot dog in her trachea. She has a respiratory rate of 60, decreased breath sounds in her lower lobes, inspiratory stridor, use of accessory muscles, and supraclavicular retractions. Her mucous membranes, nailbeds, and sclera are bluish in color.

6. What is the underlying dominant functional respiratory abnormality?
   A. obstructive lung disease
   B. restrictive lung disease
   C. ineffective gas transfer from decreased alveoli
   D. ineffective gas transfer from CNS depression

7. Amanda's cyanosis is best defined as
   A. central cyanosis from poor perfusion
   B. peripheral cyanosis from poor perfusion
   C. central cyanosis from hypoxemia
   D. peripheral cyanosis from hypoxemia

Noninvasive efforts to remove the hot dog were unsuccessful. A bronchoscopy was ordered. During the procedure, Amanda's arterial oxygen saturation decreased acutely to 40 percent, her heart rate dropped to 60, and she had a respiratory arrest. The hot dog piece was removed.

8. What intervention should be performed first?
   A. intubation
   B. bag-valve-mask ventilation with Fio_2 1.0
   C. passive flow of oxygen
   D. chest compressions

9. If Amanda requires chest compressions, what is the correct compression/ventilation ratio?
   A. 5:1
   B. 10:1
   C. 15:2
   D. 10:2

Amanda's cardiopulmonary status is stabilized. ABG results are: pH 7.32, Pao_2 80, $Paco_2$ 30, Sao_2 78 percent.

10. Amanda's ABG results can best be described as
    A. normal for a preschooler
    B. normal for a 6-month-old
    C. normal for an adult
    D. normal for a neonate

Answers: 1, D. 2, A. 3, B. 4, C. 5, B. 6, A. 7, C. 8, B. 9, A. 10, D.

PERFUSION

Section Five: Maturational Anatomy and Physiology

At the completion of this section, the learner will be able to discuss the unique characteristics of the immature cardiovascular system.

The specific role of the cardiovascular system is the same in the child as in the adult: to deliver adequate amounts of oxygen and nutrients to body tissue and organs. However, the cardiovascular system is not complete at birth and matures over time. The purpose of this section is to highlight postnatal circulatory maturation and function.

The functional differences between the neonatal and adult cardiovascular systems are, for the most part, directly related to transitional circulation. At birth, when the infant begins to breathe, placental circulation is eliminated, and fetal shunts close. Consequently, hemodynamic and anatomic changes take place. The ductus venosus and the ductus arteriosus normally constrict and become nonfunctional. The foramen ovale establishes a functional closure in response to increased left-sided heart pressure. These

three fetal shunts are usually eliminated within the first days of life, and adult circulatory patterns are established.

In contrast to the normally rapid closure of fetal shunts, there are some anatomic and hemodynamic changes that occur more gradually. Pulmonary vascular resistance (PVR) drops precipitously after birth from an increase in the diameter of the pulmonary arteries. A further decrease in PVR occurs as the medial muscle layer of the pulmonary arteries continues to thin over the first 2 to 8 weeks of life. Normal adult values of PVR are present at about 2 months of age.

Left ventricular muscle mass and ECG voltage increase over time and correspond to increasing left ventricular workload as systemic vascular resistance increases. Sympathetic innervation is incomplete at birth, suggesting vagal predominance for the first weeks of life (Hazinski and van Stralen, 1990). Table 23–9 summarizes the key maturational changes of the cardiovascular system and their clinical significance.

In summary, the immature cardiovascular system is anatomically and physiologically different. Clinical assessments and management are directly affected by these maturational differences, requiring age-appropriate modification.

TABLE 23–9. MATURATIONAL CHANGES OF THE CARDIOVASCULAR SYSTEM

Anatomy	Clinical Significance
Closure of fetal shunts	Decreased mixing of pulmonary and systemic blood; increased Sao_2[a]
PVR decreases Decreased RV workload Decreased RV dominance on ECG	Normal PVR 1st week of life: 8–10 units/m² BSA > 6 weeks of life: 1–3 units/m² BSA
SVR increases Increased LV workload LV wall thickness increases LV dominance on ECG	Normal SVR < 12 months: 10–15 units/m² BSA 12–18 months: 20–30 units/m² BSA

Physiology	Clinical Significance
Fetal Hgb replaced with adult Hgb	Oxyhemoglobin dissociation curve shifts to the right
Cardiac output (L/minute)	Increases with age Newborn: 0.8–1.0 L/minute 5 year-old: 2.5–3.0 L/minute 10-year-old: 3.8–4.0 L/minute
Cardiac index (CI)	Child's CI is slightly higher than adults Child: 3.5–4.5 L/minute/m² BSA
Heart rate	As stroke volume increases, heart rate decreases
Sympathetic innervation of the heart	Incomplete at birth; vagal effects may dominate during first weeks of life
Myocardial contraction	May be less in the newborn due to less contractile tissue per unit of myocardium

[a]PVR, pulmonary vascular resistance; SVR, systemic vascular resistance; Sao_2, arterial oxygen saturation; BSA, body surface area; Hgb, hemoglobin.

Section Six: Etiologies

At the completion of this section, the learner will be able to describe the most common etiologies of shock in the child.

Shock is a term used to describe a number of disorders that result in a common final pathway in which blood flow is unable to meet the metabolic demands of the body's tissues (Crone, 1980). Oxygen delivery, vital to cellular function, is the product of cardiac output (CO) and arterial oxygen content. In children, circulatory failure is usually due to an absolute reduction in CO. Occasionally, a severely septic or febrile child with increased metabolic demand may have circulatory failure even with a normal CO. The purpose of this section is to list the most common causes of circulatory failure in children. For an indepth discussion on the determinants of CO and in-

ternal and external controls of CO, the reader should review Module 5, *Perfusion*.

As described in Module 8, *Shock States*, the specific etiologies of shock can be grouped into one of four functional categories: hypovolemic, transport, obstructive, and cardiogenic. All etiologies grouped into one functional state have a common final pathway responsible for impaired oxygen delivery. Acute hypovolemia from a reduction in circulating blood is the most common cause of shock in children beyond the neonatal period (Perkin and Levin, 1982). The most common cause of shock in the newborn is sepsis. Table 23–10 outlines the most common etiologies of circulatory failure according to functional states.

In summary, the common final pathway of shock is inadequate oxygen delivery to the tissues. There are a vast number of potential etiologies producing this state that can be classified according to the dominant functional derangement.

TABLE 23–10. CAUSES OF CIRCULATORY FAILURE IN CHILDREN

Functional State	Etiology

Hypovolemic (decreased preload)	Whole blood loss
	  Trauma
	  Intracranial bleeding (infant)
	Plasma loss
	  Burns
	  Intestinal obstruction
	  Capillary leak syndrome
	Fluid and electrolyte loss
	  Vomiting and diarrhea
	  Sunstroke
	  Diabetes insipidus
	  Diabetes mellitus
	Relative loss
	  Vasodilating drugs, e.g., morphine
	  Positive pressure ventilation
	  Sepsis
	  Anaphylaxis

Transport	Anemia Carbon monoxide poisoning Methemoglobinemia
Obstructive	Hemopericardium Pneumopericardium Tension pneumothorax Pericardial effusion Congenital heart defects Ventricular inflow or outflow obstruction

Cardiogenic	Dysrhythmias
	Drug intoxication
	Hypoxic/ischemic episodes
	Acidemia
	Hypothermia
	Myocardiopathies
	Congenital heart defects
	  Ventricular inflow or outflow obstruction
	  Large septal defects
	  Anomalous coronary arteries

Section Seven: Clinical Manifestations

At the completion of this section, the learner will be able to list the clinical manifestations of shock in children.

As with adults, shock in children is progressive and consists of three phases: compensated, uncompensated, and irreversible. Clinical findings will vary depending on the phase and specific etiology of circulatory failure. This section compares and contrasts normal and abnormal cardiovascular parameters as they relate to the child experiencing shock.

Heart Rate

The newborn's myocardium is less compliant and has less contractile mass than the older infant and child (Friedman, 1972). Therefore, in order to increase CO, the newborn's heart is more dependent on an accelerated heart rate than on increasing contractility and altering preload and afterload. Heart rate in children normally decreases with age as stroke volume increases. The normal heart rate limits for children depend not only on age and physiologic status but on the emotional state as well. In general, the normal ranges of resting pulse are

Newborn	120–180
1 year	100–130
2 years	90–120
4 years	80–110
> 8 years	70–100

Sinus tachycardia is seen frequently in children who are experiencing stress (e.g., fever, anxiety, hypovolemia). It is a compensatory mechanism to increase CO and oxygen delivery. Sinus bradycardia is a very early sign of hypoxemia in the infant but is a late sign in the older child.

Unlike the adult, life-threatening dysrhythmias in children often are a secondary response to hypoxemia and acidosis. Once hypoxemia and acidosis are corrected, normal sinus rhythm usually resumes and is maintained. For emergency assessment and management, pediatric dysrhythmias are classified into one of three groups based on heart rate.

1. Tachydysrhythmias
2. Bradydysrhythmias
3. Disorganized or absent rhythms

Table 23–11 summarizes the most common dysrhythmias seen in children and their clinical significance.

Blood Pressure

Blood pressure is determined by CO and systemic vascular resistance. It normally increases with age. Table 23–12 lists the range of normal blood pressure for age. A simple formula can be used to quickly estimate the 50th percentile of systolic blood pressure (SBP) in children over 2 years of age (Chameides, 1988).

$$SBP = 90 + (2 \times \text{age in years})$$

Usually blood pressure will remain in a normal range despite a decrease in circulating blood volume because of circulatory compensation, e.g., vasoconstriction, increased contractility, and tachycardia. Hypotension is often a late and sudden finding in children and may not develop until the intravascular volume has been depleted by at least 25 percent

TABLE 23–11. PEDIATRIC RHYTHM DISTURBANCES

Classification	Etiology	Clinical Significance
Tachyarrhythmias	Sinus tachycardia	Related to physical/emotional stress
	Supraventricular tachycardia (SVT)	Usually caused by a reentry mechanism
	Ventricular tachycardia	Usually related to underlying structural heart disease or prolonged QT interval
		Other causes include poisons, medications, hypoxia, acidosis, electrolyte imbalance
Bradyarrhythmias	Sinus bradycardia	Most common terminal rhythms with cardiopulmonary arrest
	Sinus node arrest with escape beats	
	Atrioventricular blocks	
Absent or disorganized rhythms	Asystole	Terminal rhythm with cardiopulmonary arrest
	Ventricular fibrillation (VF)	Uncommon rhythm in children
	Electromechanical dissociation (EMD)	Exact mechanism unknown, may result from tension pneumothorax, cardiac tamponade, hypovolemia, severe acidosis, hypoxemia

TABLE 23–12. NORMAL BLOOD PRESSURE RANGES

Age	Systolic Pressure (mm Hg)	Diastolic Pressure (mm Hg)
Neonate (1 month)	85–100	51–65
Infant (6 months)	87–105	53–66
Toddler (2 years)	95–105	53–66
School age (7 years)	97–112	57–71
Adolescent (15 years)	112–128	66–80

Blood pressure tables taken from the 50th to 90th percentile ranges of the ages noted; extrapolated from graphs. Adapted from Report of the Second Task Force on Blood Pressure in Children 1987, by M.J. Horan (Chairman), 1987, *Pediatrics*. 79:5–7. Reproduced by permission of *Pediatrics* Vol. 79, p. 57, copyright 1987.

(Mayer, 1985). Systolic arterial blood pressure may be normal or elevated with an early stage of septic shock.

Peripheral Perfusion

Because sinus tachycardia may occur for numerous, nonacute reasons and blood pressure is a late sign in circulatory failure, peripheral perfusion needs to be assessed. Table 23–13 summarizes early and late clinical signs of decreased perfusion from a low CO state. In contrast to symptoms associated with a low output state, early septic shock symptoms are characterized by vascular tone abnormalities and hyperdynamic compensatory responses. Symptoms include warm extremities, bounding pulses, normal

TABLE 23–13. CLINICAL SIGNS OF DECREASED PERFUSION

	Early	Late
Pulses	Peripheral pulses decreased and central pulses present	Loss of central pulse
Skin	Capillary refill time increases 2 seconds	Capillary refill time increases with time
	Newborn: gray and ashen color	All age groups: cyanosis
	Older child: pallor	
	Cool extremities	Coolness progresses toward trunk
Brain	Altered level of consciousness	
	Infant: irritable, fretful look, weak cry, wrinkled brow	Failure to recognize parents (over 2 months)
	Child: alternating lethargy and agitation	Unresponsive to procedures
Kidneys	Decreased urine output <1 mL/kg/hour[a]	Anuric

[a] Normal urine output is 1–2 mL/kg/hour.

capillary refill, normal urine output, mild mental confusion, and wide pulse pressure.

Monitoring

In addition to physical assessment findings, continuous monitoring of cardiac function is indicated. The most useful parameters to monitor continuously include urine output, heart rate and rhythm, arterial blood pressure, central venous pressure, pulmonary artery pressure, and pulmonary artery capillary wedge pressure. Relative increases or decreases in cardiac parameters depend in part on the functional type of shock. For a review of these hemodynamic changes, the reader is referred to Module 8, *Shock States.*

In summary, circulatory failure represents inadequate perfusion of body tissues. The clinical manifestations of circulatory failure result from compensatory mechanisms and end-organ dysfunction. The key to a successful outcome is early recognition of impending circulatory failure.

Section Eight: Nursing Management

At the completion of this section, the learner will be able to describe specific interventions used to manage a child with circulatory failure.

The primary goal in the treatment of circulatory failure is to restore normal blood flow and maximize oxygen delivery immediately. The interventions needed will depend on the specific functional shock state and the degree of cardiovascular dysfunction. This section discusses initial interventions that are common to all forms of shock, as well as highlighting differential diagnosis.

Regardless of the etiology of shock, emergency management is the same. Treatment is based on the adequacy of airway, breathing, and circulation (ABCs). Management of the airway and breathing is discussed in Part I of this module. For the child with an adequate heart rate, the goal of circulatory management is early establishment of venous access for administration of fluids and medications.

Venous Access

Central cannulation is desired because of direct access to central circulation for fluid and medication administration. However, for a child who is volume depleted and vasoconstricted, the most accessible vein may be used. There are a number of peripheral sites that may be cannulated: scalp, arm, leg, hand, and foot (Rossetti et al, 1985). If IV access is impossible or significantly delays treatment in the young child (<3 years old), intraosseous cannulation should be used temporarily (Chameides, 1988). The nurse should be familiar with the technique for intraosseous cannulation so that she can assist with the procedure as needed (Table 23–14).

Fluid Administration

The two most common etiologies of shock in the child are hypovolemia and sepsis. Both of these forms of shock require volume resuscitation. Once venous access is obtained, the nurse should assist with rapid infusion of fluids (20 mL/kg) to reestablish intravascular volume. The specific type of IV fluid to use is controversial. The American Heart Association recommends a balanced crystalloid solution (normal saline, Ringer's lactate solution) for first-line volume expansion (Chameides, 1988).

The type and amount of subsequent fluid administration should be based on etiology and duration of shock and ongoing losses. For hypovolemic shock without myocardial dysfunction, an isotonic bolus may be repeated until there are clinical signs of improvement: decreased heart rate and metabolic ac-

idosis and increased pulse pressure, systemic arterial pressure, and urine output. However, central venous pressure (CVP) monitoring is generally recommended after two boluses of fluid. For a CVP greater than 10 mm Hg, subsequent fluid challenges should be administered carefully, and alternative etiologies of shock should be sought.

For cardiogenic or septic shock, volume resuscitation must be monitored carefully. Ideally, function of the right and left sides of the heart should be assessed by continuously monitoring CVP and pulmonary capillary wedge pressure (PCWP). The higher the CVP and PCWP, the smaller the amount of fluid challenge. After a fluid challenge, the CVP and PCWP should be observed for 10 minutes. Fluid challenges are repeated until there are clinical signs of improvement, the CVP exceeds the previous pressure reading by 2 mm Hg, or the PCWP exceeds the previous pressure reading by 3 mm Hg (Perkin and Levin, 1982). The specific nursing care related to CVP monitoring in the child is similar to that for the adult.

Isooncotic fluids may be indicated for patients with hypovolemia and hypoproteinemia or in patients with underlying cardiac, renal, or pulmonary disease. Because smaller amounts of oncotic fluids are necessary to expand the intravascular space and underlying disease may be present, careful monitoring of CVP and PCWP is preferred.

Medications

In addition to volume expansion, medications may be indicated to improve myocardial contractility, to correct metabolic acidosis, to correct hypoxemia, and to improve cardiac rate and rhythm (Chameides, 1988). Oxygen is a first-line medication and should be administered in the highest available concentration to the unstable child. Table 23–15 lists the first-line medications used in pediatric cardiopulmonary resuscitation. After each intervention, the nurse should reassess the patient's clinical response (e.g., heart rate and rhythm, peripheral pulses, level of consciousness).

Continuous infusions of medications also may be used to support blood pressure and maintain CO. The endogenous catecholamine response in children is variable. Little information is available regarding age-related responses to catecholamines. Therefore, catecholamine infusions in children should be titrated to individual responses while monitoring clinical and hemodynamic effects (Zaritsky and Chernow, 1984). Table 23–16 lists commonly used continuous infusions in pediatric cardiopulmonary resuscitation.

Definitive management of circulatory failure de-

TABLE 23–14. TECHNIQUE FOR INTRAOSSEOUS CANNULATION

1. Obtain equipment	16 or 18 gauge hypodermic needle 18 or 20 gauge spinal needle with stylet Bone marrow needle IV tubing IV fluid
2. Identify site	Flat anterior medial surface of the proximal tibial shaft, 2–3 cm distal to the tibial tuberosity
3. Prepare the site	Same technique for any invasive procedure
4. Insert the catheter with stylet	Penetrate the skin and advance the needle perpendicular or slightly inferiorly to avoid the epiphyseal plate[a] Apply a twisting rotary motion while advancing; a give, or release of resistance, is usually felt
5. Confirm placement	Needle stands upright without support Aspiration of bone marrow contents Free flow of fluids after infusion begun Sensation of less resistance
6. Start infusion or drug administration	

[a] If the needle becomes obstructed with bone chips or marrow, it can be replaced with a second needle inserted through the same site.

TABLE 23–15. DRUGS USED IN PEDIATRIC CARDIOPULMONARY RESUSCITATION AND POSTRESUSCITATION STABILIZATION

Drug	Dose	How Supplied	Remarks
Epinephrine hydrochloride	0.01 mg/kg 0.1 mL/kg	1:10,000 (0.1 (mg/mL)	Most useful drug in cardiac arrest; 1:1,000 must be diluted
Sodium bicarbonate	1 mEq/kg 1 mL/kg	1 mEq/mL (8.4% solution)	Infuse slowly and only when ventilation is adequate
Atropine sulfate	0.02 mg/kg 0.2 mL/kg	0.1 mg/mL	Minimum dose of 0.1 mg (1 mL); use of bradycardia after assessing ventilation Maximum dose: infants and children 1.0 mg; adolescents 2.0 mg
Calcium chloride	20 mg/kg (0.2 mL/kg)	100 mg/mL (10% solution)	Use only for hypocalcemia, calcium blocker overdose, hyperkalemia, or hypermagnesemia; give slowly
Glucose	0.5–1.0 g/kg	0.5 g/mL $D_{50}W$	Dilute 1:1 with water ($D_{25}W$): dose is then 2–4 mL/kg
Lidocaine hydrochloride	1 mg/kg	10 mg/mL (1%) (20 mg/mL (2%)	Used for ventricular arrhythmias only
Bretylium tosylate	5 mg/kg	50 mg/mL	Use if lidocaine is not effective; repeat dose with 10 mg/kg if first dose not effective

Adapted from *Textbook of pediatric advanced life support*, p. 57, by L. Chameides, 1988, Dallas: American Heart Association.

pends on the etiology. Most often, etiology can be determined based on physical examination and history. Figure 23–2 outlines guidelines for management and differential diagnosis of shock in the child.

In summary, the most common form of shock in children is hypovolemic from a total decrease in intravascular volume or from a relative decrease in intravascular volume due to vasodilation. Nursing management is based on early recognition of signs and symptoms of shock, assisting with venous access and volume expansion, and continuous reassessment.

TABLE 23–16. CONTINUOUS INFUSIONS USED IN PEDIATRIC CARDIOPULMONARY RESUSCITATION

Infusions	Dose	How Supplied	Remarks
Epinephrine infusion	0.1–1.0 μg/kg/minute	1mg/mL 1:1,000	Titrate infusion to desired hemodynamic effect
Dopamine hydrochloride	2–20 μg/kg/minute	40 mg/mL	Titrate to desired hemodynamic infusion response
Dobutamine infusion	5–20 μg/kg/minute	250 mg/vial lyophilized	Titrate to desired hemodynamic response; little vasoconstriction even at high rates
Isoproterenol infusion	0.1–1.0 μg/kg/minute	1 mg/5 mL	Titrate to desired hemodynamic effect; vasodilator
Lidocaine infusion	20–50 μg/kg/minute	40 mg/mL (4%)	Use lower infusion dose with shock, liver disease

Adapted from *Textbook of pediatric advanced life support*, p. 57, by L. Chameides, 1988, Dallas: American Heart Association.

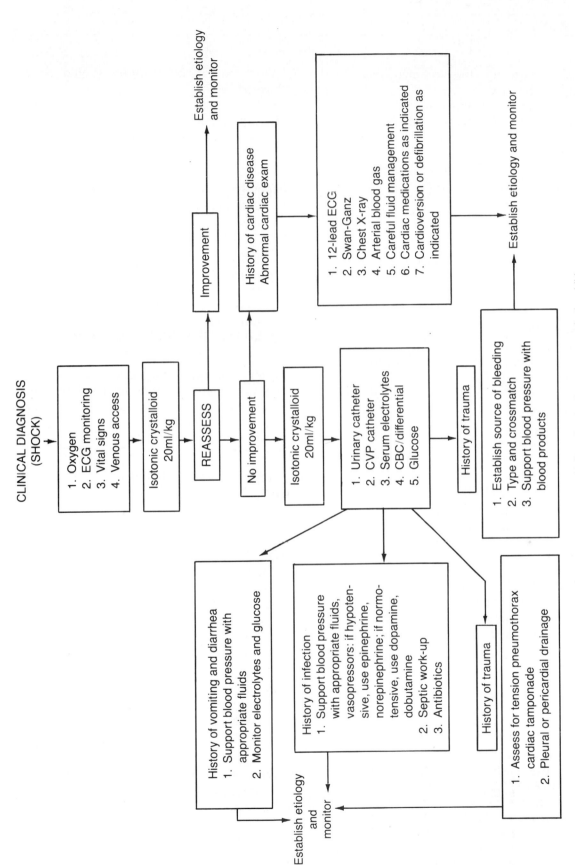

Figure 23–2. Emergency guidelines for shock management in the child.

Perfusion Review

1. Functional closure of the foramen ovale postnatally results from
   A. an increase in left atrial pressure
   B. an increase in arterial oxygen tension
   C. an increase in pulmonary artery pressure
   D. an increase in right-sided heart pressure
2. Pulmonary vascular resistance decreases to normal adult values most often by
   A. 1 week of age
   B. 2 months of age
   C. 2 years of age
   D. 6 months of age
3. In the older child, the most common functional shock state is
   A. obstructive
   B. cardiogenic
   C. hypovolemic
   D. transport
4. An early sign of circulatory failure in children is
   A. hypotension
   B. bradycardia
   C. tachycardia
   D. absent femoral pulse
5. Sinus bradycardia in the newborn is most often due to
   A. structural damage to sinoatrial node
   B. congenital heart surgery
   C. drug toxicity
   D. hypoxemia
6. The recommended first-line IV fluid for hypovolemic shock in children is
   A. lactated Ringer's solution
   B. dextrose 5% in water
   C. dextrose 5% with 0.2% normal saline
   D. fresh frozen plasma

Refer to the following case study to answer Questions 7 through 10.

Johnny is a 2-month-old, 5 kg boy admitted to the intensive care unit with a 3-day history of fever. On admission, he is lethargic and minimally responsive to noxious stimuli. Vital signs are: temperature 103.1F (39.5C), heart rate 180, respiratory rate 80, blood pressure 50 by palpation. Extremities are cool and pale in color. Lungs are clear to auscultation.

7. What nursing intervention should be performed first?
   A. IV line insertion
   B. supplemental oxygen
   C. synchronized cardioversion
   D. acetaminophen administration

Peripheral IV line insertion has been attempted for 10 minutes without success.

8. Access to the circulation should be attempted by which of the following routes?
   A. central cannulation
   B. cutdown cannulation
   C. intraosseous cannulation
   D. arterial cannulation

Access to the circulation is successful. The patient becomes unresponsive. The heart rate is 190, and the blood pressure is no longer palpable. Femoral pulses are faint.

9. How much fluid should Johnny receive as a bolus?
   A. 50 mL
   B. 150 mL
   C. 500 mL
   D. 100 mL
10. What type of IV solution should be used for the bolus?
    A. lactated Ringer's solution
    B. 5% dextrose in water
    C. 5% dextrose in 0.2 normal saline
    D. albumin

Another bolus of fluid is given. Johnny's vital signs are stabilized. A urinary catheter is inserted for urine output monitoring.

11. What should be the normal urine output per hour for Johnny?
    A. 20 mL
    B. 30 mL
    C. 10 mL
    D. 2 mL

Answers: 1,A. 2, B. 3, C. 4, C. 5, D. 6, A. 7, B. 8, C. 9, D. 10, A. 11, C.

COGNITION/PERCEPTION

Section Nine: Maturational Anatomy and Physiology

At the completion of this section, the learner will be able to discuss the unique anatomic and physiologic characteristics of the immature CNS.

Accurate assessment and management of CNS disorders in children is complicated by the fact that CNS development is incomplete at birth. In fact, for the first 3 years of life, CNS maturation continues at the same rate as in utero. Because the immature CNS is qualitatively and quantitatively different from the adult's CNS, it is commonly believed that it may respond to injuries differently. This section discusses the unique features of the immature CNS.

There are a number of developmental differences of the immature CNS that not only predispose the young child to traumatic brain injury but also are responsible for specific types of characteristic brain injuries. Table 23–17 summarizes the key developmental differences of the immature CNS. Postnatal myelination, glial cell growth, dendritic arborization, and increased synaptic connections are responsible for the rapid increase in head size and weight. The child's brain weight is approximately 70 percent of adult weight at 4 years of age and 90 percent at 6 years of age. The child's relatively large head, as well as limited supporting neck muscles, predisposes him to traumatic brain injury with multiple trauma. In addition, because the skull is thin and pliable, it offers less protection against external trauma.

Adequate cerebral blood flow (CBF) is critical for normal cellular function of the brain. Factors that control CBF (e.g., $Paco_2$, cerebral perfusion pressure, CPP) have been studied extensively in animals and in adults, but comparable research does not exist for newborns and infants. Because of the physiologic differences among newborns, infants, and adults, mechanisms that control CBF in the adult may not hold true for the young child.

In summary, there are significant anatomic and physiologic differences of the CNS between young children and adults. CNS growth occurs at a very rapid rate for the first few years of life. Age-related differences in the CNS need to be considered when assessing and managing a child with neurologic dysfunction.

TABLE 23–17. UNIQUE FEATURES OF THE IMMATURE NERVOUS SYSTEM

Myelinization	Within the CNS, myelinization progresses most rapidly in the first postnatal year and is complete by the second decade of life
Glial cell population	Cell members increase into third year of life
Dendritic arborization and synaptic connection	Occur primarily in the first and second postnatal years
Brain weight	Increases from 25% of adult weight at birth to 70% of adult weight at 4 years of age
Skull	Thin and pliable at birth with unfused suture lines (independent floating plates) Orbital roofs and floors of middle fossa smooth
Water content of cortical and white matter	Decreases from 87% and 89% at birth to 85% and 78% during first decade
Cerebral blood flow	Normal values are not known for infants and young children
Cerebrospinal fluid (CSF)	Normal volume production is not known for infants and young children A few white blood cells present in CSF; higher concentration of glucose and protein in CSF

Adapted from Head injuries in children, by P. Vernon-Levett, 1991, *Crit. Care Nursing Clin. North Am.* 3:412.

Section Ten: Etiologies

At the completion of this section, the learner will be able to list the most common types of neurologic dysfunction in children.

There are a number of potential circumstances and disease processes that can adversely affect the CNS. This section discusses the most common forms of severe neurologic dysfunction in children: status epilepticus, traumatic brain injury, and CNS infection. Defining terms and pathogenesis of each disorder are described.

Status Epilepticus

Seizures are described as abnormal electrical impulses originating from the cerebral cortex. Status epilepticus is defined as a continuing series of seizures without regaining full consciousness between seizures or one continuous seizure lasting approximately 30 minutes. The cause of status epilepticus in children is approximately 30 percent idiopathic and 60 percent to 70 percent symptomatic (Delgado, 1990). The majority of symptomatic cases are from hyperthermia (febrile seizures) and CNS infection. Less common causes of seizures include trauma, metabolic derangement, drug intoxication, and acute anoxia. Although the cause of status epilepticus may vary, the common final pathway of uncontrolled electrical activity is anoxia and cellular death.

Traumatic Brain Injury

Traumatic brain injury (TBI) is one of the leading causes of mortality and morbidity in children. TBI in children is different from TBI in adults in several important ways: mechanism of injury, specific types of injury, and response to injury. The most common cause of TBI in infancy is from falls. The older child is more often injured from a motor vehicle-related accident as a passenger, pedestrian, or cyclist.

Specific types of TBI commonly are classified according to chronologic events. CNS damage that can be attributed directly to forces at the moment of impact are primary injuries. CNS damage that develops as a consequence of the primary injury is referred to as a secondary injury. Secondary TBI most often has a common final pathway of raised ICP, which is an important feature determining outcome. Table 23–18 summarizes the most common forms of primary and secondary head injuries in children.

Although the exact mechanisms are not understood, the immature CNS responds to injury differently in children. The overall incidence of diffuse bilateral cerebral swelling and subsequent increased intracranial pressure (IICP) is much higher in children compared to adults. The incidence of focal brain injury is lower in children compared to adults (Bruce et al, 1981).

CNS Infections

The most common type of CNS infection during childhood is meningitis (inflammation of the meninges), and it is almost always bacterial in origin. The highest incidence occurs in infants less than 1 year of age. In newborns, the most common pathogens producing acute bacterial meningitis are group B streptococcus, *Escherichia coli*, and *Listeria monocytogenes*. Between 2 months and 12 years of age, the primary offending pathogens include *Streptococcus pneumoniae*, *Haemophilus influenzae*, and *Neisseria meningitidis*.

Invasion of the meninges most often results from bacteremia from a distant site of infection, such as the upper respiratory tract. Less frequently, it may develop as a consequence of direct pathogenic invasion from penetrating trauma, surgical procedures, or paranasal infections. If the bacterial infection is left untreated or progresses rapidly throughout the CNS, irreversible damage or death usually results from IICP.

In summary, the most common CNS disorders seen in the acutely ill child include status epilepticus, TBI, and CNS infection. Status epilepticus is usually a symptom of an underlying problem, TBI produces characteristic head injuries in young children, and meningitis occurs most often in the infant.

Section Eleven: Clinical Manifestations

At the completion of this section, the learner will be able to describe the key components of the neurologic examination of the child with altered mental status.

Effective nursing management of the neurologically impaired child is based on initial and serial neurologic assessments. As described in Section Nine of this module, the infant's CNS is structurally and functionally different than the older child's and adult's CNS. For these reasons, the neurologic examination of the infant varies from that of the older child and the adult. Differences in the neurologic examination do not vary in terms of the process but in terms of findings. The purpose of this section is to describe the key components and significant findings of the rapid neurologic assessment of the child with impaired CNS function. Diagnostic data used to assess the child with status epilepticus, TBI, and CNS infection are described.

Regardless of age, the clinical manifestations of neurologic dysfunction are related to the degree and duration of CNS hypoperfusion (relative or actual). Neurologic dysfunction with corresponding assessments is on a continuum. A child with a severe primary TBI may be in unresponsive coma, whereas a child with a slow growing intracranial tumor may have progressive signs of IICP. A complete neurologic examination may be inappropriate, impractical, and too time consuming for all patients. How-

TABLE 23–18. COMMON HEAD INJURIES IN CHILDREN

Primary	Minor
	Caput succedaneum[a]
	Cephalohematoma[a]
	Scalp laceration
	Scalp contusion
	Cerebral laceration
	Moderate/severe
	Concussion
	Contusion
	Skull fractures
	Simple linear
	Basilar
	Depressed
	Growing[a]
	Diffuse axonal injury
Secondary	Moderate/severe
	Expanding intracranial lesions
	Diffuse cerebral edema

[a] Usually limited to infancy.

TABLE 23–19. PERTINENT HISTORY INFORMATION

Infant	Maternal history
	Age, previous births, prepartum and intrapartum course
	Neonatal history
	Feeding, sucking, and crying patterns; presence of apnea, cyanotic spells, infection, jaundice, or seizures; Apgar score
	Developmental milestones
	Motor
	Infantile reflexes
	Verbal
	Medical history
	Psychiatric history
Child (> 2 years)	Developmental milestones
	Motor
	Verbal
	Medical history
	Psychiatric history

ever, there are key components of the neurologic assessment that must be completed for every patient: patient history, vital signs, level of consciousness, motor function, pupil signs, and brainstem function.

Patient History

The patient history can provide valuable information regarding the patient's baseline neurologic development, diagnosis, and prognosis. Pertinent history information should be individualized to the age, condition, and disposition of the child. For a traumatic injury or an acute event, the sequence of events before the injury or episode is important. For more gradual deterioration, the chief complaint and related assessments are critical to diagnosis and management. Table 23–19 lists additional pertinent history information that needs to be obtained on admission.

Vital Signs

Vital signs often are nonspecific and need to be correlated with coexisting disease states. Temperature may be abnormally elevated due to infection, drug intoxication, shock, and intracranial bleeding. It may also be low in the newborn with immature thermostatic control or a preexisting infection. Abnormal patterns of breathing associated with pathologic lesions may be difficult to differentiate in the child. Respiratory assessment should include rate and description of the pattern of breathing. Abnormal car-

diac rhythms usually are transient. However, symptomatic bradycardia often is a late sign of IICP. Another late and inconstant sign of IICP is an increase in systolic pressure, with a widened pulse pressure.

Level of Consciousness

Consciousness is a state of awareness of oneself and environment. An altered level of consciousness (LOC) results from disease states that significantly alter functioning of the cerebral hemispheres, the reticular activating system, or both. The range of LOC may vary from minor alterations to unresponsive coma. The Glasgow Coma Scale (GCS) is a widely used neurologic assessment tool to grade the depth of coma by standardizing assessments (Teasdale and Jennett, 1974). It consists of three sections, each of which measures a separate function of LOC: arousability, mentation, and motor function. The GCS has one main disadvantage in infants: it cannot accurately assess preverbal infants. As a result, a number of institutions and individuals have modified the GCS. Tables 23–20 is an example of a modified GCS for infants.

Motor Function

Motor functions can be assessed easily in the older child by using the categories outlined in the GCS. In the infant, motor function needs to be compared with developmental milestones and age-appropriate primitive reflexes. For example, a positive Babinski response is an abnormal finding in the older child and adult but a normal finding in the 6-month-old.

TABLE 23–20. MODIFIED COMA SCALE FOR INFANTS

Activity	Best Response	Score
Eye opening	Spontaneous	4
	To speech	3
	To pain	2
	None	1
Verbal	Coos and babbles	5
	Irritable cries	4
	Cries to pain	3
	Moans to pain	2
	None	1
Motor	Normal spontaneous movements	6
	Withdraws to touch	5
	Withdraws to pain	4
	Abnormal flexion	3
	Abnormal extension	2
	None	1

From *Textbook of pediatric critical care*, p. 658, by M.C. Rogers, © 1987, the Williams & Wilkins Co., Baltimore.

Pupil Signs

The integrity of the brainstem and the depth of coma can be further assessed by examining the pupils. As in the adult, the child's pupils are evaluated for size, reactivity, and shape. Abnormal findings and their clinical significance are essentially the same in the child as in the adult. Refer to Module 12, *Responsiveness,* for additional information.

Brainstem Function

In addition to pupil signs, brainstem function should be further assessed. For the comatose child, brainstem function is limited to assessment of the corneal reflex, the oculocephalic response, the oculovestibular response, and abnormal spontaneous eye movements. The presence of abnormal findings has the same clinical significance for the child as for the adult. Refer to Module 12, *Responsiveness,* for additional information.

Meningeal Irritation Signs

If meningitis is suspected, the presence of meningeal irritation should be assessed. Kernig's sign may be present and is elicited by placing the child supine with the hips flexed and passively extending the leg at the knee. With significant meningeal irritation, the child may resist and complain of back pain. Brudzinski's sign produces involuntary flexion of the knees and hips with passive flexion of the child's neck when supine. Signs of meningeal irritation may be less specific or unreliable in the infant. However, the infant may have paradoxical irritability: comforting the child by holding him may paradoxically produce more irritability.

Intracranial Pressure

Normal ICP in infants is unknown. In the toddler and older child, it is estimated to be less than 10 mm Hg and 15 mm Hg, respectively (Shapiro and Giller, 1990). Clinical signs of IICP vary depending on the age of the child. In infants with open fontanels and unfused cranial sutures, clinical signs of IICP are less acute and more nonspecific than in the older child. Table 23–21 lists the signs and symptoms of IICP in children.

Clinical evidence of IICP may not be present until significant increases in ICP have occurred. The most precise means of assessing changes in ICP and evaluating the effectiveness of pressure reduction therapy is with continuous ICP monitoring. There are a number of invasive ICP monitoring devices available, all of which have advantages and disad-

TABLE 23–21. SIGNS AND SYMPTOMS OF INCREASED INTRACRANIAL PRESSURE[a]

Infants less than 2 years of age	Lethargy
	Poor feeding
	Poor suck
	Bulging, tense anterior fontanel
	Increased head circumference
	Irritability
Older child	Nausea
	Vomiting
	Anorexia
	Headache
	Papilledema (chronic IICP)[b]
	Alteration in LOC
	Visual disturbances
	Lethargy
	Third nerve palsy (transtentorial herniation)
	Sixth nerve palsy (diffuse IICP)

[a] Clinical manifestations vary and depend on how rapidly cerebral hypertension develops.
[b] IICP, increased intracranial pressure; LOC, level of consciousness.

vantages. The most common sites for ICP monitoring are intraventricular, subdural, epidural, and parenchymal. Generally, these devices are difficult to place in the young infant because of their soft skull bones and small lateral ventricles. The reader should review Module 14, *Nursing Care of the Patient with Multiple Injuries,* for a more complete description of monitoring devices.

Neurodiagnostic Evaluation

To assist with the clinical evaluation of the neurologically impaired child, several neurodiagnostic techniques may be used. A lumbar puncture for CSF analysis is a commonly used procedure in children with suspected CNS infection. CSF values in a child with bacterial meningitis include

1. Cloudy appearance
2. WBC > 500 mm^3
3. Protein > 100 mg/100 mL
4. Glucose < $^1/_2$ to $^1/_3$ blood glucose
5. Gram stain/culture: positive
6. Polymorphonuclear leukocytes predominate

Signs and symptoms of IICP (focal neurologic deficits, papilledema, altered level of consciousness) contraindicate a lumbar puncture.

The use of skull radiographs in evaluating traumatic brain injury has been under much debate in recent years (Marshall et al, 1990). In most situations, CT remains the procedure of choice with a head injury less than 72 hours old (Snow et al, 1986). MRI is superior to CT in imaging the posterior fossa, spinal cord structures, small vascular lesions, and most brain tumors (Marshall et al, 1990). Electroencephalography (EEG) may be used as an adjunct to the clinical examination. The indications, use, and interpretation of EEG findings are similar for the child and adult.

In summary, the key components of the neurologic assessment are the same regardless of age. However, the evaluation process should be adapted to the developmental level and conditions of the child. It is essential that the examiner be able to distinguish between age-appropriate normal findings and subtle abnormal changes in neurologic function. Early detection of subtle changes with prompt treatment can improve outcome.

Section Twelve: Nursing Management

At the completion of this section, the learner will be able to discuss the nursing management of the neurologically impaired child.

The first steps in managing a child with acute neurologic dysfunction are related to the ABCs. A patient who is hypoxic or hypotensive may invalidate the neurologic assessment. Airway patency, adequacy of breathing, and perfusion must be assessed and supported if necessary. Elective intubation may be required for airway protection and controlled hyperventilation. Once oxygenation, ventilation, and circulation are adequate, attention may be directed to treating the underlying neurologic disorder. The focus of this section is to describe the management of a child with status epilepticus, TBI, and CNS infection.

Status Epilepticus

The goals in treating a child with status epilepticus are threefold: maintenance of adequate CBF, controlling seizure activity, and treatment of systemic abnormalities. Adequate CBF can be maintained with adherence to the basic principles of the ABCs. When a child is in status epilepticus, the nurse should be prepared to protect the patient from physical injury, prevent aspiration by turning the patient's head to the side, and maximize oxygenation by administering oxygen. Hypoglycemia is a common finding, precipitating a seizure in the young infant. Therefore, a rapid glucose approximation (Dextrostix/Chemostrip) should be obtained as soon as feasible. Additional laboratory studies usually are ordered by the physician when appropriate.

There are no universally accepted guidelines for the selection or order of administration of anticonvulsants. However, there are a number of general principles that are considered by the health care team when selecting appropriate drug therapy (Rosenberg, 1990).

1. The IV route is preferred.
2. Long-acting medications need to follow short-acting medications for maintenance.
3. Respiratory depression should be expected and easily controlled.

Nurses should be aware of the commonly used anticonvulsants to control seizures, as well as their side effects. For example, respiratory depression is a common side effect with many anticonvulsants. Therefore, nurses should always be prepared to assist with airway protection and supportive ventilation. Table 23–22 lists commonly used anticonvulsants to control seizures in children.

As the seizure is being controlled, it is also important to control systemic abnormalities (e.g., hypoglycemia, hyperthermia, hypoxemia) that may have caused or resulted from the seizure.

TABLE 23–22. INITIAL ANTICONVULSANTS TO CONTROL STATUS EPILEPTICUS

Drug	Dose	Rate of Administration	Time to Effect	Side Effects
Rapid-acting agents Diazepam (undiluted)	Begin 0.25 mg/kg IV and titrate to effect	<1 mg/minute	1–2 minutes	Respiratory depression; thrombophlebitis
Lorazepam 2 mg/mL	0.1 mg/kg × 4, 20 minutes apart, max. dose 4 mg	1 mg/minute	2–3 minutes	Drowsiness, confusion, ataxia
Midazolam	0.075 mg/kg IV 0.150 mg/kg IM			Same as above; respiratory arrest
Longer-acting agents Phenytoin 50 mg/mL; dilute in normal saline 1:10	15 mg/kg up to 45 mg/kg	20–50 mg/minute	~20 minutes	Heart block; hypotension
Phenobarbital 130 mg/mL	10 mg/kg up to 30 mg/kg	30 mg/minute	10–12 minutes	Respiratory depression; hypotension

From *A practical guide to pediatric intensive care*, p. 231, by J.L. Blumer, 1990, Chicago: Mosby-Year Book.

Traumatic Brain Injury

Because of the relatively low incidence of intracranial lesions in children with TBI, most injuries are nonoperable. The most common secondary injury in children is diffuse bilateral cerebral swelling. Consequently, aggressive medical management to control IICP is the guiding principle for treating TBI in children. Table 23–23 lists the independent and collaborative nursing interventions to control IICP. As a general rule, the least invasive therapy to control IICP should be initiated first. Once IICP is controlled, the last intervention to be initiated or the most invasive intervention should be discontinued while continuously monitoring ICP.

CNS Infection

The goal in treating bacterial meningitis is early recognition, early administration of antimicrobials, and control of systemic effects. Early diagnosis and treatment are dependent on the neurologic assessment discussed in Section Eleven. The selection of antimicrobials is based on the most likely pathogens for a given age group. Until cerebrospinal fluid culture results are known, broad-spectrum antibiotics are used for all suspected cases of meningitis. Advanced cases of meningitis also may cause abnormal systemic effects, such as hypotension, hyperthermia, and

IICP. Immediate attention must be given to supporting circulation and controlling IICP.

In summary, initial management of the child with an acute neurologic disorder is based on maintaining adequate cerebral blood flow by focusing on the ABCs. Beyond resuscitation, therapy should be directed to controlling systemic effects and correcting the primary disorder.

TABLE 23–23. NURSING MANAGEMENT OF INCREASED INTRACRANIAL PRESSURE

Independent nursing interventions	Elevate head of bed 30°
	Position head in midline
	Hyperventilate with bag-valve-mask; maintain $Paco_2$[a] at approximately 25 mm Hg
	Preoxygenate and hyperventilate before suctioning
	Maintain normothermia
	Organize nursing care to minimize patient stimulation
Collaborative nursing interventions	Assist with and maintain intubation and controlled hyperventilation
	Administer supplemental oxygen to keep Pao_2[b] > 80–90 mm Hg
	Administer diuretics as ordered
	Administer anticonvulsants as ordered for seizure control
	Administer barbiturate therapy as ordered; monitor serum levels, neurologic status, and hemodynamic status

[a] $Paco_2$ partial pressure of carbon dioxide; Pao_2, partial pressure of oxygen.

Cognition/Perception Review

1. Which of the following statements best explains why the young child may be predisposed to traumatic brain injury?
   A. cerebral blood flow is lower in the child, which alters sensory and motor function
   B. the ratio of brain weight/body weight is greater in the child
   C. the skull thickness is greater in the child
   D. cranial nerve function is incomplete, altering motor function and balance
2. The best description of a positive Kernig's sign is
   A. involuntary flexion of the knees and hips with passive flexion of the child's neck
   B. resistance and complaints of pain with passive flexion of the lower leg while supine with hips flexed
   C. resistance and complaints of back pain with passive extension of the leg at the knee while supine with hips flexed
   D. increased irritability while holding the child

3. Intracranial hypertension following traumatic brain injury is more common in children than adults because
   A. there is a higher incidence of focal brain injury in children
   B. loss of autoregulation is more common in children
   C. diffuse bilateral cerebral edema is more common in children
   D. children do not respond as well to osmotic diuretics
4. Bacterial meningitis most often results from
   A. direct penetrating trauma to the CNS
   B. spina bifida
   C. a paranasal infection
   D. bacteremia from a distant site of infection

5. An infant less than 2 years of age with IICP would most likely demonstrate which of the following clinical manifestations?
   A. irritability, increased head circumference, poor feeding
   B. papilledema, headache, anorexia
   C. irritability, headache, visual disturbances
   D. papilledema, increased head circumference, poor suck

Refer to the following case study to answer Questions 6 through 8.

Melanie, an 18-month-old child, is brought to the intensive care unit with a history of fever for 2 days, irritability, loss of appetite, and lethargy. Vital signs are: temperature 101.3F (38.5C), heart rate 120, respiratory rate 50, and blood pressure 80/60. Breath sounds are clear, urine culture negative, WBC 20,000. A lumbar puncture is performed. Results are: cloudy appearance, WBC 604 mm³, protein 110 mg/100 mL, gram stain positive for gram-negative rods.

6. If Melanie is not treated quickly, which of the following pathophysiologic processes may develop?
   A. decreased perfusion from cardiogenic shock
   B. decreased perfusion from hypovolemic shock
   C. increased ICP
   D. hypoxemia from CNS-induced pulmonary edema

Melanie is diagnosed with bacterial meningitis.

7. Which of the following pathogens is most likely the cause?
   A. *Escherichia coli*
   B. *Haemophilus influenzae*
   C. respiratory syncytial virus
   D. *Pseudomonas aeruginosa*
8. Which of the following nursing interventions has the highest priority?
   A. administer broad-spectrum antibiotics
   B. assess airway and breathing
   C. administer medications to prevent hypotension
   D. hyperventilate with an Ambubag
9. Which of the following interventions to control IICP would be discontinued first?
   A. hyperventilation
   B. osmotic diuretics
   C. elevation of head of bed
   D. barbiturate therapy
10. Which of the following interventions would most likely be needed following the administration of diazepam for status epilepticus?
    A. bag-valve-mask ventilation
    B. isotonic fluid bolus 20 mL/kg
    C. naloxone administration
    D. dopamine administration

Answers: 1, B. 2, C. 3, C. 4, D. 5, A. 6, C. 7, B. 8, B. 9, D. 10, A.

METABOLISM/THERMOREGULATION

Section Thirteen: Fluid and Electrolytes

At the completion of this section, the learner will be able to describe nursing management of a child with alteration in fluid and electrolytes.

Alteration in fluid and electrolyte balance is more common in the young child than in the adult. Acutely ill children are at even greater risk because of compromised compensatory mechanisms. Fluid and electrolyte disturbances can be classified into one of three groups: dehydration, water intoxication, and third space fluid shifts. The group that is most characteristic of disturbances seen in children is de-hydration. This section focuses on the management of three forms of dehydration after a brief discussion of developmental considerations and calculations of fluid and electrolyte requirements.

Homeostasis

Fluid and electrolyte intake and output vary daily, but volume and composition of body fluids are maintained within a narrow therapeutic range. Organs that are responsible for fluid and electrolyte homeostasis are the kidneys, heart and blood vessels, pituitary gland, adrenal glands, parathyroid gland, hypothalamus, and lungs. The specific ways in which these organs regulate fluids and electrolytes is discussed in Module 19, *Fluid and Electrolyte Balance.*

Because of anatomic and physiologic differences in the child, regulatory mechanisms are less efficient in maintaining balance. Young children are predisposed to fluid and electrolyte imbalances for various reasons. Table 23–24 summarizes the developmental considerations of fluid and electrolyte balance and their clinical significance.

Fluid and Electrolyte Replacement Therapy

Many acutely ill children are totally dependent on parenteral replacement therapy to maintain fluid and electrolyte balance. The two determinants of replacement therapy are maintenance and deficit fluids. Maintenance fluids represent ongoing normal physiologic losses, and deficit fluids represent abnormal fluid losses before initiation of therapy.

Because of the narrow margin of safety when administering parental fluids to infants and young children, nurses should always double check calculations for infusion rates. There are several methods for calculating daily maintenance fluid needs. Table 23–25 illustrates a commonly used method to calcu-

TABLE 23–24. FLUID AND ELECTROLYTE BALANCE: DEVELOPMENTAL CONSIDERATIONS

Anatomic Difference[a]	Clinical Significance
Greater percentage of extracellular water	More prone to fluid loss with illness
Greater percentage of water per unit of weight	Fluid requirements are greater than in adult
Greater body surface area per unit of weight	Greater loss of fluids, electrolytes, and body heat with exhaled air and through skin evaporation and radiation
Renal tubules immature, with smaller surface area	Diminished response to ADH; inefficient absorption and excretion of electrolytes
Renal nephrons have relatively short loops	Inefficient concentration of urine; increased water loss
Physiologic Difference[a]	
Metabolic rate is twice the adult rate per unit of weight	Greater fluid exchange rate per day; less reserve of fluid; urea excretion (necessary for urine concentration) is low because infants are in a high anabolic state for growth; more prone to hypoglycemia
Low glycogen stores	More prone to hypoglycemia

[a] Anatomic and physiologic differences are seen primarily in the infant and young child.

TABLE 23–25. DAILY MAINTENANCE FLUID NEEDS

Body Weight	Fluid Amount
For each kg ≤ 10 kg	100 mL/kg/24 hours
For each kg, 11–20 kg	Add 50 mL/kg/24 hours
For each kg > 20 kg	Add 20 mL/kg/24 hours

Adapted from *A practical guide to pediatric intensive care*, p. 94, by D.L. Levin, F.C. Morriss, and G.C. Moore, 1984, St. Louis: C.V. Mosby.

late maintenance fluids as determined by body weight.

The following is an example of how to calculate daily maintenance fluids for a child who weighs 24 kg.

$$First\ 10\ kg = 10 \times 100\ mL = 1{,}000\ mL$$
$$11\text{–}20\ kg = 10 \times\ \ 50\ mL =\ \ \ 500\ mL$$
$$4\ kg =\ \ 4 \times\ \ 20\ mL =\ \ \ \ \ 80\ mL$$

Total fluids in 24 hours = 1,580 mL

Replacement therapy for deficit fluids is based on the degree of dehydration. This can be determined by calculating the percentage of weight loss when the preillness weight is known. The steps for calculating the percentage of weight loss follow.

1. Subtract the child's current weight (kg) from the preillness weight (kg)
   Example: Preillness weight = 10 kg
   Current weight   = 9 kg
   Difference   = 1 kg
2. Divide the weight loss (step 1) by the preillness weight
   Example: 1 kg/10 kg = 0.10
   Percentage of weight loss = 10%

For each 1 percent of weight loss, 10 mL/kg of fluid have been lost. In the example shown, an infant with a 10 percent weight loss has a fluid loss of 100 mL/kg ($10 \times 10 = 100$). Total fluid deficit is determined by multiplying the preillness weight by the milliliters per kilogram of fluid loss. Therefore, 100 mL/kg (fluid loss) is multiplied by 10 kg (preillness weight) to give a total fluid deficit of 1,000 mL. Deficit fluids need to be added to maintenance fluids to determine the total amount of replacement therapy. If preillness weight is not known, clinical assessment data should be used to estimate the percentage of dehydration (Table 23–26).

The type of parenteral fluid to use for replacement therapy is determined by sodium, potassium, and glucose requirements. Sodium and potassium requirements are based on calorie requirements per kilogram of body weight. Established ranges for sodium are 3 to 4 mEq/kg/24 hours and for potassium are 2 to 3 mEq/kg/24 hours. Normal glucose require-

TABLE 23–26. CLINICAL ASSESSMENT DATA: DEGREES OF DEHYDRATION

Area of Assessment	Mild Infant 5% loss Children 3% loss	Moderate Infant 10% loss Children 6% loss	Severe Infant 15% loss Children 9% loss
Thirst	Slight	Moderate	Intense
Anterior fontanel	Flat	Depressed	Very sunken
Skin	Pale, cool	Grayish	Cool, pale, mottled
Blood pressure	Normal	Decreased	Low
Pulse	Slightly increased	Increased, weak	Tachycardia (rapid, thready, feeble)
Skin turgor	Decreased	Loss of elasticity	Very poor (pinch retracts very slowly)
Mucous membranes	Normal to dry	Dry	Dry, cracked
Eyes	Normal	Somewhat depressed	Grossly sunken
Tears	Present	Decreased	Absent
Urine output	Decreased	Oliguria	Prerenal azotemia
Behavior	Normal, alert, possibly some restlessness	Irritable, restless or lethargic	Hyperirritable to lethargic, limp

From *Pediatric fluids and electrolytes*, p. 24, by D. O'Donnell and J. Lathrop, 1990, Milwaukee: Maxishare Corporation.

ments are 200 to 400 mg/kg/24 hours (Perkins and Levin, 1990). Table 23–27 lists the composition of commonly used parenteral fluids in children.

Management Principles

Dehydration is a very common form of fluid loss in the infant and young child. For purposes of treatment, dehydration usually is classified into isotonic, hypertonic, or hypotonic. Isotonic dehydration refers to loss of both fluid and electrolytes with the same osmolarity of blood. Hypertonic dehydration refers to fluid loss in excess of electrolyte loss. Blood osmolality is increased. Conversely, hypotonic dehydration occurs when electrolytes are lost in excess of fluids. Because sodium is the primary osmotic force controlling fluid movement between fluid compartments, dehydration often is described in terms of serum sodium level: isonatremia (serum sodium level normal), hyponatremia (serum sodium level low), and hypernatremia (serum sodium high).

Initial management of dehydration with circulatory failure is the same for all types of fluid and electrolyte loss: rapid expansion of the extracellular space. Beyond resuscitation, replacement therapy differs depending on the amount and type of dehydration. Figure 23–3 outlines basic guidelines for the medical management of dehydration.

Nurses play an important role during all phases of rehydration therapy. They should be able to assess the circulatory status, approximate the degree of dehydration, and evaluate response to therapy. Preparation and calculation of parenteral fluids also are vital to patient care. Monitoring right-sided heart pressure and urine output is an important nursing responsibility.

In summary, almost all acutely ill children require parenteral fluid and electrolyte therapy. Regulatory mechanisms that control fluid and electrolyte homeostasis are less efficient in infants and young children. Developmental differences underscore the importance of accurate calculation and replacement of fluid and electrolyte therapy.

TABLE 23–27. COMPOSITION AND TONICITY OF PARENTERAL FLUIDS FREQUENTLY USED IN PEDIATRICS

Solution	Na⁺ mEq/L	K⁺ mEq/L	Cl⁻ mEq/L	Osmolality mOsm/Lᵃ
5% Dextrose in 0.2% sodium chloride	34	—	34	321
5% Dextrose in 0.33% sodium chloride	56	—	56	365
5% Dextrose in 0.45% sodium chloride	77	—	77	406
5% Dextrose in 0.9% sodium chloride	154	—	154	560
Ringer's lactate solution	130	4	109	261
0.45% Sodium chloride	77	—	77	280
0.9% Sodium chloride	154	—	154	292
3% Sodium chloride	513	—	513	969

From *Pediatric fluids and electrolytes*, p. 127, by D. O'Donnell and J. Lathrop, 1990, Milwaukee: Maxishare Corporation (revised edition).
ᵃNormal physiologic isotonicity range is approximately 280–310 mOsm/L.

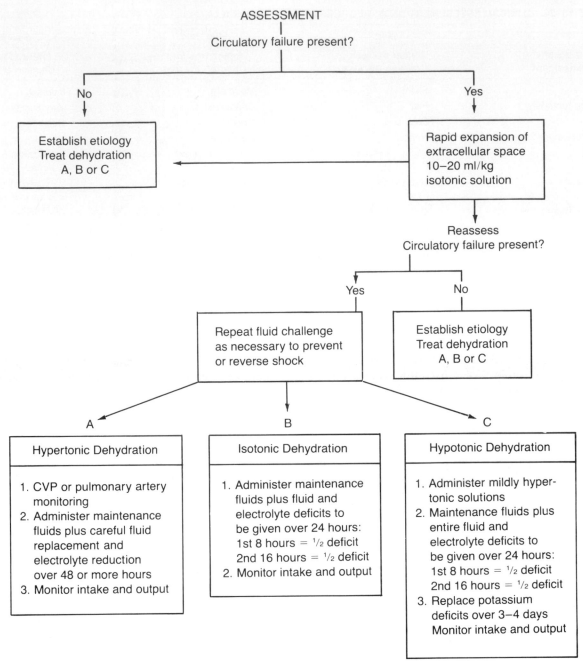

Figure 23–3. Management of dehydration. CVP, central venous pressure.

Section Fourteen: Nutrition

At the completion of this section, the learner will be able to discuss the nursing management of a child with alteration in nutritional status.

Nutrition is defined as the process by which food is converted into living tissue. This process is dependent on normal physiologic functioning of ingestion, digestion, transportation, use, and excretion of nutrients. The purpose of this section is twofold: first, to discuss how age-related factors and disease states affect the process of nutrition and, second, to discuss

nursing management of the child with increased nutritional needs.

Developmental Considerations

Unlike adults, children normally have an increased basal metabolic rate (BMR) and subsequent increased nutritional needs to support rapid growth and development. In addition, the infant has an immature digestive tract, making absorption and use of nutrients less efficient. Gastric emptying time is increased, and peristalsis is more rapid in the infant, causing less reabsorption of water. As a consequence, infant's stools usually are watery and occur more frequently than at other periods of life. Reverse peristalsis may also occur during infancy, contributing to frequent regurgitation. Digestion of all fats is not possible until approximately 1 year of age because of composition and secretion of bile and pancreatic lipase. Beyond infancy, gastrointestinal function is similar in children and adults.

Because infants have a relatively large body surface area and less subcutaneous fat, they are more prone to hypothermia. The process to increase heat production also increases glucose consumption and caloric needs. Section Fifteen provides a more detailed description of this process.

Normal Nutritional Requirements

Specific energy needs vary somewhat among children and depend on four factors: BMR, body activity, caloric loss in excreta, and dynamic action of food. The approximate kilocalorie (kcal) expenditure for each of these processes in the infant is listed (Shayevitz and Weissman, 1987).

BMR first year of life	70 kcal
Body activity and growth during childhood	20 kcal
Caloric loss in excreta	10 kcal
Dynamic action of food	5 kcal
TOTAL CALORIC EXPENDITURE	105 kcal

The three nutrients that contribute energy value (calories) are protein, carbohydrates, and fats. Recommended dietary allowances (RDA) have been published by the Committee on Food and Nutrition of the National Research Council. These guidelines make recommendations for daily intake of calories, proteins, vitamins, and minerals. Protein and caloric requirements per kilogram of body weight are highest during infancy and gradually decline throughout the childhood years. There are no specific RDA for fats and carbohydrates. The average American diet supplies an adequate amount of these nutrients. For additional information on normal nutritional requirements, the learner should review Module 16, *Nutrition*.

Alteration in Nutritional Requirements

Nutritional metabolism is a delicate balance between anabolism (physical growth of tissue) and catabolism (breakdown of tissue for energy). The acutely ill child exposed to increased metabolic stress can become catabolic very quickly. Stress factors that increase caloric needs include the following (Gorgon et al, 1988).

Fever	For every degree above 37 C, 12% increase in caloric need or expenditure
Surgery	Up to 30% increase in caloric need or expenditure
Sepsis	Up to 50% increase in caloric need or expenditure
Respiratory distress	50 to 75% increase in caloric need or expenditure

It has been shown that acutely ill adults metabolize nutrients and respond to starvation differently than patients experiencing starvation without stress (Ryan, 1976). Table 23–28 lists metabolic responses

TABLE 23–28. METABOLIC RESPONSES DURING STARVATION

	Without Stress	With Stress
Brief starvation	↓ Metabolic rate Normal body temperature ↓ Blood insulin levels ↑ Blood glucagon levels ↑ Blood free fatty acid levels ↑ Urinary nitrogen excretion	↓ Metabolic rate ↓ Body temperature ↓ Blood insulin levels ↑ Catecholamine, glucagon, cortisol levels ↑ Glucose levels ↑ Blood lactate levels ↑ Plasma free fatty acid levels ↑ Urinary nitrogen excretion
Prolonged starvation	↓ Metabolic rate ↓ Body temperature ↓ Blood insulin levels ↑ Free fatty acid levels ↑ Urinary nitrogen excretion	↑ Metabolic rate → ↓ metabolic rate ↑ Body temperature ↑ Or normal insulin levels ↑ Or normal catecholamine, glucagon, cortisol levels ↑ Or normal blood glucose levels ↑ Blood lactate levels ↑ Free fatty acid levels ↑ Urinary nitrogen excretion

From The critically ill patient: Nutritional implications, by L. Forlaw, 1983. *Nursing Clin. North Am.* 18:112.

with and without stress during starvation. The metabolic derangements that occur in children experiencing acute stress have not been well studied, and most of what is known has been adapted from adult literature.

Nutritional Management

The goals of nutritional management in the acutely ill child are to supply enough nutrients to maintain basal metabolic energy requirements, promote normal growth, and promote tissue repair.

The first step toward these goals is identifying the patient at risk. The nurse is an important member of the nutritional support team and assists with the nutritional assessment. Table 23–29 summarizes the key components of the nutritional assessment. Once the acutely ill child at risk has been identified, nutritional repletion can begin. The two modes of delivering nutrients are enteral and parenteral routes.

The preferred route of administration of nutrients is enteral. The enteral route provides more normal and homeostatic metabolism than parenteral routes and is essential for the maintenance of normal structure and function of the small intestine (Shayevitz and Weissman, 1987; Levine et al, 1974). It is also associated with a lower incidence of infection compared to a parenteral route.

There are numerous enteral formulas on the market. The nutritional team needs to consider the given osmolality and composition of the formula when selecting a product to meet the patient's individual needs. Continuous delivery of duodenal or jejunal feedings is preferred to intermittent delivery to avoid bowel distention, fluid and electrolyte shifts, and diarrhea (Forlaw, 1983).

Patients who cannot tolerate enteral feedings or require additional nutritional support, may benefit from supplementary or total nutritional support. The composition of parenteral nutritional support is individualized to the patient. The general principles of therapy are similar in the child and adult.

TABLE 23–29. SUMMARY OF METHODS OF NUTRITIONAL ASSESSMENT

Measurement of height and weight
Skinfold thickness
Arm muscle size
Creatine-height index
Total body potassium-height index
Urea nitrogen excretion
Plasma proteins
Cellular immunity

From *Textbook of pediatric intensive care*, p. 949, by M. C. Rogers, © 1987, the Williams & Wilkins Co., Baltimore.

Regardless of the type and method of nutritional support, nurses need to assist the nutrition team by maintaining accurate records of height and weight, caloric intake, and feeding tolerance. Second, nurses need to be familiar with hospital procedures for enteral and parenteral nutrition. Third, nurses need to minimize the child's energy expenditure by limiting environmental stress.

In summary, nutritional needs of the acutely ill child are increased significantly. Nutritional baseline assessment therapy needs to be initiated early in the patient's hospital course to maintain an anabolic state. Nutritional therapy needs to consider the child's increased basal energy needs, growth needs, and tissue repair needs.

Section Fifteen: Thermoregulation

At the completion of this section, the learner will be able to identify regulatory mechanisms of heat balance and discuss the nursing management of heat imbalance.

In the healthy individual exposed to normal seasonal temperatures, core temperature remains constant, within ±1°F (Guyton, 1991). There are a number of regulatory mechanisms within the body that maintain a balance between heat production and heat balance. It is the purpose of this section to discuss regulation of heat balance in the healthy and acutely ill child.

Methods of Heat Loss

Heat is being produced in the body and transferred to the environment continually. The four main methods of heat loss are radiation, evaporation, conduction, and convection. Radiation is responsible for most heat exchange and refers to the transfer of heat by infrared rays. Evaporation represents the second largest method of heat loss and occurs with the vaporization of liquid from the body. Only minute amounts of heat are lost by conduction, which represents a transfer of heat between two objects along a temperature gradient. Heat loss by convection occurs when body heat is conducted to the air and then removed by air currents.

Methods of Heat Production

Heat production is determined by the BMR, shivering thermogenesis, and chemical thermogenesis. BMR is a term used to express the rate of heat liberation with cellular chemical reactions under basal conditions. The primary motor center for shivering is located in the posterior hypothalamus. When stimulated, this center transmits impulses that increase tone of the skeletal muscle. After a critical level, shivering begins with an increase in heat production. The young infant cannot shiver to generate heat and is dependent on metabolic processes to maintain heat balance. Chemical thermogenesis, also referred to as nonshivering thermogenesis, produces heat from oxidative metabolism of brown fat. Newborns have brown fat in the interscapular space and mediastinum and around the kidneys. For the first weeks of life, it is a very important factor in thermogenesis. However, brown fat supply is limited, and the cold stressed infant can quickly deplete stores and become hypothermic.

In addition, increased consumption of glucose and oxygen to metabolize brown fat may produce acidosis, hypoxemia, and hypoglycemia. Figure 23–4 illustrates the physiologic consequences of cold stress in the neonate.

Regulatory Mechanisms

When an individual is exposed to a cold or hot state, there are several regulatory mechanisms that attempt to maintain normal body temperature. Figure 23–5 illustrates the neuroendocrine mechanisms of temperature control.

Hypothermia

Core temperatures below 95F (35C) usually are considered significant, and thermoregulatory mechanisms are activated (Brink, 1990). Uncontrolled severe hypothermia causes significant alterations in normal physiologic processes. Most notable of these are lethal dysrhythmias, apnea, and coma. Neonates are at risk for developing hypothermia because of their relatively large body surface area and limited brown fat stores. Acutely ill children also are at risk because of impaired physiologic function, poor nutri-

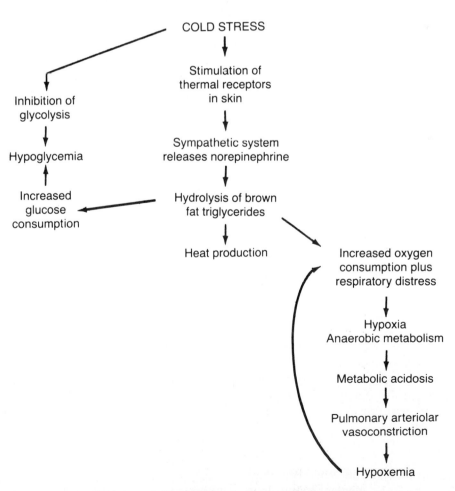

Figure 23–4. Physiological consequences of hypothermia.

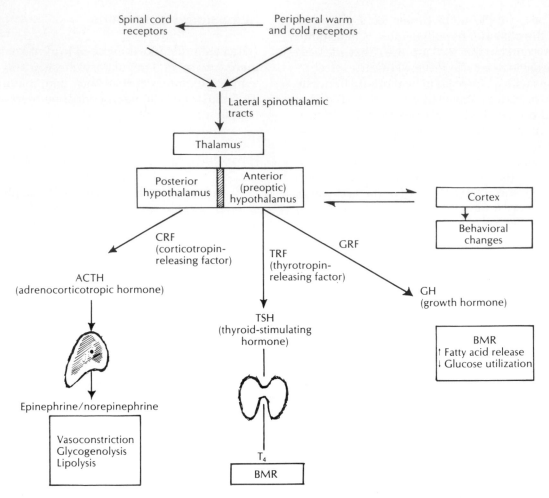

Figure 23–5. Neuroendocrine mechanisms of temperature control. BMR, basal metabolic rate. (*From* Essentials of pediatric intensive care, *p. 177, by D.L. Levin and F.C. Morriss, 1990, St. Louis: Quality Medical Publishing.*)

tional reserves, and pharmacologic agents. Trauma, submersion injuries, and drug intoxication are common etiologies producing hypothermia.

Management of hypothermia is aimed at preventing further heat loss and restoring normothermia. Children should be kept warm and dry at all times and kept in a neutral thermal environment. Drafts from windows and air conditioners should be eliminated. Blood for transfusions and supplemental oxygen should be warmed before administration. For severe hypothermia (e.g., submersion injury), the child needs to be handled with care because of ventricular irritability. To restore normal body temperature, rewarming methods must be used. In the neonate, rewarming should be gradual to prevent apnea (Williams and Lancaster, 1976). Table 23–30 summarizes three methods of rewarming.

Hyperthermia

Hyperthermia refers to a condition when the body temperature exceeds the usual normal range. It is related to one of three causes: increased environmental temperature, decreased heat elimination, or increased endogenous heat production (Brink, 1990). Common etiologies that produce hyperthermia in

TABLE 23–30. METHODS OF REWARMING

Passive external rewarming[a]	Endogenous thermogenesis, e.g., blankets
	Slowest, least invasive method
	Prevents further heat loss
Active external rewarming[a]	Application of conductive and radiant rewarming devices, e.g., heating pads, warming bottles
	Used for mild hypothermia
	Variable rate of rewarming
Active central rewarming	Rewarming occurs internally, e.g., warm IV or peritoneal fluids, warm inspired gases, mediastinal lavage
	Most invasive
	Optimal rate of rewarming is not known

[a]Problems associated with external rewarming include shock secondary to peripheral vasodilation and burns from poorly perfused areas.

children include infectious states, CNS injuries, and pharmacotherapeutics.

The treatment of fever unrelated to a hyperthermic syndrome is controversial. It is believed that the elevated temperature may support the body's normal defense against invading pathogens. Treatment usually is indicated when symptoms produced by the fever are not tolerated well by the child (e.g., dehydration, tachypnea, tachycardia). When treatment is indicated, general modes of therapy include passive and active external cooling and the use of antipyretics. Acetaminophens are used more often than aspirin because of fewer side effects, shorter duration of action, and aspirin's association with Reye's syndrome.

In summary, the balance of heat production and heat loss in the body is controlled by a number of neuroendocrine regulatory mechanisms. The acutely ill child is at risk for developing alterations in temperature regulation because of a large surface area/volume ratio and a debilitated state. The neonate is at further risk because of limited brown fat stores and limited subcutaneous fat. Alteration in heat balance needs to be prevented or controlled to prevent further impairment of the acutely ill child.

Metabolism/Thermoregulation Review

Refer to the following case study to answer Questions 1 through 6.

Christine is a 3-year-old girl admitted to the intensive care unit with a 3-day history of vomiting and diarrhea. Vital signs are: temperature 102.2F (39C), respiratory rate 40, heart rate 110, blood pressure 74/40. Additional clinical symptoms include grayish skin color, loss of skin elasticity, dry mucous membranes, and irritability. She has not voided for 7 hours. Prehospital weight is not known. Present weight is 17 kg. CBC is normal, glucose normal, serum electrolytes are Na^+ 138, K^+ 3.4, Cl^- 102.

1. Based on these data, what type of dehydration does Christine have?
   A. hypertonic
   B. hypotonic
   C. hydrotonic
   D. isotonic
2. Based on clinical symptoms, what degree of dehydration does Christine have?
   A. mild
   B. moderate
   C. severe
   D. none
3. Based on these data, which order would you initiate first?
   A. chest radiograph
   B. IV line insertion
   C. Foley catheter insertion
   D. blood culture

4. What is the hourly maintenance fluid requirement for Christine (based on hospital weight)?
   A. 26 mL
   B. 56 mL
   C. 10 mL
   D. 88 mL
5. If Christine normally weighs 19 kg, what percentage of weight loss does she have?
   A. 8
   B. 2
   C. 20
   D. 10
6. Based on Christine's temperature, what is the percentage of increase in caloric requirements?
   A. 12
   B. 24
   C. 20
   D. 10
7. The enteral route is preferred over the parenteral route for nutrition repletion because
   A. minerals are absorbed most efficiently through the small intestine
   B. there is a lower incidence of infection
   C. amino acids cannot be administered parenterally
   D. glucose is metabolized less efficiently in parenteral form
8. Cold stress can indirectly cause
   A. hyperglycemia from decreased glucose consumption
   B. hypoxemia from pulmonary arteriolar vasoconstriction
   C. decreased oxygen consumption
   D. hyperglycemia from stimulation of glycolysis

9. A potential complication of active external re-
   warming for hypothermia is
   A. hyperthermia
   B. respiratory distress
   C. hypotension
   D. hypoglycemia

10. The neonate is predisposed to hypothermia
    because of
    A. increased body surface area
    B. decreased CO
    C. decreased myelination of cortical centers
    D. increased respiratory rate

Answers: 1,D. 2, B. 3, B. 4, B. 5, D. 6, B. 7, B. 8, B. 9, C. 10, A.

IMMUNOCOMPETENCE

Section Sixteen: Risk Factors

At the completion of this section, the learner will be
able to identify age-related factors and situational
stressors that alter the immune response of the
acutely ill child.

Infections are a common problem seen in the
pediatric intensive care unit. They may develop as a
primary disorder or may be a secondary complication
of another illness. The very fact that the child is admitted to an intensive care unit places him or her at
risk for altered immune function. In addition to environmental risk factors, the child also may have an
altered immune response from a preexisting disease
state. Infancy compounds the risk factors because of
the immaturity of the immune system. The purpose
of this section is to discuss developmental aspects
and situational stressors that place the child at risk
for developing an infection.

Developmental Immunity

In the past, it was believed that the newborn had
very little immunologic function. Today, we know
that many areas of immune expression are present at
birth, and other areas are acquired with age. An understanding of the developmentally immature immune system helps to explain the infant and child's
predilection for characteristic infections. Developmental aspects of immune function are discussed in
terms of first-line defense, nonspecific immunity,
and specific cellular and humoral immunity.

The first line of defense against invasion by
pathogens is barriers, mechanical and chemical. Intact skin is a mechanical barrier and normally prevents penetration of microorganisms. The newborn's
skin is different than the adult's in terms of reduced
thickness and durability. The stratum corneum is
present in reduced amount in the newborn, resulting
in increased skin permeability. However, it rapidly

develops and is adequate by 2 weeks of age (Rosenthal, 1989).

Chemical barriers refer to secretions that assist
in host defense. Specific types of chemical barriers
include acidic surface secretions, gastric secretions,
and urine. In the infant, there is diminished sweat
production, resulting in decreased secretion of bac-
tericidal and fungicidal substances. Surface secretion
of IgA, which helps prevent attachment of pathogenic organisms, may be reduced in the gastrointestinal tract of the infant (Rosenthal, 1989; Tribett,
1989).

If mechanical or chemical barriers are altered or
bypassed, pathogenic invasion can occur, and an inflammatory response is triggered. The second line of
host defense is nonspecific defenses, which include
phagocytic cells, the complement system, and
chemical mediators. Table 23–31 summarizes specific
areas of immaturity of nonspecific mechanisms of
host defense and their clinical significance.

**TABLE 23–31. DEVELOPMENTAL ASPECTS OF
NONSPECIFIC MECHANISMS OF HOST DEFENSE**

Host Defense	Deficiency	Clinical Significance
Phagocytes	Diminished motility, adherence, and chemotaxis in newborn	May contribute to decreased ability to localize infection
	Reduced stores of neutrophils per kilogram	Neutrophils are depleted, with repeated infections or with an overwhelming infection
Complement	Complement proteins are 60–80% of normal adult levels; serum complement reaches adult levels between 3 and 6 months of age	Low levels may contribute to the neonate's afebrile and reduced leukocytosis response to infection
		Opsonization and chemotactic activity is deficient in the newborn compared with the adult

When natural and nonspecific defense are unsuccessful in eradicating or containing pathogens, an acquired immune response is triggered. Humoral immunity (B cell function) is primarily responsible for synthesis of immunoglobins. In the newborn, absolute numbers of B cells are present, but the actual synthesis of some types of immunoglobulins is limited. Table 23–32 lists the levels of immunoglobulins present at birth and when mature levels are obtained (Rosenthal, 1989). Passive transplacental transfer of IgG occurs in the last trimester. Newborns have adult serum levels of IgG at birth, but levels gradually fall over the first 4 months of extrauterine life. The infant's level of immunoglobulins is lowest at approximately 4 to 5 months of age, when passive immunity is decreasing and active immunity is still deficient (Rosenthal, 1989; Cooper and Buckley, 1982).

Age-specific cell-mediated function (T cell function) is less well understood than humoral immunity. However, it is known that in normal newborns, T cells are present in approximately the same quantity as in adults. T cells also respond to antigens to which the mother has been sensitized. Newborn T cells do, however, have decreased function in terms of gamma-interferon secretion, which activates macrophage function (Cooper and Buckley, 1982; Rosenthal, 1989).

Situational Risk Factors

In addition to developmental factors, there are also situational factors that place the acutely ill child at risk for infection. Invasive procedures that bypass epithelial barriers (e.g., IV lines, urinary catheter, inhalation therapy equipment) are the mainstay of intensive care therapy. Unfortunately, they predispose the host to opportunistic infections. Surgical trauma and burn trauma also affect immune function by altering skin barriers. Some pharmacologic agents used pre-, intra-, and postoperatively alter immune function. For example, nitrous oxide depresses bone marrow function. The child's preexisting health status may alter the immune response and function.

There are also anatomic defects that frequently are associated with opportunistic infections. Children with cardiac defects may develop subacute and acute bacterial endocarditis. Urinary tract obstructive lesions have a significant incidence of gram-negative enteric infections. Congenital dermal abnormalities of the craniospinal axis that communicate with the CNS can cause a lethal infection. Otitis media is a common problem in children with cleft palates (Cherry and Feigin, 1989).

In summary, although newborns are not completely devoid of immunologic function at birth, they are deficient in many areas. Nonspecific and acquired immunity become functional at various ages from birth to adolescence. Age-specific infections may be predicted, and prevention measures can be developed. Situational stressors of the intensive care environment, as well as therapeutic measures, also can place the child at risk. An understanding of risk factors can help the nurse develop surveillance measures and management strategies when caring for the acutely ill child.

TABLE 23–32. IMMUNOGLOBULINS: FUNCTION, LEVELS, AND CLINICAL SIGNIFICANCE

Ig	Function	% of Adult Level at Birth	Clinical Significance of Low Level	Age Mature Level Attained
IgM	First to be formed after antigen stimulation Serologic defense	10	Risk for overwhelming sepsis	1–2 years
IgD	Unknown	Small amount		1 year
IgG	Guards tissue from bacteria	110[a]	Risk for pyogenic infection, especially pulmonary Risk for reinfection	4–10 years
IgA	Defends mucosal surfaces/secretions	Small amount or none	Risk for viral and bacterial infection at mucosal surfaces, especially respiratory and sinusitis	6–15 years
IgE	Triggers immediate hypersensitivity (type I)	Small amount	Risk for parasitic infection	6–15 years

Adapted from Immunosuppression in pediatric critical care patients, by C.H. Rosenthal, 1989, *Crit. Care Nursing Clin. North Am.* 1:779.
[a]Crosses placenta.

Section Seventeen: Nursing Management

At the completion of this section, the learner will be able to state treatment strategies to prevent infection and augment host defenses in the child.

Acutely ill children are at risk for developing opportunistic infections because of a developmental predisposition and situational stressors that alter immune function. They are subjected to invasive procedures and immunosuppressive agents and reside in a location with many other patients. Nurses must consider these risk factors when developing a therapeutic plan to care for the child. The goal of therapy is to prevent or minimize infection by limiting exposure to pathogens, by early detection and monitoring of infection, and by augmenting host defenses. The first part of this section describes measures to prevent infection, followed by a discussion on augmentation of host defenses.

Prevention of Infection

One of the first steps in preventing infection is early detection. In the infant and young child, clinical manifestations often are nonspecific and variable. There are limited diagnostic criteria to confirm sepsis in the newborn. WBC with bacterial disease may be low, normal or elevated, and erythrocyte sedimentation rate and C-reactive protein also are relatively insensitive. Therefore, clinical assessment data must be correlated with the patient's history and laboratory data. If suspicion of infection exists, blood, urine, and CSF cultures should be obtained (Ackerman, 1987).

In the older infant and child, clinical manifestations and laboratory tests are more specific and diagnostic. Specific signs and symptoms depend on whether the infection is localized or systemic. Table 23–33 lists possible immunologic clues seen with altered immune function.

Limiting exposure to pathogens can help prevent infection. The importance of handwashing and strict adherence to isolation policies need no explanation. A clean environment, including room, equipment, and supplies, is critical. Liberal visitation of the child's family is important in the pediatric intensive care unit. However, visitation of the immunocompromised patient should be restricted to the immediate family, and they should adhere to isolation policies.

Augmentation of Host Defenses

Host defenses may be augmented by maintaining physical and chemical barriers, providing adequate nutrition, reducing psychologic stress, and maintain-

TABLE 23–33. IMMUNOLOGIC ASSESSMENT CLUES

System	Clues
Neurosensory	Visual changes, headaches/migraines, deafness, ataxia, and tetany
Respiratory	Wheezing and rhonchi, cough, rhinitis, hyperventilation, and bronchospasm
Cardiovascular	Hypotension, tachycardia, arrhythmias, vasculitis, and anemia
Gastrointestinal	Hepatosplenomegaly, dyspepsia, colitis, vomiting/diarrhea (chronic)
Skin/hygiene	Dermatitis, purpura, and urticaria
Mobility/comfort	Tender and swollen joints, muscle weakness, limited range of motion, lymph node enlargement and tenderness, and fever and chills
General factors	Poor nutritional status, age

From Nursing support of host defenses, by S. Esperson. Reprinted from *Critical Care Nursing Quarterly*, Vol. 9, No. 1, p. 52, with permission of Aspen Publishers Inc., © 1986.

ing comfort (Esperson, 1986). The importance of maintaining the body's first line of defense is discussed in Section Sixteen, and the importance of adequate nutrition is discussed in Section Fourteen. Prolonged or uncontrolled psychologic stress may result in depression of some components of the immune system (Schindler, 1985). Uncontrolled discomfort can add further to patient stress and indirectly alter immune function (Esperson, 1986).

Specific measures to maintain epithelial integrity (e.g., skin, oral, respiratory, urinary, bowel surfaces) are outlined in Table 23–34. Nurses should take an active role in providing nutritional support, as outlined in Section Fourteen. Stress reduction techniques need to be individualized to the age of the child. The learner should refer to Section Nineteen for a more in-depth discussion of this topic. Finally,

TABLE 23–34. ALTERATION IN SKIN BARRIERS: METHODS TO REDUCE INFECTION

Establish guidelines for invasive monitoring
IV therapy
    Use stainless steel needles for IV access (whenever possible)
    Maintain sterility with catheter insertion
    Secure IV catheters to prevent mechanical trauma to vessels
    Apply sterile dressing to IV site
    Do not prepare insertion site with acetone
Maintain adequate patient fluid intake
Promote activity
Reposition patient frequently
Use sterile technique with airway suctioning
Promote normal urinary and bowel elimination

the source of discomfort needs to be identified and eliminated. Analgesics must be individualized in terms of route, selection, and dosage. Noxious procedures need to be minimized.

In summary, acutely ill patients in the pediatric intensive care unit are at risk for developing infection. The goals of nursing management are preven-tion and augmentation of host defenses. Prevention is accomplished with close surveillance and monitoring and by limiting exposure to potential pathogens. Augmentation of host defenses includes maintaining physical and chemical barriers, nutritional support, reduction of stress, and relieving discomfort.

Immunocompetence Review

1. The infant's level of immunoglobulins is lowest between
   A. 4 and 6 years of age
   B. 4 and 5 months of age
   C. 2 and 3 weeks of age
   D. 2 and 5 years of age
2. Because complement protein levels in the infant are 60 percent to 80 percent of normal adult levels, in which of the following areas of the immune system is the infant most deficient?
   A. ability to localize infections
   B. ability to increase leukocytes in response to an infection
   C. ability to increase neutrophil stores
   D. ability to form immunoglobulins
3. Low levels of IgE place the young child at increased risk for
   A. pyogenic infections
   B. bacterial respiratory infection
   C. parasitic infection
   D. overwhelming sepsis
4. The best nursing intervention to prevent the transfer of pathogens is
   A. handwashing
   B. strict adherence to isolation
   C. bathing the patient frequently
   D. good nutrition

Refer to the following case study to answer Questions 5 and 6.

Suzanne is a 4-year-old girl admitted to the intensive care unit following open heart surgery. Postoperative monitoring devices include a right atrial catheter, radial artery catheter, and urinary catheter. On postoperative day 3, she is diagnosed with a urinary tract infection.

5. The most likely cause of the urinary tract infection is
   A. oliguria from decreased renal perfusion
   B. prophylactic antibiotics
   C. radial artery cannulation
   D. indwelling urinary catheter
6. Suzanne's immune function has been significantly altered because of
   A. low levels of IgD
   B. low levels of IgM
   C. low levels of complement proteins
   D. altered skin barriers

Answers: 1, B. 2, B. 3, C. 4, A. 5, D. 6, D.

PSYCHOSOCIAL FACTORS

Section Eighteen: Impact of Hospitalization

At the end of this section, the learner will be able to discuss age-related stressors and reactions to hospitalization.

Children often are admitted to the intensive care unit in an acute state without advance preparation. In general, childhood responses to hospitalization do not vary significantly between pediatric general and intensive care units. Furthermore, hospital-related stressors are more similar than dissimilar and are characteristically age dependent. In addition to age, the child's understanding of and reaction to hospitalization depends primarily on personality, parent–child relationship, previous separation, and characteristics of illness and treatment. On the other hand, the frequency of stressors often is greater in the intensive care unit, which may intensify the child's response. The purpose of this section is to describe age-related stressors and reactions commonly experienced by the hospitalized child.

Separation Anxiety

Separation from one's parents is a major stressor during infancy throughout the preschool years. Infants and toddlers have limited internal coping abilities and depend on significant others as their main source of coping. Three distinct stages of separation have been described in the infant: protest, despair, and detachment (Bowlby, 1969). Reactions during the stage of protest include crying, screaming for a parent, and inconsolable behavior. If separation continues, the infant goes through a stage of despair. The infant is depressed from a sense of hopelessness, demonstrated by decreased activity, no crying, and withdrawal from others. The last stage is one of detachment or denial. This is a confusing stage and often is misinterpreted by health professionals. The child outwardly appears content, but in reality, he emotionally detaches himself from the parents to avoid the emotional pain of wanting them. These stages are not always apparent in the acutely ill child who has limited ability to express emotion overtly. However, infants adapt much better to a situational crisis when one or both parents are present (Smith, 1983).

Toddlers and preschoolers also experience tremendous stress when separated from their parents, but they react to this stressor differently than the infant. The toddler is able to verbalize his displeasure with pleas for his parents to stay. He may also react with temper tantrums and uncooperative behavior. The preschooler normally can tolerate brief periods of separation from his parents. However, stress of illness and hospitalization may alter usual mechanisms of coping, and the preschooler may demonstrate reactions to separation. In general, their reactions are less intense than those seen in the toddler. Reactions include whimpering, repeatedly making requests for parents, repeatedly asking when parents will visit, and refusing to cooperate with activities and care (Smith, 1983; Whaley and Wong, 1987).

Older children generally do much better with separation from their parents, but the stress of hospitalization usually increases their desire for parental guidance. Older children also have developed support systems and relationships outside their immediate family. When alone, they may complain of boredom, isolation, and loneliness.

Loss of Control

The infant's reactions to and the effects of loss of control are not well understood. However, the older infant normally likes to explore his environment and is physically quite active. When immobilized or restricted to a bed, infants demonstrate generalized dislike by, for example, crying and screaming.

The toddler is struggling for autonomy. Therefore, any obstacle that restricts his behavior or desires will result in negativism, for example, noncompliance and temper tantrums. The toddler is struggling with self-control, which is maintained by ritualistic behavior. The hospital environment is foreign and alters the child's usual routines. Reaction to disrupted routines is principally regression, for example, asking for a bottle or wetting the bed when previously toilet-trained.

The preschooler's thought processes are characterized by egocentricity, magical thinking, and preconceptual logic. They feel all-powerful and omnipotent. In the hospital setting where many restrictions exist, the child's self-power is threatened, and self-control is lost. Reactions to loss of control include behaviors of protest, despair, detachment, aggression, and regression.

Older children may be characterized as industrious and independent. They are increasingly able to view situations objectively. They question their own perceptions, as well as those of others. When they are unable or not allowed to make decisions about their care, they feel a loss of independence and privacy. They also fear what they do not understand. Usual reactions of loss of control include frustration, hostility, and depression.

Fear of Bodily Injury and Pain

Procedures or physical disabilities that cause pain or fear of bodily injury are the last major stressors experienced by the hospitalized child. Effects of and reactions to fear of bodily injury are not known in the preverbal infant. Pain in the infant is responded to with generalized rigidity, followed by thrashing of extremities, crying, facial expression of discomfort, alteration in heart rate and respiratory rate, and physical resistance (older than 6 months).

The toddler has a poor concept of body boundaries and may react as intensely to intrusive procedure as painful ones. The preschooler has concerns about the integrity of his body. For example, they fear they will exsanguinate with cuts and needle punctures. They also have fears of castration and mutilation. The toddler and preschooler react to painful injuries or fear of bodily injury with physical aggression and uncooperative behavior (Ramsey, 1982).

The older child has fears not only of bodily injury but also of disabilities (real or imagined) that will make them different and, therefore, rejected by their friends. They are beginning to understand the need for procedures and may request why the procedure is needed, especially if it is painful. In general, the older the child, the more cooperative he or she usually is with painful procedures. They try to act brave. If they are distressed about a procedure or are experiencing pain, they usually will communicate their concerns verbally.

In summary, regardless of the inpatient setting, the hospitalized child may have very specific age-related stressors. These stressors can be categorized into three groups: separation, loss of control, and fear of bodily injury and pain. Depending on the age of the child and other significant variables, the child's reaction to these stressors may be predicted and controlled.

Section Nineteen: Nursing Management of Stressors

At the end of this section, the learner will be able to list specific methods to reduce the negative effects of hospitalization.

When a child who is acutely ill is admitted to the intensive care unit, his emotional needs frequently are given low priority. Once his condition is stabilized, he becomes increasingly more aware of the environment. Stressors are apparent to the child, and negative reactions may occur. Nursing care should encompass management of both physiologic and emotional stressors. The purpose of this section is to discuss nursing management that minimizes negative reactions to hospitalization. Specific age-related interventions are discussed in terms of separation anxiety, loss of control, and fear of bodily injury and pain.

Separation Anxiety

The intensive care environment is normally loud, hectic, frightening, and intimidating. For all age groups, it is extremely important to have liberal visitation to minimize separation anxiety. If the intensive care unit has limited visitation, the family needs a schedule of visiting times. Nursing flexibility is encouraged to meet the needs of the family and child. Whenever possible, the nurse should involve family members in patient care. Family involvement often reduces the child's separation anxiety, and the family member feels more in control. Using consistent caregivers also is important. It allows the child to develop a trusting relationship with a surrogate parent (Kidder, 1989). Table 23–35 lists additional age-

TABLE 23–35. ANXIETY RELATED TO SEPARATION: NURSING INTERVENTIONS

Infant	Toddler	Preschooler	School Age
Consistent caregiver	Consistent caregiver	Consistent caregiver	Consistent caregiver
Encourage parents to visit frequently	Encourage parents to visit frequently	Encourage parents to visit frequently	Encourage parents to visit frequently
Promote cuddling, holding when patient condition permits	Talk about parents frequently	Talk about parents frequently	Talk about parents frequently
	Place pictures of family members at bedside	Place pictures of family members at bedside	Place pictures of family members at bedside
	Allow sibling visitation when possible	Allow sibling visitation when possible	Allow sibling and peer visitation when possible
	Explain when parents will return in terms of significant events, e.g., lunch, dinner	Explain when parents will return in terms of significant events, e.g., lunch, dinner	Use a clock to explain when parents will return
	Encourage child to talk about family members	Encourage child to talk about family members	Encourage child to talk about family members
Encourage family to make tape recordings of family voices	Encourage family to make tape recordings of family voices telling favorite stories or singing a favorite song	Encourage family to make tape recordings of family voices telling favorite stories or singing a favorite song	
Allow infant to visualize parents face during procedures	Encourage expression of loneliness	Encourage expression of loneliness	Encourage expression of loneliness
	Encourage family to bring personal items	Encourage family to bring personal items	Encourage family to bring personal items
	Be honest	Be honest	Be honest
	Accept regressive behavior	Accept regressive behavior	Regressive behavior is usually absent

TABLE 23-36. POWERLESSNESS RELATED TO ENVIRONMENT: NURSING INTERVENTIONS

Infant	Toddler	Preschooler	School Age
Maintain normal routine as much as possible	Maintain normal routine as much as possible	Maintain normal routine as much as possible	Maintain normal routine as much as possible
	Allow to wear own pajamas	Allow to wear own pajamas	Allow to wear own pajamas or clothing
	Allow choices	Allow choices	Allow choices
	Promote self-care	Promote self-care	Promote self-care
Limit use of restraints when possible	Limit use of restraints when possible	Limit use of restraints when possible	
		Maintain privacy	Maintain privacy
			Allow input when scheduling nursing care
	Accept ritualistic behavior	Accept ritualistic behavior	Develop contracts to negotiate scheduling of nursing care
	Avoid questions inviting a "no" answer		

specific interventions to minimize separation anxiety.

Loss of Control

Feelings of loss of control can be minimized by limiting physical restrictions, preparing for procedures, maintaining routines, and maintaining a level of independence. Immobilizing the child for procedures is often unavoidable. However, whenever possible, the nurse should attempt to gain cooperation first to prevent restraining or allow the parent to assist with restraining. Anticipatory preparation is not always possible. When time and patient condition permit, age-appropriate preparation should be done. Promoting independence can be accomplished by allowing the child to participate in self-care, allowing the child to make decisions about care, and maintaining rituals and daily routines when possible (Wilson and Broom, 1989). Table 23–36 lists age-specific interventions to minimize feelings of loss of control.

Fear of Bodily Injury and Pain

Interventions to reduce fear of bodily injury vary depending on the age of the child and previous experiences. Again, whenever possible, advance preparation should be done. For pain management, assessment is important for recognizing pain and for evaluating the effectiveness of interventions. There are a few pain assessment tools that have been developed specifically for children to help quantify assessments (Owens, 1984; Jeans, 1983). For relieving pain, nonpharmacologic and pharmacologic management may be used. Table 23–37 lists specific interventions to minimize fears of bodily injury and reduce the pain experience.

In summary, children have age-specific reactions to their hospital experience. Despite the stresses normally associated with the intensive care unit, nurses can develop specific strategies to minimize negative reactions. Age-specific interventions to reduce separation anxiety, feelings of loss of control, and fears of bodily injury and pain have been described.

TABLE 23–37. PAIN RELATED TO INJURY AND/OR PROCEDURES: NURSING INTERVENTIONS

Infant	Toddler	Preschooler	School Age
Use restraints only when necessary	Use restraints only when necessary	Use restraints only when necessary	Use restraints only when necessary
	Use the least intrusive procedure when possible, e.g., axillary instead of rectal temperature	Use the least intrusive procedure when possible, e.g., axillary instead of rectal temperature	Use the least intrusive procedure when possible, e.g., axillary instead of rectal temperature
Allow parents to hold or be present with procedures	Allow parents to hold or be present with procedures	Allow parents to hold or be present with procedures	Allow parents to hold or be present with procedures

TABLE 23–37. PAIN RELATED TO INJURY AND/OR PROCEDURES: NURSING INTERVENTIONS (*Continued*)

Infant	Toddler	Preschooler	School Age
Keep procedure brief Comfort after procedure	Explain procedures before performing if possible a. Use simple concepts b. Explain to child how to act, e.g., "hold leg still" c. Explain procedure shortly before it begins d. Allow expression of feelings, e.g., crying	Explain procedures before performing if possible a. Explain to child he did not cause procedure and he is not being punished b. Encourage expressions of anger through play c. Explain how procedure will feel d. Allow expression of feelings; e.g., crying Suggest ways to maintain control during a procedure, e.g., deep breathing	Explain procedures before performing if possible a. Use correct medical terminology b. Allow more time for teaching (than younger children) c. Explain functioning of equipment d. Allow time for questions Suggest ways to maintain control during a procedure, e.g., deep breathing Provide privacy from peers during procedure
Assess pain Signs and symptoms	Assess pain Faces pain scale	Assess pain Numeric pain scale Color pain scale Descriptive pain scale Glasses pain scale	Assess pain Numeric pain scale Color pain scale Descriptive pain scale Glasses pain scale
Manage pain Encourage holding, cuddling Rock in wide rhythmic arc Repeat one or two words softly	Manage pain Encourage holding, cuddling Rock in wide rhythmic arc Repeat one or two words softly Distract with play	Manage pain Encourage holding, cuddling Help assume comfortable position Help with slow breathing and relaxation, e.g., limp doll Distract with play	Manage pain Encourage holding, cuddling Help assume comfortable position Help with slow breathing and relaxation, e.g., limp doll Distract with television, radio, etc.
Administer analgesics as ordered, assess effectiveness	Administer analgesics as ordered, assess effectiveness	Administer analgesics as ordered, assess effectiveness	Administer analgesics as ordered, assess effectiveness

Psychosocial Review

1. The three stages of separation anxiety in the infant are
   A. protest, despair, detachment
   B. protest, regression, detachment
   C. depression, despair, detachment
   D. protest, despair, aggression
2. The preschooler's behavior is best characterized as
   A. negative and ritualistic
   B. egocentric and magical
   C. industrious and independent
   D. quiet and modest
3. Children from which of the following age groups would most likely want a bandage for a cut or venipuncture?
   A. infant
   B. toddler
   C. preschooler
   D. school age

Refer to the following case study to answer Questions 4 through 6.

Cathy is a 2½-year-old girl admitted to the intensive care unit with epiglottitis. She is intubated and started on antibiotics. Restraints are necessary to prevent Cathy from extubating herself. Her parents are allowed to visit her every hour for 5 minutes.

4. What reaction is Cathy most likely to have to separation from her parents?
   A. withdrawal from staff
   B. complaints of boredom and loneliness
   C. temper tantrums
   D. repeated requests for parents

Cathy's IV catheter needs to be changed.

5. When preparing Cathy for the procedure, which technique would be most helpful?
   A. demonstrating an IV insertion on a doll
   B. explaining the procedure in a group with other children
   C. sedating her with diazepam
   D. restraining her
6. What intervention would be most helpful to prevent feelings of loss of control?
   A. maintain a clock at the bedside
   B. encourage her to make her own bed
   C. minimize change in normal daily routines
   D. obtain a psychiatric consult

Answers: 1, A. 2, B. 3, C. 4, C. 5, A. 6, C.

Posttest

1. The young infant is predisposed to respiratory dysfunction because of which of the following anatomic and physiologic features?
   A. relatively small tongue
   B. narrow vocal cords
   C. small airway diameter
   D. small body surface area
2. Initial signs of respiratory distress in the child are usually manifested by which of the following?
   A. unresponsive
   B. tachycardia
   C. perioral cyanosis
   D. bradypnea
3. A common cause of obstructive respiratory disease in children is
   A. epiglottitis
   B. pulmonary embolism
   C. hypoplasia of the lung
   D. pulmonary edema

4. Intracostal retractions in the infant are produced by
   A. narrowing of the nasal passages during expiration
   B. respiratory muscle fatigue
   C. premature glottic closure during expiration
   D. increased negative intrapleural pressure during inspiration

Refer to the following case study to answer Questions 5 and 6.

Sally is a 9-month-old child who is brought to the emergency room with the following history: fever for 8 hours and difficulty breathing. Clinically, she is pale, respiratory rate is 60 bpm, protruding tongue, temperature of 103F (39.5C), intercostal retractions.

5. Considering Sally's clinical presentation, which of the following orders should be initiated first?
   A. IV access
   B. chest radiograph
   C. blood culture
   D. oxygen
6. Based on these data, which of the following nursing diagnoses would you select as being appropriate in Sally's plan of care?
   A. Fluid volume deficit
   B. Ineffective airway clearance
   C. Altered tissue perfusion: renal
   D. Impaired physical mobility

Refer to the following case study to answer Questions 7 through 10.

Carlos is a 4-year-old boy admitted to the pediatric intensive care unit following a motor vehicle accident (unrestrained passenger). Clinical data: blood pressure 80/58, heart rate 120, respirations 32. Peripheral pulses slightly diminished. Hematocrit 30 and hemoglobin pending. Pulse oximeter 94 percent. Serum electrolytes normal. CT scan is positive for abdominal bleeding. Weight is 20 kg.

7. Based on these data, which of the following nursing diagnoses would you select as being appropriate in Carlos's care?
   A. Impaired gas exchange
   B. Altered cardiac output: decreased
   C. Fluid volume deficit
   D. Ineffective airway breathing

Carlos is placed on a cardiac monitor, and a urinary catheter is inserted. The one peripheral IV catheter in the left arm is infiltrated and is discontinued. An indirect blood pressure reading is 74/40, and the heart rate is 140.

8. Which of the following orders should be initiated first?
   A. IV access
   B. dopamine continuous infusion
   C. serum hematocrit and hemoglobin
   D. arterial line setup

IV access is successful.

9. What parenteral solution would you most likely prepare for Carlos's volume replacement?
   A. 5 percent dextrose in water
   B. 0.9 percent normal saline
   C. 5 percent dextrose in 0.25 percent normal saline
   D. 25 percent albumin
10. How much fluid would Carlos most likely receive as a bolus?
    A. 100 mL
    B. 40 mL
    C. 400 mL
    D. 500 mL
11. Central nervous system development is greatest during which of the following ages of life?
    A. 5 to 10 years
    B. birth to 3 years
    C. 15 to 25 years
    D. consistent throughout life
12. Which of the following is considered to be a secondary traumatic brain injury?
    A. skull fracture
    B. scalp laceration
    C. diffuse axonal injury
    D. epidural hematoma
13. CSF values for a child with bacterial meningitis would most likely include
    A. protein < 50 mg/100 mL
    B. WBC > 500 mm^3
    C. negative gram stain
    D. glucose > $\frac{1}{3}$ serum glucose

Refer to the following case study to answer Questions 14 and 15.

Maria is a 3-year-old girl admitted to the pediatric intensive care unit 2 days previously with a diagnosis of bacterial meningitis. She has been on antibiotics since admission. On the third day of admission, Maria has a generalized seizure.

14. Which of the following nursing interventions would you perform first?
    A. administer oxygen
    B. prepare an anticonvulsant
    C. call the doctor
    D. administer a fluid bolus

Diazepam (Valium) is administered. Heart rate is 102, respirations 18 and shallow, blood pressure 102/70.

---

15. Based on Maria's postseizure status, what complication should be anticipated?
    A. hypotension
    B. apnea
    C. hypertension
    D. heart block
16. Which of the following is a physiologic response to cold stress in the newborn?
    A. hypoxemia
    B. hypernatremia
    C. hypotension
    D. hyperglycemia
17. Which of the following metabolic responses may be seen in a child who has been acutely ill for 2 days without adequate parenteral or enteral nutrition?
    A. increased metabolic rate and increased blood insulin levels
    B. decreased blood insulin levels and increased urinary nitrogen excretion
    C. increased glucose levels and increased metabolic rate
    D. decreased body temperature and increased metabolic rate
18. The treatment of a moderate increase in body temperature is controversial because
    A. lowering body temperature too quickly may cause a seizure
    B. increased body temperature improves perfusion
    C. the elevated temperature may support the body's normal defense against invading pathogens
    D. antipyretics may cause hypotension in children

Refer to the following case study to answer Questions 19 through 24.

Bobby is a 3-month-old infant diagnosed with tetralogy of Fallot (ventricular septal defect and severe right ventricular outflow obstruction). He has been taking digoxin (Lanoxin) and furosemide (Lasix) since diagnosis. He is admitted to the hospital for elective cardiac surgery. Heart rate is 160, respirations 52 (at rest), blood pressure 72/50. The liver is enlarged. He has circumoral cyanosis, nasal flaring, grunting, and intercostal retractions.

---

19. Bobby has a low perfusion state from which of the following function states of shock?
    A. hypovolemic
    B. transport
    C. obstructive
    D. cardiogenic
20. Which of the following orders should be initiated first to improve Bobby's oxygenation?
    A. chest radiograph
    B. oxygen administration
    C. CBC, hemoglobin, and hematocrit determination
    D. postural drainage

Bobby's surgery is successful in correcting his heart defect, and he is admitted to the pediatric intensive care unit for postoperative management. Monitoring devices include right atrial pressure line, right radial arterial line, two peripheral venous lines, a mediastinal chest tube, and a urinary catheter. He is intubated and has assist volume ventilation.

---

21. Bobby is most at risk for infection because of
    A. a low perfusion state
    B. alteration in skin barriers
    C. abnormal WBC formation
    D. high levels of IgM

After 12 hours, Bobby is weaned off the ventilator and extubated. However, Bobby's $Paco_2$ level progressively increases over the next 24 hours, as well as his work of breathing. While waiting for a decision to reintubate, Bobby has a respiratory arrest.

---

22. What nursing intervention would you perform first?
    A. assemble intubation kit
    B. chest compressions
    C. ventilate with an Ambubag
    D. administer oxygen
23. Bobby requires ventilatory support via an endotracheal (E-T) tube. What size E-T tube would you have available?
    A. 4.0 cuffed
    B. 3.5 cuffed
    C. 5.0 uncuffed
    D. 2.5 uncuffed

Bobby's cardiopulmonary status eventually stabilizes. His invasive lines are removed, except for one peripheral IV line. He is transferred to the floor.

_____

24. Which of the following nursing interventions would be most effective in limiting Bobby's anxiety related to hospitalization?
   A. promote cuddling by parents
   B. encourage visitation of grandparents
   C. place pictures of family members in his crib
   D. talk about parents frequently

Posttest Answers

Question	Answer	Section	Table/Figure	Comment
1	C	One	Table 23–1	
2	B	Three	Table 23–7	
3	A	Two	Table 23–2	
4	D	Three	Table 23–5	
5	D	Four		
6	B	Four		The patient had an actual loss of adequate ventilation related to airway obstruction from the swollen epiglottis. The clinical data represent defining characteristics of the nursing diagnosis.
7	C	Two		The accident has produced an actual loss of intravascular volume. The normal blood pressure indicates that the patient is compensating for the volume deficit by increasing heart rate and by peripheral vaso-constriction (decreased peripheral pulses). Therefore, CO still remains within the normal range. CO will decrease if bleeding continues and compensatory mechanisms become exhausted.
8	A	Eight		
9	B	Eight		
10	C	Eight		
11	B	Nine		
12	D	Ten	Table 23–18	
13	B	Eleven		
14	A	Twelve		
15	B	Twelve		
16	A	Fifteen	Figure 23–4	
17	B	Fourteen	Table 23–29	
18	C	Fifteen		
19	D	Six	Table 23–10	
20	B	Eight		
21	B	Sixteen		
22	C	Four	Figure 23–1	
23	B	Four	Table 23–8	
24	A	Nineteen	Table 23–35	

REFERENCES

Ackerman, A.D. (1987). Conditions that predispose the critically ill child to infection. In M.C. Rogers (ed). *Textbook of pediatric intensive care*, pp. 789–842. Baltimore: Williams & Wilkins.

Bowlby, J. (1969). Patterns of attachment and contributing conditions. In J. Bowlby (ed). *Attachment and loss*, pp. 331–350. New York: Basic Books, Inc.

Brink, L.W. (1990). Abnormalities in temperature regulation. In D.L. Levin and F.C. Morriss (eds). *Essentials of pediatric intensive care*, pp. 175–185. St. Louis: Quality Medical Publishing.

Bruce, D.A., Alavi, A., Bilaniuk, L., Dolinskas, C., Obrist, W., and Uzzell, B. (1981). Diffuse cerebral swelling following head injuries in children: The syndrome of "malignant brain edema." *J. Neurosurg.* 54:170–178.

Chameides, L. (ed). (1988). *Textbook of pediatric advanced life support.* Dallas: American Heart Association.

Cherry, J.D., and Feigin, R.D. (1989). Infection in the compromised host. In E.R. Stiehm (ed). *Immunologic disorders in infants and children*, pp. 745–773. Philadelphia: W.B. Saunders Co.

Cooper, M.D., and Buckley, R.H. (1982). Developmental immunology and the immunodeficiency diseases. *JAMA.* 248:2658–2669.

Crone, R.K. (1980). Acute circulatory failure in children. *Pediatr. Clin. North Am.* 27:525–538.

Delgado, M.R. (1990). Status epilepticus. In D.L. Levin and F.C. Morriss (eds). *Essentials of pediatric intensive care*, pp. 59–63. St. Louis: Quality Medical Publishing.

Esperson, S. (1986). Nursing support of host defenses. *Crit. Care Q.* 9 (1):51–56.

Forlaw, L. (1983). The critically ill patient: Nutritional implications. *Nursing Clin. North Am.* 18 (1):111–128.

Friedman, W.F. (1972). The intrinsic physiologic properties of the developing heart. *Prog. Cardiovasc. Dis.* 15:87–111.

Gorgon, P., Kenner, C., and Schilling, S.B. (1988). Fluids, electrolytes, nutrition, and antibiotics. In C. Kenner, J. Harjo, and A. Brueggemeyer (eds). *Neonatal surgery: A nursing perspective*, pp. 263–296. New York: Grune & Stratton, Inc.

Guyton, A.C. (1987). *Human physiology and mechanism of disease*, 4th ed. Philadelphia: W.B. Saunders Co.

Hazinski, M.F., and van Stralen, D. (1990). Physiologic and anatomic differences between children and adults. In D.L. Levin and F.C. Morriss (eds). *Essentials of pediatric intensive care*, pp. 5–17. St. Louis: Quality Medical Publishing.

Jeans, M.E. (1983). The measurement of pain in children. In R. Melzack (ed). *Pain measurement and assessment*, pp. 183–219. New York: Raven Press.

Kendig, E.L., and Chernick, V. (1990). *Disorders of the respiratory tract in children*, 5th ed. Philadelphia: W.B. Saunders Co.

Kidder, C. (1989). Reestablishing health: Factors influencing the child's recovery in pediatric intensive care. *J. Pediatr. Nursing.* 4 (2):96–103.

Levin, G.M., Deren, J.J., Steiger, E., and Zinno, R. (1974). Role of oral intake in maintenance of gut mass and disaccharide activity. *Gastroenterology.* 67:975–982.

Marshall, S.B., Marshall, L.F., Vos, H.R., and Chestnut, R.M. (1990). *Neuroscience critical care.* Philadelphia: W.B. Saunders Co.

Mayer, T.A. (1985). Management of hypovolemic shock. In T.A. Mayer (ed). *Emergency management of pediatric trauma*, pp. 39–51. Philadelphia: W.B. Saunders Co.

Moore, K.L. (1988). *The developing human: Clinically oriented embryology*, 4th ed. Philadelphia: W.B. Saunders Co.

Owens, M.E. (1984). Pain in infancy: Conceptual and methodological issues. *Pain.* 20:213–230.

Perkins, R.M., and Levin, D.L. (1982). Shock in the pediatric patient. Part II. Therapy. *J. Pediatr.* 101:319–332.

Perkins, R.M., and Levin, D.L. (1990). In D.L. Levin and F.C. Morriss (eds). *Essentials of pediatric intensive care*, pp. 121–136. St. Louis: Quality Medical Publishing.

Ramsey, N.L. (1982). Effects of hospitalization on the child and the family. In M.J. Smith, J.A. Goodman, N.L. Ramsey, and S.B. Pasternack (eds). *Child and family: Concepts of nursing practice*, pp. 317–341. New York: McGraw-Hill Book Company.

Rosenberg, D.I. (1990). Status epilepticus. In J.L. Blumer (ed). *A practical guide to pediatric intensive care*, pp. 227–234. St. Louis: Mosby Year book.

Rosenthal, C.H. (1989). Immunosuppression in pediatric critical care patients. *Crit. Care Nursing Clin. North Am.* 1:775–785.

Rossetti, V.A., Thompson, B.M., Miller, J., Mateer, J.R., and Aprahamian, C. (1985). Intraosseous infusion: An alternative route of pediatric intravascular access. *Ann. Emerg. Med.* 14:885–888.

Ryan, N.T. (1976). Metabolic adaptations for energy production during trauma and sepsis. *Surg. Clin. North Am.* 56:1073–1090.

Schindler, B. (1985). Stress, affective disorders and immune function. *Med. Clin. North Am.* 69:585–597.

Shapiro, K., and Giller, C.A. (1990). Increased intracranial pressure. In D.L. Levin and F.C. Morriss (eds). *Essentials of pediatric intensive care*, pp. 49–58. St. Louis: Quality Medical Publishing.

Shayevitz, J.R., and Weissman, C. (1987). Nutrition and metabolism in the critically ill child. In M.C. Rogers (ed). *Textbook of pediatric intensive care*, pp. 943–978. Baltimore: Williams & Wilkins.

Smith, J.B. (1983). Nursing process in pediatric critical care. In J.B. Smith (ed). *Pediatric critical care*, pp. 1–20. New York: John Wiley & Sons.

Snow, R.B., Zimmerman, R.D., Gandy, S.E., and Deck, D.F. (1986). Comparison of magnetic resonance imaging and computed tomography in the evaluation of head injury. *Neurosurgery.* 18:45–52.

Teasdale, G., and Jennett, B. (1974). Assessment of coma and impaired consciousness. A practical scale. *Lancet* 2:81–84.

Tribett, D. (1989). Immune system function. *Crit. Care Nursing Clin. North Am.* 1:725–740.

Whaley, L.F., and Wong, D.L. (1987). *Nursing care of infants and children*, 3rd ed. St. Louis: C.V. Mosby Co.

Williams, J.K., and Lancaster, J. (1976). Thermoregulation of the newborn. *Maternal-Child Nursing.* 1:355–360.

Wilson, T., and Broome, M.E. (1989). Promoting the young child's development in the intensive care unit. *Heart Lung.* 18:274–280.

Zaritsky, A., and Chernow, B. (1984). Use of catecholamines in pediatrics. *J. Pediatr.* 105:341–350.

PART VII

Clinical Simulations

Module 24

A Ventilation and Perfusion Simulation

Kathleen Dorman Wagner and Pamela Stinson Kidd

Objectives

Following completion of this simulation, the learner should have gained

1. Skills in assessing a patient with a respiratory and perfusion problem
2. Skills in management of a patient with a respiratory and perfusion problem
3. Skills in altering care based on available data and patient needs
4. Skills in differentiating interventions that may be performed independently from those requiring medical orders

Directions

The case of James Rabin is a clinical problem-solving exercise, requiring application and analytic skills. It is not a comprehensive review of all of the respiratory and perfusion self-study modules, nor does it follow the patient throughout his hospitalization. The major focus of the simulation is a single, complex cardiopulmonary system problem and is confined to one isolated period during his hospitalization.

You will be asked to respond to several questions throughout the module by selecting available options. At times there are more correct answers than you are expected to select. For example, three options may be appropriate and you are asked to select two options. Nurses are constantly faced with alter-

natives of equal value. The purpose of the simulation is to assist you in making wise choices and understanding the rationale behind those choices.

This clinical simulation is designed to integrate information contained in several of the self-study modules, particularly the modules related to ventilation and perfusion. Completion of the simulation requires application of pathophysiology to use the nursing process effectively. The aims of the simulation are to promote integration and application of essential concepts in caring for the acutely ill patient.

The simulation begins by introducing a patient situation. Throughout the simulation, you will be required to focus your assessment of the patient, analyze assessment findings, prioritize nursing interventions, and evaluate patient outcomes. Select your responses as indicated throughout the module. You need only check the line at the right of the item for those items you wish to choose. Feedback on your selection and rationale for the grading of your responses is provided following each section. Make ALL of the desired choices BEFORE you examine the corresponding answers and rationales. Once your choices are marked, look at the answers and write in the point scores for each item you chose. DO NOT change or add to your original answers.

PLEASE DO NOT LOOK at the answers prior to responding; otherwise the teaching or learning as-

pects of the simulation are negated. At the end of the simulation, you can compare your score with the score ranges to examine your performance level.

Items are scored on a range of +2 to −2 points:

+2 = Essential
+1 = Facilitative
 0 = Neutral, neither facilitative nor harmful
−1 = Nonfacilitative, potentially harmful
−2 = Harmful

PLEASE COVER UP THE ANSWER SECTIONS IF VISIBLE BEFORE BEGINNING EACH INQUIRY SECTION.

Scenario

You are a registered nurse working on the night shift on a medical floor in a 300-bed community hospital. At 1:00 A.M. the Emergency Department nurse calls to notify you that you will be receiving a direct admission from a neighboring town. He is Mr. James Rabin, a 45-year-old man. He is in apparent respiratory distress. No other information is available. At 1:30 A.M. Mr. Rabin arrives by ambulance with his wife. You have placed Mr. Rabin in his bed. No physician orders have accompanied him.

Section One

Mr. Rabin has been placed in his bed. He appears to be having acute respiratory discomfort. You are now about to begin a rapid assessment of him prior to calling the physician for orders. Which of the following assessments would be best to perform at this time? (*Choose as many items as desired.*)

Item

1.1 General physical appearance _____

1.2 Pedal pulses _____

1.3 Respiratory rate and pattern _____

1.4 Color of lips and nailbeds _____

1.5 Gag reflex _____

1.6 Pupil reaction _____

1.7 Amount and color of sputum _____

1.8 Medical history _____

1.9 Color of urine _____

1.10 Deep pain response _____

1.11 Temperature _____

1.12 Medications taken at home _____

1.13 Abdominal palpation _____

1.14 Blood pressure and pulse _____

1.15 Babinski reflex _____

1.16 Auscultation of chest _____

1.17 Bowel sounds _____

1.18 Level of consciousness _____

1.19 Extremities _____

Once you have made your selection(s), read the answers to the options that you have chosen. Write down the points given for each item that you selected next to your check mark.

Section One Answers

Item	Data with Rationale
1.1 General physical appearance	Appears to be in poor nutritional state; barrel chest is noted (+1 point)

1.2 Pedal pulses	All are positive. (0 point)
1.3 Respiratory rate and pattern	Respiratory rate is 28 breaths/minute and shallow; appears dyspneic. (+2 points)
1.4 Color of lips and nailbeds	Lips appear dark and nailbeds are dusky. (+1 point)
1.5 Gag reflex	Intact; however, checking a gag reflex on this patient is inappropriate and may cause him to vomit. (−2 points)
1.6 Pupil reaction	Pupils are equal and react to light briskly. (0 point)
1.7 Amount and color of sputum	Occasional cough; no sputum has yet been produced. This is important to assess initially. It can alert nurse to potential pulmonary problems, including airway clearance. (+2 points)
1.8 Medical history	He has a 10-year history of emphysema, which is being treated by drug therapy. He has recently been diagnosed with congestive heart failure (CHF). He also has a history of insulin-dependent diabetes. (+1 point)
1.9 Color of urine	Clear yellow; this is not a priority assessment at this time. (−1 point)
1.10 Deep pain response	Yells at you to stop hurting him; this action is inappropriate in an awake patient. (−1 point)
1.11 Temperature	101° F, orally. (+1 point)
1.12 Medications taken at home	NPH insulin 15 U daily. Theo-Dur 200 mg PO every 12 hours. Digoxin 0.25 mg daily. Lasix 10 mg daily. Obtaining information concerning medication history can give a rapid picture of the patient's medical problems. (+1 point)
1.13 Abdominal palpation	Abdomen is soft and distended. This data is not a priority at this time. (0 point)
1.14 Blood pressure and pulse	BP = 146/88; P = 115/minute. These are two basic parameters that are crucial to assess early. They give a rapid baseline of hemodynamic status. (+2 points)
1.15 Babinski reflex	Normal; however, checking this reflex is inappropriate in an awake patient, causing unnecessary discomfort. (−1 point)
1.16 Auscultation of chest	Good choice; coarse crackles and expiratory wheeze heard bilaterally. Fine crackles heard over lower lung fields. Breath sounds are diminished in right lower lobe. (+2 points)
1.17 Bowel sounds	Hypoactive in all four quadrants; not a priority at this time. (−1 point)
1.18 Level of consciousness	Oriented to person and place but not to time and condition. (+1 point)
1.19 Extremities	Pitting pedal edema noted bilaterally in lower extremities. (+1 point)

Section Two

Based on the previously assessed data, what would be the most appropriate initial nursing intervention? (*Choose one item only.*)

Item

2.1 Perform tracheal suction _____

2.2 Increase head of bed to 45 degrees _____

2.3 Initiate oxygen at 2 L/minute per nasal cannula _____

2.4 Encourage patient to drink a minimum of 100 mL of fluid per hour _____

2.5 Initiate oxygen at 40% aerosol mask _____

2.6 Initiate deep breathing exercises every 1–2 hours _____

Once you have made your selection, read the answer to the option that you have chosen. Write down the points given to the item that you selected next to your check mark.

Section Two Answers

Item	Data with Rationale
2.1 Perform tracheal suction	Inappropriate; invasive procedure may not be necessary and may be harmful. (−1 point)
2.2 Increase head of bed to 45 degrees	Good choice; increasing head of bed displaces abdominal contents downward, helping diaphragm movement. (+2 points)
2.3 Initiate oxygen at 2 L/minute per nasal cannula	Respiratory Therapy is unable to comply with request—no physician's order. (0 point)
2.4 Encourage patient to drink a minimum of 100 mL of fluid per hour	While this may be appropriate for hydration of a pneumonia patient, insufficient data is available at this time to force fluids. It could be harmful if he is found to have a fluid volume overload, especially with his history of congestive heart failure and pitting edema. (−1 point)
2.5 Initiate oxygen at 40% aerosol mask	Respiratory Therapy is unable to comply—no physician's order. 40% O_2 may be harmful to this patient if he retains CO_2. (−2 points)
2.6 Initiate deep breathing exercises every 1–2 hours	Good choice; at this time, this may be the most effective means of enhancing oxygenation. (+2 points)

Section Three: Consultation

You telephone the physician to obtain a brief history and admission orders. You report the assessment data that has already been collected. You also report that you have increased the head of his bed to 45 degrees and have initiated frequent deep breathing exercises. The physician gives you the following brief history:

Mr. Rabin has a 10-year history of emphysema. He is also an insulin-dependent diabetic. He has recently been diagnosed with congestive heart failure. His last chest film, done 6 months ago, indicated the presence of cor pulmonale.

Physician Orders

1. Arterial blood gases
2. Portable chest x-ray
3. Start intravenous line of $D_5W/0.45$ normal saline at 75 mL/hour
4. Electrocardiogram (ECG)
5. CBC and electrolyte panel
6. Oxygen at 2 L/minute per nasal cannula

7. Medication orders:
   Albuterol inhaler 2 puffs every 4 hours, NPH insulin 15 U SQ daily, digoxin 0.25 mg PO daily, Lasix 10 mg PO daily, Aminophylline IV piggyback at 35 mg/hour, Kefzol (cefazolin) 500 mg IV every 8 hours
8. Sputum for culture and sensitivity

Section Four

You are now preparing to initiate collaborative interventions based on the physician orders just received. What should be your priority interventions? (*Choose two interventions.*)

Item	
4.1 Obtain complete blood cell count (CBC)	_____
4.2 Obtain portable chest x-ray	_____
4.3 Initiate IV line	_____
4.4 Obtain arterial blood gases (ABGs)	_____
4.5 Initiate oxygen at 2 L/minute per nasal cannula	_____

4.6 Initiate IV Kefzol _____

4.7 Obtain sputum culture _____

Once you have made your selection(s), read the answers to the options that you have chosen. Write down the points given to each item that you selected next to your check mark.

Section Four Answers

Item	Data with Rationale
4.1 Obtain CBC	WBC = 12,000/μL, RBC = 6.5 $\times$ 10^6/μL, Hg = 18 g/dL, Hct = 54%. CBC results can indicate presence of infection and compensatory hematopoetic responses to chronic obstructive pulmonary disease (COPD). While important, this is not the most essential data to obtain. (+1 point)
4.2 Obtain portable chest x-ray	Chest film indicates: right lower infiltrates with cardiomegaly consistent with cor pulmonale. While important, this is not the most essential data to obtain. (+1 point)
4.3 Initiate IV line	Not the best choice; while important, it is more crucial to enhance oxygenation level than to hydrate at this time. Once oxygenation has been measured and enhanced, an IV should be started as a venous access for fluids and drug therapy. (+1 point)
4.4 Obtain ABGs	Good choice. pH = 7.28, $Paco_2$ = 65 mm Hg, Pao_2 = 50 mm Hg, HCO_3 = 34 mEq, Sao_2 = 80%. Respiratory acidosis with hypoxemia. Obtaining a STAT ABG measurement will rapidly establish the acid-base balance and oxygenation status of the patient. (+2 points)
4.5 Initiate oxygen at 2L/minute per nasal cannula	Good choice; after obtaining an arterial blood sample, oxygen should be administered. Providing oxygen supplementation enhances tissue oxygenation. Observe the patient closely for adequacy of therapy. Changes may be required. (+2 points)
4.6 Initiate IV Kefzol	Unable to initiate; IV catheter has not been inserted. Obtain sputum culture prior to initiation of antibiotics. (−1 point)
4.7 Obtain sputum culture	Results pending; important to obtain before initiating antibiotic therapy. It is not the intervention of the highest priority at this time. (+1 point)

Section Five

Based on the data you have collected thus far, what action would be most appropriate to initiate immediately? (*Choose one item only.*)

Item

5.1 Place intubation tray at bedside _____

5.2 Continue to deep breathe patient vigorously _____

5.3 Increase oxygen to 6 L/minute per nasal cannula _____

5.4 Insert oral airway _____

5.5 Increase IV fluids _____

Once you have made your selection, read the answer to the option that you have chosen. Write down the points given to the item that you selected next to your check mark.

Section Five Answers

Item	Data with Rationale
5.1 Place intubation tray at bedside	Good choice; patient intubated and placed on a mechanical ventilator. (+2 points)

5.2 Continue to deep breathe patient vigorously

His ABGs show that this has not been effective in improving his respiratory status. (0 point)

5.3 Increase oxygen to 6 L/minute per nasal cannula

Not appropriate; patient may be a CO_2 retainer, relying on an hypoxic breathing drive. High concentrations of oxygen may precipitate respiratory arrest. (−2 points)

5.4 Insert oral airway

Inappropriate at this time unless tongue is blocking airway. Initiating gag reflex may precipitate vomiting with possible aspiration. Remove head pillow and perform chin lift if necessary to open airway. (−1 point)

5.5 Increase IV fluids

Inappropriate; you have no orders to do this. Also, previous assessments have shown evidence of potential for fluid volume excess and thus it could be potentially harmful. (−1 point)

Section Six: Consultation

You notify the physician of Mr. Rabin's current status and the results of the ordered tests. A summary of the test results are:

- CBC: WBC = 12,000/μL, RBC = 6.5 × 10^6/μL, Hg = 18 g/dL, Hct = 54%.
- ABG = pH 7.28, $Paco_2$ = 65 mm Hg, Pao_2 = 50 mm Hg, HCO_3 = 34 mEq, Sao_2 = 78%.
- Electrolyte panel: Na^+ = 135 mEq/L, Cl^- = 100 mEq/L, K^+ = 3.5 mEq/L, Ca^{++} = 10 mg/dL.
- ECG = Sinus tachycardia of 105/minute. Borderline first degree A-V block with P-R interval = 0.22 sec., QRS = 0.06. Unifocal ventricular premature beats (VPBs) of <5/minute. T-waves have decreased amplitude; S-T segment changes are consistent with digitalis toxicity.
- Portable chest film: right lower lobe infiltrate with right cardiac enlargement consistent with cor pulmonale.
- Sputum culture results: Positive for *Staphylococcus aureus*.

Physician Orders

1. STAT intubation per Anesthesia Department
2. Initiate mechanical ventilation (TV = 750 mL, Assist/Control Mode at 12/minute, Fio_2 = 50%)
3. Transfer to Intensive Care Unit (ICU) with routine ICU protocol
4. Repeat ABGs 30 min. following placement on ventilator
5. A.M. labs: digoxin level, theophylline level
6. Pulmonary arterial catheter tray at bedside for possible insertion

Section Seven

Mr. Rabin has been in the ICU for 24 hours. Over the past hour, the nurse has made several observations:

While intravenous intake has been maintained at a steady volume, urine output has diminished significantly. The high pressure alarm on Mr. Rabin's ventilator has triggered frequently due to coughing. His secretions are now thin, foamy, and blood tinged. Mr. Rabin's theophylline and digoxin levels have just been called in from the laboratory. Theophylline level is 18 μg/mL, and digoxin level is 2.2 ng/mL. His arterial blood pressure is 90/50 with a heart rate of 110/minute.

What data would be most essential to help analyze the changes in Mr. Rabin's status? (*Choose two items.*)

Item

7.1 Assess gag reflex   _____

7.2 Obtain STAT portable chest x-ray per ICU protocol   _____

7.3 Assess neurologic status   _____

7.4 Obtain hemodynamic readings   _____

7.5 Check urine color and specific gravity   _____

7.6 Auscultate chest   _____

7.7 Assess temperature   _____

Once you have made your selection(s), read the answers to the options that you have chosen. Write down the points given to each item that you selected next to your check mark.

Section Seven Answers

Item	Data with Rationale
7.1 Assess gag reflex	Inappropriate; unhelpful data; could cause vomiting and aspiration. (−2 points)
7.2 Obtain STAT portable chest x-ray per ICU protocol	Good choice; results show diffuse infiltrates bilaterally, consistent with pulmonary edema. The x-ray helps in rapid diagnosis of the pulmonary problem. (+2 points)
7.3 Assess neurologic status	No change in neurologic status. Changes in responsiveness level can be an early indicator of deterioration in oxygenation status. (+1 point)
7.4 Obtain hemodynamic readings	Good choice; CVP = 12 mm Hg, PAP = 36/24 mm Hg, PCWP = 22 mm Hg, C.O. = 3.1 L/minute. Readings consistent with fluid volume excess. (+2 points)
7.5 Check urine color and specific gravity	Urine is yellow, clear, and concentrated with a specific gravity of 1.017. While the specific gravity is helpful in indicating fluid status, it is not the highest priority at this time. (0 point)
7.6 Auscultate chest	You hear diffuse fine and coarse crackles throughout lung fields. (+1 point)
7.7 Assess temperature	101°F, rectally; not the highest priority at this time. However, it can be an important indicator of an acute infectious process. (+1 point)

Section Eight: Consultation

The nurse notifies the physician of the changes in Mr. Rabin's status.

Summary of new data includes:

- Chest x-ray: Bilateral diffuse pulmonary infiltrates consistent with pulmonary edema.
- Neuro status: No change.
- Hemodynamic readings: CVP = 12 mm Hg, PAP = 36/24 mm Hg, PCWP = 22 mm Hg, C.O. = 3.1 L/minute.
- Lung auscultation: Fine and coarse crackles throughout lung fields.
- Temperature: 101.0° F rectally.

Physician Orders

1. Lasix 30 mg IV push STAT
2. Decrease IV fluid to keep open rate
3. Obtain arterial blood gases STAT
4. Digoxin 0.25 mg IV daily
5. Obtain blood cultures for temperature >102°F (R)
6. Obtain STAT chest x-ray
7. Obtain STAT ECG

Section Nine

You are now preparing to begin collaborative interventions based on the physician's orders noted in Section Eight. Regarding the physician orders, which interventions will need to be performed FIRST based on Mr. Rabin's immediate needs? (*Choose two items.*)

Item

9.1 Decrease IV fluids to keep vein open   _____

9.2 Obtain STAT electrocardiogram   _____

9.3 Administer digoxin (IV)   _____

9.4 Obtain STAT arterial blood gases   _____

9.5 Obtain STAT blood cultures   _____

9.6 Administer Lasix IV push STAT   _____

9.7 Obtain STAT chest x-ray   _____

Once you have made your selection(s), read the answers to the options that you have chosen. Write down the points given to each item that you selected next to your check mark.

Section Nine Answers

Item	Data with Rationale
9.1 Decrease IV fluids to keep vein open	Since he is experiencing a fluid volume overload problem, diminishing fluid intake is an appropriate action. (+1 point)
9.2 Obtain STAT electrocardiogram	Sinus tachycardia is noted. No significant changes from previous ECG. While important, it is not the highest priority for the nurse at this point. (0 point)
9.3 Administer digoxin (IV)	Inappropriate; patient's digoxin level was reported as 2.2 ng/dL, indicating digoxin toxicity. Drug should be withheld and physician notified of digoxin level. (−2 points)
9.4 Obtain STAT arterial blood gases	Good choice; ABGs are very important in establishing acid-base balance and level of oxygenation. Pao_2 may be decreased because of lung infiltrates and fluid in lungs. Results are pending. (+2 points)
9.5 Obtain STAT blood cultures	It is inappropriate at this time. His temperature does not meet the ordered criteria. (−1 point)
9.6 Administer Lasix IV push STAT	Good choice; Lasix (furosemide) is a potent loop diuretic that promotes rapid excretion of fluid and thus is effective in the treatment of pulmonary edema/heart failure. (+2 points)
9.7 Obtain a chest x-ray	Good choice; the chest film has bilateral infiltrates indicative of moderate pulmonary edema. (+2 points)

Section Ten: Current Status Report

Ten days post admission, Mr. Rabin's status is as follows:

- Arterial blood gas readings: pH = 7.35, $Paco_2$ = 60 mm Hg, Pao_2 = 80 mm Hg, HCO_3 = 34 mm Hg, Sao_2 = 92% on ventilator settings of TV = 750 mL, synchronized intermittent mandatory ventilation (SIMV) mode at rate of 8/minute, Fio_2 = 30%.
- Hemodynamic status: CVP = 10 mm Hg, PCWP = 15 mm Hg, PAP = 28/18 mm Hg, C.O. = 6.0 L/minute.
- Urine output: 125 mL/hour.
- Most current sputum culture: Positive for pseudomonas.
- Cardiac monitor displays a normal sinus rhythm with occasional PVC.
- A current chest x-ray shows small infiltrate in right lower lobe.

Section Eleven

Based on the analysis of the patient data noted in Section Ten, which of the following nursing diagnoses is MOST IMPORTANT in the immediate management of Mr. Rabin? (*Choose one item only.*).

Item

11.1 **Fluid volume excess** _____

11.2 **Impaired gas exchange** _____

11.3 **Alteration in urinary elimination** _____

11.4 **Infection** _____

11.5 **Fluid volume deficit** _____

11.6 **Decreased cardiac output** _____

Once you have made your selection, read the answer to the option that you have chosen. Write down the points given to the item that you selected next to your check mark.

Section Eleven Answers

Item	Data with Rationale
11.1 **Fluid volume excess**	Not an active problem at this time; however, he will remain at risk for its redevelopment. (+1 point)
11.2 **Impaired gas exchange**	Not actual problem at this time; patient has chronic respiratory impairment and continues to require ventilatory assistance. Data shows his ABGs to be under reasonable control at this time. (+1 point)
11.3 **Alteration in urinary elimination**	Not actual problem at this time; since he has a urinary catheter and problems with heart failure, this will remain a risk. (0 point)
11.4 **Infection**	Good choice; this is the priority nursing diagnosis. Data confirms a pulmonary infection. (+2 points)
11.5 **Fluid volume deficit**	Inappropriate; increasing fluid intake based on this nursing diagnosis could harm this patient. (−2 points)
11.6 **Decreased cardiac output**	Inappropriate; his cardiac output is now within normal limits. (0 point)

Simulation Self-Scoring Sheet

1. On the form below, circle the point value beside the number of each response you selected on your answer sheet. (Maximum number of points in this simulation is 33.)

Response Number	Point Value	Response Number	Point Value	Response Number	Point Value
1.1	+1	2.1	−1	7.2	+2
1.2	0	2.2	+2	7.3	+1
1.3	+2	2.3	0	7.4	+2
1.4	+1	2.4	−1	7.5	0
1.5	−2	2.5	−2	7.6	+1
1.6	0	2.6	+2	7.7	+1
1.7	+2	4.1	+1	9.1	+1
1.8	+1	4.2	+1	9.2	0
1.9	−1	4.3	+1	9.3	−2
1.10	−1	4.4	+2	9.4	+2
1.11	+1	4.5	+2	9.5	−1
1.12	+1	4.6	−1	9.6	+2
1.13	0	4.7	+1	9.7	+2
1.14	+2	5.1	+2	11.1	+1
1.15	−1	5.2	0	11.2	+1
1.16	+2	5.3	−2	11.3	0
1.17	−1	5.4	−1	11.4	+2
1.18	+1	5.5	−1	11.5	−2
1.19	+1	7.1	−2	11.6	0

2. Determine your percentage score by multiplying your score by 100. Take the number obtained and divide it by 33 (the maximum number of possible points) to get your percentage.

   33 points = 100% excellent performance
   30 points = 90% good performance
   26 points = 80% average performance

Module 25

A Trauma Simulation

Pamela Stinson Kidd

Objectives

Following completion of this simulation, the learner should have gained

1. Skills in assessing a patient with a traumatic injury
2. Skills in management of a patient with traumatic injury

3. Skills in altering care based on available data and patient needs
4. Skills in differentiating interventions that may be performed independently from those requiring medical orders

---

Directions

The case of Pam Baker is a clinical problem-solving exercise requiring application and analytic skills. It is not a comprehensive review of all of the trauma self-study modules, nor does it follow the patient throughout her hospitalization. The major focus of the simulation is a single, complex trauma problem and is confined to one isolated period during her hospitalization.

You will be asked to respond to several questions throughout the module by selecting available options. At times there are more correct answers than you are expected to select. For example, three options may be appropriate and you are asked to select two options. Nurses are constantly faced with alter-

natives of equal value. The purpose of the simulation is to assist you in making wise choices and understanding the rationale behind those choices.

The simulation begins by introducing a patient situation. Throughout the simulation, you will be required to focus your assessment of the patient, analyze assessment findings, prioritize nursing interventions, and evaluate patient outcomes. Select your responses as indicated throughout the module. You need only check the line at the right of the item for those items you wish to choose. Feedback on your selection and rationale for the grading of your responses is provided following each section. Make ALL of the desired choices BEFORE you examine the

623

corresponding answers and rationales. Once your choices are marked, look at the answers and write in your point scores for each item you chose. DO NOT change or add to your original answers.

PLEASE DO NOT LOOK at the answers prior to responding; otherwise the teaching or learning aspects of the simulation are negated. At the end of the simulation, you can compare your score with the score ranges to examine your performance level.

Items are scored on a range of +2 to −2 points:

+2 = Essential
+1 = Facilitative
 0 = Neutral, neither facilitative nor harmful
−1 = Nonfacilitative, potentially harmful
−2 = Harmful

PLEASE COVER UP THE ANSWER SECTIONS IF VISIBLE BEFORE BEGINNING EACH INQUIRY SECTION.

Scenario

You are a registered nurse working in the Emergency Department (ED) of a 600-bed community hospital that is designated a Level I trauma center (by the American College of Surgeons). You have just received a radio transmission from a local Emergency Medical Services (EMS) ground crew informing you of an incoming patient.

The patient is an unrestrained driver of a vehicle involved in a two-car, T-bone (side impact) motor vehicle crash (MVC), travelling approximately 40 mph. The patient is 7 months pregnant. She did not lose consciousness. At the scene her BP was 110/70, heart rate was 96, and respiratory rate was 24. Fetal movements were reported by the patient.

Because of the patient's mechanism of injury and pregnancy, she is declared a trauma alert case. Orders are radioed to the EMS crew instructing them to start two peripheral large bore IV lines and hang Lactated Ringer's (LR) solution. Oxygen is ordered per simple face mask at 8 L/minute. The crew states that they have an estimated arrival time of 10 minutes.

Section One

Ms. Baker arrives in the ED. She is on a backboard with LR infusing wide open via #16 gauge IV cathe-

ter in the right forearm. She is complaining of pain in her right leg and chest. She has a minor forehead laceration. Based on Ms. Baker's mechanism of injury, for which of the following injuries would she be most susceptible? (*Choose as many conditions as desired.*)

Item

1.1 Posterior fracture or dislocation of the femoral head   _____

1.2 Fractured ribs   _____

1.3 Pneumothorax   _____

1.4 High cervical fracture   _____

1.5 Myocardial contusion   _____

1.6 Pelvic fracture   _____

1.7 Calcaneus fractures   _____

1.8 Ruptured bladder   _____

1.9 Lumbosacral spine fractures   _____

Once you have made your selection(s), read the answers to the options you have chosen. Write down the points given to each item that you selected next to your check mark.

Section One Answers

Item	Data with Rationale
1.1 Posterior fracture or dislocation of the femoral head	May be present in either the leg used to brake the vehicle or the leg on the side of impact. (+2 points)
1.2 Fractured ribs	May be present due to contact between chest and steering wheel in the unrestrained driver. In last trimester of pregnancy gravid uterus may be an intermediary point of contact. (+2 points)

1.3 Pneumothorax	May be present from direct forces to chest or from movement of a fractured rib in the unrestrained driver. (+2 points)
1.4 High cervical fracture	Usually associated with a closed head injury and Ms. Baker did not have a loss of consciousness. Occurs most frequently in back seat passenger position in vehicle without head seat restraints that is hit from the rear, or in a front seat passenger whose head or face impacts the windshield or dash. (0 point)
1.5 Myocardial contusion	Possible in the unrestrained driver from contact with the steering wheel and secondary forces. (+2 points)
1.6 Pelvic fracture	Usually associated with pedestrian and vehicle collisions especially when pedestrian is dragged under vehicle. Occasionally associated with seat belt use. Pelvic fractures are associated with a high incidence of placental separation and direct fetal injury (Crosby, 1983). They may occur with severe blunt trauma (Bremer and Cassata, 1986). (+1 point)
1.7 Calcaneous fractures	Fractures of the "heels" associated with falls from heights. (0 point)
1.8 Ruptured bladder	Increases with each month of pregnancy as bladder becomes an abdominal organ. (+1 point)
1.9 Lumbosacral spine fractures	Associated with falls from heights and ejection from vehicle in a MVC. (0 point)

Section Two

You are beginning a rapid assessment of Ms. Baker. Which of the following assessments would be BEST to perform at this time? (*Choose as many items as desired.*)

Item
2.1 Breath sounds   _____
2.2 Vital signs (respiratory rate [RR], blood pressure [BP], heart rate [HR])   _____
2.3 Fetal heart tones (FHT)   _____
2.4 Pedal pulses   _____
2.5 Pupillary reaction   _____
2.6 Medical history   _____
2.7 Gag reflex   _____
2.8 Pain response   _____
2.9 Allergy history   _____
2.10 Medication history   _____
2.11 Weight   _____
2.12 Genital area   _____
2.13 Temperature   _____

Once you have made your selection(s), read the answers to the options you have chosen. Write down the points given to each item that you selected next to your check mark.

Section Two Answers

Item | **Data with Rationale**
2.1 Breath sounds | Vesicular breath sounds auscultated in right lung fields. Diminished breath sounds left lung fields. (+2 points)
2.2 Vital signs (RR, BP, HR) | Respiratory rate is 28 breaths/minute. BP 108/68, Hr 100. The upward displacement of the diaphragm during pregnancy decreases the functional residual capacity and may be responsible for hyperventilation (Sorensen et al, 1986). (+2 points)

2.3 Fetal heart tones (FHT)	FHT = 140; audible with Doppler. Important to assess in patient more than 16 weeks pregnant. Early signs of maternal hypovolemia are best assessed by determining fetal status (Bremer and Cassata, 1986). (+2 points)
2.4 Pedal pulses	Left pedal pulse 2+. Right pedal pulse 1+. Important to assess secondary to complaint of right leg pain but can wait until the secondary survey. (+1 point)
2.5 Pupillary reaction	Pupils are equal and react to light briskly. (0 point)
2.6 Medical history	Negative medical history. Gravida 1 Para 0 AB 0. (+1 point)
2.7 Gag reflex	Intact; however, checking a gag reflex on this patient is inappropriate because she is conscious and may cause her to vomit. (−2 points)
2.8 Pain response	Yells at you for "pinching" her. This is inappropriate in an awake patient. (−1 point)
2.9 Allergy history	Allergic to penicillin. This information can wait until the secondary survey. (+1 point)
2.10 Medication history	Prenatal vitamins with iron; obtaining information concerning medications can provide a rapid picture of existing medical problems. You are thankful that Ms. Baker's medication history is nonsignificant. (+1 point)
2.11 Weight	Not important to weigh Ms. Baker at the present time. A self-reported weight might be useful later for comparison purposes. (0 point)
2.12 Genital area	Important to assess for presence of vaginal bleeding and drainage since separation of placenta from uterine wall is a possibility in any pregnant patient following an injury. She is not bleeding at present. (+2 points)
2.13 Temperature	May be useful information later for comparison purposes. (0 point)

Section Three

Based on the previously assessed data, what would be the MOST appropriate initial nursing intervention? (*Choose one item.*)

Item

3.1 Mark Ms. Baker's fundus   _____

3.2 Place a wedge under the backboard on Ms. Baker's right side   _____

3.3 Date and time the IV tubing started in the prehospital setting   _____

3.4 Encourage Ms. Baker to breathe slowly and deeply   _____

3.5 Place the automatic external BP cuff on Ms. Baker's arm   _____

3.6 Cover Ms. Baker's forehead laceration   _____

Once you have made your selection, read the answer to the option you have chosen. Write down the points given to the item that you selected next to your check mark.

Section Three Answers

| **Item** | **Data with Rationale** |
| 3.1 Mark Ms. Baker's fundus | Measuring fundal height will provide a quick way of estimating gestational age. Serial measurement may indicate uterine bleeding (Gatrell, 1987). This is a good choice but can wait until the secondary survey. (+1 point) |

3.2 Place a wedge under the backboard on Ms. Baker's right side

Excellent choice; all women more than 20 weeks pregnant are at risk for supine hypotension and reduced uterine blood flow. Since the inferior vena cava is located on the right side, positioning Ms. Baker on her left side can increase her cardiac output by 25%. Make sure she is adequately strapped to the backboard first! (+2 points)

3.3 Date and time the IV tubing started in the prehospital setting

Not necessary at this time; can be performed later. (0 point)

3.4 Encourage Ms. Baker to breathe slowly and deeply

The gravid woman has a reduced oxygen reserve. Encouraging her to breathe slowly and deeply will help prevent hypoxia. (+1 point)

3.5 Place the automatic external BP cuff on Ms. Baker's arm

BP falls during the second trimester of pregnancy but increases to near normal in the last trimester. Because of Ms. Baker's mechanism of injury, she is susceptible for a hemothorax and internal bleeding. BP monitoring is important but should be done after you position Ms. Baker correctly. (+1 point)

3.6 Cover Ms. Baker's forehead laceration

Not necessary at this time. (0 point)

Section Four: Consultation

After assessing Ms. Baker, in consultation with you, the trauma surgeon orders the following interventions.

1. Oxygen 8 to 10 L/minute non-rebreathing mask post obtaining arterial blood gases (ABGs)
2. Third peripheral IV line with LR 1000 mL at keep vein open (KVO) rate
3. Complete blood count (CBC)
4. Type and cross match for 4 units of blood
5. Fetal monitor
6. Electrocardiogram (ECG)
7. Chest x-ray
8. Cervical spine films
9. Right leg x-ray
10. Nasogastric tube to low wall suction
11. Urinary catheter
12. Pulse oximeter
13. Pelvic x-ray

Section Five

You are now preparing to initiate collaborative interventions based on the trauma surgeon's orders.

What should be your priority interventions? (*Choose two priority interventions.*)

Item

5.1 Initiate 40% oxygen per face mask post ABGs _____

5.2 Initiate peripheral IV line _____

5.3 Obtain CBC _____

5.4 Obtain type and crossmatch _____

5.5 Apply fetal monitor _____

5.6 Obtain ECG _____

5.7 Obtain portable chest x-ray _____

5.8 Obtain cervical spine films _____

5.9 Obtain right leg x-ray _____

5.10 Insert nasogastric tube _____

5.11 Insert urinary catheter _____

5.12 Apply pulse oximeter _____

5.13 Pelvic x-ray _____

Once you have made your selection(s), read the answers to the options you have chosen. Write down the points given to each item that you selected next to your check mark.

Section Five Answers

Item	Data with Rationale
5.1 Initiate oxygen 8–10 L/minute per non-rebreather mask post ABGs	Pregnancy is associated with marked increase in oxygen consumption and reduced oxygen reserves. Ms. Baker may also have a pulmonary injury based on her history of chest pain, non-restrained driver, and respiratory rate of 28. The fetus is sensitive to maternal hypoxia. Switching from a simple face mask to a non-rebreather mask will decrease CO_2 retention and the possibility of respiratory acidosis. Excellent choice. (+2 points)
5.2 Initiate peripheral IV line	Venous access in the pregnant trauma patient includes placement of two or three large-bore peripheral IV lines if a central IV line is unavailable. Even though Ms. Baker already has two IV lines in, blood samples can be obtained during the insertion of the third IV line for laboratory testing. In case Ms. Baker experiences blood loss from her injuries, venous access is extremely important. (+2 points)
5.3 Obtain CBC	Baseline hemoglobin and hematocrit values are important for monitoring blood loss. However, this is not the best choice at this time since this may be obtained at the same time as initiating the IV. Because plasma blood volume increases by 50% during pregnancy, the hemoglobin decreases to approximately 11 grams. Therefore a hemoglobin of less than 11 grams is a significant finding. (+1 point)
5.4 Obtain type and crossmatch	Should be done in conjunction with initiation of IV line to expedite care. This is an important procedure in case blood administration is necessary. (+1 point)
5.5 Apply fetal monitor	It is important to monitor fetal heart rate particularly if Ms. Baker experiences contractions. However, mother should be cared for first since maternal oxygenation and circulation is directly related to fetal well-being. (+1 point)
5.6 Obtain ECG	Can postpone this briefly; it is important because of Ms. Baker's history of chest pain and being an unrestrained driver. Ectopic beats are more prevalent during pregnancy. Promoting Ms. Baker's oxygenation and circulation may alleviate the chest pain. (+1 point)
5.7 Obtain portable chest x-ray	This should be done after the airway, breathing, and circulation are addressed. The test may indicate the source of Ms. Baker's chest pain and increased respiratory rate. (+1 point)
5.8 Obtain cervical spine films	As long as Ms. Baker is properly anchored and positioned on the backboard and the backboard is elevated on the right side, this can wait until chest and pelvic x-rays are done. (0 point)
5.9 Obtain right leg x-ray	Important but can wait until later. Right pedal pulse is diminished (+1 point) in comparison to the left but it is present. (0 point)
5.10 Insert nasogastric tube	Important because aspiration is a possibility in any supine, trauma patient secondary to catecholamine response. In pregnancy, there is a delay in gastric emptying and increased gastric reflux, thus predisposing to vomiting. (+1 point)
5.11 Insert urinary catheter	Urine output can be used as an indirect measure of renal blood flow and maternal circulation. This can be inserted later for monitoring purposes. (+1 point)
5.12 Apply pulse oximeter	This can provide data about gas exchange until ABG results are available. Adjustments can be made in the maternal oxygen therapy based on this data. (+1 point)

5.13 Obtain pelvic x-ray

This may be done in conjunction with the chest x-ray and cervical spine films. This x-ray will confirm or rule out a hip fracture or dislocation or pelvic fractures, which are the cause of a significant number of fatal injuries for the gravid trauma patient. (+1 point)

Section Six

Ms. Baker was admitted to the Intensive Care Unit for 24 hours for observation. Her x-rays have been completed. Cervical spine films were normal. She has a fractured right femur, which was pinned in the Operating Room. Her right pedal pulse is 2+ and sensation is intact. Vital signs at present are: BP = 100/60, HR = 100, RR = 18, temperature = 99.1° F. The chest film revealed a left pneumothorax. She has a #32 gauge chest tube inserted in her left anterior chest and connected to −20 cm water suction. Her peripheral intravenous lines have been converted to heparin locks. She is tolerating a clear liquid diet. She is transferred to the floor. Ms. Baker is at risk for developing complications of immobility. Which of the following data supports her susceptibility? (*Choose all that apply.*)

Item

6.1 Prolonged bedrest greater than 3 days   _____

6.2 Pregnancy   _____

6.3 Traumatic injury of the right leg   _____

6.4 Absence of tidaling in the chest tube drainage system   _____

6.5 Presence of multiple IV sites   _____

Once you have made your selection(s), read the answers to the options you have chosen. Write down the points given to each item that you selected next to your check mark.

Section Six Answers

Item	Data with Rationale
6.1 Prolonged bedrest greater than 3 days	Good choice; research has demonstrated that after 3 days of bedrest, venous stasis increases and muscle atrophy begins. (+2 points)
6.2 Pregnancy	Another good choice; pregnancy is considered a hypercoagulable state because clotting factors increase while circulating plasminogen activator decreases. Therefore, immobility may further increase her susceptibility for thrombus formation. (+2 points)
6.3 Traumatic injury of the right leg	This is relevant since the injury has created the decreased mobility. Local tissue inflammation and postoperative edema may further increase the chance for thrombus formation. (+2 points)
6.4 Absence of tidaling in the chest tube drainage system	Not pertinent; this sign may indicate that lung reexpansion has occurred, thereby decreasing Ms. Baker's susceptibility for pneumonia, another complication of immobility. (0 point)
6.5 Presence of multiple IV sites	Bad choice; the presence of multiple IV sites increases the chance for infection regardless of Ms. Baker's mobility status. (0 point)

Section Seven

You are developing a nursing care plan for Ms. Baker. Below are a list of nursing diagnoses. Select the three most appropriate nursing diagnoses for Ms. Baker based on existing data. (*Choose three.*)

Item

7.1 **Impaired physical mobility**   _____

7.2 **High risk for infection**   _____

7.3 **Impaired gas exchange**   _____

7.4 **High risk for fluid volume deficit**   _____

7.5 **High risk for injury of fetus**   _____

7.6 **Alteration in nutrition: Less than body requirements**   _____

Once you have made your selection(s), read the answers to the options you have chosen. Write down the points given to each item that you selected next to your check mark.

Section Seven Answers

Item	Data with Rationale
7.1 **Impaired physical mobility**	Good choice; her mobility will be decreased due to her fractured right femur. (+2 points)
7.2 **High risk for infection**	Because of Ms. Baker's facial lacerations, pneumothorax, and multiple IV sites, she has an increased risk of infection. (+2 points)
7.3 **Impaired gas exchange**	Inappropriate; ABG results have not been provided. You cannot validate that she is unable to compensate for the pneumothorax or that the chest tube is not effective. (0 point)
7.4 **High risk for fluid volume deficit**	Ms. Baker has not demonstrated any sign of hypovolemia. During pregnancy 25% or greater blood loss will produce tachycardia and hypotension. (0 point)
7.5 **High risk for injury of fetus**	This is a possibility. Emotional and physiological stressors can initiate labor. The emotional stress of the injury and hospitalization as well as the physiological stress of surgery may initiate labor. Ms. Baker is 7 months pregnant. The fetal respiratory system may not be mature enough to maintain oxygenation needs upon delivery without invasive assistance. (+2 points)
7.6 **Alteration in nutrition: Less than body requirements**	Inappropriate; not enough data to justify this diagnosis—PO intake, albumin and transferrin levels, and maternal weight have not been provided. (0 point)

Simulation Self-Scoring Sheet

1. On the form below, circle the point value beside the number of each response you selected on your answer sheet. (Maximum number of points for this exercise is 40.)

Response Number	Point Value	Response Number	Point Value	Response Number	Point Value
1.1	+2	3.1	+1	6.1	+2
1.2	+2	3.2	+2	6.2	+2
1.3	+2	3.3	0	6.3	+2
1.4	0	3.4	+1	6.4	0
1.5	+2	3.5	+1	6.5	0
1.6	+1	3.6	0	7.1	+2
1.7	0	5.1	+2	7.2	+2
1.8	+1	5.2	+2	7.3	0
1.9	0	5.3	+1	7.4	0
2.1	+2	5.4	+1	7.5	+2
2.2	+2	5.5	+1	7.6	0
2.3	+2	5.6	+1		
2.4	+1	5.7	+1		
2.5	0	5.8	0		
2.6	+1	5.9	0		
2.7	−2	5.10	+1		
2.8	−1	5.11	+1		
2.9	+1	5.12	+1		
2.10	+1	5.13	+1		
2.11	0				
2.12	+2				
2.13	0				

2. Determine your percentage score by multiplying your score by 100. Take the number obtained and divide it by 40 (the maximum number of possible points) to get your percentage.
   40 = 100% excellent performance
   36 = 90% good performance
   32 = 80% average performance

REFERENCES

Bremer, C., and Cassata, L. (1986). Trauma in pregnancy. *Nurs. Clin. N. Am.* 21: 705–716.

Crosby, W. (1983). Traumatic injuries during pregnancy. *Clin. Obstet. Gynecol.* 26: 903–912.

Gatrell, C. (1987). Trauma and pregnancy. *Trauma Quarterly* 4:67–85.

Sorensen, V., Bivins, B., Obeid, F., and Horst, M. (1986). Trauma in pregnancy. *Henry Ford Hosp. Med. J.* 34(2): 101–104.

A Metabolism Simulation

Kathleen Dorman Wagner and Pamela Stinson Kidd

Objectives

Following completion of this simulation, the learner should have gained

1. Skills in assessing a patient with a metabolic problem

2. Skills in management of a patient with a metabolic problem

3. Skills in altering care based on available data and patient needs

4. Skills in differentiating interventions that may be performed independently from those requiring medical orders

---

Directions

The case of Katy W. is a clinical problem-solving exercise, requiring application and analytic skills. It is not a comprehensive review of all of the metabolic self-study modules, nor does it follow the patient throughout the hospitalization. The major focus of the simulation is a single, complex metabolic problem and is confined to one isolated period during her hospitalization.

You will be asked to respond to several questions throughout the module by selecting available options. At times there are more correct answers than you are expected to select. For example, three options may be appropriate and you are asked to select only two options. Nurses are constantly faced with alternatives of equal value. The purpose of the simulation is to assist you in making wise choices and in understanding the rationale behind those choices.

The simulation begins by introducing a patient situation. Throughout the simulation, you will be re-

quired to focus your assessment of the patient, analyze assessment findings, prioritize nursing interventions, and evaluate patient outcomes. Select your
responses as indicated throughout the module. You
need only check the line at the right of the item for
those items you wish to choose. Feedback on your
selection and rationale for the points assigned to
your responses is provided following each section.
Make ALL of the desired choices BEFORE you examine the corresponding answers and rationales. Once
your choices are marked, look at the answers and
write in your point scores for each item you chose.
DO NOT change or add to your original answers.

PLEASE DO NOT LOOK at the answers prior to

indicating your responses, or the teaching and learning aspects of the simulation are negated. At the end
of the simulation, you can compare your score with
the score ranges to examine your performance level.

Items are scored on a range of +2 to −2 points:

+2 = Essential
+1 = Facilitative
 0 = Neutral, neither facilitative or harmful
−1 = Nonfacilitative, potentially harmful
−2 = Harmful

PLEASE COVER UP THE ANSWER SECTIONS
IF VISIBLE BEFORE BEGINNING EACH INQUIRY
SECTION.

Scenario

Katy W. is an 82-year-old resident of the Golden Days
Nursing Home. Her level of responsiveness has been
decreasing over the last 24 hours. She is admitted to a
450-bed university hospital on a general medical
floor for a diagnostic workup. Katy W. has a history
of Type I diabetes. She is disoriented but easily awakened.

You are working the 7 P.M. to 7 A.M. shift on the
general medical floor. Katy W. was admitted at 6 P.M.
and physician orders accompanied her.

Section One

You have just completed listening to the previous
shift status report on your patients. It is now time to
make your initial shift assessments. Since Katy W. is
the newest admission, you decide to assess her first.
Upon approaching her bedside you note that she is
resting quietly with her eyes closed. When verbally
stimulated, she is easily awakened but is disoriented
to place, time, and condition. Assuming that you
have the necessary orders for collaborative-type actions and assuming that no lab work has been drawn
thus far, which of the following assessments would
be best to obtain as soon as possible? (*Choose as many
items as desired.*)

Item
1.1 Color of lips and nailbeds   _____

1.2 Respiratory rate and pattern   _____

1.3 Gag reflex   _____

1.4 Height and weight   _____

1.5 Ability to swallow   _____

1.6 Level of consciousness   _____

1.7 Moro reflex   _____

1.8 Temperature   _____

1.9 Serum glucose and ketone
     levels   _____

1.10 Blood pressure and apical
      pulse   _____

1.11 Medical history   _____

1.12 Pupil reaction   _____

1.13 Medications taken at
      nursing home   _____

1.14 Serum BUN and creatinine   _____

1.15 Skin turgor and mucous
      membranes   _____

1.16 Visual acuity   _____

1.17 Pedal pulses   _____

Once you have made your selection(s), read the
answers to the options that you have chosen. Write
down the points given to each item that you selected
next to your check mark.

Section One Answers

Item	Data with Rationale
1.1 Color of lips and nailbeds	Lips and nailbeds are pale but pink. (+1 point)
1.2 Respiratory rate and pattern	Respirations are regular and deep at 24/minute. (+1 point)
1.3 Gag reflex	Intact; however, checking a gag reflex on this patient is inappropriate and may cause harm. (−2 points)
1.4 Height and weight	Height = 64 inches and weight = 130 pounds. (+1 point)
1.5 Ability to swallow	Intact; her decreased responsiveness level may alter her ability to swallow. Evaluation of this prior to giving oral nutrition or medications is important. (+1 point)
1.6 Level of consciousness	She is drowsy and oriented to her name only. She is able to follow simple commands. This is a crucial assessment since mentation changes were the cause for admission. (+2 points)
1.7 Moro reflex	An inappropriate assessment in this patient. (0 point)
1.8 Temperature	99° F orally, using an electronic thermometer. (+1 point)
1.9 Serum glucose and ketone levels	Her serum glucose is 530 mg/dL and ketones are strong. With her history of diabetes, early evaluation of these levels is crucial to rule out complications of diabetes. (+2 points)
1.10 Blood pressure and apical pulse	BP = 92/70 and P = 104/minute. (+2 points)
1.11 Medical history	She has a 20-year history of Type I diabetes mellitus. She also has a long history of mild congestive heart failure and peripheral vascular disease, which limits her mobility. She is normally well-oriented and talkative. (+2 points)
1.12 Pupil reaction	Pupils are equal at 2.0 mm and sluggish to react. In the elderly, chronic visual problems such as cataracts or glaucoma may alter normal pupil reaction. (0 point)
1.13 Medications taken at nursing home	Insulin: NPH 20 U in the A.M. and 10 U in the P.M. Lasix 10 mg daily PO. Digoxin 0.125 every other day PO. Potassium supplement daily. (+1 point)
1.14 Serum BUN and creatinine	BUN − 20 mg/dL and creatinine = 1.5 mg/dL. (+1 point)
1.15 Skin turgor and mucous membranes	Mucous membranes are dry and skin turgor is poor. (+1 point)
1.16 Visual acuity	She is unable to cooperate for testing at this time. (0 point)
1.17 Pedal pulses	Pulses are not palpable. Katy's history of peripheral vascular disease invalidates the use of pedal pulses as an indicator of cardiac output. (0 point)

Section Two

Based on the previously assessed data, what would be the most appropriate initial independent nursing intervention? (*Choose one item only.*)

Item

2.1 Oxygen at 4 L/minute _____

2.2 Intake and output _____

2.3 Force fluids _____

2.4 Bedrest _____

2.5 Initiate IV access _____

2.6 Fingerstick glucose level _____

2.7 Urine sugar and acetone levels _____

Once you have made your selection, read the answer to the option that you have chosen. Write down the points given to the item that you selected next to your check mark.

Section Two Answers

Item	Data with Rationale
2.1 Oxygen at 4 L/minute	Inappropriate; there is nothing in assessment supporting the need for oxygen supplementation at this time. Also, in many facilities, oxygen requires a physician's order outside of critical care areas. (−1 point)
2.2 Intake and output	Appropriate; careful monitoring of intake and output is indicated to better assess her fluid and renal status. Her presenting symptoms are suspicious of fluid volume deficit (dehydration). (+1 point)
2.3 Force fluids	Inappropriate without further data; with history of congestive heart failure, this intervention could be harmful. (−2 points)
2.4 Bedrest	Appropriate. (0 point)
2.5 Initiate IV access	Inappropriate outside of critical care areas—no physician orders. (−1 point)
2.6 Fingerstick glucose level	Appropriate, if hospital policy allows the nurse to initiate this action. Glucose level is 360 mg/dl. (+2 points)
2.7 Urine sugar and acetone levels	Appropriate; however, urine sugar and acetone levels do not reflect current status and are, therefore, of limited usefulness. (+1 point)

Section Three: Consultation

Following your assessment of Katy, the physician calls for a status report.

The physician orders the following:

1. STAT laboratory tests

   - CBC
   - Electrolyte panel
   - Glucose and ketone levels
   - Urine analysis
   - BUN and creatinine levels

2. Repeat electrolytes, glucose, BUN, and creatinine levels
3. Arterial blood gases (ABGs) in A.M.
4. Indwelling urinary catheter
5. Initiate IV of dextrose 5%/0.45 normal saline at 150 mL/hour.
6. Chest x-ray
7. Electrocardiogram (ECG)
8. 1800 calorie ADA diet
9. Oxygen at 2 L/minute per nasal cannula

Section Four

You are now preparing to initiate collaborative interventions based on the physician orders just received. What should be your priority interventions? (*Choose two interventions.*)

Item

4.1 Initiate 1800 calorie ADA diet _____

4.2 Insert Foley catheter _____

4.3 Obtain serum glucose and ketone levels _____

4.4 Obtain chest x-ray _____

4.5 Obtain electrolyte panel _____

4.6 Obtain ECG _____

4.7 Obtain ABGs _____

4.8 Initiate IV with fluids _____

Once you have made your selection(s), read the answers to the options that you have chosen. Write down the points given to each item that you selected next to your check mark.

Section Four Answers

Item	Data with Rationale
4.1 Initiate 1800 calorie ADA diet	Inappropriate; diet is often held until serum glucose and ketone levels normalize to better control medical interventions. (−1 point)
4.2 Insert Foley catheter	Appropriate; urine output is 200 mL, light yellow, with a specific gravity of 1.002. Accurate urine output measurement is important in evaluation of fluid volume status. (+1 point)
4.3 Obtain serum glucose and ketone levels	Good choice; serum glucose is 420 mg/dL and ketones = large. Serum glucose and ketone levels are a more sensitive indicator of glucose and acidosis problems than fingersticks or urine specimens. (+2 points)
4.4 Obtain chest x-ray	Chest x-ray is clear. Not a priority action; while an important diagnostic aid, her assessments thus far do not indicate a need for chest x-ray as a priority. (0 point)
4.5 Obtain electrolyte panel	Na = 148 mEq/L, K = 5.8 mEq/L, and Cl = 112 mEq/L. Electrolyte levels are consistent with dehydration. Elevated potassium may be indicative of an acidotic state as well as dehydration. (+1 point)
4.6 Obtain ECG	ECG shows normal sinus rhythm with changes consistent with digoxin therapy; not the highest priority at this time. (0 point)
4.7 Obtain ABGs	Good choice; results are pH = 7.30, $Paco_2$ = 32 mm Hg, Pao_2 = 84, HCO_3 = 16. Rapid evaluation of arterial pH and bicarbonate is important in evaluating acid-base status. (+2 points)
4.8 Initiate IV with fluids	Good choice; a venous access is necessary to deliver fluid to relieve fluid volume deficit and possible IV medications, such as insulin or bicarbonate. (+2 points)

Section Five: Consultation

You notify the physician of Katy's current status.

Katy's urine specific gravity is dilute at 1.002, possibly indicative of diuresis. Serum glucose and ketones are elevated and serum pH and bicarbonate are both acidotic. Her elevated electrolytes are consistent with dehydration and acidosis. This cluster of data is consistent with diabetic ketoacidosis.

Once you have completed your report, the physician orders the following:

1. NPH Insulin 12 U SQ every 12 hours
2. Regular insulin 10 U SQ now
3. Sliding scale insulin coverage:

Glucose Level	Regular Insulin
200–250 mg/dL	5 U
251–300 mg/dL	10 U
301–350 mg/dL	15 U
>351 mg/dL	Call Physician

4. Laboratory tests: Serum ketones and osmolality; repeat BUN and creatinine.
5. Fingerstick glucose every 6 hours
6. Continue IV fluid rate as ordered

Section Six: Update

Katy has been receiving her new insulin regimen for the past 24 hours. She was scheduled for a radiographic test and, consequently, was placed on a nothing by mouth (NPO) status at midnight. At 8:00 A.M. she received her NPH insulin. At 9:00 A.M., she complained of nausea. It is now noon, and she continues to be nauseated and is more confused and restless. She presently has no IV. As her nurse, you must decide what should be done first. (*Choose one item only.*)

Item

6.1 Continue to observe   _____

6.2 Start an IV of D$_5$W _____   6.6 Administer glucagon _____

6.3 STAT fingerstick glucose _____   6.7 Call the physician _____

6.4 Check urine for glucose and
     ketones _____   Once you have made your selection, read the
                                                answer to the option that you have chosen. Write
6.5 Administer 12 oz of orange   down the points given to the item that you selected
     juice _____   next to your check mark.

Section Six Answers

Item   **Data with Rationale**

6.1 Continue to observe   Inappropriate; observation without appropriate intervention could
                                                   lead to a severe glucose imbalance. (−2 points)

6.2 Start an IV of D$_5$W   Inappropriate; no physician's order. (−1 point)

6.3 STAT fingerstick glucose   Glucose = 60 mg/dL. Good choice; provides a means of rapid
                                                   evaluation of approximate glucose level. (+2 points)

6.4 Check urine for glucose and   Urine is negative for glucose and ketones. Testing the urine can
     ketones   help rule out hyperglycemia. (+1 point)

6.5 Administer 12 oz of orange   Inappropriate for two reasons: the patient has been nauseated all
     juice   day, and also, she has been made NPO for a test. There are other
                                                   alternatives available. (−1 point)

6.6 Administer glucagon   Inappropriate; there is no physician's order. (−1 point)

6.7 Call the physician   You could call the physician first; however, it would be better to
                                                   gather more data before calling. (+1 point)

Section Seven

Based on the analysis of the current assessment data
noted in Section Six, which of the following nursing
diagnoses is MOST important in the immediate management of Katy? (*Select one option only.*)

Item

7.1 **Fluid volume deficit** _____

7.2 **Alteration in nutrition: less
     than body requirements** _____

7.3 **High risk for injury:
     Physiologic related to
     electrolyte disturbances** _____

7.4 **High risk for injury:
     Physiologic related to
     hypoglycemia** _____

7.5 **Anxiety** _____

   Once you have made your selection, read the
answer to the option that you have chosen. Write
down the points given to the item that you selected
next to your check mark.

Section Seven Answers

Item   **Data with Rationale**

7.1 **Fluid volume deficit**   Inappropriate; there is no current indication of fluid volume deficit.
                                                   (−1 point)

7.2 **Alteration in nutrition: less than body requirements**	Her NPO status has interfered with two meals, yet she received her insulin as usual. This problem should have been avoided. First, because of her diabetes, her test should have been specifically scheduled for early morning; or second, if the test delay was unavoidable, the physician should have been made aware of the delay. A light diet may be ordered early in the day, or insulin dosage may require adjustment. Remember, NPH insulin peaks in 8 to 12 hours; therefore, her risk of hypoglycemia peaks at 4 to 8 P.M. (+1 point)
7.3 **High risk for injury: Physiologic related to electrolyte disturbances**	Inappropriate; there is no current data to indicate that an electrolyte disturbance exists. (0 point)
7.4 **High risk for injury: physiologic related to hypoglycemia**	Good choice; Katy's symptoms and serum glucose are typical of hypoglycemia. Rather than administering the morning NPH insulin, as usual, the nurse should have clarified the order with the physician based on the anticipated NPO status. This problem needs to be addressed immediately, before it worsens. (+2 points)
7.5 **Anxiety**	Inappropriate; while Katy may be anxious about her impending test or some other aspect of her hospitalization, her symptoms are typical of a glucose abnormality. (−1 point)

Simulation Self-Scoring Sheet

1. On the form below, circle the point value beside the number of each response you selected on your answer sheet. (Maximum number of points in this simulation is 26)

Response Number	Point Value	Response Number	Point Value	Response Number	Point Value
1.1	+1	2.3	−2	6.7	+1
1.2	+1	2.4	0	7.1	−1
1.3	−2	2.5	−1	7.2	+1
1.4	+1	2.6	+2	7.3	0
1.5	+1	2.7	+1	7.4	+2
1.6	+2	4.1	−1	7.5	−1
1.7	0	4.2	+1		
1.8	+1	4.3	+2		
1.9	+2	4.4	0		
1.10	+2	4.5	+1		
1.11	+2	4.6	0		
1.12	0	4.7	+2		
1.13	+1	4.8	+2		
1.14	+1	6.1	−2		
1.15	+1	6.2	−1		
1.16	0	6.3	+2		
1.17	0	6.4	+1		
2.1	−1	6.5	−1		
2.2	+1	6.6	−1		

2. Determine your percentage score by multiplying your score by 100. Take the number obtained and divide it by 26 (the maximum number of possible points) to get your percentage.
   26 = 100 excellent performance
   24 = 90% good performance
   21 = 80% average performance

Index

Page numbers in *italics* refer to illustrations; page numbers followed by t refer to tables.

High Acuity Nursing

Preparing for Practice in
Today's Health Care Settings

By Pamela Stinson Kidd
and Kathleen Dorman Wagner

Earn Nursing CE Credits!

AACN Category A CEU's

Companion test modules are available
through Buchanan and Associates
for self-paced study. Order all six tests
for a total of 46 CE Hours or 4.6 CEUs
and save $10!

Check Box(es)

☐ Test #1	Ventilation Module Chapters 1–4	7 Hrs. or 0.7 CEU	$10
☐ Test #2	Perfusion Module Chapters 5–9	11 Hrs. or 1.1 CEU	$10
☐ Test #3	Trauma Module Chapters 10–14	8 Hrs. or 0.8 CEU	$10
☐ Test #4	Metabolism Module Chapters 15–20	13 Hrs. or 1.3 CEU	$10
☐ Test #5	Psychosocial Concepts Module Chapter 21	2 Hrs. or 0.2 CEU	$10
☐ Test #6	Caring for Special Patients Module Chapters 22–23	4 Hrs. or 0.4 CEU	$10

Name _____ Credentials _____

Address _____

City _____ State _____ Zip _____

Make check or money order (in US dollars) payable
to Buchanan & Associates.

☐ Please send me _____ tests at $10.00 per test.
☐ Please send me all 6 tests for $50.00

Mail order form to:
Buchanan and Associates
13223 Black Mountain Road #351
San Diego, CA 92129-2674

(619) 484-9264

Buchanan and Associates is accredited as a provider of continuing education credit by the
American Nurses Credentialing Center Commission on Accreditation.